Veterinary Allergy

In memory of my dear colleague and friend Stefano Toma, who is greatly missed. (CN)

I dedicate this book to Susan Shaw in recognition of her great enthusiasm and ability to share with me, as for many vets, her considerable knowledge and understanding of veterinary medicine and dermatology. (AF)

To my cherished friend and mentor, Peter Ihrke, who first introduced me to this wonderful specialty and continues to be an inspiration to all. (WR)

Veterinary Allergy

Edited by

Chiara Noli (canine) (Italy)

Aiden Foster (feline, large animals, exotics) (UK)

Wayne Rosenkrantz (equine) (USA)

WILEY Blackwell

This edition first published 2014

Registered office: John Wiley & Sons, Ltd, The Atrium, Southern Gate, Chichester, West Sussex, PO19 8SQ, UK

Editorial offices: 9600 Garsington Road, Oxford, OX4 2DQ, UK
The Atrium, Southern Gate, Chichester, West Sussex, PO19 8SQ, UK
111 River Street, Hoboken, NJ 07030-5774, USA

For details of our global editorial offices, for customer services and for information about how to apply for permission to reuse the copyright material in this book please see our website at www.wiley.com/wiley-blackwell

Library of Congress Cataloging-in-Publication Data

Veterinary allergy / edited by Chiara Noli, Aiden Foster, Wayne Rosenkrantz.
pages cm.
Includes bibliographical references and index.
ISBN 978-0-470-67241-9 (pbk. : alk. paper) – ISBN 978-1-118-73881-8 – ISBN 978-1-118-73889-4 (epub) – ISBN 978-1-118-73890-0 (emobi) – ISBN 978-1-118-73891-7 (epdf) 1. Allergy in dogs. 2. Allergy in cats. 3. Allergy in animals. I. Noli, Chiara, editor of compilation. II. Foster, Aiden P., editor of compilation. III. Rosenkrantz, Wayne, editor of compilation.
[DNLM: 1. Hypersensitivity–veterinary. 2. Allergens–immunology. 3. Dermatitis–veterinary. 4. Immune System Diseases–veterinary. 5. Veterinary Medicine–methods. SF 757.2]
SF992.A44V48 2014
636.089'6975–dc23

2013026498

A catalogue record for this book is available from the British Library.

Wiley also publishes its books in a variety of electronic formats. Some content that appears in print may not be available in electronic books.

Cover images: dog and horse – courtesy of Wayne Rosenkrantz; alpaca – courtesy of Natalie Jewell and the AHVLA library, Crown Copyright 2013; cat – courtesy of Karen Clifford; centre image – courtesy of Valerie A. Fadok
Cover design by Steve Thompson

Set in 10.5/12.5 pt Minion by Toppan Best-set Premedia Limited, Hong Kong
Printed and bound in Singapore by Markono Print Media Pte Ltd

1 2014

Contents

Acknowledgments

We are grateful to Wiley for taking on this publishing project and for bringing it to fruition so quickly and efficiently. We are particularly grateful to Rupert Cousens, Jessica Evans and Nancy Turner for setting up and running the project; to Elizabeth Paul and Ruth Swan for sorting out the production issues including copyediting and typesetting.

A book project of this size is time consuming for all concerned and as editors we have been delighted at the speed and enthusiasm of authors to provide their chapters and agree to revisions and changes. Inevitably the editing has taken us away from our families and everyday work, and we are grateful to our spouses for their support and understanding and to our colleagues for their patience and advice.

It has taken three years to bring the original concept to print, and we hope that readers will find this book useful; as editors it has been an enjoyable learning experience, working together and with the authors.

Contributors

Emmanuel Bensignor
Dermatology Referral Practice
Rennes-Cesson
France

Kerstin Bergvall
Swedish University of Agricultural Sciences
Department of Clinical Sciences
Uppsala
Sweden

Ross Bond
Department of Clinical Sciences and Services
Royal Veterinary College
Hatfield
UK

Mona J. Boord
Animal Dermatology Clinic
San Diego, CA
USA

Stewart T.G. Burgess
Moredun Research Institute
Pentlands Science Park
Edinburgh, Midlothian
UK

Marie-Christine Cadiergues
Toulouse Veterinary School
Toulouse
France

Didier N. Carlotti
Service de Dermatologie
Aquivet Clinique Vétérinaire
Eysines, Bordeaux
France

Nick J. Cave
Institute of Veterinary, Animal and Biomedical Sciences
Massey University
Palmerston North
New Zealand

Michael J. Day
School of Veterinary Sciences
University of Bristol
Langford, North Somerset
UK

Douglas J. DeBoer
Department of Medical Sciences
School of Veterinary Medicine
University of Wisconsin–Madison
Madison, WI
USA

Alison B. Diesel
Department of Small Animal Clinical Sciences
College of Veterinary Medicine and Biomedical Sciences
Texas A&M University
College Station, TX
USA

Michael W. Dryden
Department of Diagnostic Medicine and Pathobiology
Kansas State University
Manhattan, KS
USA

Valerie A. Fadok
North Houston Veterinary Specialists
Spring, TX
USA

Claude Favrot
Vetsuisse Faculty
University of Zurich
Zurich
Switzerland

Aiden P. Foster
Animal Health and Veterinary Laboratories Agency
Shrewsbury
Shropshire
UK

Vinzenz Gerber
Swiss Institute of Equine Medicine (ISME)
Vetsuisse Faculty
University of Bern
and ALP-Haras Avenches
Switzerland

Paola Gianella
Dipartimento di Scienze Veterinarie
Università degli Studi di Torino
Grugliasco
Italy

Craig E. Griffin
Animal Dermatology Clinic
San Diego, CA
USA

Joya Griffin
Animal Dermatology Clinic
Louisville, KY
USA

Richard E.W. Halliwell
Royal (Dick) School of Veterinary Studies
University of Edinburgh
Easter Bush Veterinary Centre
Roslin, Midlothian
UK

Bruce Hammerberg
Center for Comparative Medicine and Translational Research
College of Veterinary Medicine
North Carolina State University
Raleigh, NC
USA

Eman Hamza
Clinical Immunology Group
Department of Clinical Research and Veterinary Public Health
Vetsuisse Faculty
University of Bern
Bern
Switzerland

Peter Hill
Companion Animal Health Centre
School of Animal and Veterinary Sciences
University of Adelaide
Roseworthy, SA
Australia

Hilary A. Jackson
Dermatology Referral Service Ltd
Glasgow
UK

Janet D. Littlewood
Veterinary Dermatology Referrals
Landbeach, Cambridge
UK

David H. Lloyd
Department of Clinical Sciences and Services
Royal Veterinary College
Hatfield
UK

Anette Loeffler
Royal Veterinary College
University of London
London
UK

Dawn Logas
Veterinary Dermatology Center
Maitland, FL
USA

Gwendolen Lorch
The Ohio State University
College of Veterinary Medicine
Columbus, OH
USA

Rosanna Marsella
Department of Small Animal Clinical Sciences
College of Veterinary Medicine
University of Florida
Gainesville, FL
USA

Eliane Marti
Clinical Immunology Group
Department of Clinical Research and Veterinary Public Health
Vetsuisse Faculty
University of Bern
Bern
Switzerland

Karen A. Moriello
Department of Medical Sciences
School of Veterinary Medicine
University of Wisconsin–Madison
Madison, WI
USA

Daniel O. Morris
School of Veterinary Medicine
University of Pennsylvania
Philadelphia, PA
USA

Ralf S. Mueller
Centre for Clinical Veterinary Medicine
Ludwig Maximilian University
Munich
Germany

Masahiko Nagata
ASC Dermatology Service
Tokyo;
Synergy Animal General Hospital Dermatology Service
Saitama
Japan

Claudia S. Nett-Mettler
Vetderm.ch-Dermatologie und Allergologie fuer Tiere
c/o Ennetsee Klinik für Kleintiere AG
Huenenberg
Switzerland

Koji Nishifuji
Department of Veterinary Medicine
Tokyo University of Agriculture and Technology
Fuchu, Tokyo
Japan

Chiara Noli
Servizi Dermatologici Veterinari
Peveragno
Italy

James O. Noxon
Hixson-Lied Small Animal Hospital
Department of Veterinary Clinical Sciences
College of Veterinary Medicine
Iowa State University
Ames, IA
USA

Tim Nuttall
Royal (Dick) School of Veterinary Studies
University of Edinburgh
Easter Bush Veterinary Centre
Roslin, Midlothian
UK

William E. Oldenhoff
Department of Medical Sciences
School of Veterinary Medicine
University of Wisconsin–Madison
Madison, WI
USA

Laura Ordeix
Department of Animal Medicine and Surgery
Veterinary School
Autonomous University of Barcelona;
Dermatology Service
Hospital Ars Veterinaria
Barcelona
Spain

Annette D. Petersen
Department of Small Animal Clinical Sciences
College of Veterinary Medicine
Michigan State University
East Lansing, MI
USA

Pascal Prélaud
Clinique Advetia
Paris
France

Chris Reeder
Animal Dermatology Clinic
Louisville, KY
USA

Carol R. Reinero
Department of Veterinary Medicine and Surgery
University of Missouri
Columbia, MO
USA

Petra J. Roosje
Division of Clinical Dermatology
Department of Clinical Veterinary Medicine
Vetsuisse Faculty
University of Bern
Bern
Switzerland

Wayne Rosenkrantz
Animal Dermatology Clinic
Tustin, CA
USA

Edmund J. Rosser Jr
Department of Small Animal Clinical Sciences
College of Veterinary Medicine
Michigan State University
East Lansing, MI
USA

Ian Sayers
South Devon Exotics
% Silverton Veterinary Practice Ltd
Paignton, Devon
UK

Harold C. Schott II
Department of Large Animal Clinical Sciences
College of Veterinary Medicine
Michigan State University
East Lansing, MI
USA

Adri van den Broek
Royal (Dick) School of Veterinary Studies
University of Edinburgh
Easter Bush Veterinary Centre
Roslin, Midlothian
UK

Bettina Wagner
College of Veterinary Medicine
Cornell University
Ithaca, NY
USA

Stephen White
School of Veterinary Medicine
University of California
Davis, CA
USA

Anthony A. Yu
Yu of Guelph Veterinary Dermatology
Guelph Veterinary Specialty Hospital
Guelph, ON
Canada

Foreword

The term 'allergy' was introduced by the Austrian physician Clemens von Pirquet in 1906 [1], however with a somewhat different meaning to that of today. He was studying the immune response to tuberculosis and diphtheria, and was thus working at the interface between immunity and hypersensitivity. He proposed the use of the term 'allergy' to imply 'altered reactivity' in the host. Thus allergy was not a disease *per se*, but rather a state that would result in a hypersensitivity reaction if appropriately challenged. This concept was gradually discarded despite some attempts to keep it alive. Tremendous advances in the understanding of the science behind allergy in man—now used synonymously with hypersensitivity, were made between 1920 and 1940. Notable were the studies by Prausnitz and Küstner [2] who described the skin-sensitizing antibody that was responsible for many allergic reactions. Then in the 1930s Coca [3] introduced the term 'atopy' which was derived from the Greek and translated literally as 'strange disease', to encompass the triad of the familial diseases of allergic asthma, allergic rhinitis, and atopic dermatitis. They also applied the term 'reagin' to the skin-sensitizing antibody of Prausnitz and Küstner. Anyone who reads these early publications cannot but marvel at the painstaking and insightful work, undertaken without the aid of modern-day techniques and at the generally sound conclusions that were reached. The next major step forward was the demonstration by Ishizaka and colleagues that the reagin belonged to a hitherto undescribed antibody class that they termed 'IgE' [4].

Over the years, a wide range of diseases of man mediated by diverse immunological mechanisms were described that could be ascribed to hypersensitivity reactions; Gell and Coombs believed that it was necessary to introduce a system of classification [5]. They proposed four categories, namely Type 1 hypersensitivity (IgE mediated), Type 2 (cytotoxic), Type 3 (immune complex), and Type 4 (cell-mediated). Robin Coombs was in fact a veterinarian, and although he never practised, he was responsible for training a number of veterinary immunologists who passed through his laboratory in Cambridge. However useful this classification undoubtedly was, it has become clear that few allergic diseases are caused exclusively by one type of hypersensitivity and most result from a combination. In the last three decades, and aided by the advent of molecular biological techniques, the science of allergy has advanced exponentially to become a highly sophisticated science and a major branch of human medicine.

In contrast, veterinary allergy (now defined as 'a hypersensitivity reaction initiated by a specific immunological response to an allergen and mediated by antibodies or cells' [6]) was slower to emerge as a recognized discipline. In large measure this can be ascribed to fewer resources for research, but also to the fact that we are concerned with multiple species, each one of which requires the development of species-specific reagents. And, of course, no formal specialist status exists for the discipline in any country. Nonetheless, its importance in everyday veterinary practice is unquestioned—indeed it is unlikely that a day will pass by in the life of a busy practitioner, no matter what the species of emphasis, without allergy being involved in one or a number of cases.

Much of the early work on veterinary allergy was undertaken by physicians who were largely concerned with the characterisation of potential animal models for allergic diseases of man. The lack of full veterinary involvement did lead to some incorrect deductions—including one that what we now know as canine atopic dermatitis was primarily a respiratory disease, with any dermatological signs being of secondary significance [7]. But the last three decades have witnessed significant advances, all of which are detailed in this text. These have been the result of single individuals or small groups who have made in-depth studies of systems in specific species of veterinary interest. These advances however have been patchy, rather than on a broad front, and significant knowledge gaps still exist in some major body systems of important species.

The current state of knowledge on this increasingly important subject is beautifully described in this, the first truly comprehensive text of allergic diseases affecting the major veterinary species. It will be an invaluable guide to students, clinicians and researchers alike. However, most importantly, whilst it quite naturally concentrates on what is known, it also draws attention to what is not yet known. In so doing it will hopefully provide the necessary stimulus for future research so that this fascinating subject will continue to advance.

Richard E.W. Halliwell
Edinburgh, 2013

References

1. Von Pirquet C. Allergie. *Munchener Medizinische Wochenschrift* 1906; **53**: 1457–1458.
2. Prausnitz C, Küstner H. Studien über Uberempfindlicht. *Centrablatt Bakteriologie* 1921; **86**: 160–169.
3. Coca AF. Specific sensitiveness as a cause of symptoms in disease. *Bulletin of the New York Academy of Medicine* 1930; **6**: 593–604.
4. Ishizaka K, Ishizaka T. Identification of gamma-E-antibodies as a carrier of reaginic activity. *Journal of Immunology* 1967; **99**: 1187–1198.
5. Coombs RRA, Gell PGH. Classification of allergic reactions responsible for clinical hypersensitivity and disease. In: Gell PGH, Coombs RRA, eds. *Clinical Aspects of Immunology*. Oxford: Blackwell Scientific, 1975: 761–770.
6. Halliwell R, and the International Task Force on Atopic Dermatitis. Revised nomenclature for veterinary allergy. *Veterinary Immunology and Immunopathology* 2006; **114**: 207–208.
7. Patterson R, Sparks DB. The passive transfer to normal dogs of skin reactivity, asthma and anaphylaxis from a dog with spontaneous ragweed pollen hypersensitivity. *Journal of Immunology* 1962; **88**: 262–268.

Introduction: the immunological basis of allergic diseases

Michael J. Day

School of Veterinary Sciences, University of Bristol, Langford, North Somerset, UK

Introduction

In 1963, P.G.H. Gell and R.A.A. Coombs published their seminal text *Clinical Aspects of Immunology*, in which they described and classified immunological hypersensitivity reactions [1]. The Gell and Coombs classification of hypersensitivity remains the cornerstone for modern human and veterinary clinical immunology. It is significant that Robin Coombs (1921–2006), one of the founding fathers of this discipline, was a veterinary surgeon [2].

Hypersensitivity, as described classically, involves the immunological sensitization of an individual (man or animal) by repeated exposure to the causative antigen (allergen) over time. A sensitized individual may, on subsequent exposure to the allergen, react in an immunologically excessive or inappropriate manner, leading to tissue pathology and clinical changes of hypersensitivity or allergic disease. The allergens involved are often ubiquitous environmental substances to which only genetically susceptible individuals will react in an inappropriate fashion.

The Gell and Coombs classification describes four major forms of hypersensitivity reaction [1]:

1 type I (immediate) hypersensitivity involving tissue inflammation mediated by mast cell degranulation subsequent to cross-linking of surface membrane immunoglobulin (Ig) E molecules by allergen;
2 type II (cytotoxic) hypersensitivity involving destruction of a target cell via the effects of antibody (generally IgG or IgM) and molecules of the complement pathway;
3 type III (immune complex) hypersensitivity in which immune complexes of antigen and antibody form locally in tissue (when antibody is in excess) or circulate systemically (when antigen is in excess), leading to local or multisystemic inflammatory pathology; and
4 type IV (delayed-type) hypersensitivity (DTH) mediated not by antibody, but by sensitized mononuclear inflammatory cells (particularly T lymphocytes and macrophages) releasing specific proinflammatory and regulatory, soluble signalling proteins (cytokines).

Now, 50 years since this classification scheme was proposed, there is much greater understanding of the molecular basis of the fundamental mechanisms involved in these key immunological reactions. Although we most often consider these hypersensitivity mechanisms in the context of immune-mediated disease, in evolutionary terms they most likely developed in order to make appropriate immune responses to coevolving pathogens. For example, the type I reaction also underpins the host immune response to parasitic infestation and the type IV reaction is intrinsic to the control of obligate intracellular bacterial or protozoal pathogens. Therapeutic management of allergic disease should therefore ideally be allergen-specific in order not to impair appropriate immune responses to infectious challenge.

This book will review in great detail the immunopathology, clinical presentation, and management of allergic diseases of the skin, respiratory tract, and gut of dogs, cats, and horses. It is the aim of this introductory chapter to overview the fundamentals of the allergic immune response. Many of the basic concepts presented here will be expanded in the pages that follow.

The multifactorial nature of allergy

Immune-mediated diseases (allergic, autoimmune, immunodeficiency, or neoplastic diseases) are by definition complex and multifactorial in nature. Allergic diseases will only become expressed clinically in individual people or animals in which there is an optimum combination of underlying predisposing and triggering factors at play. The key factors are genetic background, environmental influences, and immunological dysregulation (Figure 0.1).

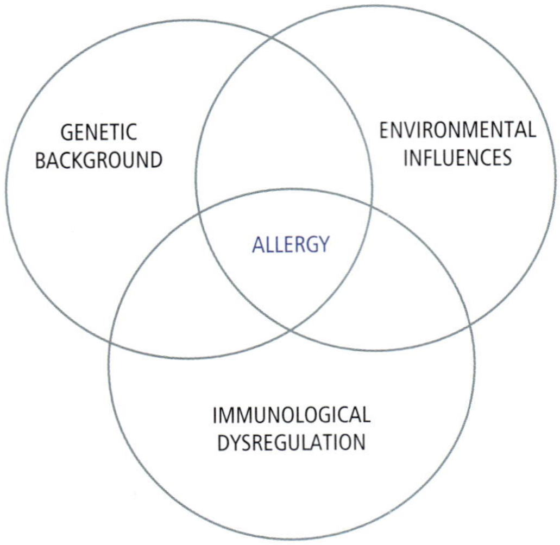

Figure 0.1 The multifactorial nature of allergy. Clinical manifestations of allergy will only become apparent when an individual person or animal has in place an optimum number of background predisposing and triggering factors. The three most important of these are genetic background, environmental influences, and immunological dysregulation.

Genetic background

There is no doubt that allergic disease runs through human families and therefore has a heritable component. Given that we now live in the 'postgenomic era', it might be assumed that the genetic basis of human allergy is well defined and that polymorphisms in specific allergy-associated genes are fully characterized. However, despite intensive research, the precise genetic basis of allergic diseases of man is not yet understood [3,4]. It is also clear that allergic disease has greater prevalence in certain breeds of dog and runs through canine pedigrees [5,6]. Clear examples of this phenomenon come from observations of the predisposition of the West Highland white terrier [7] and golden retriever [8] to atopic dermatitis. Again, despite publication of the canine genome in 2005 [9], the genetic basis of allergy in this species is not yet defined. Gene expression microarrays applied to samples of atopic dog skin have indicated a range of likely candidate genes [10] but early genome-wide association studies (GWAS) [11] and candidate gene investigations [12] have not provided clear data. At the time of writing, we await the outcome of GWAS of canine atopic dermatitis performed under the European Union-funded 'LUPA' project [13].

There is far less evidence for a genetic predisposition to allergy in the cat and the best example of breed-associated equine allergic disease is the predisposition of the Icelandic pony to *Culicoides* spp. hypersensitivity ('insect bite hypersensitivity' (IBH), 'sweet itch') [14].

Environmental influence

Simply inheriting a susceptibility genotype does not guarantee that an individual will go on to develop allergic disease. It is now very clear that the environment and personal lifestyle factors impact strongly on predisposition to allergy. At the simplest level, contact with potential allergens, to allow sensitization and subsequent hypersensitivity, is important. Allergen exposure may be geographical (e.g. the global distribution of particular plants and their pollens; the climatic influence on the distribution of ectoparasites) or related to the balance between an indoor and outdoor lifestyle. For example, in most developed nations the dominant allergens responsible for canine atopic dermatitis are traditionally indoor in nature (particularly of house dust mite origin); however, in some areas there is anecdotal suggestion that the prevalence of pollens as causative allergens may be increasing subsequent to climate change and more accessible outdoor lifestyle. Icelandic ponies do not develop IBH unless they are exported from Iceland where *Culicoides* spp. midges do not exist, but even then only 50% of exported horses are susceptible, suggesting a genetic component to susceptibility [14].

Of greatest impact in this area of allergy research has been discussion of the 'hygiene hypothesis' [15]. The hygiene hypothesis seeks to explain the fact that the prevalence of allergic (and autoimmune) disease in the human population of developed nations has increased exponentially since the 1960s. This epidemiological observation has been linked to changes in human lifestyle and the impact of these changes on the immune system. In the past five decades, people (and particularly children in whom allergy is particularly prevalent) live an increasingly indoor and 'sanitized' lifestyle based around modern technology. Numerous such lifestyle factors are implicated in the hygiene hypothesis, including: indoor carpeting, central heating or air-conditioning; frequency of use of indoor cleaning agents; ingestion of highly processed diets; increased use of childhood vaccination; smaller family size; and lack of exposure to infectious agents in the natural environment. Immunologically, these effects are collectively believed to impair the number or function of 'natural regulatory T cells' (natural Tregs; see section 'Immunological basis') that are important in the suppression of allergen-specific or autoantigen-specific T cells that may promote allergic or autoimmune disease [16]. Other investigations have demonstrated the protective effects of exposure to environmental infectious agents or the ability of such agents to modulate allergic disease. For example, it is clear that living in a rural environment on a farm is protective from developing allergic disease [17] and that this protective effect may also impact on the fetus *in utero* [18]. One of the most potent means of stimulating or restoring Treg function is by intestinal exposure to probiotic bacteria or helminth parasites, and human clinical trials support use of these novel therapies [19–21].

It is clear that some elements of the 'hygiene hypothesis' might also potentially impact on the prevalence of allergic disease in indoor dogs and cats that have contemporaneously been exposed to more widespread use of processed diets, vaccination, and endoparasite control. The latter serves an important role in human public health, but the link between parasitism, Treg amplification, and control of allergic disease has not been lost on the veterinary research community, where already clinical trials of 'parasite therapy' have been performed in atopic dogs [22].

Immunological basis

The chapters that follow will describe the major allergic diseases of dogs, cats, and horses as they affect the skin (e.g. canine and feline atopic dermatitis and flea allergy dermatitis, equine atopic dermatitis, and IBH), respiratory tract (e.g. feline asthma and equine recurrent airway obstruction), and intestinal tract (e.g. dietary hypersensitivity). Immunologically, the majority of these disorders are suggested to have an underlying type I hypersensitivity pathogenesis, although there remain unproven, suggestions that other mechanisms might sometimes be involved (e.g. type III and IV reactions in dietary hypersensitivity [23]). True 'contact allergic dermatitis' is relatively uncommon in animals, but involves a classical type IV hypersensitivity reaction. Following is a generic summary of type I hypersensitivity as it might be applied to many of the specific diseases discussed throughout this text.

Immunological sensitization to allergen of a susceptible individual living in an appropriate environment is a complex affair (Figure 0.2). Sufficient environmental loads of allergen must be present and placed in contact with the cutaneous, respiratory, or intestinal surface. It is generally presumed that some form of 'barrier defect' affects the covering epithelium and that this permits greater access of the allergen to deeper levels of the epithelial barrier [24]. For example, many human atopic patients have mutations in the profilaggrin gene (*FLG*), which encodes a precursor of the filaggrin protein that is important in maintaining structural integrity of the upper epidermis [25]. Both human and canine atopic patients have now been shown to have increased transcription of genes encoding antimicrobial peptides (e.g. cathelicidins, β-defensins) within lesional skin, although the significance of this finding remains undetermined [26]. Defects in epithelial adhesion molecules forming interepithelial tight junctions (e.g. E-cadherin, claudins, and α-catenin) have been proposed as mechanisms of mucosal epithelial barrier dysfunction in airway or intestinal disease; however, it is not always clear whether these defects are pre-existing or a consequence of the inflammatory response. For example, the *Dermatophagoides pteronyssinus* cysteine protease allergen Der p 1 is known to enzymatically disrupt respiratory epithelial tight junctions [27]. Once allergen

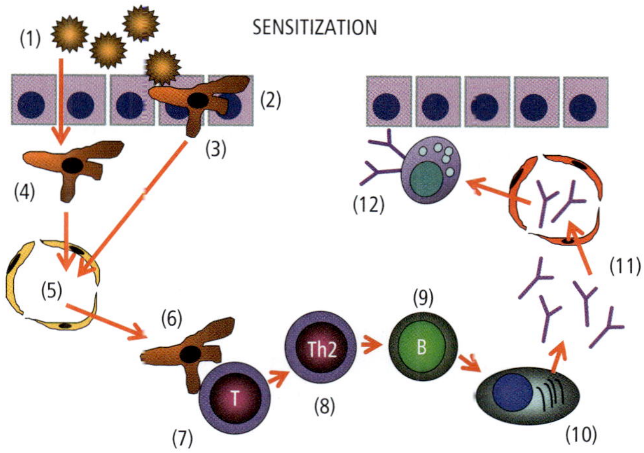

Figure 0.2 The sensitization phase of type I hypersensitivity.
(1) Allergen is deposited onto or into the epithelial barrier (i.e. epidermis, bronchial, or intestinal mucosa).
(2) Loss of barrier integrity permits penetration of the allergen.
(3) Allergen encounters an epithelial resident dendritic cell (e.g. epidermal Langerhans cell).
(4) Allergen encounters a subepithelial dendritic cell. These encounters may involve conserved allergenic structures and dendritic cell pattern-recognition receptors.
(5) Dendritic cells migrate within lymphatic vessels to the regional draining lymph node.
(6) Dendritic cells localize to the paracortex of the lymph node and present allergenic peptide in the context of MHC class II molecules.
(7) A naïve T cell recognizes the combination of allergenic peptide and MHC via its T-cell receptor.
(8) Dendritic cell co-stimulation directs differentiation towards the Th2 phenotype.
(9) The activated Th2 cell enters the lymph node follicle to provide co-stimulation to the allergen-specific B cell.
(10) The activated B cell differentiates to become a plasma cell, likely committed to the synthesis of allergen-specific IgE or IgG subclass.
(11) Plasma cells secrete allergen-specific antibodies that enter the circulation.
(12) Allergen-specific IgE (or IgG subclass) binds Fcε receptors on circulating basophils or tissue mast cells. At this stage the individual is 'sensitized' by allergen and primed to mount a hypersensitivity reaction on subsequent exposure to the allergen.

penetrates the barrier it must come into contact with an epithelial-resident (e.g. cutaneous Langerhans dendritic cell) or subepithelial dendritic cell. In the case of the intestinal tract, dendritic cells that lie immediately beneath the enterocyte monolayer may extend cytoplasmic processes between adjacent enterocytes and into the intestinal lumen to achieve antigen sampling. The recognition of allergen by the dendritic cell may have specificity if the allergen bears some form of conserved molecular sequence ('pathogen-associated molecular pattern'; PAMP) that interacts with ligands on the dendritic cell surface ('pattern recognition receptors', PRRs; or 'Toll-like receptors', TLRs).

Dendritic cells capture antigen and transport it via lymphatics to the nearest organized secondary lymphoid tissue (i.e. subcutaneous, bronchial, or mesenteric lymph nodes) where these cells largely remain within the T-cell areas of the tissue (i.e. the paracortex). Such dendritic cell migration has been shown in murine models in which fluorochromes are painted onto the skin and labelled dendritic cells detected subsequently in draining lymph nodes [28]. Concomitant with migration, dendritic cells also 'process' their captured exogenous antigen through a lysosomal compartment within the cytoplasm of the cell. Allergen processing involves enzymatic degradation of the allergen to small peptide fragments and 'loading' of these peptides to the antigen-binding region of a class II molecule of the major histocompatibility complex (MHC). Antigen-loaded MHC II molecules are then expressed on the surface of the dendritic cell during 'antigen presentation' for repeated inquisition by different T lymphocytes (via their T-cell receptors, TCRs) that pass by the relatively stationary dendritic cell.

In a clinically normal individual, the 'default' immune response to allergens (and autoantigens) is to ignore them (immunological tolerance). Tolerance may be achieved through the combination of particular forms of tolerogenic or 'immature' dendritic cell, activated via particular PRR events to deliver signals that stimulate and maintain populations of Treg cells. Dendritic cells expressing the molecule CD103 have tolerogenic function at mucosal sites [29]. Natural Tregs are characterized by the production of the cytokine interleukin (IL)-10 and expression of the transcription factor Foxp3. Should any allergen-specific T cells be inappropriately activated in the normal individual, they would be largely controlled by the circulating complement of natural Tregs that are designed to prevent allergic or autoimmune pathology. Allergic individuals of many species have now been shown to lack adequate numbers of Tregs and this is believed to be a key immunological feature of the allergic response [30].

Therefore, in the presence of a significant allergen load, a barrier defect, a non-tolerogenic dendritic cell, and lack of Treg inhibition, presentation of allergenic peptides by dendritic antigen presenting cells (APCs), together with provision of appropriate co-stimulatory cytokines and surface molecular interactions, may permit the inappropriate activation of $CD4^+$ helper T cell (Th) subsets that promote the allergic response; in particular, the Th2 cell characterized by production of IL-4, IL-5, IL-9, and IL-13 and expression of the transcription factors signal transducer and activator of transcription (STAT)-6, suppressor of cytokine signalling (SOCS)-3 and GATA binding protein (GATA)-3.

In parallel to the dendritic cell–T cell interaction, intact allergen particles must be translocated to the same lymph node to enter the B-cell areas of the tissue (the follicles) and interact with the B-cell receptor (BCR) or surface membrane Ig (SmIg). Allergen-specific B cells cannot be fully activated until they receive co-stimulatory signals (e.g. IL-4, IL-13) from allergen-specific Th2 cells that migrate from the paracortex into the follicles to permit this interaction. Activated allergen-specific B cells with high affinity receptors will divide and undergo genetic rearrangement of genes known as the 'immunoglobulin class switch'. In the case of allergen-specific B cells the outcome of this process is that the cell commits to production of IgE or IgG antibodies of particular subclasses (in dogs most allergen-specific IgG antibodies are either IgG1 or IgG4) and transforms to become an antibody-secreting plasma cell.

In the final stages of immunological sensitization, this allergen-specific IgE (and to a lesser extent the IgG subclasses) circulates in the bloodstream and engages with Fcε receptors on the surface of circulating basophils, and, more importantly, on the surface of tissue mast cells. The IgE-coated mast cells are most often resident immediately beneath (or sometimes within) the epithelial surface of the skin, respiratory tract, or gut. They are generally located in close proximity to small capillaries in the subepithelial matrix. At this stage, the individual is classically 'sensitized' to allergen. Of note is the fact that concentrations of serum allergen-specific IgE or IgG do not necessarily correlate with clinical allergy, as shown repeatedly for atopic cats [31] and dogs with atopic dermatitis [32] and dietary hypersensitivity [33].

The clinical manifestation of allergy becomes apparent on the next occasion that the sensitized individual is exposed to the same allergen (Figure 0.3). At this time, allergen that penetrates the epithelial barrier encounters IgE-coated mast cells. Where adjacent membrane IgE molecules bind epitopes on the same allergenic particle, those IgE molecules are said to be 'cross-linked'. The process of cross-linking leads to physical movement of

Fcε receptors and initiation of complex intracellular signal transduction pathways. The end result of this is classical rapid (within minutes) mast cell degranulation with release of preformed bioactive mediators, resulting in the combination of vasodilation, local tissue oedema, leucocyte exocytosis, interaction with neural receptors, and the induction of cutaneous pruritus, and, in the case of airway disease, bronchoconstriction following smooth muscle contraction.

Although regarded as an 'immediate' phenomenon it is now clear that this early pathology is followed by the subsequent 'late-phase response' (between 4 and 24 hours) during which there is infiltration of eosinophils, macrophages, and Th2 $CD4^+$ T lymphocytes into the inflamed tissue microenvironment (Figure 0.3). Plasma cells (presumptively allergen-specific) may also be present within lesional tissue and expression of Th2-related genes (e.g. IL-4, IL-13) has been shown in early-stage canine atopic skin. It is also apparent that in many patients, allergic disease becomes chronic in nature and compounded by other immunological events (Figure 0.4). This is particularly the case in atopic dermatitis which may become complicated by the secondary effects of staphylococcal or yeast infections.

Microbial 'superantigens' (e.g. staphylococcal toxins) may non-specifically activate leucocytes and amplify tissue pathology; microbe-specific Th1 or Th17 effector immune responses may be engendered with infiltration of these T cells into the affected tissue. Th1 cells are characterized by the production of the cytokine interferon (IFN)-γ and expression of transcription factors STAT-4, SOCS-5, and T-bet. Th17 cells are characterized by production of IL-17 and IL-22 and use of the transcription factors STAT-3 and retinoic acid receptor-related orphan receptor (Ror) γt and Rorα and are proposed to amplify innate immune and inflammatory responses in allergic disease [34]. It has also been proposed that a separate Th subset, the IL-9-producing

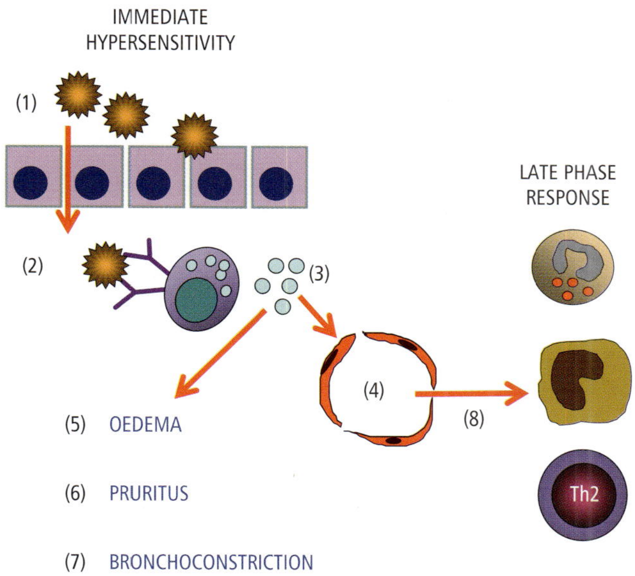

Figure 0.3 The immediate and late-phase hypersensitivity response.
(1) Allergenic re-exposure occurs to a sensitized individual.
(2) Allergen penetrates the epithelial barrier and encounters allergen-specific IgE on the surface of a subepithelial mast cell. Two IgE molecules are cross-linked by binding to epitopes on one allergen molecule.
(3) Signal transduction leads to mast cell degranulation and release of potent preformed biological mediators.
(4) There is vasodilation of capillaries. Other effects of mast cell degranulation include: (5) tissue oedema, (6) cutaneous pruritus, and (7) airway bronchoconstriction (depending upon the anatomical location of allergen challenge).
(8) Between 4 and 24 hours later there is an influx of eosinophils, macrophages, and lymphocytes comprising the 'late-phase response'.

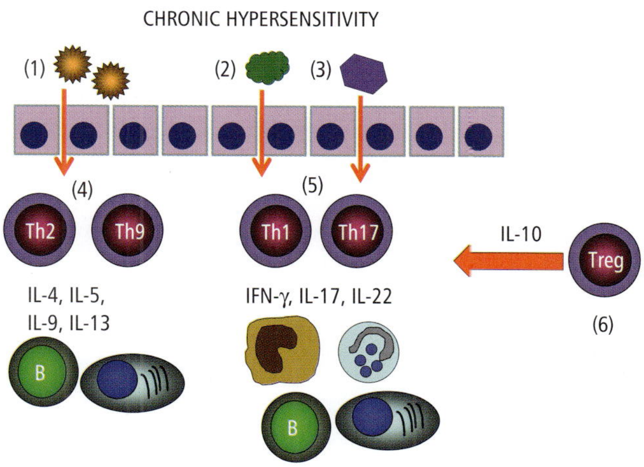

Figure 0.4 The chronic phase of type I hypersensitivity.
(1) Continued exposure to allergen may be compounded by secondary infection by (2) bacteria and (3) yeasts.
(4) Allergen exposure drives Th2 cells producing IL-4, IL-5, IL-9, and IL-13 to expand B cell and plasma cell activity. In chronic allergy there may also be differentiation of a population of Th9 cells that preferentially produce IL-9.
(5) Additional exposure to microbial pathogens now induces a Th1 and Th17 response with recruitment of macrophages and neutrophils. Th1 cells may provide help for antibody responses of a different IgG subclass to those subclasses involved in the immediate phase.
(6) Although IL-10 producing Tregs are recognized at sites of chronic hypersensitivity, they are unable to successfully down-regulate the active immune response.

Th9 cell (which uses PU.1 as a transcription factor), may play a role in perpetuating the chronic stages of the cutaneous and respiratory allergic response [35,36]. Some studies have suggested that there is a dominance of Th1-related genes (IFN-γ, IL-12, IL-18) in canine chronic atopic skin, but, in reality, in most canine lesional skin there is a complex mix of Th1, Th2, and Treg cells, as indicated by gene expression studies [37]. A complex immunopathology is also suggested for canine cutaneous lesions of adverse food reactions in which there are more $CD8^+$ T cells than $CD4^+$ cells and expression of genes encoding IL-4, IL-13, Foxp3, and SOCS-3 [38].

Future progress

Although we have come a long way in the understanding of allergic disease, there remain many areas for future research in human and animal allergy. Knowledge of susceptibility genotypes may allow controlled breeding programmes in predisposed canine breeds, although it is likely that allergic diseases will prove to be complex multigenic disorders. Recognition of the contribution of the environment and lifestyle factors might permit recommendations to be made for avoidance of triggering factors and further definition of immunological pathways will lead to development of targeted therapeutic approaches that affect only the allergen-specific elements of the host immune system. In this respect, it is now known that the likely mechanism underlying allergen-specific immunotherapy (ASIT) is amplification of the effects of Tregs to control the aberrant immune response [39–41]. Further approaches targeting deficient Treg activity (e.g. the use of parasite-derived molecules [42], development of refined ASIT using recombinant allergens [43] or DNA vaccines [44], administration of ASIT via novel approaches such as sublingual delivery [45]) should be a focus of future developments.

References

1. Gell PGH, Coombs RAA. *Clinical Aspects of Immunology*. Oxford: Blackwell, 1963.
2. Packman CH. The spherocytic haemolytic anaemias. *British Journal of Haematology* 2001; **112**: 888–899.
3. Vercelli D. Discovering susceptibility genes for asthma and allergy. *Nature Reviews in Immunology* 2008; **8**: 169–182.
4. Holloway JW, Koppelman GH. Identifying novel genes contributing to asthma pathogenesis. *Current Opinion in Allergy and Clinical Immunology* 2007; **7**: 69–74.
5. Jaeger K, Linek M, Power HT, *et al.* Breed and site predispositions of dogs with atopic dermatitis: a comparison of five locations in three continents. *Veterinary Dermatology* 2010; **21**: 119–123.
6. Wilhem S, Kovalik M, Favrot C. Breed-associated phenotypes in canine atopic dermatitis. *Veterinary Dermatology* 2010; **22**: 143–149.
7. DeBoer DJ, Hill PB. Serum immunoglobulin E concentrations in West Highland white terrier puppies do not predict development of atopic dermatitis. *Veterinary Dermatology* 1999; **10**: 275–281.
8. Shaw SC, Wood JLN, Freeman J, *et al.* Estimation of heritability of atopic dermatitis in Labrador and golden retrievers. *American Journal of Veterinary Research* 2004; **65**: 1014–1020.
9. Lindblad-Toh K, Wade CM, Mikkelsen TS, *et al.* Genome sequence, comparative analysis and haplotype structure of the domestic dog. *Nature* 2005; **438**: 803–819.
10. Merryman-Simpson AE, Wood SH, Fretwell N, *et al.* Gene (mRNA) expression in canine atopic dermatitis: microarray analysis. *Veterinary Dermatology* 2008; **19**: 59–66.
11. Wood SH, Ke X, Nuttall T, *et al.* Genome-wide association analysis of canine atopic dermatitis and identification of disease related SNPs. *Immunogenetics* 2009; **61**: 765–772.
12. Wood SH, Ollier WE, Nuttall T, *et al.* Despite identifying some shared gene associations with human atopic dermatitis the use of multiple dog breeds from various locations limits detection of gene associations in canine atopic dermatitis. *Veterinary Immunology and Immunopathology* 2010; **138**: 193–197.
13. Lequarre A-S, Andersson L, Andre C, *et al.* LUPA: a European initiative taking advantage of the canine genome architecture for unravelling complex disorders in both human and dogs. *Veterinary Journal* 2011; **189**: 155–159.
14. Marti E, Wilson AD, Lavoie JP, *et al.* Report of the 3rd Havemeyer workshop on allergic diseases of the horse, Holar, Iceland, June 2007. *Veterinary Immunology and Immunopathology* 2008; **126**: 351–361.
15. Strachan DP. Hay fever, hygiene, and household size. *British Medical Journal* 1989; **299**: 1259–1260.
16. Okada H, Kuhn C, Feillet H, *et al.* The 'hygiene hypothesis' for autoimmune and allergic diseases: an update. *Clinical and Experimental Immunology* 2010; **160**: 1–9.
17. Von Mutius E, Vercelli D. Farm living: effects on childhood asthma and allergy. *Nature Reviews in Immunology* 2010; **10**: 861–868.
18. Holt PG, Strickland DH. Soothing signals: transplacental transmission of resistance to asthma and allergy. *Journal of Experimental Medicine* 2010; **206**: 2861–2864.
19. Summers RW, Elliott DE, Urban JF, *et al.* *Trichuris suis* therapy for active ulcerative colitis: a randomized controlled trial. *Gastroenterology* 2005; **128**: 825–832.
20. Buning J, Homann N, von Smolinkski D, *et al.* Helminths as governors of inflammatory bowel disease. *Gut* 2008; **57**: 1182–1183.
21. Abraham C, Medzhitov R. Interactions between the host innate immune system and microbes in inflammatory bowel disease. *Gastroenterology* 2011; **140**: 1729–1737.
22. Mueller RS, Specht L, Helmer M, *et al.* The effect of nematode administration on canine atopic dermatitis. *Veterinary Parasitology* 2011; **181**: 203–209.
23. Ishida R, Masuda K, Kurata K, *et al.* Lymphocyte blastogenic responses to inciting food allergens in dogs with food hypersensitivity. *Journal of Veterinary Internal Medicine* 2004; **18**: 25–30.
24. Marsella R, Olivry T, Carlotti DN, International Task Force on Canine Atopic Dermatitis. Current evidence of skin barrier dysfunction in human and canine atopic dermatitis. *Veterinary Dermatology* 2011; **22**: 239–248.
25. Novak N, Leung DYM. Advances in atopic dermatitis. *Current Opinion in Immunology* 2011; **23**: 778–783.
26. Santoro D, Marsella R, Bunick D, *et al.* Expression and distribution of canine antimicrobial peptides in the skin of healthy and atopic beagles. *Veterinary Immunology and Immunopathology* 2011; **144**: 382–388.

27. Gregory LG, Lloyd CM. Orchestrating house dust mite-associated allergy in the lung. *Trends in Immunology* 2011; **32**: 402–411.
28. Randolph GJ, Angeli V, Swartz MA. Dendritic-cell trafficking to lymph nodes through lymphatic vessels. *Nature Reviews in Immunology* 2005; **5**: 617–628.
29. Scott CL, Aumeunier AM, Mowat AM. Intestinal CD103+ dendritic cells: master regulators of tolerance? *Trends in Immunology* 2011; **32**: 412–419.
30. Heimann M, Janda J, Sigurdardottir OG, *et al.* Skin-infiltrating T cells and cytokine expression in Icelandic horses affected with insect bite hypersensitivity: a possible role for regulatory T cells. *Veterinary Immunology and Immunopathology* 2011; **140**: 63–74.
31. Diesel A, DeBoer DJ. Serum allergen-specific immunoglobulin E in atopic and healthy cats: comparison of a rapid screening immunoassay and complete-panel analysis. *Veterinary Dermatology* 2010; **22**: 39–45.
32. Roque JB, O'Leary CA, Kyaw-Tanner M, *et al.* High allergen-specific serum immunoglobulin E levels in nonatopic West Highland white terriers. *Veterinary Dermatology* 2011; **22**: 257–266.
33. Zimmer A, Bexley J, Halliwell REW, *et al.* Food allergen-specific serum IgG and IgE before and after elimination diets in allergic dogs. *Veterinary Immunology and Immunopathology* 2011; **144**: 442–447.
34. Wang Y-H, Liu Y-J. The IL-17 cytokine family and their role in allergic inflammation. *Current Opinion in Immunology* 2008 **20**: 697–702.
35. Soroosh P, Doherty TA. Th9 and allergic disease. *Immunology* 2009; **127**: 450–458.
36. Lloyd CM, Hessel EM. Functions of T cells in asthma: more than just Th2 cells. *Nature Reviews in Immunology* 2010; **10**: 838–848.
37. Schlotter YM, Rutten VPMG, Riemers FM, *et al.* Lesional skin in atopic dogs shows a mixed type-1 and type-2 immune responsiveness. *Veterinary Immunology and Immunopathology* 2011; **143**: 20–26.
38. Veenhof EZ, Knol EF, Schlotter YM, *et al.* Characterisation of T cell phenotypes, cytokines and transcription factors in the skin of dogs with cutaneous adverse food reactions. *Veterinary Journal* 2011; **187**: 320–324.
39. Keppel KE, Campbell KL, Zuckermann FA, *et al.* Quantitation of canine regulatory T cell populations, serum interleukin-10 and allergen-specific IgE concentrations in healthy control dogs and canine atopic dermatitis patients receiving allergen-specific immunotherapy. *Veterinary Immunology and Immunopathology* 2008; **123**: 337–344.
40. Maggi E. T cell responses induced by allergen-specific immunotherapy. *Clinical and Experimental Immunology* 2010; **161**: 10–18.
41. Sabatos-Peyton CA, Verhagen J, Wraith DC. Antigen-specific immunotherapy of autoimmune and allergic diseases. *Current Opinion in Immunology* 2010; **22**: 609–615.
42. Grainger JR, Smith KA, Hewitson JP, *et al.* Helminth secretions induce de novo T cell Foxp3 expression and regulatory function through the TGF-β pathway. *Journal of Experimental Medicine* 2010; **207**: 2331–2341.
43. Schaffartzik A, Marti E, Torsteinsdottir S, *et al.* Selective cloning, characterization, and production of the *Culicoides nubeculosus* salivary gland allergen repertoire associated with equine insect bite hypersensitivity. *Veterinary Immunology and Immunopathology* 2011; **139**: 200–209.
44. Masuda K. DNA vaccination against Japanese cedar pollinosis in dogs suppresses type I hypersensitivity by controlling lesional mast cells. *Veterinary Immunology and Immunopathology* 2005; **108**: 185–187.
45. Berin MC, Sicherer S. Food allergy: mechanisms and therapeutics. *Current Opinion in Immunology* 2011; **23**: 794–800.

Part 1

Canine Allergy

(Editor: Chiara Noli)

Section 1

Canine Atopic Dermatitis

1

Introduction: canine atopic dermatitis as an evolving, multifactorial disease

Douglas J. DeBoer

Department of Medical Sciences, School of Veterinary Medicine, University of Wisconsin–Madison, Madison, WI, USA

Conflict of interest: none declared.

Canine atopic dermatitis (CAD) has been defined as a genetically predisposed, inflammatory and pruritic, allergic skin disease with characteristic clinical features, most commonly associated with IgE antibodies to environmental allergens [1]. However, this rather simplistic definition belies our incomplete understanding of the complex pathogenesis of the disease and its varied clinical features. In fact, as knowledge increases, CAD is increasingly viewed as a clinical description or syndrome, with a variety of manifestations and potential underlying causes that vary from patient to patient.

Historically, the commonly diagnosed skin disease termed 'eczema' in humans was recognized as having allergic origins, and as early as the 1930s veterinarians understood that a similar syndrome also existed commonly in dogs [2]. The exact allergens responsible for 'canine eczema' were undefined but often were thought to be either food or parasite related, as with fleas in 'summer eczema' [3]. In 1941, a physician allergist named F.W. Wittich provided the first description of a dog with seasonal pollen allergy [4], with successful treatment by desensitization via injections of pollen extracts. Subsequent work in dogs focused on respiratory signs associated with pollen allergy and the possible use of dogs as a model for allergic respiratory disease in human beings. Patterson (also a physician allergist) developed a colony of pollen-sensitive dogs in the 1960s, which were reported to have allergic rhinitis and dermatitis [5]. The same dogs could be induced to display asthmatic signs if high concentrations of allergen were introduced into the airways. This emphasis on respiratory signs prompted investigators to deem the disease 'allergic inhalant dermatitis', as it was assumed that the dermatitis was caused principally by allergen that entered via the respiratory route. The disease in dogs became known by this name, or sometimes by the more general 'atopic disease' or 'atopy'.

On the human front, by the late 1960s, continuing research on the pathogenesis of 'eczema' and allergic respiratory disease was pointing to involvement of a newly described and very different type of immunoglobulin, termed immunoglobulin E (IgE), which was capable of binding to the surface of mast cells. Following exposure to the relevant allergen the IgE induced mast cell degranulation, mediator release, and the familiar inflammatory signs. Though Patterson and colleagues [6] were the first to demonstrate that allergic reactivity could be transferred from a sensitive dog to a normal dog with injections of serum—suggesting mediation by an immunoglobulin—it was Halliwell *et al.* who made the final connection, publishing a series of papers in the early 1970s confirming the existence of canine IgE, its antigenic relationship to human IgE, its localization in canine skin, and a complete description of canine atopic disease, including detection of allergen-specific IgE in sera of affected dogs [7–10].

Veterinary Allergy, First Edition. Edited by Chiara Noli, Aiden Foster, and Wayne Rosenkrantz.

It seems that for many years, we were blissfully content to view 'canine atopy' as a rather straightforward disorder of the immune system: simply an IgE-mediated, immediate-type hypersensitivity reaction, caused by exposure to environmental allergens via the inhalant route. Students for decades were taught this mechanism as gospel, in spite of many dogs presenting with extreme dermatitis *without* respiratory signs, reports of human atopic patients with no demonstrable IgE involvement, and 'classically' atopic dogs with negative allergy tests. In the 1990s, a new generation of veterinary investigators began to view 'atopy' in the light of the explosion in knowledge about the immune system and its complex regulatory mechanisms and to use the more preferred and specific term of 'canine atopic dermatitis'. The role of cutaneous IgE-bearing antigen presenting cells [11], expression of cytokines by different T-helper lymphocyte populations in the skin [12], and other immunologic details of CAD were uncovered and found to remarkably parallel those of the human atopic disease. From here, a large number of studies extending to the present day have examined such factors as epidermal barrier function and percutaneous allergen penetration as the actual main route of allergen exposure in CAD [13], the important role of skin infections, genetic and environmental influences, and countless other immunologic and molecular details.

The details of these many investigations, and how they fit in the framework of our current understanding, will be the subject of the following chapters in this book. New knowledge about pathogenesis has a direct impact on how we diagnose and treat CAD, and is the basis of new treatments that will arrive on our pharmacy shelves in the future.

In proceeding through these chapters it will be useful for the reader to be aware of some definitions and terminology that describe AD and associated phenomena. This 'standard terminology' was originally proposed by the ACVD Task Force on Canine Atopic Dermatitis in 2001 [1] and has been updated since to more accurately express our current understanding [14]. The most common terms that are important to understand, with their current definitions, include the following:

- **Atopy.** Strictly, a genetically predisposed tendency to develop IgE-mediated allergy to environmental allergens. *Atopy* is a term originally and literally meaning 'strange disease', reflecting the historical lack of understanding of the disease process. It is a general term that in its adjective form *atopic* can indicate disease of various organ systems, for example *atopic rhinitis*, *atopic asthma*, or *atopic dermatitis*. Though in casual conversation we may refer to a dog as *atopic* or *having atopy*, it is important to understand (and to explain to students) that the correct and preferred name for the skin disease in dogs is *atopic dermatitis*.
- **Atopic disease.** Any clinical manifestation of atopy. In the dog, *atopic dermatitis* is the most commonly diagnosed atopic disease. Other, less common atopic diseases include *atopic rhinitis*, *atopic conjunctivitis*, etc.
- **Atopic dermatitis.** A genetically predisposed inflammatory and pruritic allergic skin disease with characteristic clinical features, associated with IgE antibodies most commonly directed against environmental allergens.
- **Atopic-like dermatitis.** An inflammatory and pruritic skin disease with clinical features identical to those seen in CAD, but in which an IgE response to environmental or other allergens cannot be documented with serological or intradermal methods. From a practical standpoint, this term describes dogs that fit all the clinical criteria for CAD, but who are negative on all allergy tests.

Though these definitions are not perfect and will no doubt be revised again, they represent our best current efforts to describe atopic diseases in dogs in a way that is clinically useful and enables us to establish uniform diagnostic criteria, evaluation schemes and formulate appropriate management plans.

References

1. Olivry T, DeBoer DJ, Griffin CE, *et al.* The ACVD Task Force on Canine Atopic Dermatitis: forewords and lexicon. *Veterinary Immunology and Immunopathology* 2001; **81**: 143–146.
2. Schnelle GB. Eczema in dogs—an allergy. *North American Veterinarian* 1933; **14**: 37–40.
3. Kissileff A. The dog flea as a causative agent in summer eczema. *Journal of the American Veterinary Medical Association* 1938; **83**: 21–24.
4. Wittich FW. Spontaneous allergy (atopy) in the lower animal. *Journal of Allergy* 1941; **12**: 247–257.
5. Patterson R, Chang WW, Pruzansky JJ. The Northwestern colony of atopic dogs. *Journal of Allergy and Clinical Immunology* 1963; **34**: 455–459.
6. Patterson R, Sparks DB. The passive transfer to normal dogs of skin test reactivity, asthma and anaphylaxis from a dog with spontaneous ragweed pollen hypersensitivity. *Journal of Immunology* 1962; **88**: 262–268.
7. Halliwell REW, Schwartzman RM. Atopic disease in the dog. *Veterinary Record* 1971; **89**: 209–213.
8. Halliwell REW, Schwartzman RM, Rockey LH. Antigenic relationship between human and canine IgE. *Clinical and Experimental Immunology* 1972; **10**: 399–407.
9. Halliwell REW. The localization of IgE in canine skin: an immunofluorescent study. *Journal of Immunology* 1973; **110**: 422–430.
10. Halliwell REW, Kunkle GA. The radioallergosorbent test in the diagnosis of canine atopic disease. *Journal of Allergy and Clinical Immunology* 1978; **62**: 236–244.

11. Olivry T, Moore PF, Affolter VK, *et al.* Langerhans cell hyperplasia and IgE expression in canine atopic dermatitis. *Archives of Dermatological Research* 1996; **288**: 579–585.
12. Nuttall TJ, Knight PA, McAleese SM, *et al.* Expression of Th1, Th2 and immunosuppressive cytokine gene transcripts in canine atopic dermatitis. *Clinical and Experimental Allergy* 2002; **32**: 789–795.
13. Marsella R, Nicklin C, Lopez J. Studies on the route of access of allergen exposure in high IgE-producing beagle dogs sensitized to house dust mites. *Veterinary Dermatology* 2006; **17**: 306–312.
14. Halliwell R. Revised nomenclature for veterinary allergy. *Veterinary Immunology and Immunopathology* 2006; **114**: 207–208.

2

Canine immunoglobulin E

Bruce Hammerberg

Center for Comparative Medicine and Translational Research, College of Veterinary Medicine, North Carolina State University, Raleigh, NC, USA

Conflict of interest: none declared.

Introduction

The details of the discovery of canine immunoglobulin E (IgE), as recently reviewed [1], illustrate how both canine and human IgE were linked to the most common clinical manifestations of allergic disease more or less simultaneously in the first 70 years of the past century. Atopic dermatitis was described as part of seasonal 'hay fever'-like signs in a fox terrier in 1941 by a physician [2], on evidence that when serum from this dog was injected into the skin of a human volunteer it demonstrated a wheal and flare response to mixed weed pollens in a classic Prausnitz and Küstner (P-K assay) reaction measurement of reaginic antibodies. Rhinitis and asthma occurring spontaneously in dogs were considered to be allergic responses as early as 1937 [3] in a human medical textbook on clinical allergy.

Similarly, the isolation and characterization of canine IgE [4–6] followed closely the timeline for identical work on human IgE. Only after the discovery of a human myeloma that provided a ready source of human IgE [7] did work on canine IgE lag behind, particularly in the development of reagents for measurement of IgE applying to clinical diagnosis. Even in the absence of a readily accessible source of canine IgE, Halliwell [8] generated highly specific rabbit antibodies against canine IgE that revealed the role of IgE at tissue sites such as skin and mucosal surfaces and in activating mast cells to respond to allergens. This observation and his proposal that local tissue site production of IgE by plasma cells, rather than production in splenic tissue or bone marrow, were important to the understanding of the role of IgE in the pathogenesis of allergic diseases for both human and veterinary medicine.

In this chapter, four areas will be addressed: (1) the role of IgE in atopic disease as compared to other possible aetiologies; (2) IgE interaction with immune and inflammatory cells; (3) the network of soluble receptors and serum proteins bound by IgE; and (4) evidence from the clinical use in humans of monoclonal antibodies against IgE (omalizumab) for the role of IgE in the pathophysiology of atopic diseases and the status of the same therapeutic approach for dogs.

The role of immunoglobulin E in atopic disease

The gold standard for establishing the aetiology of atopic disease has been the identification of the allergen(s) that triggers onset of clinical signs, by use of selective exposure to the allergen by cutaneous contact, inhalation, or ingestion. Risk of severe reaction and the inconvenience of repetitions of exposure or avoidance for multiple candidate allergens has encouraged the use of serological testing for allergen-specific IgE. Unfortunately, there is often a lack of strong correlation between serum allergen-specific IgE and clinical signs or controlled allergen-challenge test results [9]. However in practice, intradermal testing and measurement of serum allergen-

Veterinary Allergy, First Edition. Edited by Chiara Noli, Aiden Foster, and Wayne Rosenkrantz.

specific IgE perform equally well in identifying allergens for immunotherapy or avoidance [10,11].

Strong association of inherited skin barrier function defects [12], as well as several innate and adaptive immune system components, with increased risk for developing AD [13] bring into question the role of IgE, which at present lacks a clearly inherited association. As in human atopic dermatitis, the question remains as to whether IgE is a co-factor of allergic disease or does it directly influence pathways to disease [14]? There is precedence for confounding the mere presence of high IgE levels with cause and effect in the long-standing assumption that because helminth infections are associated with induction of IgE responses, IgE must be essential in protection against helminthes; however, this has often been shown not to be the case [15,16]. On the other hand, the recent high level of success of therapy for allergic diseases using parenteral administration of a blocking monoclonal antibody specific for IgE, known as omalizumab (trade name Xolair®, Novartis), in humans is evidence for a direct role for IgE in the pathogenesis of allergic diseases, including atopic dermatitis [17,18] as presented below.

Canine atopic dermatitis (CAD) is distinctly different from human atopic dermatitis in the lack of correlation between total [19] or allergen-specific serum IgE [9] and clinical signs. The reason for relatively higher levels of serum IgE in normal dogs compared to humans remains unknown; however, infections with helminth parasites, particularly the enteric nematodes *Toxocara canis* and *Ancylostoma caninum* that infect *in utero* and at birth, respectively, have been proposed to be responsible agents. Indeed, in human populations where neonatal enteric nematode infections are endemic serum IgE levels in non-allergic individuals are often comparable to the levels measured in dogs [20].

The long-standing question remains as to why individuals, either human or canine, with similar levels of allergen-specific serum IgE measured by *in vitro* assays, but different in inherited risk background, should show markedly different responses by basophils and mast cells upon cross-linking cell-bound IgE, based upon their clinical status [21,22]. Halliwell *et al.* [23] observed functional heterogeneity in IgE measured by P-K tests, that differentiated cats responding to vaccination from those demonstrating spontaneous response to allergen exposure.

Although there seems to be little support for a genetic basis to proposed functional IgE constant region heterogeneity, effective functional heterogeneity may be the result of different levels of allergen-binding affinity by the variable regions of IgE antibodies directed against the same allergen. Affinity maturation is the increase in binding affinity of antibodies for an allergen epitope that occurs during B cell clonal selection as a function of hypermutation in the immunoglobulin gene variable region. Thus, in studies of human IgE, binding repertoires that defined affinity to house dust mite allergen Der p 2, it was found that IgE repertoire greatly influenced basophil degranulation [24] as well as IgE-facilitated antigen presentation [25]. Recent reports in humans and mice describe affinity maturation by IgE committed B cells that is distinct from IgG affinity maturation. Immunoglobulin E affinity maturation was dependent on tissue site [26,27] and commonly associated with helminth parasite infection [20], as well as being observed in responses to environmental allergens [26].

Typically, IgG antibodies develop higher levels of affinity through the process of somatic hypermutation of the variable region gene and multiple iterations of clonal selection. This process is associated with cell interactions within germinal centres [28]. Sequence analysis in humans of variable region complementarity determining regions (CDR) comparing evidence for numbers of mutation events between IgG and IgE antibodies indicate that IgE B cells undergo substantially fewer mutations and consequently lack the level of affinity maturation observed in IgG B cells [20,26]. This is proposed to be due to the inefficient processing of mRNA for membrane IgE, which makes up the allergen-binding component of the B cell receptor (BCR) of IgE committed cells, thus limiting the ability of IgE B cells to undergo antigen-driven clonal selection [29]. Class switching from IgM μ gene usage directly to IgE ε gene generates low-affinity serum IgE, due to limited opportunity for somatic hypermutation and clonal selection, whereas the less frequently occurring switch from IgG1 to IgE allows affinity maturation that has occurred in IgG1 B cells to be registered in IgE B cells and their IgE product, as demonstrated in mice [27,30]. Whether the strength of IgE affinity for an allergen, rather than the concentration of allergen-specific IgE measured (regardless of affinity), can be useful in more accurate identification of trigger allergens may be an important consideration for improving serologic testing in AD and in establishing a prognosis in allergic diseases [31].

Immunoglobulin E interaction with immune and inflammatory cells

The physiological and pathophysiological effects of IgE are manifested through interactions with specific receptors on cells that respond with: (1) release of inflammatory mediators and cytokines, foremost being mast cells and basophils but also including eosinophils and human neutrophils; (2) regulated changes in antibody production by B cells and plasma cells; (3) antigen presentation by B cells and dendritic cells; and (4) IgE and allergen complex transport from the intestinal lumen to the submucosa by enterocytes [32]. The principle receptors, both membrane bound and soluble forms, responsible for the interactions between IgE and effector cells are the high-affinity Fc epsilon receptor (FcεRI) and the so-called low-affinity IgE receptor (CD23) [33]. Beyond these primary receptors there are additional proteins that interact with IgE by direct binding, such as galactin-3 [33], or indirectly by IgE binding to CD23, which can in turn bind the B-cell complement receptor, CD21, in humans but not rodents [34]. To this author's knowledge there have been no reports of canine CD23 binding to CD21.

The interaction between human IgE and FcεRI has been the subject of intense study for many years, at the level of defining intermolecular binding sites [35], IgE conformational changes [36,37], and signal pathways to mast cell degranulation [38]. FcεRI is a heterotetrameric receptor composed of the ligand (IgE epsilon chain) binding alpha chain, one signal-enhancing beta chain, and two cytoplasmic signalling, disulphide-linked, gamma chains (Figure 2.1). Only just recently have sequence data for canine IgE epsilon chain and FcεRI alpha chain permitted extending molecular studies to include dogs as one of the few well-characterized animal models that manifests spontaneous allergic disease in outbred individuals. This is somewhat ironic in that more than 35 years ago Halliwell [8] demonstrated the presence of IgE on canine mast cells and localized production of IgE at mucosal and skin sites almost in concert with identical studies in humans [39,40].

Although human IgE does not bind canine FcεRI, canine IgE does bind to human FcεRI [41]. Using canine × human chimeras of IgE with constant regions Cε2, Cε3, and Cε4 interchanged between the two sources, Hunter *et al.* [41] explored the role of each canine constant domain in binding canine FcεRI, while maintaining the basic structure of IgE with substituted species-specific, non-reactive human Cε regions. The results confirmed that canine Cε3 bears the site that binds FcεRI alpha chain and that, just as in humans, canine Cε2 prevents dissociation after binding, thereby allowing very high affinity due to slow dissociation rates. Most recently, more precise measurements of the conformational changes occurring in human IgE constant region dimeric $(C\varepsilon2\text{-}C\varepsilon4)_2$ during binding to FcεRI revealed that the degree of bending in IgE is substantially greater than previously reported, and reinforces the role of Cε2 in stabilizing this binding [37]. The bending of IgE to accommodate FcεRI binding by Cε3 and subsequent locking down of that binding with movement of Cε2 in closer proximity to Cε3 and Cε4 regions is essential to this uniquely high-affinity interaction [37].

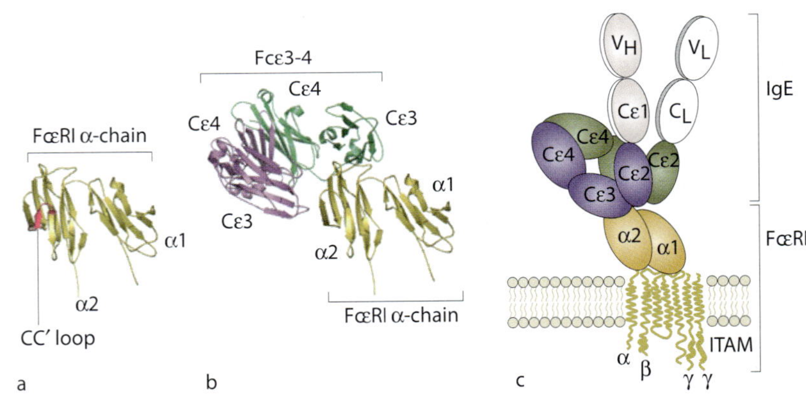

Figure 2.1 The structure of the FcεRIα-chain and its complex with I gE. (a) The structure of the extracellular domains of the FcεRIα-chain (Protein Data Bank (PDB) ID: 1F6A), taken from the crystal structure of the Fcε3-4–FcεRIα-chain complex, with the superimposed structure of free FcεRIα-chain (PDB ID: 1J87) showing only the region (in red) in which the structures differ. This is the CC′ loop region, which displays conformational flexibility even within uncomplexed structures determined in different crystal forms. The structural change involves the edge β-strand moving from one face of the immunoglobulin fold to the other. (b) The structure of the high-affinity complex between Fcε3-4 and the extracellular domains of the FcεRIα-chain, showing the extensive interaction surface and engagement of both Cε3 domains in the 'open' conformation (PDB ID: 1F6A). The connection to the membrane is at the C-terminal end of the α2 domain. (c) Schematic representation of the entire IgE molecule bound to the extracellular domains of the FcεRIα-chain, according to the structural information from the Fcε3-4 complex and the bent IgE-Fc structure. The β- and γ-chains of FcεRI, with their immunoreceptor tyrosine-based activation motifs (ITAMs), are also shown. Reproduced with permission from Gould HJ, Sutton BJ. IgE in allergy and asthma today. *Nature Reviews in Immunology* 2008; **8**: 205–217.

Expression of the canine FcεRI on rat basophilic leukaemia cells RBL-2H3, that have functional secretory pathways responsive to cross-linking of canine IgE chimeras, demonstrated that the chimera composed of canine Cε3 and Cε4 with human Cε2 was necessary for maximal degranulation response compared to canine Cε2 and Cε3 with human Cε4. This confirmed that stimulation of degranulation, as measured by β-hexosaminidase release, is more dependent on the orientation of IgE for FcεRI recognition, as influenced by Cε4, than on affinity based on Cε2, delaying release of IgE from FcεRI after binding [41]. Development of new therapies for both dogs and humans that operate by blocking or modulating IgE interactions with FcεRI will be facilitated by this deeper understanding of the interactions at a protein structural level.

In addition to the essential role that IgE binding to FcεRI plays in mast cell and basophil inflammatory mediator and cytokine release, there is yet another role that IgE binding to FcεRI plays in dendritic cell (DC) function in humans [42,43] and dogs [44,45], which is apparently absent in rodents because their dendritic cells lack constitutive expression of this receptor [32,46]. As in human AD [47], in dogs the presence of IgE bound to epidermal Langerhans cells (LC) and dermal DC significantly correlated with AD lesional skin, distinct from normal or non-allergic inflammatory skin [44]. It is likely that the proposed role of FcεRI-bearing human DC as a highly potent antigen presenter to T cells [48,49] and as the source of cytokines driving Th2 responses as well as inflammation [50,51] is also a role played by canine DC in the pathogenesis of CAD.

Adding still more layers of complexity to the understanding of the pathophysiological relevance of circulating IgE levels are the recent reports of a circulating soluble form of FcεRI (sFcεRI) in humans [33,52]. This form of FcεRI has been characterized as the 40-kDa alpha chain of FcεRI, which functionally inhibits IgE binding to cells bearing FcεRI [52]. Although the source of sFcεRI has not yet been determined, evidence suggests it is released from cells bearing FcεRI when these receptors are cross-linked [52]. This may be a negative feedback mechanism to limit further membrane-bound FcεRI-mediated signalling in the cell. In addition to playing a role in mechanisms modulating IgE-mediated inflammation, sFcεRI may well reduce the sensitivity of commercial serology measurements of IgE that employ FcεRI-based detection or antibodies specific for the FcεRI-binding epitope.

The other major receptor that binds IgE, CD23, is less directly linked to allergic disease pathogenesis than FcεRI. CD23, or FcεRII as it is also known, is found as two isoforms in humans, CD23a and CD23b; where CD23a is mainly expressed on B cells and regulates IgE production, and CD23b is present on a variety of cells including T cells, DC, and intestinal epithelial cells. The regulatory role of CD23a on B cells is complex and multifaceted [33,53]. Soluble monomeric CD23 and a modified form of soluble trimeric CD23 lacking the carboxy terminal binding site for CD21 inhibit IgE production by IgE bearing B cells when these forms of CD23 bind membrane IgE [54,55] but not CD21.

In contrast to inhibiting IgE production, in humans, but not mice, soluble, full length, trimeric CD23 can stimulate IgE production when it cross-links IgE and CD21 on the surface of B cells [55–57]. Phase I trials of an anti-CD23 monoclonal antibody, lumiliximab, in humans with mild to moderate allergic asthma demonstrated reduced serum IgE [58], suggesting that on balance removal of soluble CD23 in humans results in decreased stimulation of IgE-committed B cells. Mice lack the carboxy terminal portion of CD23 that binds directly to C21 [34]. Consequently, it has been proposed that the reason outbred mice typically do not manifest spontaneous allergic disease is because of the lack of this mechanism for trimeric CD23 upregulation of IgE production [32]. However, from the published sequence data for canine CD23 [59], it is likely that dogs also lack the sequence responsible for CD23/CD21 binding. Thus, speculation that lack of direct binding of CD23 to CD21 precludes spontaneous allergic disease may be premature.

The immunoglobulin E network of soluble receptors and autoantibody complexes

As outlined above, IgE is bound by the alpha chain of the high-affinity receptor that is present in cell surface tetrameric FcεRI on mast cells and basophils, and in trimeric FcεRI (lacking beta chain) present on eosinophils, antigen presenting cells such as dendritic cells and Langerhans cells, and on epithelial cells. However, it is only within the last two years that examination of serum for sFcεRI, composed of the alpha chain alone, revealed its presence in free form and in complex with IgE, in humans with and without allergic disease manifestation [52]. The possibility of naturally occurring sFcεRI modulating the pathogenic role of IgE in allergic diseases is just beginning to be explored [33].

Soluble CD23 is the proteolytic cleavage product of surface membrane-expressed CD23, primarily from B cells; however, CD23 is also found on a large variety of cells including T cells, NK cells, monocytes, macrophages, follicular dendritic cells, Langerhans cells, neutrophils, eosinophils, and epithelial cells [54]. CD23, as described above, binds IgE at a site distinct from the FcεRI binding site, and all of the several proteolytically generated forms of sCD23 bind IgE, although with different physiological outcomes. Binding of membrane-expressed IgE on B cells by sCD23 that cross-links CD21 drives increased production of IgE. The increase in IgE is proportional to the size of the aggregate of IgE and CD21 on the B cell mediated by sCD23 [34], and this is related to the oligomerization of CD23 through its proteolytically vulnerable stalk region [33].

Immune complexes of IgE bound by autoantibodies of the IgG subclass have been well documented to be elevated in sera from allergic and parasite-infected humans [60–62] and dogs [63]. Human anti-IgE IgG antibodies have been shown to be mainly of the IgG1 subclass and recognize most often an epitope on the IgE epsilon chain, which includes amino acids 341–355 [64]. This sequence includes part of the site bound by the FcεRI alpha chain (amino acids 343–353) and thus may inhibit IgE binding to FcεRI [64]. Epitope specificities of the canine IgG autoantibodies against IgE have not yet been determined. However, proteins complexed with IgE, in the serum from a dog with high anti-IgE IgG levels isolated by affinity chromatography with IgE-specific monoclonal antibody [63] coated beads, and analysed by mass spectroscopy sequencing of polyacrylamide gel electrophoresis separated proteins, demonstrated sequenced fragments found in canine IgGB to be predominant, followed by canine IgE sequences (Hammerberg, unpublished data). Interestingly, and suggesting the possibility of complement fixing properties of canine IgGB [65], most of the remaining sequences of bands were identified as coming from complement C1q. It remains to be determined whether these IgG anti-IgE antibodies have a protective or pathogenic function in dogs. The possibility of enhancing a naturally occurring protective function in allergic individuals by immunizing to boost IgG specific for epsilon chain epitopes that would prevent IgE binding to FcεRI is a long-standing goal in human allergic disease research [62].

Therapeutic anti-immunoglobulin E

The most convincing evidence for IgE being a key component in the pathogenesis of allergic disease comes from the highly successful add-on treatment of human allergic asthma and rhinitis with the humanized monoclonal antibody omalizumab, made against the epitope on IgE that is bound by FcεRI. This therapeutic monoclonal antibody, known by the trade name Xolair®, has been in clinical use since being approved by the Federal Drug Agency in the USA in 2003 and has been demonstrated to be highly effective in reducing the frequency of administration and amount of anti-inflammatory drugs needed to control allergic asthma and rhinitis [66]. This clinical evidence for the role of IgE in allergic asthma is supported by measurements of inflammatory marker reduction during therapy with omalizumab [67]. Given the success and safety of Xolair® in humans, it is not surprising that identical therapies are being pursued for use in canine allergic diseases. A USA patent described the ability of a caninized mouse monoclonal antibody against the canine IgE epitope, analogous to that bound by omalizumab on human IgE, to reduce total serum IgE to undetectable levels for several months after multiple injections in a two-dog trial [68].

More recently, we have developed an antibody that binds canine IgE at an epitope distinct from the Cε3 site where FcεRI binds. This antibody shows the same efficacy as omalizumab in blocking IgE binding to cells bearing FcεRI, without causing release of inflammatory mediators, and, in a single dog trial, one subcutaneous injection reduced serum IgE levels by more than 80% for a period of 60 days (Hammerberg, unpublished data). These results suggest that the complexity of the binding interaction between IgE and FcεRI may allow it to be disrupted by anti-IgE binding to allosteric sites.

The past 15 years of work on developing and implementing omalizumab for clinical use in humans have revealed much about the relationship of IgE to allergic symptom induction [69]. Four humoral response parameters define the relationship of IgE to clinical allergic symptoms [24]: (1) concentration of allergen-specific IgE antibody; (2) affinity of IgE binding to the allergen; (3) specificity of the IgE to an allergen epitope, or IgE clonality; and (4) the ratio of allergen-specific IgE to total IgE, or IgE specific activity. All of these response parameters are instructive to the diagnostic power of serological measurements; however, the last one, IgE specific activity, is also predictive of clinical responses to omalizumab therapy [68]. When the amount of disease-related, allergen-specific IgE antibody is small in comparison to total IgE, then the efficacy of omalizumab treatment is higher [70].

Prior to the results of omalizumab in clinical trials, human asthma was not often treated as, or considered to be, an allergic disease [71]. The role of IgE in asthma was confirmed after 15 Phase II and III clinical studies with anti-IgE [72]. Omalizumab use has been similarly important in the understanding of the pathogenesis of human allergic rhinitis, where the rapidity of its effect on reducing basophil FcεRI expression and activation was clearly faster than its effect on these same parameters on tissue mast cells. Symptom relief closely correlated with the former, thus incriminating basophils in rhinitis pathogenesis [73]. From these observations it is anticipated that anti-IgE therapy for atopic dermatitis will require longer periods of time to demonstrate clinical improvement, due to the stability of IgE resident on skin mast cells [74]. In a limited number of proof-of-concept trials involving human AD a majority of patients showed good responses to omalizumab treatment [75–77].

Because of the success of omalizumab and its general acceptance as an add-on therapy for human asthma, highly relevant studies are being undertaken with patients being administered anti-IgE therapy for clinical purposes, that reveal the role of IgE in early pathways of the immune response leading to allergic disease. Key among the pathways leading to outcomes of allergen sensitization of course is antigen presentation. *In vitro* findings have incriminated IgE-mediated presentation of antigens to professional antigen-presenting cells, bearing the trimeric ($\alpha\gamma_2$) form of FcεRI, in driving Th2 responses correlated with allergic diseases [49]. Early on in the clinical experience with omalizumab, it was found that FcεRI expression on both plasmacytoid (pDC) and myeloid (mDC) dendritic cells in blood of treated patients was markedly reduced [78]. The consequences of this effect on DC function has just recently been demonstrated in cat-allergic subjects where allergen-induced proliferation of T cells in co-culture with DC was reduced 20–40% from pretreatment levels, and pDC/T-cell co-culture supernatants showed significant decreases in IL-5, IL-10, and IL-13 but no changes in IL-2 or IFN-γ [79].

Conclusion

Assigning a pre-eminent role to IgE in the pathogenesis of CAD, as well as human AD, has been questioned based on serological measurements of total and allergen-specific IgE that fail to correlate with clinical disease manifestation. Recent detailed characterization of the influence of IgE repertoire, including affinity, clonality of allergen epitope recognition, and disease-related allergen-specific activity in human allergic disease, indicates that current commercial measurements of IgE lacking these defining components have limited ability to differentiate clinical disease patients from non-allergic individuals. Fortunately, this suggests that for both human and canine patients improved serology in the future that measure these components will provide a more robust diagnostic tool.

The complexity of the relationships between IgE and the immune and inflammatory systems influences both the adaptive antigen-presenting mechanisms of dendritic cells as well as the responses of T cells and IgE committed B cells. Newly discovered interactions between IgE and soluble FcεRI, in addition to long-recognized IgE interactions with anti-IgE IgG autoantibodies and soluble CD23, form a network of IgE interacting serum proteins. The balance of their effects on clinical allergic disease has yet to be worked out. What is clear, however, is that the clinical outcomes from the therapeutic use in asthma and rhinitis of the anti-IgE monoclonal antibody, omalizumab, in humans demonstrate that blocking IgE binding to FcεRI markedly reduces development of allergic diseases. The degree of this reduction in AD specifically, is encouraging but yet to be fully described.

References

1. Hammerberg B. Canine immunoglobulin E. *Veterinary Immunology and Immunopathology* 2009; **132**: 7–12.
2. Wittich FW. Spontaneous allergy (atopy) in the lower animal. *Journal of Allergy* 1941; **12**: 147–151.
3. Tuft L, ed. *Clinical Allergy*, 1st edn. Philadelphia: WB Saunders Company, 1937.
4. Rockey JH, Schwartzman RM. Skin sensitizing antibodies: a comparative study of canine and human PK and PCA antibodies and a canine myeloma protein. *Journal of Immunology* 1967; **98**: 1143–1151.
5. Schwartzman RM, Rockey JH, Halliwell RE. Canine reaginic antibody. Characterization of the spontaneous anti-ragweed and induced anti-dinitrophenylreaginic antibodies of the atopic dog. *Clinical and Experimental Immunology* 1971; **9**: 549–569.
6. Halliwell RE, Schwartzman RM, Rockey JH. Antigenic relationship between human IgE and canine IgE. *Clinical and Experimental Immunology* 1972; **10**: 399–407.
7. Johansson SG, Bennich H. Immunological studies of an atypical (myeloma) immunoglobulin. *Immunology* 1967; **13**: 381–394.
8. Halliwell RE. The sites of production and localization of IgE in canine tissues. *Annals of the New York Academy of Science* 1975; **254**: 476–488.
9. Roque JB, O'Leary CA, Kyaw-Tanner M, *et al.* High allergen-specific serum immunoglobulin E levels in nonatopic West Highland white terriers. *Veterinary Dermatology* 2011; **22**: 257–266.
10. Park S, Ohya F, Yamashita K, *et al.* Comparison of response to immunotherapy by intradermal skin tetst and antigen-specific IgE in canine atopy. *Journal of Veterinary Medical Science* 2000; **62**: 983–988.
11. Foster AP, Littlewood JD, Webb P, *et al.* Comparison of intradermal and serum testing for allergen-specific IgE using FcεRIα-based assay in atopic dogs in the UK. *Veterinary Immunology and Immunopathology* 2003; **93**: 51–60.
12. Marsella R, Olivry T, Carlotti D-N. Current evidence of skin barrier dysfunction in human and canine dermatitis. *Veterinary Dermatology* 2011; **22**: 239–248.
13. Bussmann C, Weidinger S, Novak N. Genetics of atopic dermatitis. *Journal der Deutschen Dermatologischen Gesellschaft* 2011; **9**: 670–676.
14. Novak N, Leung DYM. Advances in atopic dermatitis. *Current Opinion in Immunology* 2011; **23**: 778–783.
15. Finkelman FD, Shea-Donohue T, Morris SC, *et al.* Interleukin-4- and interleukin-13-mediated host protection against intestinal nematode parasites. *Immunology Reviews* 2004; **201**: 139–155.
16. Zhao A, Urban JF, Jr, Anthony RM, *et al.* Th2 cytokine-induced alterations in intestinal smooth muscle function depend on alternatively activated macrophages. *Gastroenterology* 2008; **135**: 217–225.

17. Sheinkopf LE, Rafi AW, Do LT, *et al.* Efficacy of omalizumab in the treatment of atopic dermatitis: a pilot study. *Allergy and Asthma Proceedings* 2008; **29**: 530–537.
18. Kopp MV. Omalizumab: Anti-IgE therapy in allergy. *Current Allergy and Asthma Reports* 2011; **11**: 101–106.
19. de Weck AL, Mayer P, Stumper B, *et al.* Dog allergy, a model for allergy genetics. *International Archives of Allergy and Immunology* 1997; **113**: 55–57.
20. Wang Y, Jackson KJL, Chen Z, *et al.* IgE sequences in individuals living in an area of endemic parasitism show little mutational evidence of antigen selection. *Scandinavian Journal of Immunology* 2011; **73**: 496–504.
21. Altin J, Shen C, Liston A. Understanding the genetic regulation of IgE production. *Journal of Allergy and Clinical Immunology* 2010; **24**: 163–169.
22. Rogue JB, O'Leary CA, Duffy DL, *et al.* IgE responsiveness to Dermatophagoides farina in West Highland white terrier dogs is associated with region on CFA35. *Journal of Heredity* 2011; **102** (SI): S74–S80.
23. Halliwell RE, Gilbert SM, Lian TM. Induced and spontaneous IgE antibodies to *Dermatophagoides farina* in dogs and cats: evidence of functional heterogeneity of IgE. *Veterinary Dermatology* 1998; **9**: 179–184.
24. Christensen LH, Holm J, Lund G, *et al.* Several distinct properties of the IgE repertoire determine effector cell degranulation in response to allergen challenge. *Journal of Allergy and Clinical Immunology* 2008; **122**: 298–304.
25. Holm J, Willumsen N, Wurtzen PA, *et al.* Facilitated antigen presentation and its inhibition by blocking IgG antibodies depends on IgE repertoire complexity. *Journal of Allergy and Clinical Immunology* 2011; **127**: 1029–1037.
26. Kerzel S, Rogosch T, Struecker B, *et al.* IgE transcripts in the circulation of allergic children reflect a classical antigen-driven B cell response and not a superantigen-like activation. *Journal of Immunology* 2010; **185**: 2253–2260.
27. Xiong H, Dolpady J, Wabl M, *et al.* Sequential class switching is required for the generation of high affinity IgE antibodies. *Journal of Experimental Medicine* 2012; **209**: 353–364.
28. Talay O, Yan D, Brightbill HD, *et al.* IgE$^+$ memory B cells and plasma cells generated through a germinal-center pathway. *Nature Immunology* 2012; **13**: 396–404.
29. Karnowski A, Achatz-Straussberger G, Klockenbusch C, *et al.* Inefficient processing of mRNA for the membrane form of IgE is a genetic mechanism to limit recruitment of IgE-secreting cells. *European Journal of Immunology* 2006; **36**: 1917–1925.
30. Wesemann DR, Magee JM, Boboila C, *et al.* Immature B cells preferentially switch to IgE with increased direct Sμ to Sε recombination. *Journal of Experimental Medicine* 2011; **208**: 2733–2746.
31. Turcanu V, Stephens AC, Chan MH, *et al.* IgE-mediated facilitated antigen presentation underlies higher immune responses in peanut allergy. *Allergy* 2010; **65**: 1274–1281.
32. Gould HJ, Sutton BJ. IgE in allergy and asthma today. *Nature Reviews in Immunology* 2008; **8**: 205–217.
33. Platzer B, Ruiter F, van der Mee J, *et al.* Soluble IgE receptors — elements of the IgE network. *Immunology Letters* 2011; **141**: 36–44.
34. Hibbert RG, Teriete P, Grundy GJ, *et al.* The structure of human CD23 and its interactions with IgE and CD21. *Journal of Experimental Medicine* 2005; **202**: 751–760.
35. Nissim A, Jouvin M-H, Eshhar Z. Mapping of the high affinity Fcε receptor bining site to the third constant region domain of IgE. *EMBO Journal* 1991; **10**: 101–107.
36. Wurzburg BA, Jardetzky TS, Conformational flexibility in immunoglobulin E-Fc$_{3\text{-}4}$ revealed in multiple crystal forms. *Journal of Molecular Biology* 2009; **393**: 176–190.
37. Hunt J, Keeble AH, Dale RE, *et al.* A fluorescent biosensor reveals conformational changes in human Immunoglobulin E Fc: implications for mechanisms of receptor binding, inhibition and allergen recognition. *Journal of Biological Chemistry* 2012; **287**: 17459–17470.
38. Lee JH, Kim JW, Kim DK, *et al.* The Src family kinase Fgr is critical for activation of mast cells and IgE-mediated anaphylaxis in mice. *Journal of Immunology* 2011; **187**: 1807–1815.
39. Tada T, Ishizaka K. Distribution of gamma E-forming cells in lymphoid tissues of the human and monkey. *Journal of Immunology* 1970; **104**: 377–387.
40. Gerber MA, Paronetto F, Kochwa S. Immunohistochemical localization of IgE in asthmatic lungs. *American Journal of Pathology* 1971; **62**: 339–352.
41. Hunter MJ, Vratimos TP, Housden JEM, *et al.* Generation of canine-human chimeric Fc IgE antibodies for the determination of the canine IgE domain of interaction with FcεRIα. *Molecular Immunology* 2008; **45**: 2262–2268.
42. Maurer D, Fiebiger E, Ebner C, *et al.* Peripherial blood dendritic cells express FcεRI as a complex composed of FcεRIα- and FcεRIγ-chains and can use this receptor for IgE-mediated allergen presentation. *Journal of Immunology* 1996; **157**: 607–616.
43. Sallmann E, Reininger B, Brandt S, *et al.* High-affinity IgE receptors on dendritic cells exacerbate Th2-dependent inflammation. *Journal of Immunology* 2011; **187**: 164–171.
44. Ricklin ME, Roosje P, Summerfield A. Characterization of canine dendritic cells in healthy, atopic, and non-allergic inflamed skin. *Journal of Clinical Immunology* 2010; **30**: 845–854.
45. Olivry T, Moore PF, Affolter VK, *et al.* Langerhans cell hyperplasia and IgE expression in canine atopic dermatitis. *Archives of Dermatology Research* 1996; **288**: 579–585.
46. Dehlink E, Fiebiger E. The role of the high-affinity IgE receptor, FcepsilonRI, in eosinophilic gastrointestinal diseases. *Immunology and Allergy Clinics of North America* 2009; **29**: 159–170.
47. Guttman-Yassky E, Lowes MA, Fuentes-Duculan J, *et al.* Major differences in inflammatory dendritic cells and their products distinguish atopic dermatitis from psoriasis. *Journal of Allergy and Clinical Immunology* 2007; **119**: 1210–1217.
48. Stingl G, Maurer D. IgE-mediated allergen presentation via Fc epsilon RI on antigen-presenting cells. *International Archives of Allergy and Immunology* 1997; **113**: 24–29.
49. Bieber T. The pro- and anti-inflammatory properties of human antigen-presenting cells expressing the high affinity receptor for IgE (FcεRI). *Immunobiology* 2007; **212**: 499–503.
50. Novak N, Peng W, Yu C. Network of myeloid and plasmacytoid dendritic cells in atopic dermatitis. *Advances in Experimental Medical Biology* 2007; **601**: 97–104.
51. Chu C-C, Meglio PD, Nestle FO. Harnessing dendritic cells in inflammatory skin diseases. *Seminars in Immunology* 2011; **23**: 28–41.
52. Dehlink E, Platzer B, Baker AH, *et al.* A soluble form of the high affinity IgE receptor, Fc-epsilon-RI, circulates in human serum. *PLoS One* 2011; **6**: e19098.
53. Burton OT, Oettgen HC. Beyond immediate hypersensitivity: evolving roles for IgE antibodies in immune homeostasis and allergic diseases. *Immunological Reviews* 2011; **242**: 128–143.
54. Acharya M, Borland G, Edkins AL, *et al.* CD23/FcεRII: molecular multi-tasking. *Clinical and Experimental Immunology* 2010; **162**: 12–23.

55. Bowles SL, Jaeger C, Ferrara C, *et al.* Comparative binding of soluble fragments (derCD23, sCD23, and exCD23) of recombinant human CD23 to CD21 (SCR 1-2) and native IgE, and their effect on IgE regulation. *Cellular Immunology* 2011; **271**: 371–378.
56. Cooper AM, Hobson PS, Jutton MR, *et al.* Soluble CD23 controls IgE synthesis and homeostasis in human B cells. *Journal of Immunology* 2012; **188**: 3199–3207.
57. McCloskey N, Hunt J, Beavil RL, *et al.* Soluble CD23 monomers inhibit and oligomers stimulate IgE synthesis in human B cells. *Journal of Biological Chemistry* 2007; **282**: 24083–24091.
58. Rosenwasser LJ, Meng J. Anti-CD23. *Clinical Reviews in Allergy and Immunology* 2005; **29**: 61–72.
59. Weber ER, McCall CA. *Canine low affinity IgE receptor (CD23) nucleic acid molecules and uses* (USA, Heska). Patent No. 6,410,714, 2002.
60. Koike T, Tsutsumi A, Nawata Y. Prevalence and role of IgG anti-IgE antibody in allergic disorders. *Monographs in Allergy* 1989; **26**: 165–175.
61. Shakib F, Pritchard DI, Walsh EA, *et al.* The detection of autoantibodies to IgE in plasma of individuals infected with hookworm (*Necatoramericanus*) and the demonstration of a predominant IgG1 anti-IgE autoantibody response. *Parasite Immunology* 1993; **15**: 47–53.
62. Shakib F, Smith SJ, Pritchard DI. Do autoantibodies to IgE play a role in IgE-mediated events? *Immunology and Cellular Biology* 1995; **73**: 109–112.
63. Hammerberg B, Bevier D, DeBoer DJ, *et al.* Auto IgG anti-IgE and IgG x IgE immune complex presence and effects on ELISA-based quantitation of IgE in canine atopic dermatitis, demodecticacariasis and helminthiasis. *Veterinary Immunology and Immunopathology* 1997; **60**: 33–46.
64. Shakib F, Hooi DSW, Smith SJ, *et al.* Identification of peptide motifs recognized by a human IgGautoanti-IgE antibody using a phage display library. *Clinical and Experimental Allergy* 2000; **30**: 1041–1046.
65. Tang L, Sampson C, Dreitz J, *et al.* Cloning and characterization of cDNAs encoding four different canine immunoglobulin γ chains. *Veterinary Immunology and Immunopathology* 2001; **80**: 259–270.
66. Pelaia G, Gallelli L, Renda T, *et al.* Update on optimal use of omalizumab in management of asthma. *Journal of Asthma and Allergy* 2011; **4**: 49–59.
67. Holgate S, Smith N, Massanari M, *et al.* Effects of omalizumab on markers of inflammation in patients with allergic asthma. *Allergy* 2009; **64**: 1728–1736.
68. Krah ER, Lawton R. *Methods and compositions for inhibiting binding of IgE to a high affinity receptor* (USA, IDEXX Laboratories, Inc.). Patent No. 7,931,898, B2, 2011.
69. Hamilton RG, MacGlashan DW, Saini SS. IgE antibody-specific activity in human allergic disease. *Immunological Research* 2010; **47**: 273–284.
70. Johansson SGO, Nopp A, Oman H, *et al.* The size of the disease relevant IgE antibody fraction in relation to 'total-IgE' predicts the efficacy of anti-IgE (Xolair®) treatment. *Allergy* 2009; **64**: 1472–1477.
71. Chang TW, Wu PC, Hsu CL, *et al.* Anti-IgE antibodies for the treatment of IgE-mediated allergic diseases. *Advances in Immunology* 2007; **93**: 63–119.
72. Holgate S, Casale T, Wensel S, *et al.* The anti-inflammatory effects of omalizumab confirm the central role of IgE in allergic inflammation. *Journal of Allergy and Clinical Immunology* 2005; **115**: 459–465.
73. Eckman JA, Sterba PM, Kelly K, *et al.* Effects of omalizumab on basophil and mast cell responses using intranasal cat allergen challenge. *Journal of Allergy and Clinical Immunology* 2010; **125**: 889–895.
74. Beck LA, Marcotte GV, MacGlashan DW, *et al.* Omalizumab induced reductions in mast cell Fc epsilon RI expression and function. *Journal of Allergy and Clinical Immunology* 2004; **114**: 527–530.
75. Lane JE, Cheyney JM, Lane TN, *et al.* Treatment of recalcitrant atopic dermatitis with omalizumab. *Journal of the American Academy of Dermatology* 2006; **54**: 68–72.
76. Vigo PG, Girgis KR, Pfuetze BL, *et al.* Efficacy of anti-IgE therapy in patients with atopic dermatitis. *Journal of the American Academy of Dermatology* 2006; **55**: 168–170.
77. Belloni B, Ziai M, Lim A, *et al.* Low-dosing anti-IgE therapy in patients with atopic eczema with high serum IgE levels. *Journal of Allergy and Clinical Immunology* 2007; **120**: 1223–1225.
78. Prussin C, Griffith DT, Boesel KM, *et al.* Omalizumab treatment down regulates dendritic cell FcepsilonRI expression. *Journal of Allergy and Clinical Immunology* 2003; **112**: 1147–1154.
79. Schroeder JT, Bieneman AP, Chichester KL, *et al.* Decreases in human dendritic cell-dependent T_H2-like responses after acute *in vivo* IgE neutralization. *Journal of Allergy and Clinical Immunology* 2010; **125**: 896–901.

3

The aberrant immune system in atopic dermatitis

Rosanna Marsella
Department of Small Animal Clinical Sciences, College of Veterinary Medicine, University of Florida, Gainesville, FL, USA

Conflict of interest: none declared.

The literature on immune abnormalities in atopic dermatitis (AD) is quite extensive. Despite this body of research, it is somewhat unclear whether these abnormalities have a causative effect in determining the disease or whether they are a consequence of other impairments such as the one involving the skin barrier function. Over the years, various theories have been proposed, ranging from the 'outside-in', which stresses the importance of the skin barrier defect as the primary cause, to the 'inside-out', which emphasizes the primary role of immune system aberrations. There is evidence to support both views. Thus, it is very likely that both aspects play a role and affect each other in a very delicate and complex way. It is also likely that, since AD is a clinical syndrome rather than a specific disease, different aberrations play a role in different subsets of patients. While the majority of patients with AD are considered allergic, a smaller subset (in humans this comprises approximately 10–15% of patients) have a dermatitis that is not allergy driven (so called intrinsic or atopic-like). In veterinary medicine the majority of the work has been done to elucidate the allergic subgroup of AD and consideration of the intrinsic subgroup is quite recent.

In terms of the allergic response and the immune aberrations, our understanding of AD has greatly evolved over the years. While in the past most of the emphasis had been placed on the role of IgE, mast cells, and mediators released by mast cells (e.g. histamine, leukotrienes), over time a robust body of evidence has been built to emphasize the role of T cells and cytokines' imbalances. Studies to characterize the cutaneous inflammatory infiltrate in canine AD (CAD) [1] have described mast cells, dendritic antigen-presenting cells, memory helper T lymphocytes (Th), and low numbers of eosinophils and neutrophils. It is important to point out that even the non-lesional skin in atopic dogs is not normal but shows subclinical inflammation.

Atopic dermatitis as a type I hypersensitivity: the role of mast cells, histamine, IgE, and leukotrienes

For a long time, most of the interest was focused on the role of mast cells and aberrations in their reactivity. Results of these studies in CAD have been mixed. A study that measured total cell histamine from leukocyte preparations found no significant differences between atopic and non-atopic dogs [2]. However, histamine release in response to anti-IgE and to allergen stimulation was significantly greater in atopic dogs than in the normal controls [2]. In the same study, no statistically significant difference in total serum IgE was found between the groups, leading the authors to conclude that the leukocytes of atopic dogs have a greater tendency to

Veterinary Allergy, First Edition. Edited by Chiara Noli, Aiden Foster, and Wayne Rosenkrantz.

release histamine than those of normal dogs and that this is independent of the concentration of total serum IgE or antigen-specific IgE.

Another study reported a lack of difference in the percentage of mast cell histamine release between atopic and non-atopic dogs [3]. A different study, aiming to characterize the histamine secretory pattern of mast cells enzymatically dispersed from the skin of dogs with CAD, reported that the total histamine content per isolated skin mast cell was higher in the allergic dogs than in healthy controls [4]. This result, in combination with the higher number of skin mast cells in CAD lesions, was proposed as an explanation for the observed increase in local histamine concentration. The authors also reported that atopic dog-derived mast cells were highly reactive to both non-immunological and immunological-like stimuli, and concluded proposing a role for mast cells through enhanced sensitivity or releasability with the open question of whether this was a primary or a secondary change.

The clinical relevance of the increased cutaneous histamine in the canine disease is unclear, due to the often unsatisfactory clinical response to antihistamines and histamine receptor blocking agents [5]. Even so, the increased histamine in the skin of atopic patients may lead to a variety of effects, including recruitment of leukocytes, because histamine enhances the secretion of proinflammatory cytokines (IL-1 and IL-6) and chemokines (RANTES and IL-8) and promotes the activation of dendritic cells. In humans, it has been shown that histamine participates in the activation of dendritic cell precursors and that dendritic cells express all four histamine receptors [6–8].

Leukotrienes (LT) have been investigated in the past as possible mediators in CAD, as their production usually accompanies the production of histamine. In humans, LT play a huge role in asthma [9] but their role in AD is not prominent and LT inhibitors seem to have only a modest clinical effect [10]. A role for LT in pruritus has been found in experimental mouse models [11]. In dogs, however, LT do not seem to be key mediators in AD. In one study using dogs with naturally occurring CAD no increase in sulphide-LT (s-LT) and no correlation with severity of clinical signs and cutaneous concentrations was found [12]. Additionally, the few attempts made to use LT inhibitors as treatment for CAD have given only moderate response [13,14].

Enzymes involved in the production of prostaglandin E(2) (PGE2) and LTB4 have also been investigated in non-lesional and lesional skin from atopic dogs and in healthy skin [15]. In that study it was found that significantly higher mRNA expression of key enzymes such as 5-lipoxygenase (5-LO), 5-LO activating protein, LTA4 hydrolase, and PGE synthase 1 and their receptors (PGE receptors 2 and 3) were present. Whether these enzymes can be suitable future targets for treatment of CAD is not known at this time.

The role of dendritic cells

In human patients with AD several populations of dendritic cells have been characterized, and the different subgroups play a role in the various phases of the immune response [16,17]. Epidermal Langerhans cells express a high-affinity receptor for IgE (FcεRI), which allows Langerhans cells to carry out Fc receptor-mediated uptake of allergens. Once the allergen is presented to lymphocytes and the inflammatory response has been triggered, inflammatory dendritic epidermal cells (IDEC) are recruited to the epidermis. These cells play an important function in the progression and maintenance of the inflammatory process.

Cytokines and chemokines have major effects on determining changes of dendritic cells subtype in the epidermis and dermis in the various phases of AD, in response to allergen challenge [18]. In humans and mice, thymic stromal lymphopoietin (TSLP) and histamine have been shown to contribute to the disease process by specifically modulating the function of dendritic cells [19–21]. SLP is an interleukin 7-like cytokine, which can trigger dendritic cell-mediated Th2 inflammatory responses. In humans, TSLP polymorphisms are associated with susceptibility to asthma and AD. Currently, TSLP is considered key in the initiation of allergic and adaptive inflammation through innate pathways at the epithelial cell–DC interface and is considered a prime target for treatment of allergic diseases [22].

A recent study in dogs with CAD reported that TSLP expression in keratinocytes is increased after allergen stimulation with *Dermatophagoides farinae* [23]. This study also found a significantly higher expression of TSLP in canine atopic skin compared to healthy control skin, suggesting that this cytokine may have a role also in CAD. Thus, it is reasonable to propose that the initial allergen exposure stimulates keratinocytes to release TSLP which, in turn, will activate antigen presenting cells and promote a Th2 response.

In terms of dendritic cells, important similarities exist between atopic dogs and humans. In dogs, Langerhans cells express the high-affinity IgE receptor, FcεRI [24]. In atopic dogs higher numbers of epidermal and dermal dendritic cells have been described compared to normal controls, with the highest numbers in lesional skin [25]. IgE^+ dendritic cells are present in lesional atopic epidermis and dermis, also in non-lesional atopic dermis, but not in normal control skin. These findings support a role for Langerhans cells in facilitating allergen capture after epicutaneous exposure. A study aiming to determine the frequency and phenotype of dendritic cells in dogs with AD [26] reported a main population of canine skin dendritic cells identified as $CD1c^+$ $CD11c^+$ $CD14^-$ $CD80^+$ $MHCII^+$ $MAC387^-$ cells, with dermal dendritic cells but not Langerhans cells expressing CD11b.

Dendritic cells contribute to inflammatory processes through the activation of antigen-specific T cells. Both the type of dendritic cells and the inflammatory environment in which dendritic cells become activated can influence the type of T cell response that is elicited [27]. By presenting IgE-bound allergens, Langerhans cells are thought to hyperstimulate a Th2 cell response. Th2 response is also favoured by exposure to allergen in the presence of skin barrier damage [28]. Thus, a significant amount of research has been focused on the role of different subsets of Th cells and the cytokines produced by those lymphocytes with particular emphasis on a Th2 polarized response.

T cells: different populations and cytokine response

As research in CAD progressed, it became clear that T lymphocytes play a fundamental role and great effort was made to investigate whether an imbalance in Th populations was present. In humans, a biphasic response has been described where Th2 predominate in the acute phase (producing IL-4, IL-5, IL-13) and Th1 predominate in the chronic phase (producing gamma-IFN and IL-2) [29,30]. This is particularly evident in atopy patch test studies [31]. In the early phase, IL-4 production by Th2 cells is predominant while in the later phases interferon-gamma production by Th1 prevails with IL-12 playing an important role in the switching of this polarization.

In dogs, cytokine kinetics in atopy patch tests showed a similar dynamic response. A study of atopy patch testing with house dust mites in *an experimental model* for CAD found that mRNA expression for gamma-IFN, IL-6, IL-12p35, IL-13, IL-18, and thymus and activation-regulated chemokine (TARC) significantly increased during the allergen challenge compared to baseline [32]. Interestingly, no appreciable alteration in expression for tumour necrosis factor-alpha (TNF-alpha), IL-12p40, IL-10, regulated on activation normal T-cell expressed and secreted (RANTES), IL-5, IL-2, IL-4, and IL-8 was found. Importantly, IL-6 peaked in early reactions followed by an increase of TARC and IL-13, while IL-18 increased in later reactions. The same study also reported on a progressive accumulation of $CD1c^+$ epidermal Langerhans cells with cluster formation and dermal dendritic cell infiltration.

When studying cytokine profiles in the skin of dogs *with naturally occurring disease*, the results are mixed. One study reported that approximately one-quarter of atopic samples exhibited clear type-2 cytokine profiles while the rest of the samples showed a mixed profile [33]. The reason for these mixed results may lie in the fact that dogs with naturally occurring disease have skin lesions at different immunological stages (some in acute and some in more chronic phases) and that different cytokines are predominant in different phases. One study specifically reported increased production of IL-4 and reduced expression of TGF-beta in the skin of atopic dogs compared to controls [34]. The decreased expression of TGF-beta may be consistent with a lack of tolerance to allergens in atopic dogs. This is supported by the fact that dogs responding successfully to immunotherapy have an increase in TGF-beta and in T regulatory cells (Tregs) [35]. A study aiming to evaluate the cytokine profile of chronic AD lesions showed that *both Th1- and Th2-type as well as T regulatory cells* are present in atopic skin [36] and that IL-12p40 mRNA was lower in lesional skin when compared to healthy controls. In the same study, the expression of signal transducer and activator of transcription 4, a transcription factor required for the development of Th1 cells, was higher in atopic lesional skin compared to non-lesional skin and healthy controls. Additionally, increased IL-13 and suppressor of cytokine signalling 3, a cytokine-inducible suppressor of cytokine signalling, were found in atopic skin (lesional and non-lesional) compared to healthy controls. Also, IL-10 expression was higher in atopic skin (lesional and non-lesional) compared to healthy controls and it was particularly abundant in lesional skin.

Over the years, new Th1 and Th2 cytokines (IL-16, IL-21, IL-23, IL-27, IL-31, IL-33, IL-35) have been identified and their role in human AD is currently under investigation [37,38]. Of interest is IL-21, a Th1 cytokine, which has been found to be dramatically decreased in children with severe AD [39]. IL-21 is produced by activated human $CD4^+$ T cells and its receptor is expressed on the surface of T, B, and natural killer (NK) cells. IL-21 is a cytokine that has potent regulatory effects on NK cells and cytotoxic T cells. In a mouse model for rhinitis IL-21 was shown to be successful in controlling allergic responses and decreasing proinflammatory cytokines in addition to decreasing IgE levels [40]. At this time no studies are available on IL-21 in atopic dogs.

Another cytokine that is attracting a lot of attention is IL-31. The structure of IL-31 places it in the IL-6 family of cytokines. Binding of IL-31 to its receptor activates JAK/STAT, PI3K/AKT, and MAPK pathways. IL-31 acts on a broad range of immune and non-immune cells. Receptors for IL-31 are found on a variety of cells, including keratinocytes. A study in normal human keratinocytes showed that several chemokine genes are induced upon stimulation with human IL-31, including those encoding GRO1α (CXCL1), TARC (CCL17), MIP-3β (CCL19), MDC (CCL22), MIP-3 (CCL23), MIP-1β (CCL4), and I-309 [41]. These data suggest a potential function for IL-31 in regulating immune responses through modulation of keratinocytes, antigen-presenting cells, or more directly T cell themselves. IL-31 is able to induce dermatitis in mice [41] and its mRNA expression in NC/Nga mice, an animal modal of AD, was significantly higher in animals with scratching behaviour than that in NC/Nga mice without scratching behaviour [42], suggesting an important role for pruritus. IL-31 has been linked to AD in humans and higher levels of IL-31 expression have been found in biopsy specimens taken from patients with AD compared to those from healthy individuals [43,44]. In one study in humans, it was found that atopic samples had many IL-31-producing T cells, which co-produced IL-13 and to lesser extent IL-22, but rarely produced gamma-IFN or IL-17 [45]. IL-31 activates eosinophils and has pruritogenic effects [46].

In terms of dogs, one initial study investigated this cytokine in AD and did not find IL-31 to be increased in the skin of atopic dogs [47]. However, more recent investigations demonstrated an important role for IL-31 in pruritus and in CAD [48]. In these studies, research beagles were administered recombinant IL-31 by several routes and it was found that the injection of IL-31, regardless of the route, induced transient and dose-dependent pruritus. Additionally, serum levels of IL-31 were detectable in more that half of the dogs with naturally occurring AD while they were below detection limits in healthy controls [48]. IL-31 was able to activate JAK/STAT and MAPK signal transduction pathways in a dose-dependent way in canine cell cultures [48]. Another study reported on the increased release of IL-31 by Th2 cells secondary to stimulation with *D. farinae* and demonstrated the presence of IL-31 receptor alpha chain on the dorsal root ganglia [49]. These two findings support a role of IL-31 in atopic inflammation and pruritus. A strong expression of IL-31 receptor alpha was confirmed in another report that examined multiple dorsal root ganglia per dog. These authors also suggested that these receptors may be involved in the neural transmission of itch in dogs [50]. Furthermore, a model of IL-31-induced pruritus has been developed with intravenous injections of IL-31 [51]. In this model prednisolone was effective in decreasing pruritus. Importantly, a janus kinase inhibitor called oclacitinib was also effective in reducing pruritus [51]. All together, these studies demonstrate an important role for IL-31 in both pruritus and CAD in dogs, thus making this cytokine an attractive target for treatment.

In recent years, other effector Th cell subsets besides Th1 and Th2 have also been documented. Of particular interest are Th17 and Th22 cells [52].

Th17 cells differentiate under a specific cytokine environment. A major factor in the development of Th17 cells is IL-23, which is primarily secreted by activated dendritic cells, monocytes, and macrophages. Other cytokines that contribute to Th17 formation include TGF-beta, IL-6, and IL-21. Both gamma-IFN and IL-4, the main stimulators of Th1 and Th2 differentiation, respectively, have been shown to inhibit Th17 differentiation. Th17 cells serve a very important function in antimicrobial immunity at epithelial/mucosal barriers and play an important role in autoimmune diseases. They produce IL-17A and IL-17F, which are involved in the recruitment, activation, and migration of neutrophils. These cells also secrete IL-21 and IL-22, which stimulate epithelial cells to produce antimicrobial proteins. IL-17 is over-expressed in AD patients and aggravates the severity of the inflammatory response by stimulating keratinocytes to produce proinflammatory cytokines [53]. Interestingly, mice with filaggrin deficiency exhibit Th17-dominated skin inflammation [54] and Th17 cells are induced by epicutaneous sensitization with protein antigens [55]. Thus, it could be speculated that in individuals with impaired skin barrier, which allows increased allergen penetration and enhances the activation of dendritic cells with subsequent release of IL-23, Th17 cells are promoted and contribute to the inflammatory response. Currently, no data exist on the role of Th17 in dogs with CAD but preliminary information is available in dogs with osteoarthritis [56].

IL-22 is a cytokine expressed not only by Th17 cells but also by NK cells and a subset of T cells that express IL-22 independently of IL-17 [57,58]. These T cells are called Th22 cells and their development is under the control of Langerhans cells. IL-22 belongs to the IL-10 family and binds to a receptor that is shared with IL-10. Despite the shared receptor, the signalling of IL-22 is independent from IL-10 and triggers 3 MAPK pathways. The receptor for IL-22 is present on epithelial cells such as keratinocytes. Th22 cells also secrete TNF-alpha and have the main function to enable innate immune responses. In the skin Th22 cells mediate keratinocytes proliferation, promote epidermal hyperplasia, and stimulate antimicrobial peptides. Th22 cells play a role in chronic skin diseases such as psoriasis and AD by promoting the synthesis of proinflammatory cytokines [59]. No data are available at this time for dogs.

T regulatory cells or Tregs

It is important to highlight that, while in the past AD was mainly seen as an imbalance between Th2 and Th1 response, currently, AD is more viewed as a disease of defective regulatory immune response. Tregs, previously called suppressor T cells (Ts), are a subpopulation of T cells which modulates the immune system maintaining tolerance to self-antigens, and abrogating autoimmune disease. Increased susceptibility to allergy is thought to result from impaired development and function of Tregs. Tregs may be present in different forms but the ones expressing CD4, CD25, and Foxp3 have been the most studied. Th2 response to allergens is normally suppressed by both $CD4^+$ $CD25^+$ Tregs, and IL-10 Tregs and this suppression is decreased in allergic individuals. Changes in the Treg subpopulations have been described in human patients with AD [60] showing increased numbers of circulating $CD4^+$ CD25(high) $FoxP3^+$ compared to healthy controls. A strong positive correlation also exists between this subset of T cells and the severity of clinical signs in AD patients [60]. Importantly, even if AD patients have significantly increased numbers of peripheral blood Treg cells with normal immunosuppressive activity, after stimulation with staphylococcal superantigens, Treg cells lose their immunosuppressive activity [61], highlighting the complex relationship between these cells and bacteria in the development of AD. Dendritic cells also modulate the function of Tregs and can reverse the suppressive effect of Tregs independent of cytokine production [62]. There is also emerging evidence to suggest that Treg cells can convert to Th2 cells and that this pathway is bidirectional [63,64]. Thus, the role of Tregs in the development of AD is complex and dynamic and regulated by multiple factors.

Allergen-specific immunotherapy has been used for the therapy of allergic disease, and this treatment may induce IL-10 Tregs, leading to the suppression of Th2 responses. In dogs, as mentioned above, CAD lesions have a mixed profile of both Th and Tregs [36]. No significant difference in the number of circulating Tregs has been found between CAD dogs and healthy controls [35]. Dogs with CAD undergoing allergen-specific immunotherapy significantly increased the number of Tregs over a course of 12 months, confirming a protective effect of these cells against allergies [35].

Keratinocytes: an active player in the immune response

Keratinocytes had previously been viewed as passive bystanders; it is now apparent that keratinocytes play an active role in the response to allergens and microbes, both by providing a physical and chemical barrier as well as interacting with the immune system. A variety of cytokines and chemokines can be produced by keratinocytes (TNF-alpha, IL-12p35, IL-18, GM-CSF, TGF-beta, IL-8/CXCL8, TARC/CCL17, CTACK/CCL27, and MEC/CCL28) even in the absence of an allergic response [65]. Of great interest is TARC/CCL17, which has been shown to be over-expressed in both human AD and CAD [66,67]. TARC is important in the trafficking of Th2 cells, which express the ligand for TARC (CC chemokine receptor 4 or CCR4). A study in dogs with CAD demonstrated that CCR4 mRNA was preferentially expressed in lesional skin of atopic dogs [68], highlighting a role in the pathogenesis of this disease. TARC is induced by other cytokines (TNF-alpha, IL-1beta, or gamma-IFN) in canine keratinocytes, thus leading to a progressively increasing cycle of inflammation [69].

The cutaneous cytokine milieu affects the skin barrier [70], and both affect proteins involved in keratinization, such as filaggrin [71], and antimicrobial peptides [72], which are important components of the innate immune response [73]. Alterations of antimicrobial peptides have been documented in dogs with CAD [74,75], which may help contribute to the increased frequency of staphylococcal infections. Antimicrobial peptides are small molecules produced by a variety of cells, including epithelial cells. The most studied are beta defensins (BD) and cathelicidin (Cath). In keratinocytes antimicrobial peptides are stored in lamellar bodies [76,77] and released in the upper layers of the epidermis in the course of keratinization. As atopic individuals are prone to staphylococcal infections and have a disturbed process of lamellar body extrusion, it is reasonable to expect decreased expression of some antimicrobial peptides in AD [78]. In dogs, so far, the results of the studies on antimicrobial peptides in CAD have been mixed [74,75], with some showing increase, others reporting decrease, and a most recent one describing no significant differences in mRNA levels for cBD1, cBD103 in healthy, non-infected atopic or infected atopic skin [79]. Thus, this is an area that requires additional investigation to understand the clinical relevance of the reported findings.

The role played by bacteria in AD is complex and has attracted great interest for a variety of reasons. In the past, *Staphylococcus* has been viewed as a secondary invader that would aggravate AD, and effort has been placed on studying the mechanisms underlying the increased colonization by *Staphylococcus* on AD patients. There is now evidence that *Staphylococcus* has the ability to actually induce AD *by itself* and not just as a secondary aggravating factor. The keratinocytes of individuals with AD react differently, compared to healthy controls, to staphylococcal superantigens and it is believed that the increased proinflammatory cytokine production

(IL-1alpha, IL-1beta, and TNF-alpha secretion) is one of the many ways that *Staphylococcus* actually induces AD [80]. Another pathway to AD lesions is the superantigenic activation of T lymphocytes and the subsequent induction of the skin homing receptor CLA on activated cells [81]. Superantigens are effectively able to promote Th2 polarized skin inflammation, IgE production, T-regulatory cell subversion, expansion and migration of skin-homing T cells, and IgE antisuperantigen production. In humans, it has been shown that application of staphylococcal enterotoxin B (SEB) on intact skin can induce clinical lesions of AD [82]. From all subjects, both healthy and patients with AD, skin biopsy specimens from SEB-treated areas demonstrated selective accumulation of T cells expressing SEB-reactive T cell receptor (TCR) Vbeta12 and 17 [83]. The difference between normal and AD patients as far as staphylococcal superantigens lays in the preferential production of cytokines. SEB favours Th1 type cytokine production in SEB-reactive (TCRVbeta3$^+$ or Vbeta12$^+$ or Vbeta17$^+$) CD4$^+$ T cells from healthy subjects and Th2 cytokines in those from AD patients [84]. Thus, addressing the staphylococcal component is a crucial step in dealing with the aberrant immunological response found in AD. A detailed discussion of the role of bacteria in CAD can be found in Chapter 7.

Summary of proposed pathogenesis

Over the past few decades, incredible progress has been made in our understanding of the complex immune aberrations of AD. As our understanding improves it becomes evident that no one single aberration is responsible for this multifaceted syndrome and that many abnormalities, which were at some point thought to be primary, may actually be secondary and linked to others, making the identification of one single culprit impossible. As we learn more about this disease, we realize that the relationship between the immune system and skin barrier is very complex and interconnected.

With our current knowledge, it is reasonable to propose that atopic dogs may, at least in part, have some genetically inherited defect of skin barrier, which increases the risk for allergic sensitization. The allergens are captured by Langerhans cells, which process and present them to T lymphocytes with resulting Th2 polarization. Under the influence of Th2 cytokines, an overproduction of allergen-specific IgE and an enhancement of eosinophilic response occur. The combination of mast cell degranulation and release of chemokines by hyper-reactive keratinocytes stimulates the inflammatory response, leading to the recruitment of Th2 lymphocytes and eosinophils at the site of allergen exposure. Th2 cells upon allergenic stimulation release pruritogenic cytokines such as IL-31, leading to self trauma and further deterioration of the skin barrier. As modulation of cytokine profile in the dendritic cells occurs (e.g. release of IL-12), the development of a chronic Th1-driven response ensues. The chronic inflammation leads to additional skin damage both by promoting pruritus and self trauma and by negatively affecting the synthesis of proteins and lipids important for proper skin barrier and protection against allergen penetration and bacterial colonization. These changes in the epidermis favour the establishment of secondary infections and precipitate vicious cycles of allergic sensitization. Importantly, a deficiency in T regulatory mechanisms significantly impairs the establishment of tolerance toward common allergens and the shutting down of the inflammatory response.

References

1. Olivry T, Naydan DK, Moore PF. Characterization of the cutaneous inflammatory infiltrate in canine atopic dermatitis. *American Journal of Dermatopathology* 1997; **19**: 477–486.
2. Jackson HA, Miller HA, Halliwell RE. Canine leukocyte histamine release: response to antigen and anti-IgE. *Veterinary Immunology and Immunopathology* 1996; **53**: 195–206.
3. Brazís P, Queralt M, de Mora F, *et al.* Comparative study of histamine release from skin mast cells dispersed from atopic, ascaris-sensitive and healthy dogs. *Veterinary Immunology and Immunopathology* 1998; **66**: 43–51.
4. DeMora F, Garcia G, Puigdemont A, *et al.* Skin mast cell releasability in dogs with atopic dermatitis. *Inflammation Research* 1996; **45**: 424–427.
5. Bäumer W, Stahl J, Sander K, *et al.* Lack of preventing effect of systemically and topically administered histamine H(1) or H(4) receptor antagonists in a dog model of acute atopic dermatitis. *Experimental Dermatology* 2011; **20**: 577–581.
6. Caron G, Delneste Y, Roelandts E, *et al.* Histamine polarizes human dendritic cells into Th2 cell-promoting effector dendritic cells. *Journal of Immunology* 2001; **167**: 3682–3686.
7. Gutzmer R, Langer K, Lisewski M, *et al.* Expression and function of histamine receptors 1 and 2 on human monocyte-derived dendritic cells. *Journal of Allergy and Clinical Immunology* 2002; **109**: 524–531.
8. Dijkstra D, Stark H, Chazot PL, *et al.* Human inflammatory dendritic epidermal cells express a functional histamine H4 receptor. *Journal of Investigative Dermatology* 2008; **128**: 1696–1703.
9. Glowacka E, Jedynak-Wasowicz U, Sanak M, *et al.* Exhaled eicosanoid profiles in children with atopic asthma and healthy controls. *Pediatric Pulmonology* 2013; **48**: 324–335.
10. Yanase DJ, David-Bajar K. The leukotriene antagonist montelukast as a therapeutic agent for atopic dermatitis. *Journal of American Academy of Dermatology* 2001; **44**: 89–93.
11. Andoh T, Haza S, Saito A, *et al.* Involvement of leukotriene B4 in spontaneous itch-related behaviour in NC mice with atopic dermatitis-like skin lesions. *Experimental Dermatology* 2011; **20**: 894–898.
12. Marsella R, Nicklin CF. Sulphido-leukotriene production from peripheral leukocytes and skin in clinically normal dogs and house dust mite positive atopic dogs. *Veterinary Dermatology* 2001; **12**: 3–12.

13. Senter DA, Scott DW, Miller WH Jr. Treatment of canine atopic dermatitis with zafirlukast, a leukotriene-receptor antagonist: a single-blinded, placebo-controlled study. *Canadian Veterinary Journal* 2002; **43**: 203–206.
14. Crow DW, Marsella R, Nicklin CF. Double-blinded, placebo-controlled, cross-over pilot study on the efficacy of zileuton for canine atopic dermatitis. *Veterinary Dermatology* 2001; **12**: 189–195.
15. Schlotter YM, Riemers FM, Rutten VP, *et al.* Enzymes involved in the conversion of arachidonic acid to eicosanoids in the skin of atopic dogs. *Experimental Dermatology* 2010; **19**: e317–319.
16. Gros E, Novak N. Cutaneous dendritic cells in allergic inflammation. *Clinical and Experimental Allergy* 2012; **42**: 1161–1175.
17. Novak N. An update on the role of human dendritic cells in patients with atopic dermatitis. *Journal of Allergy and Clinical Immunology* 2012; **129**: 879–886.
18. Gros E, Bussmann C, Bieber T, *et al.* Expression of chemokines and chemokine receptors in lesional and nonlesional upper skin of patients with atopic dermatitis. *Journal of Allergy and Clinical Immunology* 2009; **124**: 753–760.
19. Schäkel K, Hänsel A. News from dendritic cells in atopic dermatitis. *Current Opinion in Allergy and Clinical Immunology* 2011; **11**: 445–450.
20. Vanbervliet B, Akdis M, Vocanson M *et al.* Histamine receptor H1 signaling on dendritic cells plays a key role in the IFN-γ/IL-17 balance in T cell-mediated skin inflammation. *Journal of Allergy and Clinical Immunology* 2011; **127**: 943–953.
21. Akdis CA. Immune regulation by histamine H4 receptors in skin. *Journal of Investigative Dermatology* 2008; **128**: 1615–1616.
22. Wang WL, Li HY, Zhang MS, *et al.* Thymic stromal lymphopoietin: a promising therapeutic target for allergic diseases. *International Archives of Allergy and Immunology* 2012; **160**: 18–26.
23. Klukowska-Rotzler J, Chevret L, Muller EJ, *et al.* Expression of thymic stromal lymphopoietin in canine atopic dermatitis. *Veterinary Dermatology* 2012: **23**: 6–7.
24. Bonkobara M, Miyake F, Yagihara H, *et al.* Canine epidermal langerhans cells express alpha and gamma but not beta chains of high-affinity IgE receptor. *Veterinary Research Communications* 2005; **29**: 499–505.
25. Olivry T, Moore PF, Affolter VK, *et al.* Langerhans cell hyperplasia and IgE expression in canine atopic dermatitis. *Archives of Dermatology Research* 1996; **288**: 579–585.
26. Ricklin ME, Roosje P, Summerfield A. Characterization of canine dendritic cells in healthy, atopic and non-allergic inflamed skin. *Journal of Clinical Immunology* 2010; **30**: 845–854.
27. Johnson-Huang LM, McNutt NS, Krueger JG, *et al.* Cytokine-producing dendritic cells in the pathogenesis of inflammatory skin diseases. *Journal of Clinical Immunology* 2009; **29**: 247–256.
28. Onoue A, Kabashima K, Kobayashi M, *et al.* Induction of eosinophil- and Th2-attracting epidermal chemokines and cutaneous late-phase reaction in tape-stripped skin. *Experimental Dermatology* 2009; **18**: 1036–1043.
29. Böhm I, Bauer R. Th1 cells, Th2 cells and atopic dermatitis. *Hautarzt* 1997; **48**: 223–227.
30. Jenmalm MC, Van Snick J, Cormont F, *et al.* Allergen-induced Th1 and Th2 cytokine secretion in relation to specific allergen sensitization and atopic symptoms in children. *Clinical and Experimental Allergy* 2001; **31**: 1528–1535.
31. Thepen T, Langeveld-Wildschut EG, Bihari IC, *et al.* Biphasic response against aeroallergen in atopic dermatitis showing a switch from an initial TH2 response to a TH1 response in situ: an immunocytochemical study. *Journal of Allergy and Clinical Immunology* 1996; **97**: 828–837.
32. Marsella R, Olivry T, Maeda S. Cellular and cytokine kinetics after epicutaneous allergen challenge (atopy patch testing) with house dust mites in high-IgE beagles. *Veterinary Dermatology* 2006; **17**: 111–120.
33. Olivry T, Dean GA, Tompkins MB, *et al.* Toward a canine model of atopic dermatitis: amplification of cytokine-gene transcripts in the skin of atopic dogs. *Experimental Dermatology* 1999; **8**: 204–211.
34. Nuttall TJ, Knight PA, McAleese SM, *et al.* T-helper 1, T-helper 2 and immunosuppressive cytokines in canine atopic dermatitis. *Veterinary Immunology and Immunopathology* 2002; **87**: 379–384.
35. Keppel KE, Campbell KL, Zuckermann FA, *et al.* Quantitation of canine regulatory T cell populations, serum interleukin-10 and allergen-specific IgE concentrations in healthy control dogs and canine atopic dermatitis patients receiving allergen-specific immunotherapy. *Veterinary Immunology and Immunopathology* 2008; **123**: 337–344.
36. Schlotter YM, Rutten VP, Riemers FM, *et al.* Lesional skin in atopic dogs shows a mixed Type-1 and Type-2 immune responsiveness. *Veterinary Immunology and Immunopathology* 2011; **143**: 20–26.
37. Noh G, Lee JH. Atopic dermatitis and cytokines: the immunoregulatory and therapeutic implications of cytokines in atopic dermatitis—part ii: negative regulation and cytokine therapy in atopic dermatitis. *Recent Patents on Inflammation and Allergy Drug Discovery* 2012; **6**: 248–261.
38. Lee J, Noh G, Lee S, *et al.* Atopic dermatitis and cytokines: recent patients in immunoregulatory and therapeutic implications of cytokines in atopic dermatitis—part i: cytokines in atopic dermatitis. *Recent Patents on Inflammation and Allergy Drug Discovery* 2012; **6**: 222–247.
39. Lin SC, Chuang YH, Yang YH, *et al.* Decrease in interleukin-21 in children suffering with severe atopic dermatitis. *Pediatric Allergy and Immunology* 2011; **22**: 869–875.
40. Tamagawa-Mineoka R, Kishida T, Mazda O, *et al.* IL-21 reduces immediate hypersensitivity reactions in mouse skin by suppressing mast cell activation or IgE production. *Journal of Investigative Dermatology* 2011; **131**: 1513–1520.
41. Dillon SR, Sprecher C, Hammond A, *et al.* Interleukin 31, a cytokine produced by activated T cells, induces dermatitis in mice. *Nature Immunology* 2004; **5**: 752–760.
42. Takaoka A, Arai I, Sugimoto M, *et al.* Expression of IL-31 gene transcripts in NC/Nga mice with atopic dermatitis. *European Journal of Pharmacology* 2005; **516**: 180–181.
43. Sonkoly E, Muller A, Lauerma AI, *et al.* IL-31: a new link between T cells and pruritus in atopic skin inflammation. *Journal of Allergy and Clinical Immunology* 2006; **117**: 411–417.
44. Raap U, Weißmantel S, Gehring M, *et al.* IL-31 significantly correlates with disease activity and Th2 cytokine levels in children with atopic dermatitis. *Pediatric Allergy and Immunology* 2012; **23**: 285–288.
45. Szegedi K, Kremer AE, Kezic S, *et al.* Increased frequencies of IL-31-producing T cells are found in chronic atopic dermatitis skin. *Experimental Dermatology* 2012; **21**: 431–436.
46. Wong CK, Leung KM, Qiu HN, *et al.* Activation of eosinophils interacting with dermal fibroblasts by pruritogenic cytokine IL-31 and alarmin IL-33: implications in atopic dermatitis. *PLoS One* 2012; **7**: e29815.
47. Mizuno T, Kanbayashi S, Okawa T, *et al.* Molecular cloning of canine interleukin-31 and its expression in various tissues. *Veterinary Immunology and Immunopathology* 2009; **131**: 140–143.
48. Gonzales A, Humphrey W, Teel J, *et al.* IL-31: its role in canine pruritus and prevalence in naturally occurring canine atopic dermatitis. *Veterinary Dermatology* 2012; **23**: 6.

49. McCandless EE, Messamore J, Rugg C, *et al.* Production of IL-31 by canine Th2 cells and identification of inflammatory and neuronal target cells. *Veterinary Dermatology* 2012; **23**: 52.
50. Rossbach K, Bäumer W. Expression of different receptors possibly involved in pruritus in canine dorsal ganglia. *Veterinary Dermatology* 2012; **23**: 98–99.
51. Humphrey W, Fleck T, Aleo M, *et al.* Development of a model of IL-31 induced pruritus in beagle dogs. *Veterinary Dermatology* 2012; **23**: 35.
52. Souwer Y, Szegedi K, Kapsenberg ML, *et al.* IL-17 and IL-22 in atopic allergic disease. *Current Opinion in Immunology* 2010; **22**: 821–826.
53. Koga C, Kabashima K, Shiraishi N, *et al.* Possible pathogenic role of Th17 cells for atopic dermatitis. *Journal of Investigative Dermatology* 2008; **128**: 2625–2630.
54. Oyoshi MK, Murphy GF, Geha RS. Filaggrin-deficient mice exhibit TH17-dominated skin inflammation and permissiveness to epicutaneous sensitization with protein antigen. *Journal of Allergy and Clinical Immunology* 2009; **124**: 485–493.
55. Wang LF, Chiu HC, Hsu CJ, *et al.* Epicutaneous sensitization with a protein antigen induces Th17 cells. *Journal of Dermatological Science* 2009; **54**: 192–197.
56. Maccoux LJ, Salway F, Day PJ, *et al.* Expression profiling of select cytokines in canine osteoarthritis tissues. *Veterinary Immunology and Immunopathology* 2007; **118**: 59–67.
57. Eyerich S, Eyerich K, Pennino D, *et al.* Th22 cells represent a distinct human T cell subset involved in epidermal immunity and remodeling. *Journal of Clinical Investigation* 2009; **119**: 3573–3585.
58. Fujita H, Nograles KE, Kikuchi T, *et al.* Human Langerhans cells induce distinct IL-22-producing $CD4^+$ T cells lacking IL-17 production. *Proceedings of the National Academy of Sciences USA* 2009; **106**: 21795–21800.
59. Fujita H. The role of IL-22 in the pathogenesis of skin diseases. *Nihon Rinsho Meneki Gakkai Kaishi* 2012; **35**: 168–175.
60. Samochocki Z, Alifier M, Bodera P, *et al.* T-regulatory cells in severe atopic dermatitis: alterations related to cytokines and other lymphocyte subpopulations. *Archives of Dermatological Research* 2012; **304**: 795–801.
61. Ou LS, Goleva E, Hall C, *et al.* T regulatory cells in atopic dermatitis and subversion of their activity by superantigens. *Journal of Allergy and Clinical Immunology* 2004; **113**: 756–763.
62. Ahn JS, Krishnadas DK, Agrawal B. Dendritic cells partially abrogate the regulatory activity of $CD4^+CD25^+$ T cells present in the human peripheral blood. *International Immunology* 2007; **19**: 227–237.
63. Robinson DS, Larché M, Durham SR. Tregs and allergic disease. *Journal of Clinical Investigation* 2004; **114**: 1389–1397.
64. Agrawal R, Wisniewski JA, Woodfolk JA. The role of regulatory T cells in atopic dermatitis. *Current Problems in Dermatology* 2011; **41**: 112–124.
65. Maeda S, Maeda S, Shibata S, *et al.* House dust mite major allergen Der f 1 enhances proinflammatory cytokine and chemokine gene expression in a cell line of canine epidermal keratinocytes. *Veterinary Immunology and Immunopathology* 2009; **131**: 298–302.
66. Hon KL, Leung TF, Ma KC, *et al.* Serum levels of cutaneous T-cell attracting chemokine (CTACK) as a laboratory marker of the severity of atopic dermatitis in children. *Clinical and Experimental Dermatology* 2004; **29**: 293–296.
67. Maeda S, Fujiwara S, Omori K, *et al.* Lesional expression of thymus and activation-regulated chemokine in canine atopic dermatitis. *Veterinary Immunology and Immunopathology* 2002; **88**: 79–87.
68. Maeda S, Okayama T, Omori K, *et al.* Expression of CC chemokine receptor 4 (CCR4) mRNA in canine atopic skin lesion. *Veterinary Immunology and Immunopathology* 2002; **90**: 145–154.
69. Shibata S, Maeda S, Maeda S, *et al.* Augmentation of CCL17 and CCL28 gene expression by TNF-alpha, IL-1beta, or IFN-gamma in cultured canine keratinocytes. *Research in Veterinary Science* 2010; **88**: 422–426.
70. Vestergaard C, Hvid M, Johansen C, *et al.* Inflammation-induced alterations in the skin barrier function: implications in atopic dermatitis. *Chemical Immunology and Allergy* 2012; **96**: 77–80.
71. Gutowska-Owsiak D, Schaupp AL, Salimi M, *et al.* IL-17 downregulates filaggrin and affects keratinocyte expression of genes associated with cellular adhesion. *Experimental Dermatology* 2012; **21**: 104–110.
72. Alase A, Seltmann J, Werfel T, *et al.* Interleukin-33 modulates the expression of human beta defensin 2 in human primary keratinocytes and may influence the susceptibility to bacterial superinfection in acute atopic dermatitis. *British Journal of Dermatology* 2012; **167**: 1386–1389.
73. Leonard BC, Affolter VK, Bevins CL. Antimicrobial peptides: agents of border protection for companion animals. *Veterinary Dermatology* 2012; **23**: 177–e36.
74. van Damme CM, Willemse T, van Dijk A, *et al.* Altered cutaneous expression of beta-defensins in dogs with atopic dermatitis. *Molecular Immunology* 2009; **46**: 2449–2455.
75. Santoro D, Marsella R, Bunick D, *et al.* Expression and distribution of canine antimicrobial peptides in the skin of healthy and atopic beagles. *Veterinary Immunology and Immunopathology* 2011; **144**: 382–388.
76. Braff MH, Di Nardo A, Gallo RL. Keratinocytes store the antimicrobial peptide cathelicidin in lamellar bodies. *Journal of Investigative Dermatology* 2005; **124**: 394–400.
77. Oren A, Ganz T, Liu L, *et al.* In human epidermis, β-defensin 2 is packaged in lamellar bodies. *Experimental Molecular Pathology* 2003; **74**: 180–182.
78. Yamasaki K, Gallo RL. Antimicrobial peptides in human skin disease. *European Joruna1 of Dermatology* 2008; **18**: 11–21.
79. Mullin J, Carter S, Williams N, *et al.* Transcription of canine toll-like receptor 2, β-defensin 1 and β-defensin 103 in infected atopic skin, non-infected atopic skin, healthy skin and the CPEK cell line. *Veterinary Microbiology* 2013; **162**: 700–706.
80. Kim KH, Han JH, Chung JH, *et al.* Role of staphylococcal superantigen in atopic dermatitis: influence on keratinocytes. *Journal of Korean Medical Science* 2006; **21**: 315–323.
81. Davison S, Allen M, Vaughan R, *et al.* Staphylococcal toxin-induced T cell proliferation in atopic eczema correlates with increased use of superantigen-reactive Vbeta-chains in cutaneous lymphocyte-associated antigen (CLA)-positive lymphocytes. *Clinical and Experimental Immunology* 2000; **121**: 181–186.
82. Strange P, Skov L, Lisby S, *et al.* Staphylococcal enterotoxin B applied on intact normal and intact atopic skin induces dermatitis. *Archives of Dermatology* 1996; **132**: 27–33.
83. Skov L, Olsen JV, Giorno R, *et al.* Application of Staphylococcal enterotoxin B on normal and atopic skin induces up-regulation of T cells by a superantigen-mediated mechanism. *Journal of Allergy and Clinical Immunology* 2000; **105**: 820–826.
84. Lin YT, Wang CT, Hsu CT, *et al.* Differential susceptibility to staphylococcal superantigen (SsAg)-induced apoptosis of $CD4^+$ T cells from atopic dermatitis patients and healthy subjects: the inhibitory effect of IL-4 on SsAg-induced apoptosis. *Journal of Immunology* 2003; **171**: 1102–1108.

4

Allergens and environmental influence

Pascal Prélaud

Clinique Advetia, Paris, France

Conflict of interest: none declared.

Introduction

Historically, canine atopic dermatitis (CAD) was first described in dogs allergic to ragweed pollens [1,2]. These early descriptions led to the definition of atopic dermatitis as a pruritic dermatitis due to allergy to environmental allergens (aeroallergens) [3]. These allergens include dust and storage mites, pollens, mould spores, epithelium, insects, and, historically, miscellaneous antigens like kapok or wool. Today, knowledge about the pathogenesis of the disease is substantial and complex. Environmental allergens still play a major role in most cases, but the improved knowledge on the specificity of the immune response to these allergens has allowed a more targeted diagnostic approach.

Sources of allergens

House dust and storage mites

House dust as a whole is no longer classed as an allergen but rather each constituent is considered separately. It is a mixture of danders, moulds, and mites, the latter being the most potent allergens.

Dust mite biology

House dust and storage mites eat protein-rich substrates, like dandruffs and moulds. *Dermatophagoides* spp. (300 μm) live where keratinized fragments (dandruff, hair, nail, feathers) are abundant, including mattresses, cushions, pillows, couches, and beds. Two days of dandruff production from one human or one dog (250 mg) can feed thousands of mites for 3 months. They can be found in very high concentration on carpets (several thousands/m^2). The optimal microclimate for most domestic mites is 20–30°C and 80–90% humidity [4]. *Dermatophagoides pteronyssinus* (Dp) is vulnerable to fluctuations in humidity [5] and is more common in humid, maritime climates in temperate (e.g. UK) [6] and tropical (e.g. Taiwan) countries [7]. *D. farinae* (Df) is more frequent in dryer environments; in most studies, skin test reactions are much more frequent to Df extracts (18–80%) than to Dp (2–22%) [8].

The presence of a dog does not appear to influence the number of mites in house dust [9].

Euroglyphus maynei is a house dust mite often associated with *Dermatophagoides* in temperate climates. Its role in canine allergic diseases is unclear. In tropical climates, *Blomia tropicalis* (Bt), *D. microceras*, and *D. siboney* are the main house dust mites [7,10,11]. Sensitization to Bt is frequent in atopic dogs in these areas.

Storage mites

The main storage mites involved in allergy in human and animals are *Acarus siro*, *Glycyphagus destructor*, *Tyrophagus putrescentiae* (Tp), and *Lepidoglyphus* sp. These mites are usually found in stored hay, straw, grains, or dry feed stuffs, and use moulds as their main nutritional source; therefore, they can be the main

Veterinary Allergy, First Edition. Edited by Chiara Noli, Aiden Foster, and Wayne Rosenkrantz.

Table 4.1 Minor and major allergens of main aeroallergens of dogs and humans

	Major allergens in human	Major allergens in the dog	Minor allergens in the dog	Molecular weight	Family, function
Acarus siro	Aca s 13	?	?	15	Fatty acid-binding protein
Blomia tropicalis	Blo t 1	? Unnamed	?	39 52 and 76	Cysteine protease ?
Dermatophagoides farinae	Der f 1	–	–	27	Cysteine protease
	Der f 2	Der f 2**	Der f 2*	15	NPC2 family
		Der f 15	–	98/109	Chitinase
		Der f 18	–	60	Chitinase
		Zen 1	–	188	?
Dermatophagoides microceras	Der m 1	?	?	25	Cysteine protease
Dermatophagoides pteronyssinus	Der p 1	?	?	24	Cysteine protease
	Der p 2	?	?	15	NPC2 family
	Der p 15	?	?	59–61	Chitinase
	Der p 18	?	?	49	Chitinase
Euroglyphus maynei	Eur m 1	?	?		Cysteine protease
	Eur m 2	?	?		NPC2 family
Glycyphagus domesticus	Gly d 2	?	?	15	Cysteine protease
Lepidoglyphus destructor	Lep d 2	?	?	16	NPC2 family
Tyrophagus putrescentiae	Tyr p 2	?	?	16	NPC2 family
Cryptomeria japonica (pollen)	Cry j 1	Cry j 1	–	41–45	Pectate lyase
	Cry j 2	–	Cry j 2	45	Polygalacturonase
	–	Cry j 3	–		Thaumatin-like protein
Ambrosia artemisiifolia	Amb a 1	Amb a 1	–	38	Pectate lyase

*In USA and Europe; **in Japan; ?, no data available; –, no major or minor allergen for this species.

constituents of house dust in very humid environments (>80%) [12]. By contrast, the development of storage mites in dry dog food is minimal at low temperature in a dry environment (68%) [13]. When food bags are open in a humid (71%) and warm (23°C) environment almost all dry food is contaminated after 5 weeks [13].

Atopic dogs are more often sensitized to storage mites than human beings. Different European studies report the following frequency of positive intradermal test (IDT) reactions in atopic dogs: *Acarus siro* 35–66%, *Glycyphagus domesticus* 25%, *Tyrophagus putrescentiae* 33–54%, *Lepidoglyphus* 23% [14–17]. The frequency of sensitization is higher with *in vitro* tests, sometimes over 90% [18,19]. It is difficult to know if this high frequency of test reactions is due to cross-sensitization with house dust mites (HDM) or is a result of their regular contact with storage mites (i.e. contaminated dry food). *In vitro* inhibition of HDM-specific IgE showed strong cross-reactions between *D. farinae, A. siro,* and *T. putrescentiae* and also between *D. pteronyssinus* and *L. destructor* [17]. Major allergens of storage mites for the dog are probably high molecular weight proteins (>80 kDa) [18].

In humans, most storage mite allergens have been isolated, sequenced, and cloned. Most of these allergens have homologous structure and functions with *Dermatophagoides* allergens (Table 4.1) [20], supporting the cross-reactivity hypothesis between HDM and storage mites. Sensitization only to storage mites is very rare.

In the dog, the specificity of storage mites sensitization is poorly understood, partly because the prevalence of positive skin test reactions in healthy dogs has been reported as high [15,16].

Cross-sensitization

Cross-sensitization between mite allergens is considered to be highly frequent. In practice, two phenotypes of HDM sensitization are observed in atopic dogs: sensitization to *D. farinae* and *Euroglyphus maynei* alone and polysensitization to most domestic mites, which is probably due to cross-sensitization. Cross-sensitization between *Dermatophagoides* mites and numerous parasite mites was described in the dog: *Sarcoptes scabiei, Cheyletiella* sp., and *Otodectes cynotis* [21–23]. This can lead to false-positive results in skin testing or IgE determination in infested dogs. On the other hand sensitization to HDM in atopic dogs does not significantly influence the results of *Sarcoptes scabiei* serology [24].

Human, feline, canine, equine, and other dandruffs

Human, feline, canine, equine, rodent, or horse dandruff or hair are often incorporated into allergen test panels for the dog. However, cases of true allergy to these components have never been described. To date, *in vitro* testing for this type of sensitization still lacks positive controls and the interpretation of such results must be made with caution.

Feathers

Feathers are often incriminated through bedding, but in these cases they act as a reservoir for domestic mites. Mites living in pigeon feathers (*Diplaegidia columbae*) can represent 10% of the feathers' protein weight. In humans, cross-reactions with *Dermatophagoides* sp. exists, and have provoked anaphylactic reactions in pigeon breeders in Australia. One study from Greece showed a high incidence of positive intradermal test results to pigeon feathers in atopic dogs. However, additional studies on cross-sensitization are missing. Consequently, the use of such allergenic extracts is now rare in veterinary dermatology.

Cockroach

Different species can be found in the canine environment: *Blatella germanica, B. orientali, Suppela suppelectillium,* and *Periplaneta americana*, depending on the geographical area. Their cross-antigenicity with different types of insects is high and up to 50% for *B. germanica* and *Ctenocephalides felis felis* [25]. The frequency of sensitization is highly variable, from 0%, 16% in Marseille, to 60% in New York. However, prospective studies are necessary to provide evidence of the clinical usefulness of such allergen extracts.

Pollens

Allergenic pollens must be airborne and produced in large amounts to be able to sensitize humans and animals. Therefore entomophilic pollens are theoretically poor allergens (i.e. fruit trees flowers, daisy flowers) [26].

As dogs are closer to the ground the sensitizing pollens may be different to those observed 1.5 m higher in humans. Pollens, which are present in large amounts on the ground, like grass pollens, can sensitize atopic dogs all year round [27].

The most frequent sensitizing pollens are those of ragweed in North America and Eastern Europe, grasses in most European countries, birch in northern Europe, and Japanese cypress in Japan. Three families of allergenic pollens are classically described with specific pollination seasons:

- trees (early and late spring);
- grasses (late spring and early summer);
- weeds (summer and early autumn).

The pollination season is influenced by the climate and varies depending on the year and geographical location (see the websites given below for pollen calendars of various countries).

Tree pollens

This group is heterogeneous. The most commonly involved tree pollen in Europe is birch, the cypress and olive tree in the Mediterranean area, and the Japanese cypress in Japan. The most important trees and tree families involved in allergic sensitization in dogs are:

- Plane tree (*Platanus acerifolia*) is often involved in human allergy, but no sensitization has been described in dogs.
- Betulacea family (birch, alder, hazel, hornbeam) is the main family of tree pollens sensitizing allergic dogs in Europe.
- Pinacea (i.e. pine trees, *Pinus pinaster*) sensitizations are not described in the dog.
- Oleacea are mainly composed of olive tree (*Olea europaea*) and ash tree (*Fraxinus excelsior*). Cross-antigenicity is described, which enables the use of mixtures or only one species in routine diagnosis.
- Cupressacea are one of the most allergenic tree pollens around the world, with Japanese cypress (*Cryptomeria japonica*) in Japan, red cedar (*Juniperus virginiana)* in North America, and cypress (*Cupressus* sp.) in Europe.
- Moracea (mulberry, *Morus* sp.), leguminous plants (locust tree, *Robinia pseudoacacia*, mimosa, *Mimosa* sp.), Fagacea (oak, *Quercus* sp.), chestnut (*Castanea* sp.), Salicacea (willow, *Salix babylonica*, poplar, *Populus* sp.), and lime tree can be identified in large intradermal or serological screening tests but their clinical significance is not known.

Grass pollens

Grasses are the main pollens involved in pollen allergy in animals in most countries. They include many different species with broad common allergenicity, e.g. Bermuda grass (*Cynodon dactylon*), Timothy grass

(*Phleum pratense*), Kentucky blue grass (*Poa pratensis*), Johnson grass (*Sorghum halepense*), orchard grass (*Dactylis* sp.), oat grass (*Arrhenaterum* sp.), ryegrass (*Lolium* sp.), and cultivated rye (*Secale cereale*). Cross-sensitization is so common that human allergists routinely use mixtures of only two, five or seven grass pollens.

Pollination occurs in late spring until midsummer. They produce very large amounts of pollens, which can be on the ground the whole year round. A study in Europe showed that dogs can be in contact with these pollens even out of the pollination season [27]. Accordingly, it could be considered in atopic dogs with non-seasonal clinical signs. The indoor environment can also be rich in grass pollen allergens the whole year round [28]. This is why grass pollens can be considered as non-seasonal allergens in some atopic dogs.

Weed pollens

The weed family of pollens is also very heterogeneous.

The English plantain (*Plantago lanceolata*) is rarely involved in the dog and sensitization is often associated with sensitization to grasses.

Ragweed (*Ambrosia* sp.) and *Artemisia* are the main members of the Composacea family. Ragweed is an invasive weed, which produces a very allergenic pollen. It is involved mainly in North America and in areas of Europe, especially the Rhône valley in France, northern Italy, and central and eastern Europe (Austria, Hungary, Romania, Serbia, Slovenia, and Croatia). In these areas, sensitization of atopic dogs is as frequent as 5–27% [29] and ragweed is often the second most frequent allergen implicated after Df in atopic dogs. Signs in allergic animals are typically seasonal (late summer, autumn).

The nettle (*Urtica* sp.) and the pellitory (*Parietaria judaica, P. officinalis*) are well-known sources of clinically relevant allergens in the family Urticaceae. Pellitory is the most allergenic Urticacea pollen, pollinating from April to October in the Mediterranean area. However, it can provoke clinical flares in any season and the pollens contain enzymes that are able to disrupt the skin barrier [29].

The clinical importance of Chenopodiacea, Amarantacea, and Polygonacea is not known despite occasional sensitization.

Airborne allergy to ornamental plants (aster, daisy, or sunflower family) is increasingly being described in humans [29] but such sensitization has not been described in animals.

Mould spores

Allergy to mould spores is controversial in canine medicine because numerous false positive reactions have been observed *in vivo* and *in vitro*. These spores can be found in humid habitats (*Alternaria, Aspergillus, Penicillium*) or dry habitats (*Cladosporium* sp.), depending on the sporulation season.

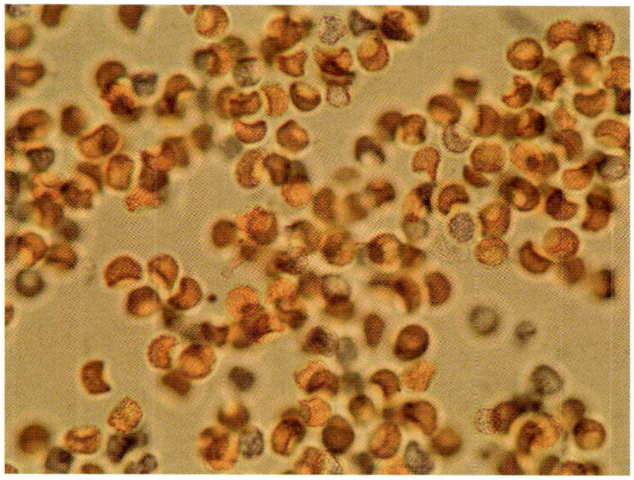

Figure 4.1 Spores of *Ustilago* sp. in the coat of a dog.

Some moulds that parasitize plants, like *Ustilago* sp., can produce very large amounts of spores, which can be easily found in dogs hair and provoke hypersensitivity reactions (personal observation) (Figure 4.1).

To date more than 150 mould allergens have been identified; however, no definitive study has been published on mould allergy in the dog.

Environment and canine atopic dermatitis

Several epidemiological studies have highlighted the potential role of the environment in the development of CAD. One retrospective study from Sweden on three predisposed breeds—boxer, bull terrier, and West Highland white terrier—showed that dogs developing CAD spent significantly more time indoors [30]. In a larger study of Labradors and retrievers in Germany and Switzerland, Meury *et al.* [31] identified some environmental predisposing factors, suggesting again the importance of the indoor environment. In this study, living in a rural environment, with other dogs and cats or walking regularly in a forest was associated with a lower risk of developing CAD. On the contrary, living in an indoor environment was a predisposing factor for CAD. However, these associations do not prove causality or the potential role of aeroallergens.

Another way to explore the link between environmental allergens and CAD is to evaluate the presence of allergens in the environment of allergic and non-allergic dogs. A study comparing the environment of HDM-sensitive dogs to that of healthy controls showed a higher density of HDM in the dog's sleeping area in both groups. However, such results do not prove causality (i.e. HDM concentration could have been different when the dog was initially sensitized) [9]. Another study did not show any association of HDM exposure in beddings or living rooms of Labrador dogs that developed CAD [32]. Interestingly, in this study there were higher levels of Der p 1 and mould glucans on carpeted floors compared to smooth floors; however, levels of these two compounds were not increased in the coats and bedding of dogs living in carpeted living rooms [32]. This study also showed that endotoxin exposure was inversely associated with CAD, suggesting a protective effect of high indoor endotoxin exposure towards the development of the condition [32]. This protective effect of Gram-negative endotoxins could be due to their immunomodulatory properties, as seen in humans [33].

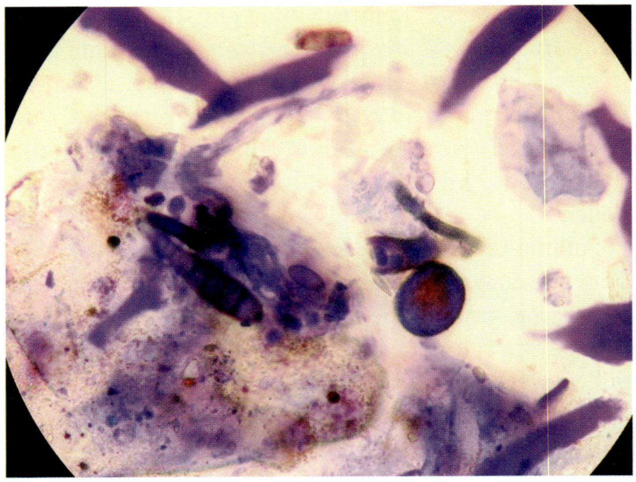

Figure 4.2 Numerous pollens and mould spores from the interdigital area of a dog (stained with RAL555, ×100).

Mites as triggers of canine atopic dermatitis flares and route of sensitization

Dust and storage mite exposure can provoke flare ups in dogs with atopic dermatitis and sensitized to *D. farinae*. In experimentally sensitized dogs, the epicutaneous application, via occluded patch tests or painting of allergen extracts, resulted in visible inflammation as early as 2 hours after provocation, and it increases in severity with time [34,35]. Such provocation can be done with Df or Tp extracts in Df-sensitized dogs [34–36].

It is now well recognized that the route of sensitization to most environmental allergens is epicutaneous in cases of atopic dermatitis [37,38]. In a lineage of atopic dogs, weekly epicutaneous applications of HDM extracts led to increased HDM-specific IgE and provoked localized and generalized pruritic dermatitis resembling spontaneous CAD [35]. Skin barrier defects can enhance this propensity to induce sensitization because the removal of the stratum corneum enhances IgE-dependant epicutaneous sensitization to HDM in the dog [35]. No data have been published on pollen sensitization, but a similar pathomechanism is very probably implicated, because high amounts of pollens are isolated quite frequently from the face and interdigital areas in the dog (Figure 4.2).

Environmental allergen avoidance as a therapeutic tool

In experimental conditions, the confinement of atopic dogs in an environment without house dust mites can control pruritus in almost 66% of the dogs in 1 week [39]. However, such measures are difficult or impossible to reproduce in practice. Reducing mite allergens is possible when using environmental flea control or benzoyl benzoate spray. In an open clinical trial, the use of the latter was associated with a reduction of clinical signs of CAD in mite-hypersensitive dogs [40]. However, there is a need for controlled blinded studies to prove such an efficacy. If mite avoidance measures were to be attempted, as for human patients, a combination of measures would be performed: acaricides, impermeable pet mattress covers, frequent vacuuming and frequent cleaning of mattresses, and bathing the dog. The latter is very important in practice. Frequent shampooing or bathing can help removing environmental allergens, bacteria, and yeasts and help control skin barrier defects and pruritus [41]. More details on allergen avoidance can be found in Chapter 11.

Choosing environmental allergens for allergen-specific immunotherapy (ASIT)

When sensitization is limited to one or two aeroallergens, choosing allergens for ASIT is easy. In cases of polysensitization, this choice is more complex. In human medicine, there is an ongoing debate as to whether polysensitized patients are best treated with many allergens simultaneously (chosen according to the sensitization profile, a predominantly North American approach) or a single allergen (chosen according to the most clinically problematic allergy, a predominantly European approach) [42]. Such a debate cannot exist in the dog, because cross-sensitization between house dust mites is highly frequent and the quality of storage mite extracts is inconsistent.

One study in the dog compared a *D. farinae* 100% extract to a placebo in ASIT of polysensitized dogs [43].

Table 4.2 Examples of proposed restricted ASIT according to the results of intradermal or serology tests and cross-reactivity to antigens

Positive allergen tests	ASIT composition
Df	Df
Df, Dp	Df, Dp
Df, Dp, Tp, As, Ld	Df, Dp
Grass pollens	Grasses mix (2, 4, 5, or 7)
Df, Dp, Tp, As, Ld , grasses	Df, Dp, grasses mix (2, 4, 5, or 7)
Df, Dp, Tp, As, Ld, tree or weed pollen	Df, Dp, pollens (if season of pollination is linked to AD flare)
Df, Dp, Tp, As, Ld, *Alternaria* or other mould spores	Df, Dp
Df, Dp, flea	Df, Dp

No significant difference was observed; however, no studies compared *D. farinae* to a mixture of domestic mites in polysensitized dogs.

Both approaches (restricted choice of allergens and 'all included') can be justified. However, an approach close to single ASIT (restricted choice) allows the use of allergen extracts for human use that are often significantly less expensive than veterinary products in most countries (Table 4.2). More detail on ASIT can be found in Chapter 12.

Another very important way to limit the number of allergens is to follow recommendations on allergen mixtures [44]. This can lead to exclusion of insects or mould extracts if pollens or HDM are included, because these extracts can have protease activity.

Allergen specificities

Major and minor allergens

Major allergens are defined as those that are recognized by more than 50% of atopic patients' sera and minor allergens as those recognized by less than 50% [45]. By convention, major and minor allergens are named by the first three letters of the genus and first letter of the species of the allergen and end with a progressive number, which is often determined by human major allergens (Table 4.1). To date, there are only three major aeroallergens defined in the dog, which are structurally very different from those of the humans. They are derived from the house dust mite *D. farinae* (Df) and the pollen of Japanese cypress trees (Table 4.1).

Most major allergens for the dog are high molecular weight proteins. This has been demonstrated for *D. farinae* and is highly suspected for *D. pteronyssinus, A. siro,* and *T. putrescentiae* [4,8,46,47].

The major Df allergens in dogs worldwide are Der f 15, Der f 18, and Zen 1, as 80–90% of dogs sensitized to Df extracts recognize these fractions [4,8,46,47]. The Der f 2 allergen seems to be a major allergen in Japan [48] and not in the USA and Europe. Such a difference could be due to genetic variations between dog populations in these countries. Interestingly, Der f 1, the major Df allergen in humans, is almost never recognized by dogs sensitized to Df (0–14%)[49].

The description of major allergens Der f 15 and 18 in the dog led to the discovery of new major allergens in humans, Der p 15 and 18, which have high sequence homology with their Df counterpart [50]. Some major allergens of house dust mites have proteolytic activity, which could enhance skin barrier defect [51]. This is now largely substantiated for Der p 1, but the role of such proteases is not known in the dog.

Panallergens

Panallergens are evolutionarily conserved, ubiquitous components of several complex sources of allergens, which usually act as minor allergens; however, their presence has important clinical implications in establishing the phenomenon of food–pollen cross-reactivity in humans. This phenomenon is very rare in canine medicine and only one case of cross-reactivity, between tomato and Japanese cypress, has been described [52]. The Cry j 3 allergen is hypothesized to be the responsible panallergen, a thaumatin-like protein categorized in the PR-5 protein family [53]. Cross-sensitization to birch pollen and fruits or house dust mites and sea food (tropomyosin) is not described in veterinary medicine.

Non-allergenic mode of action

Most mite allergens have an enzymatic activity and/or can interfere with the innate immune response (i.e. through toll-like receptors, TLR). In canine *in vitro* experimental models, *Dermatophagoides* and storage mites species are able to elicit cytokine secretion (IL-1alpha, IL-1 receptor antagonist, IL-6, IL-8, cutaneous T cell-attracting chemokine, transforming growth factor-alpha, granulocyte/macrophage, and macrophage colony-stimulating factors) from keratinocytes or fibroblasts in culture [54–56].

Pollens can also act directly on the immune system through release of water-soluble phytoprostanes that display Th2-polarizing capacities *in vivo* [57]. These observations are one of the arguments for regular shampooing of atopic dogs sensitized to environmental allergens.

Conclusion

The environment is probably important in the development of CAD, as shown in epidemiological studies, but we do not know if this is linked to exposure to aeroallergens. Furthermore, the frequency of sensitization is not systematically higher in atopic dogs than in healthy ones in predisposed breeds [19,58] and some dogs can develop atopic dermatitis without known sensitization to common potential allergens (atopic-like dermatitis) [59,60].

Sensitization to environmental allergens is predominantly to HDM in atopic dogs. Knowledge of the specificity of the canine IgE response to these antigens has shown some significant differences from that in humans. Therefore, a standardization of allergenic extracts adapted to each species (human, dog, cat, horse) is necessary, because the current standardization of allergenic extracts is mainly based on the concentration of human major allergens.

This standardization could allow the production of more efficient allergenic extracts for the diagnosis and treatment of atopic dermatitis. Furthermore, this would enable a big step forward in clinical and basic science research of this complex disease.

Internet sites

Pollen calendars and alerts:

- Europe: www.medaeronet.net
- Australia: www.allergy.org.au
- United States: www.pollen.com
- Japan: www.tenki.jp (then click on 花粉)

Allergens nomenclature:

- www.allergen.org

References

1. Wittich FW. Spontaneous allergy in the lower animal. *Journal of Allergy* 1941; **62**: 236–242.
2. Patterson R. Ragweed allergy in the dog. *Journal of the American Veterinary Medical Association* 1959; **135**: 178–180.
3. Halliwell RE. Atopic disease in the dog. *Veterinary Record* 1971; **89**: 209–214.
4. Nuttall TJ, Hill PB, Bensignor E, *et al.* House dust and forage mite allergens and their role in human and canine atopic dermatitis. *Veterinary Dermatology* 2006; **17**: 223–235.
5. Arlian LG, Morgan MS. Biology, ecology, and prevalence of dust mites. *Immunology and Allergy Clinics of North America* 2003; **23**: 443–468.
6. Colloff MJ. Mites from house dust in Glasgow. *Medical and Veterinary Entomology* 1987; **1**: 163–168.
7. Tsai HHL, Chen C, Chen K-H, *et al.* Detection of specific serum IgE in dog with allergic dermatitis and the identification of major brewer's yeast allergens. *Taiwan Veterinary Journal* 2012; **38**: 138–152.
8. Noli C, Bernadina WE, Willemse T. The significance of reactions to purified fractions of *Dermatophagoides pteronyssinus* and *Dermatophagoïdes farinae* in canine atopic dermatitis. *Veterinary Immunology and Immunopathology* 1996; **52**: 147–157.
9. Farmaki R, Saridomichelakis MN, Leontides L, *et al.* Presence and density of domestic mites in the microenvironment of mite-sensitive dogs with atopic dermatitis. *Veterinary Dermatology* 2010; **21**: 469–476.
10. Prélaud P. *Allergologie Canine*. Paris: Masson-PMCAC, 2008.
11. Cunha VES, Silva MH, Faccini JLH. Serological identification of house dust mite allergens in dogs with atopic dermatitis. *Pesquisa Veterinaria Brasileira* 2012; **32**: 917–921.
12. Canfield MS, Wrenn WJ. *Tyrophagus putrescentiae* mites grown in dog food cultures and the effect mould growth has on mite survival and reproduction. *Veterinary Dermatology* 2010; **21**: 57–62.
13. Brazis P, Serra M, Selles A, *et al.* Evaluation of storage mite contamination of commercial dry dog food. *Veterinary Dermatology* 2008; **19**: 209–214.
14. Vollset I. Immediate type hypersensitivity in dogs induced by storage mites. *Research in Veterinary Science* 1986; **40**: 123–127.
15. Bensignor E, Carlotti DN. Sensitivity patterns to house dust mites and forage mites in atopic dogs: 150 cases. *Veterinary Dermatology* 2002; **13**: 37–42.
16. Mueller RS, Fieseler KV, Rosychuk RA, *et al.* Intradermal testing with the storage mite *Tyrophagus putrescentiae* in normal dogs and dogs with atopic dermatitis in Colorado. *Veterinary Dermatology* 2005; **16**: 27–31.
17. Saridomichelakis MN, Marsella R, Lee KW, *et al.* Assessment of cross-reactivity among five species of house dust and storage mites. *Veterinary Dermatology* 2008; **19**: 67–76.
18. Arlian LG, Schumann RJ, Morgan MS, *et al.* Serum immunoglobulin E against storage mite allergens in dogs with atopic dermatitis. *American Journal of Veterinary Research* 2003; **64**: 32–36.
19. Roque JB, O'Leary CA, Kyaw-Tanner M, *et al.* High allergen-specific serum immunoglobulin E levels in nonatopic West Highland white terriers. *Veterinary Dermatology* 2011; **22**: 257–266.
20. Fernandez-Caldas E, Iraola V, Carnes J. Molecular and biochemical properties of storage mites (except *Blomia* species). *Protein and Peptide Letter* 2007; **14**: 954–959.
21. Prélaud P, Guaguère E. Sensitisation to the house dust mite *Dermatophagoides farinae* in dogs with Sarcoptic mange. *Veterinary Dermatology* 1995; **6**: 205–209.
22. Saridomichelakis MN, Koutinas AF, Gioulekas D, *et al.* Sensitization to dust mites in cats with Otodectes cynotis infestation. *Veterinary Dermatology* 1999; **10**: 89–94.
23. White SD, Rosychuk RA, Fieseler KV. Clinicopathologic findings, sensitivity to house dust mites and efficacy of milbemycin oxime treatment of dogs with *Cheyletiella* sp. infestation. *Veterinary Dermatology* 2001; **12**: 13–18.
24. Buckley LM, Schmidt VM, McEwan NA, *et al.* Positive and negative predictive values of a sarcoptes specific IgG ELISA in a tested population of pruritic dogs. *Veterinary Dematology* 2012; **23** (Suppl. 1): 36.
25. Pucheu-Haston CM, Grier TJ, Bevier DE. Allergenic cross-reactivities in flea-reactive canine serum samples. *American Journal of Veterinary Research* 1996; **57**: 1000–1005.
26. Prélaud P. Traitement de la dermatite allergique par piqûres de puces. *Pratique Médicale et Chrirurgicale de l'Animal de Compagnie* 2011; **46**: 411–418.

27. Fraser MA, Caulton E, McNeil PE. Examination of faecal samples as a method of identifying pollen exposure in dogs. *Veterinary Record* 2001; **149**: 424–426.
28. Fahlbusch B, Hornung D, Heinrich J, *et al.* Quantification of group 5 grass pollen allergens in house dust. *Clinical and Experimental Allergy* 2000; **30**: 1645–1652.
29. D'Amato G, Cecchi L, Bonini S, *et al.* Allergenic pollen and pollen allergy in Europe. *Allergy* 2007; **62**: 976–990.
30. Nodtvedt A, Bergvall K, Sallander M, *et al.* A case-control study of risk factors for canine atopic dermatitis among boxer, bullterrier and West Highland white terrier dogs in Sweden. *Veterinary Dermatology* 2007; **18**: 309–315.
31. Meury S, Molitor V, Doherr MG, *et al.* Role of the environment in the development of canine atopic dermatitis in Labrador and golden retrievers. *Veterinary Dermatology* 2011; **22**: 327–334.
32. Looringh van Beeck FA, Hoekstra H, Brunekreef B, *et al.* Inverse association between endotoxin exposure and canine atopic dermatitis. *Veterinary Journal* 2010; **190**: 215–219.
33. Caramalho I, Lopes-Carvalho T, Ostler D, *et al.* Regulatory T cells selectively express toll-like receptors and are activated by lipopolysaccharide. *Journal of Experimental Medicine* 2003; **197**: 403–411.
34. Olivry T, Deangelo KB, Dunston SM, *et al.* Patch testing of experimentally sensitized beagle dogs: development of a model for skin lesions of atopic dermatitis. *Veterinary Dermatology* 2006; **17**: 95–102.
35. Pucheu-Haston CM, Jackson HA, Olivry T, *et al.* Epicutaneous sensitization with *Dermatophagoides farinae* induces generalized allergic dermatitis and elevated mite-specific immunoglobulin E levels in a canine model of atopic dermatitis. *Clinical and Experimental Allergy* 2008; **38**: 667–679.
36. Marsella R, Saridomichelakis MN. Environmental and oral challenge with storage mites in beagles experimentally sensitized to *Dermatophagoides farinae. Veterinary Dermatology* 2010; **21**: 105–111.
37. Olivry T, Hill PB. The ACVD task force on canine atopic dermatitis (IX): the controversy surrounding the route of allergen challenge in canine atopic dermatitis. *Veterinary Immunology and Immunopathology* 2001; **81**: 219–225.
38. Marsella R, Sousa CA, Gonzales AJ, *et al.* Current understanding of the pathophysiologic mechanisms of canine atopic dermatitis. *Journal of the American Veterinary Medical Association* 2012; **241**: 194–207.
39. Fujimura M. The study of canine atopic dermatitis involving the isolation of dogs. *Polish Journal of Veterinary Science* 2011; **14**: 273–277.
40. Swinnen C, Vroom M. The clinical effect of environmental control of house dust mites in 60 house dust mite-sensitive dogs. *Veterinary Dermatology* 2004; **15**: 31–36.
41. Olivry T, DeBoer DJ, Favrot C, *et al.* Treatment of canine atopic dermatitis: 2010 clinical practice guidelines from the International Task Force on Canine Atopic Dermatitis. *Veterinary Dermatology* 2010; **21**: 233–248.
42. Calderon MA, Cox L, Casale TB, *et al.* Multiple-allergen and single-allergen immunotherapy strategies in polysensitized patients: Looking at the published evidence. *Journal of Allergy and Clinical Immunology* 2012; **129**: 929–934.
43. Willemse T, Bardagi M, Carlotti DN, *et al. Dermatophagoides farinae*-specific immunotherapy in atopic dogs with hypersensitivity to multiple allergens: a randomised, double blind, placebo-controlled study. *Veterinary Journal* 2009; **180**: 337–342.
44. Esch RE. Allergen immunotherapy: what can and cannot be mixed? *Journal of Allergy and Clinical Immunology* 2008; **122**: 659–660.
45. Berrens L. What is a major allergen? *Clinical and Experimental Allergy* 1994; **24**: 606–609.
46. McCall C, Hunter S, Stedman K, *et al.* Characterization and cloning of a major high molecular weight house dust mite allergen (Der f 15) for dogs. *Veterinary Immunology and Immunopathology* 2001; **78**: 231–247.
47. Weber E, Hunter S, Stedman K, *et al.* Identification, characterization, and cloning of a complementary DNA encoding a 60-kd house dust mite allergen (Der f 18) for human beings and dogs. *Journal of Allergy and Clinical Immunology* 2003; **112**: 79–86.
48. Masuda K, Tsujimoto H, Fujiwara S, *et al.* IgE sensitivity and cross-reactivity to crude and purified mite allergens (Der f 1, Der f 2, Der p 1, Der p 2) in atopic dogs sensitive to Dermatophagoides mite allergens. *Veterinary Immunology and Immunopathology* 1999; **72**: 303–313.
49. Olivry T, Dunston SM, Favrot C, *et al.* The novel high molecular weight *Dermatophagoides farinae* allergen Zen-1 is a major allergen in North American and European mite-allergic dogs with atopic dermatitis. *Veterinary Dermatology* 2009; **20**: 215.
50. O'Neil SE, Heinrich TK, Hales BJ, *et al.* The chitinase allergens Der p 15 and Der p 18 from *Dermatophagoides pteronyssinus. Clinical and Experimental Allergy* 2006; **36**: 831–839.
51. Nakamura T, Hirasawa Y, Takai T, *et al.* Reduction of skin barrier function by proteolytic activity of a recombinant house dust mite major allergen Der f 1. *Journal of Investigative Dermatology* 2006; **126**: 2719–2723.
52. Fujimura M, Ohmori K, Masuda K, *et al.* Oral allergy syndrome induced by tomato in a dog with Japanese cedar (*Cryptomeria japonicum*) pollinosis. *Journal of Veterinary Medical Science* 2002; **64**: 1069–1070.
53. Kubotaa S, Miyajia K, Shimoa Y, *et al.* IgE reactivity to a Cry j 3, an allergen of Japanese cedar (*Cryptomeria japonica*) pollen in dogs with canine atopic dermatitis. *Veterinary Immunology and Immunopathology* 2012; **149**: 132–135.
54. Arlian LG, Morgan MS. Immunomodulation of skin cytokine secretion by house dust mite extracts. *International Archives of Allergy and Immunology* 2011; **156**: 171–178.
55. Boasen J, Chisholm D, Lebet L, *et al.* House dust extracts elicit Toll-like receptor–dependent dendritic cell responses. *Journal of Allergy and Clinical Immunology* 2005; **116**: 185–191.
56. Kimura T, Sekido M, Chimura N, *et al.* Production of GM-CSF mediated by cysteine protease of Der f 1 in canine keratinocytes. *Journal of Veterinary Medical Science* 2012; **131**: 298–302.
57. Gutermuth J, Bewersdorff M, Traidl-Hoffmann C, *et al.* Immunomodulatory effects of aqueous birch pollen extracts and phytoprostanes on primary immune responses in vivo. *Journal of Allergy and Clinical Immunology* 2007; **120**: 293–299.
58. Laubera B, Molitorb V, Meuryc S, *et al.* Total IgE and allergen-specific IgE and IgG antibody levels in sera of atopic dermatitis affected and non-affected Labrador and Golden retrievers. *Veterinary Immunology and Immunopathology* 2012; **149**: 112–118.
59. Prélaud P, Cochet-Faivre N. A retrospective study of 21 cases of canine atopic-like dermatitis. *Veterinary Dermatology* 2007; **18**: 385.
60. Halliwell REW. Revised nomenclature for veterinary allergy. *Veterinary Immunology and Immunopathology* 2006; **114**: 207–208.

5

The genetics of canine atopic dermatitis

Tim Nuttall

Royal (Dick) School of Veterinary Studies, University of Edinburgh, Easter Bush Veterinary Centre, Roslin, Midlothian, UK

Conflict of interest: none declared.

Introduction

Both human and canine atopic dermatitis (AD) have a genetic component. Family history is a major risk factor for human AD [1]. Strong breed predispositions, with high prevalences in some dog breeds (e.g. up to 25% in West Highland white terrier dogs), suggest that this is also true in canine AD (CAD) [2–4]. In British guide dogs (mostly Labrador and golden retriever cross bred dogs) the mean heritability is 0.47 (range 0.13 to 0.81), suggesting that the genetic background accounts for almost 50% of the risk of developing CAD [5]. Experimental laboratory colonies of dogs with conditions that mimic clinical CAD have also been established [6–9]. Despite this, the risk of developing CAD, the severity, and the response to treatment are highly variable. This may be explained by complex genotypes, but it also likely that environmental influences are important [3,10,11]. These may be important in the development of allergic and inflammatory responses, tolerance, and skin barrier function. The balance of genetic and environmental influences, however, varies with breed. For example, environmental factors do not appear to affect the prevalence of CAD in West Highland white terrier dogs [11].

Historically, studies have been limited to observations of breed predispositions, and heritability and linkage studies. Advances in genomics now allow us to study the genetics of AD in more detail. The aim of this chapter is to review these techniques, the current evidence for the genetic basis of CAD, and future opportunities.

Investigating atopic dermatitis-associated genotypes

Genome-wide linkage studies

Genome-wide linkage studies have been widely used to investigate human AD [1]. These are family-based approaches using affected individuals, their parents, and non-affected family members. The inheritance of the disease is compared to the inheritance of microsatellite markers.

This technique evaluates the whole genome, avoiding the limitations of candidate-gene approaches. Microsatellite markers have been used to identify chromosomal loci associated with human AD [1]. However, the usefulness of this approach has been questioned, as there has been little overlap in the results from published studies. The linked loci extend over large areas of each chromosome that span several genes, making it difficult to identify a candidate gene without either extensive chromosomal sequencing or further genotyping of additional microsatellite markers clustered around the loci of interest. In addition to these problems, it has proved difficult to amass enough affected individuals and unaffected relatives to perform powerful genome-wide linkage studies in CAD.

Candidate gene association studies

It is possible to genotype markers specifically associated with candidate genes of interest. This allows the use of relatively simple markers such as single nucleotide polymorphisms (SNPs), insertions, deletions, and repeats. In addition, candidate gene approaches are not

Veterinary Allergy, First Edition. Edited by Chiara Noli, Aiden Foster, and Wayne Rosenkrantz.

limited to families, making it easier to recruit large numbers of affected individuals and controls [1]. However, case–control studies can be confounded by population stratification effects such as ethnicity or breed and geography. A major disadvantage of this approach is that it is hypothesis-dependent in that the genetic analysis is restricted to genes that have been previously implicated in the pathogenesis of AD. Novel genes may therefore be missed.

Genome-wide association studies

Genome-wide association studies (GWASs) are a hypothesis-free way to discover disease-associated SNPs [1]. This avoids the limitations of using candidate genes while retaining the advantages of the case–control approach. Genome sequencing has identified large numbers of genetic variants that can be read on SNP arrays. This allows identification of SNPs that are more frequent in affected individuals than controls. These disease-associated SNPs mark regions of the genome that may be involved in the pathogenesis of AD (Figure 5.1). Depending on the number and distribution of SNPs, GWASs can interrogate the entire genome. However, fine mapping relies on having many SNPs evenly distributed throughout the genome. In addition, disease-associated SNPs may be located in unknown areas of the genome. Further sequencing and functional studies are therefore required to confirm whether the disease association is causal. The functional effects, moreover, may depend on the specific combinations of SNPs within a gene and/or interactions with SNPs in other genes, or both. Another weakness of this approach is that GWASs are limited to identifying common SNPs with small effects. Rare SNPs with large effects, untyped SNPs, and structural variations (e.g. microsatellites, variable number tandem repeats, insertions, deletions, and duplications) may be missed.

GWASs in dogs can take advantage of their strong linkage disequilibrium (LD). In humans, LD is relatively weak (extending over about 10–100 kb), necessitating high-density arrays (up to 1.6×10^6 SNPs) and large cohorts (at least 1000 cases and controls) [12]. Dog breeds are of recent origin and are highly inbred with LD over long distances (0.8–5 Mb) [13,14], meaning that fewer genetic markers and smaller sample sizes can be used. For example, complete coverage of the canine genome only requires 5000 to 30 000 SNPs [15]. However, low numbers of SNPs can result in incomplete coverage

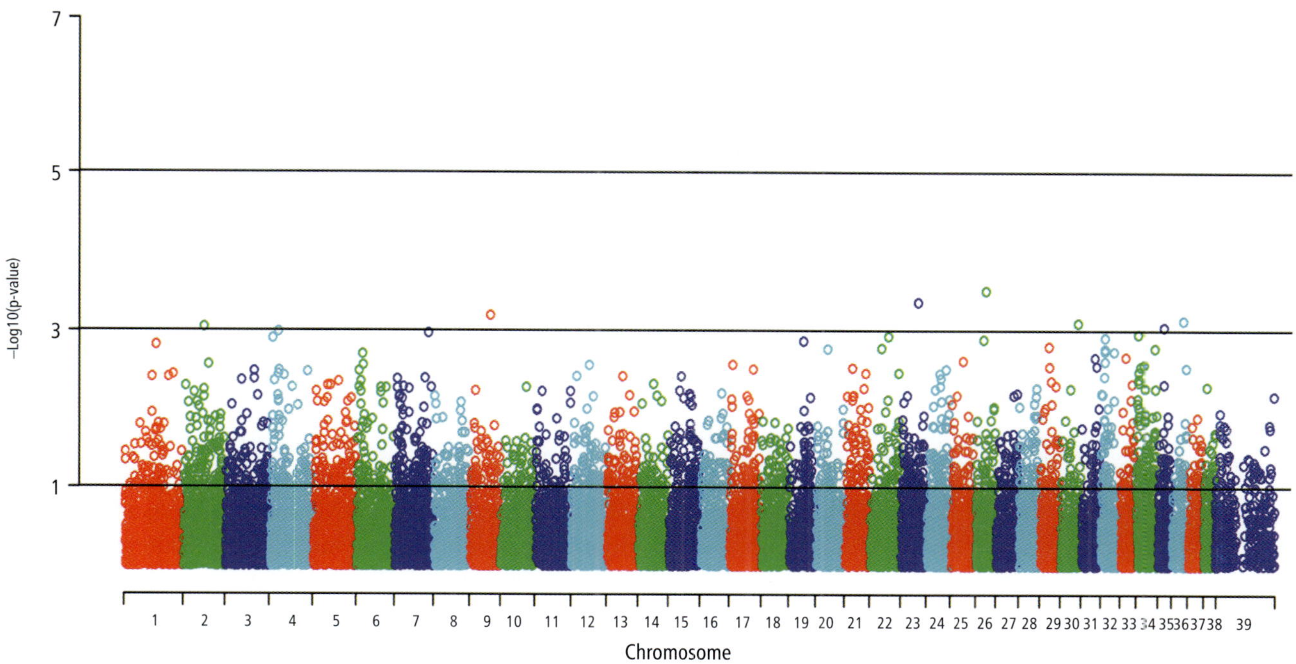

Figure 5.1 Whole-genome association plot of significance for CAD after Wood *et al.* [16]. This study used a chip with approximately 22 000 SNPs to study their frequency in atopic and healthy control dogs. The SNPs are plotted on the x-axis according to their position on each chromosome, with their association with CAD on the y-axis shown as $\log_{10}$ *P*-value. The circles represent individual SNPs, which are grouped by chromosome. Individual SNPs that are statistically more frequent in the atopic compared to the control population are found above the great mass of SNPs coalescing nearer the x-axis. These identify potentially AD-associated genes or loci for further studies. (Reprinted with permission from [16]. © 2009 Springer Science+Business Media.)

that could miss important genes. For example, the first GWAS in CAD [16] used the Illumina Canine SNP20 chip (San Diego, California, USA). This included 22 362 canine SNPs from the CanFam 2.0 assembly based on the boxer dog with the partial sequence of a standard poodle dog and 100 000 sequence reads from nine other breeds. Despite this, many genes of interest (e.g. filaggrin) were not included. These gaps should be covered by continued development of the Dog Genome Project.

Quantitative reverse transcription polymerase chain reaction (RT-PCR)

Quantification of mRNA can identify genes that are differentially regulated in affected individuals compared to controls. Single-chip microarrays can be used for hypothesis-free evaluation of very large numbers of genes in any tissue [17]. Gene transcription, however, does not necessarily imply causality, as the change may be secondary to the disease process. Despite this, gene expression studies help identify candidate genes and confirm involvement of genes associated with AD in genomic studies. Genome-wide microarrays can produce a hypothesis-free transcriptome of all known genes in any tissue, but the high cost and complexity of the results are barriers to widespread use at present [1].

Bias and false results

Genomic studies are prone to bias and error that reduce the power of the analyses and affect replication of the results. Accurate phenotyping is critical, as any variation will have a profound impact on determining associations with AD. Other issues include failing to account for population stratification in case–control studies. Studies with relatively low numbers of cases are vulnerable to type II (i.e. false-negative) errors. Type I (i.e. false-positive) errors can occur following multiple testing unless corrections are used to reduce the false discovery rate. Most analyses, furthermore, assume Hardy–Weinberg equilibrium (i.e. allele and genotype frequencies in a population remain in equilibrium), but non-random mating, mutations, selection, small population effects, genetic drift, etc. mean that this may not be true in canine populations.

Genomic studies in canine atopic dermatitis

Canine atopic dermatitis is a complex disease

Early observations of atopic West Highland white terriers concluded that the inheritance patterns were consistent with a common fully penetrant dominant or recessive major locus [18–20]. However, later studies in other breeds suggest that CAD is a multifactorial and polygenic condition with a complex mode of inheritance [5,7,9,21]. Recent haplotype analysis of 15 dog breeds with an increased risk of CAD revealed that they had a common genetic origin with susceptible breeds clustered in specific clades [22].

Genomic studies in dogs have now implicated numerous genes in the pathogenesis of CAD (Table 5.1), although whether these are associated with cause or effect is not always clear. These include genes involved in innate and adaptive immunity, inflammation, cell cycle, apoptosis, skin barrier formation, and transcription regulation. Many of these genes have also been implicated in human AD [1].

Microarray studies

An initial paper reported that 54 of 22 000 genes (Agilent 22K oligonucleotide canine array, Agilent Technologies, Palo Alto, CA, USA) showed significantly different transcription in skin from atopic dogs compared to healthy controls (Table 5.1) [17]. The affected genes broadly grouped into inflammation/immunity, cell cycle/apoptosis/repair, barrier formation, transport/regulation, and transcription pathways. Most of the inflammation or immunology markers were up-regulated in atopic, particularly lesional, skin. Other genes were generally under-expressed, especially in non-lesional atopic skin. A large number of these down-regulated genes are involved in the transport of calcium, potassium, and other ions, which may affect expression and function of mediators involved in inflammation and barrier function. The most dysregulated gene was S100 calcium binding protein A8 (*S100A8*). This is an important proinflammatory molecule located on the epidermal differentiation complex, and *S100A8* expression has been correlated with the clinical severity of CAD [23]. Release is stimulated by TNF-alpha, the levels of which also correlate with clinical severity [24]. The epidermal differentiation complex comprises genes such as profilaggrin, loricrin, involucrin, and S100, essential for keratinocyte and epidermal barrier differentiation [25]. These genes were not available on the canine microarray and GWAS chips used in earlier studies [16,17], but since then canine and human AD have been associated with loss-of-function filaggrin mutations and altered filaggrin expression [26–29]. The initial microarray study [17] provided a rapid, wide-ranging assessment of many genes, identifying novel targets and pathways for further investigation. However, it was limited by the omission of key epidermal barrier and inflammatory cytokine genes. In addition, there were relatively few dogs, reducing the power to detect small changes. Using multiple breeds may have also confounded the results and reduced the power of the study.

Table 5.1 Genes that have been implicated in CAD by candidate gene quantitative PCR (qPCR), microarrays, genome-wide linkage studies (GWLS), candidate gene single nucleotide polymorphism studies (SNP), or genome-wide association studies (GWAS). Genes that were differentially expressed in atopic skin compared to healthy controls are indicated by: (+) = up regulated and (–) = down regulated

Gene	Study	Potential relevance to CAD
Inflammation/immunology		
S100A8(+), *S100A9*(+), *S100P*(+), *S100A3*(–), *TNF*(+)	Microarrays [17,30] GWLS [20] qPCR [31]	Proinflammatory; correlate with clinical severity
ARG1(+)a, *CCL2*(+), *CCL7*(+), *CCL8*(+)b, *CCL17*(+), *CHI3L1*(+), *CLEC4G*(+), *AMSN1*(*HACS1*)(+), *TFEC*(+)	Microarray [30]	Markers for alternatively activated macrophages, MCP gene family
INPPL1(+), *ARTS-1*(–), *PTPN22*, *PKP2*(+), *DPP4*(–), TSLP-receptor, Sushi-repeat-containing protein *SRPX*(–)	Microarray [17] qPCR [31] SNP [34]	Allergen-specific IgE responses, allergen presentation and uptake, regulation of B- and T-cell receptor signalling, and innate immune responses; cytokine signalling
SAA(+), *SAA3*(+), Serum amyloid A protein(+)	Microarray [17]	Expressed in inflammation
TIMP1(+), *SCCA-2*(+), *ADAMTS20*(–), *ELA1*(+), *KLK2*(–), *KLK4*(–), *KLK8*(+), *KLK13*(+), *MMP1*(+), *MMP7*(+), *MMP9*(–/+), *MMP13*(+), *NLN*(–), *PI16*(–), *SERPINA3*(+), *SERPINA7*(–), *SERPINB4*(+), *SERPINB13*(–), *SERPINE1*(+), *SPINK4*(+), *TIMP1*(+), *TMPRSS3*(–), *S6K-alpha 6*(–), *PH* domain leucine-rich repeat protein phosphatase-like(–)	Microarrays [17,30] qPCR [31]	Matrix metalloproteinases and their inhibitors; promote cell proliferation; antiapoptosis
CD83, *LY75*(–), *LY9*(+), *LY86*(+), *LY96*(+)	GWAS [36] Microarray [30]	Lymphocyte antigens; antigen presentation and humoral immunity
CMA1, *CPA3*(+), *FCER1A*(+), *FCER1G*(+), *LOC448801*(Mastin)(+), *SRGN*(+), *SYK*(+), *MS4A2*	GWAS [16] Microarray [30] SNP [34]	Mast cell associated IgE receptor, enzymes and other markers
NOD1, *CLEC4G*(+), *CLEC4M*(+), *MSR1*(+), *MST1R*(+), *NLRC5/P1/P3*(+), *NLRP9*(–)	GWAS [16] Microarray [30]	Intracellular microbial pattern recognition receptor; innate and adaptive immunity
SELP (p-selectin)(+), *CADM1*(–), *ITGB2*(+), *ITGB6*(+), *SELE*(+), *SELL*(+)	GWAS [16] Microarray [30]	Leukocyte recruitment, cell adhesion
CCL19(+), *CCL28*(+), *CCR1*(+), *CCR3*(+), *CXCL10*(+), *IL1B*(+), *IL1F8*(+), *IL1F10*(–), *IL6*(+)d, *IL8*(+), *IL20*(+), *IL26*(+), *IL1RAPL1*(+), *IL12RB2*(–), *IL13RA2*(+), *IL18BP*(+)	Microarrays [17,30]	Chemokines, interleukins and receptors
C3(+), *C5AR1*(+), *CFP*(+)	Microarray [30]	Complement associated
GBP1(+), *IFI44*(+), *IFITM2*(+), *ISG15*(+), *ISG20*(+), *MNDA*(+), *MX1*(+), *MX2*(+), *OAS1*(+), *OAS2*(+)	Microarray [30]	Interferon induced, microbial defence, and innate immunity
LILRB2(+), *LILRB3*(+)	Microarray [30]	Inhibit MHC1 activation
Cell cycle/apoptosis/repair/lesion formation		
SDC1 (syndecan 1)(–), *POSTN*(+)/(–), Cadherin-13(–)	Microarray [17] qPCR [31]	Cell signalling, cell proliferation, cell migration and cell-matrix interaction
ANGPTL4, *BCL2L15* (BCL2-like 15)(+), *CIDE-3*(–), Cullin 4A(–)	GWAS [16,19] Microarray [30] qPCR [3]	Apoptosis, survival and tolerance, wound healing, keratinocyte migration
RAD50 homologue isoform 1(+), *DCLRE1B*	Microarray [17] GWAS [19]	Unknown

(Continued)

Table 5.1 (*Continued*)

Gene	Study	Potential relevance to CAD
Transport/regulation		
Kinectin 1(+), Myosin Va(+), A-kinase anchor protein 9 isoform 2(+), Sperm-associated antigen 5(+), *Canis familiaris* ret proto-oncogene(–), Nucleoprotein TPR(–), Phospholipase C, zeta 1(–), Potassium channel tetramerization(–), ATP-binding cassette C12e(–), *FERM*, *RhoGEF*, pleckstrin domain protein 2(–), *SFXN5* sideroflexin 5	Microarray [17]	Unknown
EXOC6B exocyst complex component 6B, *AP4B1*, *ABCC3*, *SYT6* synaptotagmin VI	GWAS [19]	Endocytosis, protein transport, and drug efflux
Barrier formation		
GOLGA4 subfamily a5(+)/a4(+), *PPAR* gamma(–), *RAB3C*, cytochrome P450 26B1, *FABP9*(–), *FADS1*(–), *LPCAT1*(+), *PLA2G2E*(–), *PLA2G4D*(+)/*4E*(+)/*4F*(+)/*6*(–), *PLCB4*(–), *PTGDS*(–)	Microarray [17,30] qPCR [31] GWAS [16,19]	Golgi body function; glycosylation and transport of proteins and lipids, lamellar body formation
FLG (Filaggrin), *SPINK5*(+), *SGPL1*(+)	qPCR [31] SNP [34]	Skin barrier regulation, proteolysis and keratinocyte differentiation; filaggrin function; Th2 polarization, antimicrobial
Tight junction protein 3(–), Mucin-2(–), Mucin-15(+)	Microarray [17]	Cell adhesion and signalling
COL7A1(–), *COL10A1*(+), *COL11A2*(–), *COL13A*(–), *COL29A1* (*COL6A5*)(+)	Microarray [30]	Collagens
KRT2(+), *KRT5/26/27/28/31/32/33B/35/37/39/72/81/82/85*(–)	Microarray [30]	Keratins
Transcription and translation regulation		
eIF-5B(+), empty spiracles homolog 1, *CGGBP1*(–), FUSE binding protein 2(–), *PAIP2B*, *PHTF1*, *HIPK1*, *TRIM33*	Microarray [17] GWAS [19]	Unknown
STAT2(–), *FOXO4* (foxhead box)(–)	Microarray [17]	Cell growth, survival and differentiation; inflammation and immunity; tolerance
ZNF638, *ZBTB22*(–), *ZC3H12A*(+)m, *ZFP106*(–), *ZNF208*(+), *AFF3*(+), *BNC2*(–), *FOXF1*(–), *GLI1*(–), *GRHL3*(–), *HOXB3*(–), *HOXC12*(+), *HOXC13*(–)k, *KLF7*(+), *MKX*(–), *NFAM1*(+)l , *NFE2*(+), *NR0B2*(–), *PDX1*(–), *SPI1*(*PU.1*)(+), *TAL1*(+), *TBX1*(–), *TFEC*(+)	GWAS [19] Microarray [30]	Transcription factors and zinc finger proteins
CCR3(+), *EMR1*(+)/*3*(+), *RHGEF12*(+), *ARHGEF4*(+), *GALR1*(+), *GPR65*(+), *GPR98*(+), *GPR112*(–), *GPR143*(–), *GPRC5D*(–), *GPSM3*(+), *PROKR2*(–)	Microarray [30]	Cell signalling and activation
Miscellaneous		
RAB7A	GWAS [16]	Melanocyte function and melanogenesis
SORCS2	GWAS [16]	Neuropeptide receptor activity
INDO(*IDO1*)(+), *INDOL1*(*IDO2*)(–), *KMO*(+)	Microarray [30]	L-tryptophan metabolism
EEA1(+), *CG15747-PA*(+), *HIF1a* (Hypoxia-induced gene 1a)(+), *C6orf142*(–), *RING-H2* protein(–), *ATRX1*(–), *C1orf163*(–), *FBXL10*(–), *FOLH1*(–), mSin3A-associated protein 130(–), Spag6(–), ecotropic viral integration site 1(–), SPR sepiapterinreductase, DYSF dysferlin, NAGK N-acetylglucosamine kinase, *RSBN1L*, *OLFML3*, *PROM1*	Microarray [17] GWAS [19]	Unknown

In another microarray study of 13 atopic and control dogs using the Affymetrix Canine 2 Genome May 2005 assembly (Affymetrix Inc., Santa Clara, CA, USA) 764 genes were differentially expressed between acute lesional and non-lesional atopic skin, 1070 between acute lesional and healthy skin, and 312 between non-lesional and healthy skin [30]. The transcription data sets from the atopic dogs shared common network pathways with human AD and asthmatic chronic rhinosinusitis with nasal polyps (aCRSwNP). These included altered IgE (increased *FCER1A* and *FCER1G*), Th2 (increased *IL13RA2*), Th1 (decreased *IL12RB2*), and eosinophil (increased *CCR3*) associated genes. There was also increased transcription of genes associated with alternatively activated monocyte-derived cells (aaMDCs) such as *ARG1* and the monocyte chemotactic protein (MCP) gene cluster, which are associated with human eosinophil-associated allergic diseases. Other changes included increased transcription of proinflammatory and decreased transcription of anti-inflammatory IL-1 family genes similar to human AD, and altered calcineurin/NFAT, cytokine gene promoter, keratin regulation and transcription, oxidative damage repair, eosinophil (*EMR1* and *3*) activation, and interferon up-regulation pathways. This study, however, used a low-stringency *P*-value increasing the risk of false-positive associations. In addition, this was a small study without matching for age, sex, breed, biopsy site, or concurrent medication.

Candidate gene studies

One study using atopic and healthy skin quantified mRNA for 20 genes identified in earlier studies [17,31]. Significant differences were seen for 11 genes, involving immune responses, regulation, and skin barrier function. Seven of these have been associated with human AD. *S100A8* was again the most dysregulated gene. Three genes correlated with CADESI-03 scores (*S100A8*, *SAA-1*, and *PKP2*) and four genes correlated with intradermal test results (*CMA1*, *SAA-1*, *SPINK5*, and *S100A8*); these have been associated with inflammation, T-cell survival, and skin barrier function [23,32,33]. Weaknesses of this study included the small sample size, multiple dog breeds, and variable time scale of the lesions.

Analysis of 97 SNPs in 25 candidate genes in 659 dogs of eight breeds from the UK, USA, and Japan found that six were significantly associated with CAD [34]. A SNP in the thymic stromal lymphopoietin (TSLP)-receptor, which has been implicated in allergic inflammation [35], was seen in all eight breeds. Other CAD-associated SNPs, however, were restricted to certain dog breeds and locations (e.g. filaggrin with UK Labrador retriever, and *INPPL1* and *MS4A2* with Japanese shiba inu).

A linkage study in West Highland white terrier dogs [18] using specific microsatellite markers to fine map the filaggrin locus did not find any haplotypes that significantly associated with CAD. This makes a primary role for filaggrin defects in these dogs unlikely, although this has been implicated in other breeds [26–28].

Genome-wide linkage studies

A genome-wide family-based linkage approach using microsatellites (256 markers from the Minimal Screening Set 2 [MSS-2] that covered the genome with an average intermarker distance of 8.59 cM) in 90 West Highland white terrier dogs from families with CAD did not detect any chromosomal regions significantly linked to CAD [20]. However, some chromosomal regions were not covered at high density, reducing the power of this study. The highest linkage score was for a region on CFA7 that contains the *S100A8* gene, which has been associated with CAD [17,23,31]. This study excluded linkage to the filaggrin locus, again suggesting that primary defects in filaggrin expression are not important in the pathogenesis of CAD in West Highland white terrier dogs [18,34,36].

Genome-wide association studies

The first GWAS in CAD [16] evaluated DNA from 242 atopic and 417 control dogs of eight breeds from the UK, US, and Japan, with the top 40 SNPs selected for validation. Nine chromosomes expressed multiple SNPs, suggesting a haplotype effect. Subsequent quantitative PCR with quality assurance testing, and corrections for the false discovery rate and population structure revealed that 13 SNPs had a significant association with CAD. However, a number were intergenic with unknown functions and interactions.

Two independent intergenic SNPs were linked with CAD in all eight breeds; rs22114085 (CFA10) was associated with susceptibility while rs23472497 (CFA29) was protective. These may represent novel loci for sequencing and fine mapping [16]. There was a lack of interbreed correspondence between the CAD-associated SNPs, suggesting that the atopic genotype varies among breeds. However, the numbers of each individual breed in this study were relatively low. The relevance of the intergenic SNPs, furthermore, is unclear and further study of these areas on the genome is required.

Some breed-specific gene-associated SNPs were identified. Atopic dermatitis in golden retriever dogs was associated with SNPs in *RAB3C* (rs22859255) and *PROM1* (rs23602938). This *RAB3C* SNP also formed a significant haplotype with another *RAB3C* SNP (rs22784610). Atopic Labrador retriever dogs and West Highland white terrier dogs from the UK showed

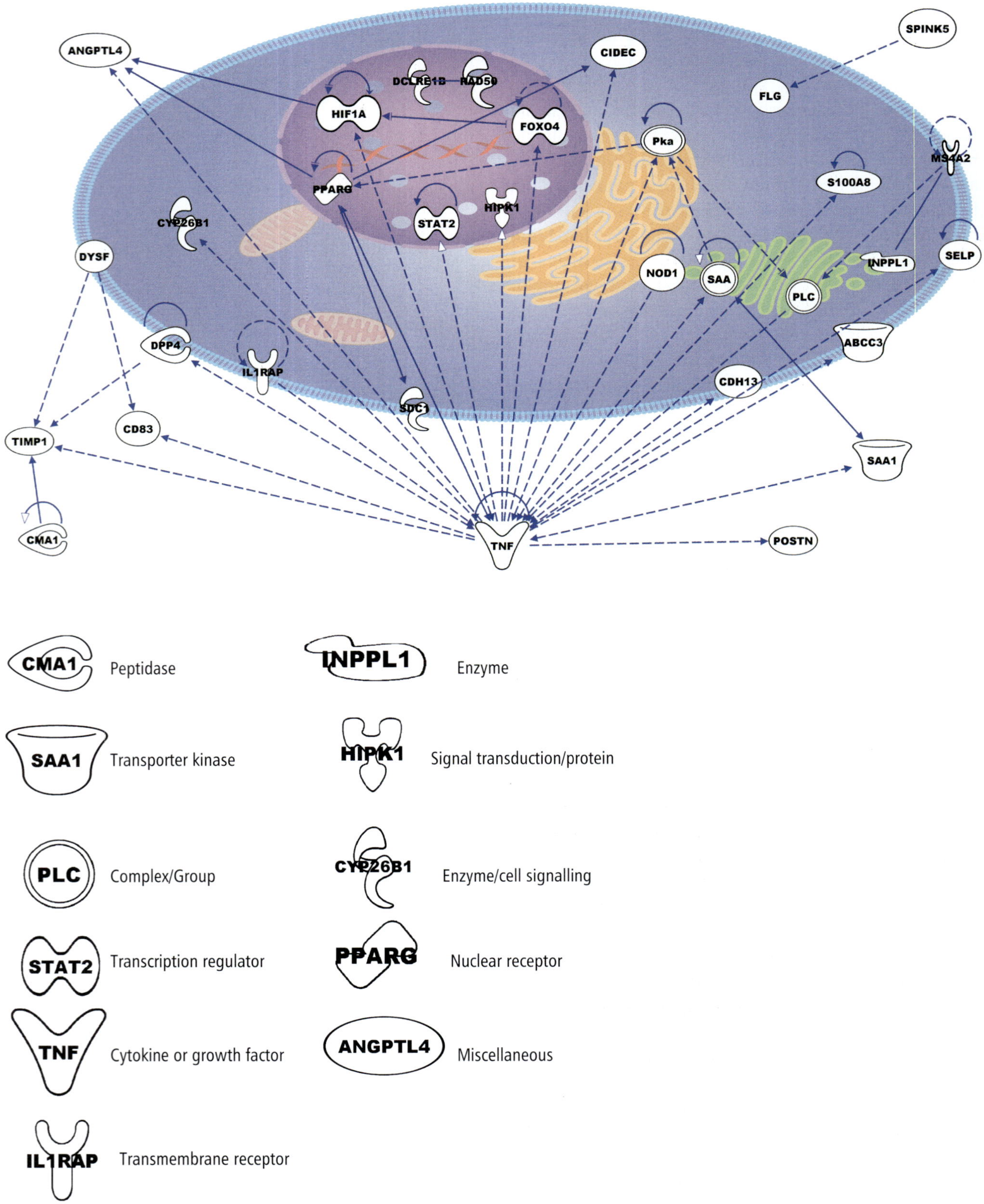

Figure 5.2 Network pathway of genes associated with CAD supported by at least one reference from the literature or from canonical information stored in the Ingenuity Knowledge Base (IPA; Ingenuity Systems, www.ingenuity.com) [40]. Nodes are displayed using various shapes that represent the functional class of the gene product. This is only a partial network to illustrate the complexity of the potential interactions between mediators implicated in canine atopic dermatitis. At present, the functional identity of many mediators implicated in dogs is unknown. Further data will improve the detail and accuracy of the network pathways in CAD. This will be useful in studying the pathogenesis of the disease, identifying novel therapeutic targets, and in understanding how an individual's genotype contributes to their clinical expression of CAD. (Reprinted from [40], © 2013, with the permission of John Wiley & Sons, Inc.)

associations with an SNP within *RAB7A* (rs22915894) as well as the intergenic SNP rs8806978, which is downstream of *RAB7A*. German shepherd dogs from the UK showed an association with *SORCS2*. Significant associations were, however, variable between breeds and within breeds from different geographical locations. However, the fact that a SNP is associated with CAD in one breed but not another does not necessarily mean that the SNP is not a risk factor for CAD, as a SNP may have different levels of penetrance in different breeds [37]. However, breed variation in genotype may explain breed-specific phenotypes in CAD [2].

A further GWAS was performed on 35 atopic and 25 non-atopic West Highland white terrier dogs using an Affymetrix Canine SNP V2 array with approximately 42 800 SNPs [19]. This reported significant association with a locus on CFA17. Nineteen genes less than 0.5 Mb from this region were identified. Two other main linkage peaks for CAD were also found on CFA6 and CFA9. These candidate genes covered a range of functions including innate and adaptive immunity, skin barrier function, and transcription and regulation. Another GWAS using this array found a significant association between serum *Dermatophagoides farinae*-specific IgE levels in West Highland white terriers and a 2.3-Mb area on CFA35 [36]. *CD83*, a gene closely associated with this region, is important in antigen presentation and humoral immunity. Sequencing detected an intronic polymorphic repeat sequence, but this did not explain the GWAS association in these dogs.

Finally, a very recent GWAS used allergen-specific immunoglobulin levels (IgE, IgG1, and IgG4 specific for *Dermatophagoides farinae*, and IgE specific for *D. pteronyssinus*, *Tyrophagus putrescentiae*, *Lepidoglyphus destructor*, *Acarus siro*, *Alternaria alternata*, *Cladosporium herbarum*, *Aspergillus fumigatus*, *Penicillium*, cat epithelium, flea saliva, and *Blatella germanica*) as phenotypic markers for CAD in Labrador retriever dogs [38]. The GWAS analysed 113 021 SNPs in 135 affected dogs and 24 controls, with correction for false discovery rate, population stratification, and relatedness. Three SNPs on CFA5 (79–82.5 Mb) were significantly associated with serum specific IgE levels: two (BICF2S2297212 and BICF2P1022237) with *A. siro* and one (BICF2G630182288) with *T. putrescentiae*. However, no genes involved in IgE regulation are known to reside in this area. These results may therefore indicate the presence of a novel gene, and these loci warrant further investigation and fine-mapping. However, the relevance of *Acarus- and Tyrophagus*-specific serum IgE in the pathogenesis of CAD is unclear [39], and the use of surrogate markers, such as serum IgE levels, will only identify a subset of atopic dogs.

Conclusion

These studies have greatly improved our understanding of CAD. Despite this, the genetic background for CAD is still far from clear. There has been little correlation between the studies published so far. This variation could be due to the complexity of the genotype, although it is also likely to reflect environmental factors, phenotypic differences between dogs in the studies, different study techniques, mutations with low penetrance, and incomplete genome coverage. Genome-wide association studies appear to be the most powerful technique to study the genotype of CAD, but future studies will require larger cohorts of individual breeds from defined geographical areas.

Atopic dermatitis involves a complex network of many genes with multiple variants affecting gene function and expression (Figure 5.2). The effect of any one polymorphism is likely to be relatively small, and the final phenotype will depend on their interactions across the genome. These findings also suggest that the genetic background to CAD varies between breeds and geographical gene pools. This could explain variations in clinical phenotype and response to treatment between individuals and breeds.

This complexity, and the high prevalence of CAD, means that a screening and breeding programme to eliminate the condition is unlikely to succeed. Despite this, the genomics revolution has huge potential. These techniques will allow identification of target molecules for novel treatments. In addition, we should be able to genotype atopic dogs and relate this to their phenotype. Understanding the genotype will enable better targeting of treatment options—for example, some dogs may respond well to skin barrier therapy whereas other would benefit more from allergen-specific immunotherapy. We should also be able to identify dogs that may have a poor response or an increased risk of adverse effects to certain anti-inflammatory drugs. Finally, it may be possible to discover atopic genotypes in young dogs and manage environmental and other factors to minimize their risk of developing clinical CAD. However, we must be careful to avoid misuse of genomic data in diagnosis and by breeders or insurance companies.

Glossary

Allele: One of two or more forms of a gene or DNA sequence on a chromosome that may be associated with a phenotypic trait. Diploid organisms can be *homozygous* (i.e. two copies of the same allele) or *heterozygous* (i.e. two different alleles).

Exon: DNA sequences within a gene that make up the final RNA transcript. Exons are usually separated by one or more introns in a gene.

Genotype: The specific genetic makeup of an individual. The genotype, epigenetic factors (i.e. changes in gene expression not associated with the DNA sequence) and environmental influences determine the phenotype.

Haplotype: A combination of alleles at adjacent loci on the chromosome that are inherited together. Haplotype also refers to a set of SNPs on a single chromosome that are statistically associated.

Intron: DNA sequences within a gene that are removed during transcription to produce the final RNA sequence.

Linkage disequilibrium: Non-random association of alleles at two or more loci, which may be on the same or different chromosomes.

Locus: The specific location of a gene or DNA sequence on a chromosome.

Microsatellite markers (simple sequence repeats [SSRs] or short tandem repeats [STRs]): Highly polymorphic repeating sequences of 2–6 base pairs throughout the genome used in inheritance studies.

Penetrance: The proportion of individuals with a particular genotype that develop the associated phenotype.

Phenotype: An individual's observable characteristics or traits. These may include morphology, development, physiology, behaviour, and/or disease states.

Population stratification: Differences in allele frequencies between groups in a study population that are associated with ancestry (e.g. race, breed, geography, etc.) rather than a disease condition.

Single nucleotide polymorphisms (SNPs): A difference in single nucleotide (A, T, C or G) in a DNA sequence—for example AGC**C**TA and AGC**T**TA.

References

1. Barnes KC. An update on the genetics of atopic dermatitis: Scratching the surface in 2009. *Journal of Allergy and Clinical Immunology* 2010; **125**: 16–29.
2. Wilhem S, Kovalik M, Favrot C, *et al.* Breed-associated phenotypes in canine atopic dermatitis. *Veterinary Dermatology* 2011; **22**: 143–149.
3. Picco F, Zini E, Nett C, *et al.* A prospective study on canine atopic dermatitis and food-induced allergic dermatitis in Switzerland. *Veterinary Dermatology* 2008; **19**: 150–155.
4. DeBoer DJ, Hill PB. Serum immunoglobulin concentrations in West Highland White Terriers do not predict development of atopic dermatitis. *Veterinary Dermatology* 2000; **10**: 275–281.
5. Shaw SC, Wood JLN, Freeman J, *et al.* Estimation of heritability of atopic dermatitis in Labrador and Golden Retrievers. *American Journal of Veterinary Research* 2004; **65**: 1014–1020.
6. Marsella R, Olivry T, Nicklin CF, *et al.* Pilot investigation of a model for canine atopic dermatitis: environmental house dust mite challenge of high-IgE-producing beagles, mite hypersensitive dogs with atopic dermatitis and normal dogs. *Veterinary Dermatology* 2006; **17**: 24–35.
7. Marsella R, Girolomoni G. Canine models of atopic dermatitis: a useful tool with untapped potential. *Journal of Investigative Dermatology* 2009; **129**: 2351–2357.
8. Olivry T, Deangelo KB, Dunston SM, *et al.* Patch testing of experimentally sensitized beagle dogs: development of a model for skin lesions of atopic dermatitis. *Veterinary Dermatology* 2006; **17**: 95–102.
9. Schiessl B, Zemann B, Hodgkin-Pickart LA, *et al.* Importance of early allergen contact for the development of a sustained immunoglobulin E response in a dog model. *International Archives of Allergy and Immunology* 2003; **130**: 125–134.
10. Nodtvedt A, Guitian J, Egenvall A, *et al.* The spatial distribution of atopic dermatitis cases in a population of insured Swedish dogs. *Preventive Veterinary Medicine* 2007; **78**: 210–222.
11. Nodtvedt A, Bergvall K, Sallander M, *et al.* A case-control study of risk factors for canine atopic dermatitis among boxer, bullterrier and West Highland white terrier dogs in Sweden. *Veterinary Dermatology* 2007; **18**: 309–315.
12. Esparza-Gordillo J, Weidinger S, Fölster-Holst R, *et al.* A common variant on chromosome 11q13 is associated with atopic dermatitis. *Nature Genetics* 2009; **41**: 596–601.
13. Lindblad-Toh K, Wade CM, Mikkelsen TS, *et al.* Genome sequence, comparative analysis and haplotype structure of the domestic dog. *Nature* 2005; **438**: 803–819.
14. Sutter NB, Ostrander EA. Dog star rising: The canine genetic system. *Nature Reviews Genetics* 2004; **5**: 900–910.
15. Starkey MP, Scase TJ, Mellersh CS, *et al.* Dogs really are man's best friend—canine genomics has applications in veterinary and human medicine! *Briefings in Functional Genomics and Proteomics* 2005; **4**: 112–128.
16. Wood SH, Ke XY, Nuttall T, *et al.* Genome-wide association analysis of canine atopic dermatitis and identification of disease related SNPs. *Immunogenetics* 2009; **61**: 765–772.
17. Merryman-Simpson AE, Wood SH, Fretwell N, *et al.* Gene (mRNA) expression in canine atopic dermatitis: microarray analysis. *Veterinary Dermatology* 2008; **19**: 59–66.
18. Barros Roque J, O'Leary CA, Kyaw-Tanner M, *et al.* Haplotype sharing excludes canine orthologous Filaggrin locus in atopy in West Highland White Terriers. *Animal Genetics* 2009; **40**: 793–794.
19. Roque JB, O'Leary CA, Duffy DL, *et al.* Atopic dermatitis in West Highland white terriers is associated with a 1.3-Mb region on CFA 17. *Immunogenetics* 2012; **64**: 209–217.
20. Salzmann CA, Olivry TJM, Nielsen DM, *et al.* Genome-wide linkage study of atopic dermatitis in West Highland White Terriers. *BMC Genetics* 2011; **12**: 37.
21. Schwartzman RM. Immunologic studies of progeny of atopic dogs. *American Journal of Veterinary Research* 1984; **45**: 375–378.
22. Mazrier H, Vogelnest LJ, Taylor RM. Comparative analysis of dogs with atopic dermatitis identifies a clade of susceptible breeds (abstract). *Veterinary Dermatology* 2012; **23** (Suppl. 1): 57.
23. Chung T-H, Oh J-S, Lee Y-S, *et al.* Elevated serum levels of S100 calcium binding protein A8 (S100A8) reflect disease severity in canine atopic dermatitis. *Journal of Veterinary Medical Science* 2010; **72**: 693–700.
24. Nuttall TJ, Knight PA, McAleese SM, *et al.* Expression of T-helper 1 cytokine mRNA in canine atopic dermatitis correlates with clinical severity. *Advances in Veterinary Dermatology* 2004; **5**: 17–27.
25. Candi E, Schmidt R, Melino G. The cornified envelope: A model of cell death in the skin. *Nature Reviews Molecular Cell Biology* 2005; **6**: 328–340.

26. Chervet L, Galichet A, McLean WHI, *et al.* Missing C-terminal filaggrin expression, NFkappaB activation and hyperproliferation identify the dog as a putative model to study epidermal dysfunction in atopic dermatitis. *Experimental Dermatology* 2010; **19**: E343–E346.
27. Marsella R, Olivry T, Carlotti D-N. Current evidence of skin barrier dysfunction in human and canine atopic dermatitis. *Veterinary Dermatology* 2011; **22**: 239–248.
28. Marsella R, Samuelson D, Harrington L. Immunohistochemical evaluation of filaggrin polyclonal antibody in atopic and normal beagles. *Veterinary Dermatology* 2009; **20**: 547–554.
29. O'Regan GM, Sandilands, A, Irvine, AD. Filaggrin in atopic dermatitis. *Journal of Allergy and Clinical Immunology* 2008; **122**: 689–693.
30. Plager DA, Torres SMF, Koch SN, *et al.* Gene transcription abnormalities in canine atopic dermatitis and related human eosinophilic allergic diseases. *Veterinary Immunology and Immunopathology* 2012; **149**: 136–142.
31. Wood SH, Clements DN, Ollier WE, *et al.* Gene expression in canine atopic dermatitis and correlation with clinical severity scores. *Journal of Dermatological Science* 2009; **55**: 27–33.
32. Moffatt MF. SPINK5: A gene for atopic dermatitis and asthma. *Clinical and Experimental Allergy* 2004; **34**: 325–327.
33. Ding Y, Shen S, Lino AC, *et al.* Beta-catenin stabilization extends regulatory T cell survival and induces anergy in nonregulatory T cells. *Nature Medicine* 2008; **14**: 162–169.
34. Wood SH, Ollier WE, Nuttall T, *et al.* Despite identifying some shared gene associations with human atopic dermatitis the use of multiple dog breeds from various locations limits detection of gene associations in canine atopic dermatitis. *Veterinary Immunology and Immunopathology* 2010; **138**: 193–197.
35. Liu YJ. Thymic stromal lymphopoietin: master switch for allergic inflammation. *Journal of Experimental Medicine* 2006; **203**: 269–273.
36. Roque JB, O'Leary CA, Duffy DL, *et al.* IgE Responsiveness to *Dermatophagoides farinae* in West Highland white terrier dogs is associated with a region on CFA35. *Journal of Heredity* 2011; **102**: S74–S80.
37. McCarthy MI, Hirschhorn JN. Genome-wide association studies: potential next steps on a genetic journey. *Human Molecular Genetics* 2008; **17**: R156–R165.
38. Owczarek-Lipska M, Lauber B, Molitor V, *et al.* Two loci on Chromosome 5 are associated with serum IgE levels in Labrador retrievers. *PLoS ONE* 2012; **7**: e39176.
39. Nuttall TJ, Hill PB, Bensignor E, *et al.* House dust and forage mite allergens and their role in human and canine atopic dermatitis. *Veterinary Dermatology* 2006; **17**: 223–235.
40. Nuttall TJ. The genomics revolution. Will canine atopic dermatitis become preventable and predictable? *Veterinary Dermatology* 2013; **24**: 10–18.

6

Skin barrier and its role in the pathophysiology of atopic dermatitis

Koji Nishifuji

Department of Veterinary Medicine, Tokyo University of Agriculture and Technology, Fuchu, Tokyo, Japan

Conflict of interest: none declared.

Introduction

The skin, which covers the entire body surface of mammals, acts as an enclosing barrier to protect the body from physical, chemical, and biological injury, and to prevent loss of water and solutes essential for physiological homeostasis. The stratum corneum (SC) is the outermost layer of the epidermis and is composed of 'bricks', represented by flattened corneocytes, and 'mortar', represented by extracellular lipids ('bricks and mortar' structure)[1]. It is generally accepted that ceramides (CERs) are the major constituents of the extracellular lipids in the SC and play a key role in preventing transepidermal water loss (TEWL). The intracellular proteins of corneocytes, such as filaggrin (FLG) and keratin, provide mechanical strength to the cells and may hamper percutaneous entry of foreign bodies. It has been reported that an aberrant expression of the extracellular lipids or of the various intracellular proteins in the SC and stratum granulosum (SG) might be associated with disturbed cutaneous barrier function, which leads to increased TEWL and enhanced percutaneous allergen entry through the SC in human and canine atopic dermatitis (CAD) (Figure 6.1, Table 6.1).

Methods to determine impairment of barrier function of the canine skin

In human medicine, impairment of permeability barrier function and water holding capacity of the skin are analysed by measuring TEWL and the skin hydration. Although skin hydration is decreased in the skin of humans with AD, the values in dogs with CAD are comparable to those in healthy dog skin [2]. This difference is probably due to the higher density of hair follicles in canine skin compared to human skin. The secretions from hair follicle appendages (e.g. epitrichial sweat glands, sebaceous glands) may diffuse onto the surface of the SC and mask the decreased skin hydration caused by the impairment of the permeability barrier function in canine skin.

To date, there are only a few studies that have investigated the changes of TEWL in atopic skin in dogs. Shimada *et al.* reported that TEWL, measured by a closed chamber device, becomes higher with increased frequency of tape stripping on canine skin, suggesting that elevated TEWL values reflect impairment of cutaneous permeability barrier function [3]. The same group also reported that the TEWL value in visibly non-lesional skin of dogs with spontaneous CAD was significantly higher than that in healthy dog skin [2]. When the TEWL value was compared between lesional

Veterinary Allergy, First Edition. Edited by Chiara Noli, Aiden Foster, and Wayne Rosenkrantz.

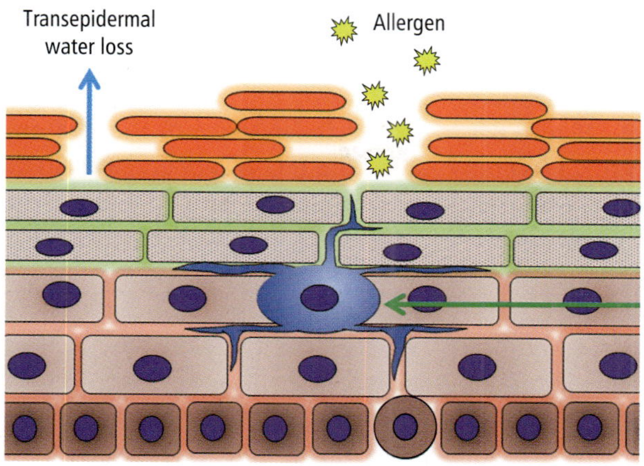

Figure 6.1 Schematic representation of the epidermal components crucial to maintain cutaneous barrier function and their aberration in atopic dermatitis (AD). Decreased ceramides (CERs) and sphingosine-1-phosphate (S1P) have been recognized in the skin of humans and dogs with AD. In addition, aberrant expression of filaggrin (FLG), kallikrein-related peptidase 7 (KLK7), and tight junction protein claudin-1 (CLDN1) has been recognized in humans with AD. These changes might be responsible for increased transepidermal water loss and/or enhanced percutaneous entry of allergens, which could be captured by dendrites of Langerhans cells and provoke immune responses.

Table 6.1 Skin molecules associated with aberrant cutaneous barrier function in human and canine atopic dermatitis

Human atopic dermatitis
Lipids and related enzymes
Ceramides
Sphingosine-1-phosphate lyase (SGPL1)
Structural or functional proteins
Filaggrin (FLG)
Kallikrein-related peptidase 7 (KLK7)
Claudin-1
Canine atopic dermatitis
Lipids and related enzymes
Ceramides
Sphingosine-1-phosphate lyase (SGPL1)
Structural or functional proteins
Filaggrin?

and visibly non-lesional skin of dogs with CAD, the value was significantly higher in lesional skin (K. Shimada, personal communication). Similarly, Hightower *et al.* reported that TEWL measured by an open chamber device was significantly higher in the skin of atopic beagles than that in healthy dog skin, especially in predilection sites for CAD, including pinna, periocular region, axilla, and antebrachium [4]. After house dust mite exposure, TEWL was significantly increased in atopic beagles but did not markedly change in healthy dogs [4].

There is, however, some debate regarding the usefulness of TEWL measurements for the assessment of cutaneous permeability barrier function in dogs. Although open chamber devices were used in previous studies [4,5], another paper described the superiority of closed chamber devices for measuring TEWL in dog skin, with less variability of the values than those measured by open chamber devices [6]. The possible explanation might be that the closed chamber device is less affected by air turbulence owing to movement of the dog or moisture in the fur [6]. On the other hand, a previous study reported that a closed chamber device (Vapometer® SWL-5, Delfin Technologies Ltd, Kuopio, Finland) exhibited very high interoperator variance, as well as day-to-day, site-to-site, and dog-to-dog variability in TEWL values [7]. The variability of the TEWL data has not been determined when using other devices available worldwide.

In summary, TEWL is believed to reflect impairment of cutaneous barrier function in human and possibly canine skin; it is increased in visibly normal skin of dogs with CAD compared with healthy dog skin. However, it should be noted that the TEWL values may also be influenced by factors other than impaired barrier function, such as oedema or excoriation of inflamed skin.

Extracellular lipids in the stratum corneum and atopic dermatitis

Structure and metabolic pathway of ceramides in the epidermis

In the mammalian SC there are three major lipid constituents of the extracellular lipid lamellae (ELL): CERs, cholesterol, and free fatty acids [8]. It is generally accepted that CERs are the main constituent of the SC lipids and that they play an important role in maintaining cutaneous permeability barrier function [9,10].

CERs are sphingoids consisting of sphingoid bases that are amide-linked to fatty acids (Figure 6.2). Figure 6.3 summarizes the possible metabolic pathway of CERs and their degradation products in the epidermis [11–15]. In the stratum spinosum CERs are synthesized by the *de novo* pathway and then converted to glucosylceramides and sphingomyelins by glucosylceramide synthase and sphingomyelin synthase, respectively. The glucosylceramides and sphingomyelins are then packed into lamellar granules. During the differentiation of keratinocytes, lamellar granules move to the apex of granular cells, fuse with the plasma membrane, and secrete the contents into the extracellular space of the stratum granulosum–stratum corneum (SG-SC) boundaries. In the boundaries, the glucosylceramides and sphingomyelins are converted back to CERs by β-glucocerebrosidase and sphingomyelinase, respectively. The importance of a well-functioning glucosylceramide-CER pathway in permeability barrier function of the skin has been analysed by using two lines of gene knock-out mice [14,16,17] and naturally occurring hereditary diseases in humans [18,19]. Deficiency of β-glucocerebrosidase causes increased TEWL, increased glucosylceramides, decreased SC CERs, and incompetent structure of ELL in Gaucher mice [14,16] and type II Gaucher disease in humans [18]. In addition, deficiency of ATP binding cassette subfamily A member 12 (ABCA12), which is a lipid transporter and plays an important role in the incorporation of glucocylceramides into lamellar granules, causes severe skin fissures, neonatal death, and decreased CERs or glucosylceramides in

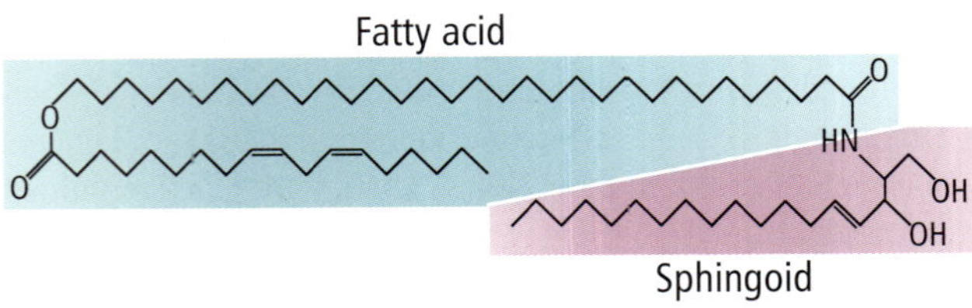

Figure 6.2 Structure of free ceramides (CERs) in the stratum corneum. CERs consist of sphingoid bases that are amide-linked to fatty acids. The figure represents the structure of CER[EOS].

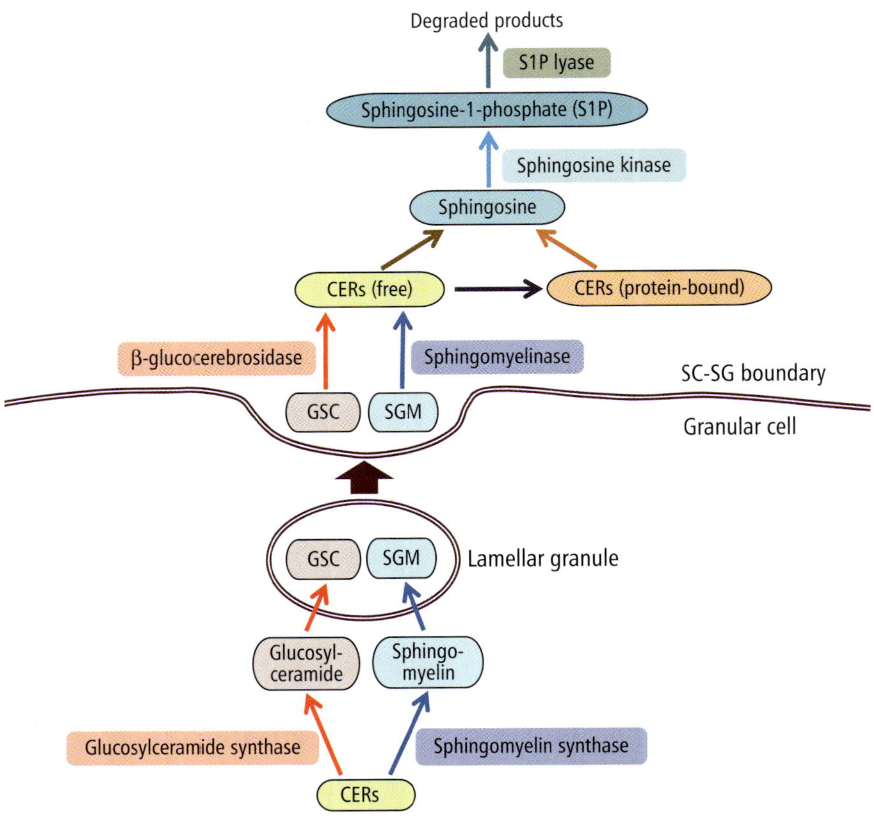

Figure 6.3 Metabolic pathway of ceramides (CERs) and their degradation products in the epidermis. Ceramides synthesized in keratinocytes are converted into glucosylceramides (GSCs) and sphingomyelins (SGMs) and then packed into lamellar granules (LGs). When the LG contents are secreted into the extracellular spaces in the stratum corneum–stratum granulosum (SC-SG) boundaries, GSCs and SGMs are converted back to free-extractable CERs. Some free-extractable CERs are degraded into protein-bound CERs. The CERs are then degraded into sphingosine then sphingosine-1-phosphate (S1P) and irreversibly inactivated by S1P lyase.

the SC in *Abca12*$^{-/-}$ mice [17] and humans with harlequin ichthyosis [19].

Ceramides in the SC initially are formed as free-extractable CERs, but some are subsequently degraded to protein-bound CERs [20]. The free-extractable and protein-bound CERs are cleaved to generate sphingosine, which is subsequently phosphorylated to sphingosine-1-phosphate (S1P) by sphingosine kinase. It is thought that S1P has anti-inflammatory activity. S1P is irreversibly digested to degradation products by S1P lyase (SGPL1) [21,22].

Liquid chromatography–mass spectrometry has revealed that free-extractable CERs in human and canine SC can be divided into 11 groups according to their sphingoid and fatty acid structures (Figure 6.4) [23,24]. These free-extractable CERs, together with cholesterols and free fatty acids, form the ELL in the extracellular space of the SC, and are thought to maintain the water holding capacity of the SC (Figure 6.5) [8]. In humans, seven out of the 11 CER classes, including esterified ω-hydroxyceramides (CER[EOS], CER[EOP], and CER[EOH]) are expressed exclusively in the SC,

Fatty acids / Sphingoids	Esterified ω–hydroxy fatty acid [EO]	α–hydroxy fatty acid [A]	Non-hydroxy fatty acid [N]
6-hydroxy sphingosine [H]	CER[EOH]	CER[AH]	CER[NH]
Phytosphingosine [P]	CER[EOP]	CER[AP]	CER[NP]
Sphingosine [S]	CER[EOS]	CER[AS]	CER[NS]
Dihydrosphingosine [DS]	Not detected	CER[ADS]	CER[NDS]

Figure 6.4 Ceramide classes recognized in human and canine stratum corneum (SC). The SC CERs are divided into 11 classes according to their sphingoid and fatty acid structure. Purple cells represent CER classes recognized exclusively in human SC and the orange cell represents a CER class recognized in human SC and hairs. CER[EODS] has not been detected in mammalian SC.

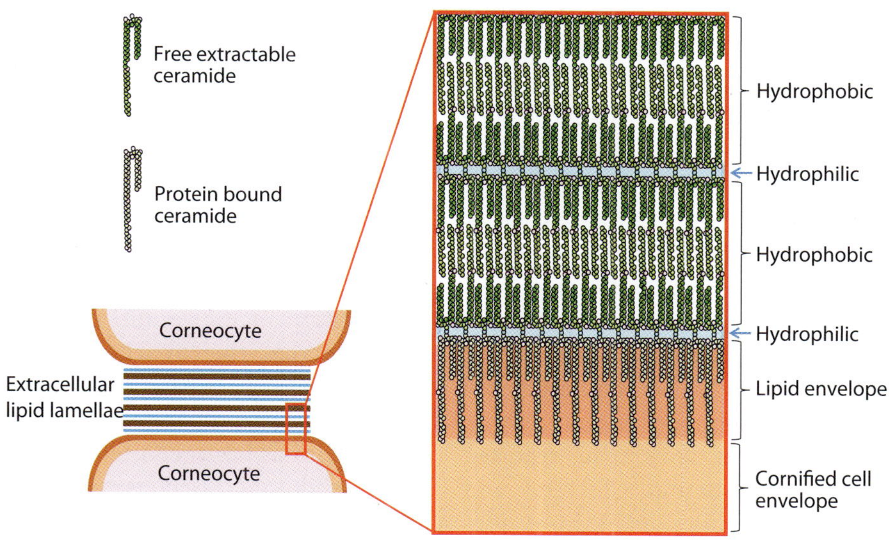

Figure 6.5 Schematic representation of the extracellular lipid lamellae (ELL) and lipid envelope. The extracellular lipids, including free-extractable CERs, are thought to form the multiple lamellae structure that is called the ELL and hold the water within hydrophilic layers. The lipid envelope, including protein-bound CERs, covalently binds to the cornified cell envelope, which consists of a multiple protein complex and is located on the inner surface of the plasma membrane and acts as scaffold for the ELL.

whereas CER[ADS] is expressed in the SC and hairs but not in other organs (Figure 6.4) [25]. Although the composition ratios of the esterified ω-hydroxyceramides are relatively low among all SC CER classes, the esterified ω-hydroxyceramides are thought to play important roles in cutaneous barrier function owing to their extremely long carbon chains in fatty acid moieties [23,24,26–28]. Moreover, non-esterified ω-hydroxyceramides (CER[OS], CER[OP], and CER[OH]), the degradation products of the esterified ω-hydroxyceramides, form the lipid envelope that binds covalently to CCE and acts as a scaffold for ELL (Figure 6.5) [20]. It has been reported that CER[OS] and CER[OP] are two major protein-bound CERs in canine SC[29].

Reduction of ceramides in the stratum corneum in dogs with atopic dermatitis

Several studies have described that CERs are decreased in the SC of dogs with CAD, as is seen in humans with AD [30–34]. Electron microscopy revealed that the continuity and thickness of the ELL were reduced in non-lesional skin of dogs with spontaneous CAD [35,36]. Similar ultrastructural observations were also reported in a previous study using atopic beagles sensitized with house dust mites [37].

A reduction in free-extractable and protein-bound CERs in the SC of dogs with naturally occurring CAD has been reported in three publications [2,24,38]. Reiter *et al.* reported that the relative amounts of CER1 (probably CER[EOS]) and CER9 (probably CER[EOP]) were lower in non-lesional skin of dogs with spontaneous CAD than in that from breed- and age-matched healthy dogs [38]. Similarly, Yoon *et al.* reported that the quantities of total free-extractable CERs and some CER classes (CER[EOS], CER[EOP], CER[NP], mixtures of CER[NDS/NS], and CER[AS/NH]) were significantly lower in visibly non-lesional skin in dogs with spontaneous CAD than that in breed- and age-matched healthy dogs [24]. In that study, the differences in the quantities of CER[EOS], CER[EOP], and a mixture of CER[AS/NH] were ≥2.2-fold, while the differences in the quantities of the other CER classes were ≤1.6-fold. Furthermore, Shimada *et al.* reported that the relative amounts of free-extractable CERs, but not those of cholesterol or free fatty acids, in the SC were negatively correlated with TEWL in dogs with spontaneous CAD [2].

Besides free-extractable CERs, Popa *et al.* reported that the amounts of protein-bound CER[OS] and CER[OP] were decreased in non-lesional skin of dogs with CAD compared to healthy dogs [39]. Moreover, Bäumer *et al.* reported that S1P in the skin, plasma and serum is decreased in dogs with CAD [22]. It has also been reported that transcription of a gene encoding SGPL1 was up-regulated in both non-lesional and lesional skin of dogs with spontaneous CAD [40], while the expression level of sphingosine, the precursor of S1P, was not altered [22].

In summary, there is evidence that free-extractable and protein-bound CERs are reduced in the SC of dogs with CAD. In addition, the reduction of free-extractable CERs in the SC appears to be associated with increased water permeability in dogs with CAD. Moreover, the amount of the anti-inflammatory product S1P in the skin and plasma is decreased in dogs with CAD and this change is probably associated with up-regulation of *SGPL1* gene transcription.

Current evidence for aberrant filaggrin expression in dogs with atopic dermatitis

Structure and function of filaggrin in the epidermis and its role in humans and mice

Profilaggrin, the precursor protein of FLG, is the major constituent in keratohyalin granules [41–43]. It is encoded by the *FLG* gene, and is a large, insoluble, highly phosphorylated, histidine-rich protein which contains tandemly arranged FLG repeats flanked on either side by two partial FLG repeats, and with N- and C-terminal domains [42,43]. In humans, there are 10–12 FLG repeats in one profilaggrin molecule, and each FLG repeat consists of 324 amino acids and shares significant amino acid identity between the repeats [44–46]. In contrast, dot matrix analysis revealed that canine profilaggrin appeared to have four FLG repeats, which include three FLG repeats of 549 amino acids and one shorter repeat of 507 amino acids [47]. In response to increased intracellular calcium concentration, the keratohyalin granules are degranulated, their content is released to the cytoplasm, and profilaggrin is broken down into FLG molecules at the SG-SC boundary (Figure 6.6) [41–43,48]. The N- and C-terminal domains in profilaggrin are hypothesized to be important in processing profilaggrin to FLG monomers [42,49,50].

The major role of FLG monomers in the SC is in the aggregation of the keratin intermediate filaments into tight bundles, thereby leading to collapse of the cells, which then have a flattened appearance, and providing mechanical strength to the cells (Figure 6.6) [41–43,48]. Indeed, it has been reported that *Flg* knock-out ($Flg^{-/-}$) mice exhibit increased desquamation under mechanical stress [51]. Previous studies demonstrated that genetic mutations in the *FLG* gene, which encode N- to C-terminal FLG repeats, appear to be associated with AD or contact dermatitis in humans [48,52–55]. Finally, topical application of foreign materials (e.g.

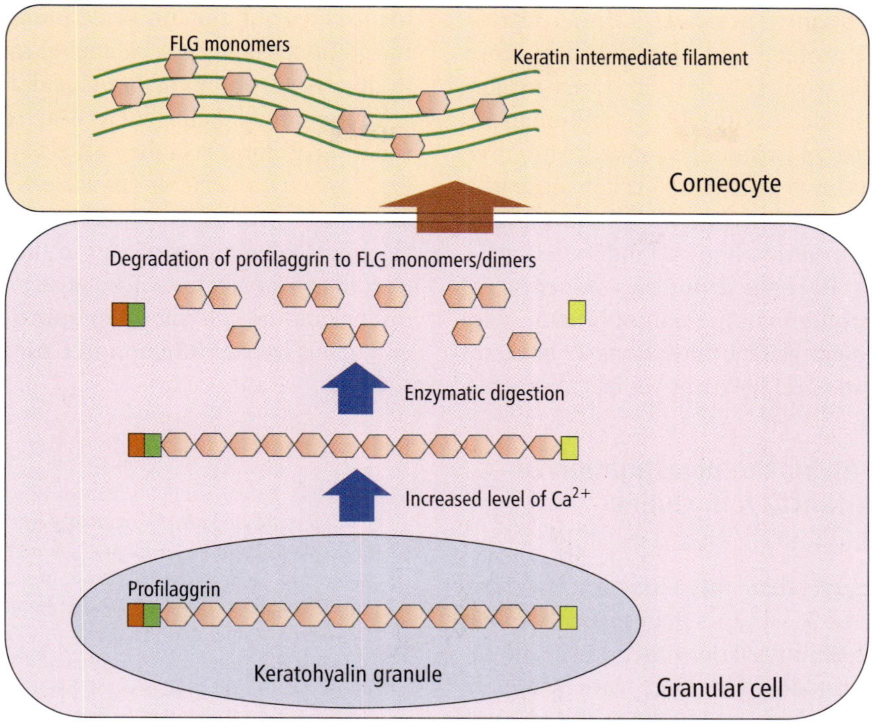

Figure 6.6 Structure and function of filaggrin (FLG) in the epidermis. In granular cells, profilaggrin is released from keratohyalin granules in response to increased intracellular calcium level and solubilized into FLG monomers or dimers by proteases. The FLG monomers aggregate keratin intermediate filaments into tight bundles in corneocytes.

haptens, *Dermatophagoides pteronyssinus*) to *Flg*$^{-/-}$ mice [51] or flaky-tail mice [56], in which a 1-bp deletion (5303delA) in the murine *Flg* gene is recognized, enhanced the antigen-specific humoral immune response (IgE production) and a dermatitis phenotype. Thus, it is suggested that aberrant expression of FLG monomers allows percutaneous sensitization by foreign materials and leads to development of AD or contact dermatitis.

Conventionally, it is thought that pyrrolidone carboxylic and urocanic acids, the degraded products of FLG monomers, act as natural moisturizing factors (NMF) in the upper SC [42,57,58]. In contrast, even if NMF levels were decreased in the SC of *Flg*$^{-/-}$ mice, SC hydration and TEWL were comparable to those in wild-type mice [51].

In summary, FLG appears to play a role in providing mechanical strength to corneocytes and hampering percutaneous entry of foreign materials through the SC. However, it is debatable whether the FLG degradation products (NMF) provide water holding capacity to the SC, and this needs further investigation.

Aberrant expression of filaggrin in canine atopic dermatitis—what we know so far

To date, there is only limited evidence for an association of FLG with CAD. Marsella *et al.* reported that atopic beagles had significantly less positive FLG epidermal immunostaining than control dogs [59]. The immunostaining was recognized diffusely in all epidermal layers in this study [59], whereas another study showed that rabbit antisera raised against canine FLG peptide stained only the SG in canine epidermis with a dotted pattern [47]. Chervet *et al.* reported that the immunostaining of the C-terminal of FLG in the epidermis was lacking, but that of the N-terminal of FLG was present in four out of 18 dogs with spontaneous CAD [60], suggesting a truncation mutation in a gene encoding canine FLG in those dogs. The immunostaining of the C-terminal of FLG appeared in all 16 healthy dogs. Genome wide analyses revealed that a single nucleotide polymorphism within the *FLG* gene is associated with CAD only in UK Labradors [61]. The association with *FLG* gene has not been reported in other breeds (e.g. West Highland white terrier, boxer, German shepherd dog, golden retriever, shiba inu, shih tzu, and pit bull terrier) or Labradors in other regions [61–63].

Other barrier abnormalities in human atopic dermatitis

A mutation in the gene encoding kallikrein-related peptidase 7 (KLK7), which is a family of trypsin- or chymotrypsin-like serine proteases that degrade corneodesmosomal proteins in the SC, has been identified in humans with AD [64]. Increased protein expression and enzymatic activity of KLKs in human AD have also been reported in two studies [65,66]. Moreover, transcription of claudin-1 gene, a major constituent in tight junctions, was down-regulated in the skin of humans with AD compared to non-AD individuals [67]. This finding might be related to the reduction of claudin-1 immunoreactivity in the skin of humans with AD [67]. However, such genetic mutations or aberrant protein expressions in CAD have not yet been reported.

Future perspectives for the investigation of cutaneous barrier function in canine atopic dermatitis

Several studies suggest that the reduction of free-extractable CERs in the SC appears to be associated with impairment of permeability barrier function (inside-to-outside barrier dysfunction) in dogs with CAD. In contrast, it has not yet been proven that the changes in CERs are associated with outside-to-inside barrier dysfunction that leads to percutaneous invasion of microorganisms or allergens, and that this accelerates percutaneous entry of allergens through the SC in CAD. Also, it is still a mystery whether the reduction of CERs is the primary factor that causes AD or whether it is secondary to AD. Stahl *et al.* reported that in an experimental dog model of atopic dermatitis sensitized to house dust mite allergen, total SC CERs and some fractions were decreased in postchallenge lesional and non-lesional SC compared with prechallenge samples, while there were no marked changes in the contents of cholesterols or free fatty acids in the postchallenge samples [68]. Although the study provided evidence that SC CERs are decreased, at least in part, secondary to inflammation, the data do not provide an argument for the theory that CER deficiencies are the primary cause of CAD, because the investigators did not compare the CER contents in prechallenged skin in naturally occurring CAD dogs with age- and breed-matched healthy dogs that do not develop CAD when challenged with an allergen.

In human medicine, two possible mechanisms that underlie decreased SC CERs have been proposed: decreased epidermal acid sphingomyelinase activity [69] and hydrolysis of sphingomyelin and glucosylceramide into degradation products by sphingomyelin- and glucosylceramide-deacylases [70–72]. In addition, it has been reported that bacterial ceramidases also cause reduction of SC CERs [73]. Further studies will be expected to determine the exact mechanisms causing the reduction of CERs in the SC of dogs with CAD. Moreover, involvement of the anti-inflammatory product S1P in the pathophysiology of cutaneous inflammation in CAD in dogs needs to be further elucidated.

In human medicine, it has been reported that loss-of-function mutations in the *FLG* gene, decreased claudin-1 expression, as well as increased KLK7 activity, are associated with AD. Future studies to investigate the genetic abnormalities related to the aberrant expression of epidermal proteins will be expected to provide a better understanding of the pathophysiology of impaired cutaneous barrier function in CAD.

References

1. Elias PM. Epidermal lipids, barrier function, and desquamation. *Journal of Investigative Dermatology* 1983; **80**: 44s–49s.
2. Shimada K, Yoon JS, Yoshihara T, *et al.* Increased transepidermal water loss and decreased ceramide content in lesional and non-lesional skin of dogs with atopic dermatitis. *Veterinary Dermatology* 2009; **20**: 541–546.
3. Shimada K, Yoshihara T, Yamamoto M, *et al.* Transepidermal water loss (TEWL) reflects skin barrier function of dog. *Journal of Veterinary Medical Science* 2008; **70**: 841–843.
4. Hightower K, Marsella R, Flynn Lurie A. Effects of age and allergen exposure on transepidermal water loss in a house dust mite-sensitized beagle model of atopic dermatitis. *Veterinary Dermatology* 2010; **21**: 88–95.
5. Watson A, Fray T, Clarke S, *et al.* Reliable use of the ServoMedEvaporimeter EP-2 to assess transepidermal water loss in the canine. *Journal of Nutrition* 2002; **132**: 1661S–1664S.
6. Yoshihara T, Shimada K, Momoi Y, *et al.* A new method of measuring the transepidermal water loss (TEWL) of dog skin. *Journal of Veterinary Medical Science* 2007; **69**: 289–292.
7. Lau-Gillard PJ, Hill PB, Chesney CJ, *et al.* Evaluation of a hand-held evaporimeter (VapoMeter) for the measurement of transepidermal water loss in healthy dogs. *Veterinary Dermatology* 2010; **21**: 136–145.
8. Bouwstra JA, Ponec M. The skin barrier in healthy and diseased state. *Biochimica et Biophysica Acta* 2006; **1758**: 2080–2095.
9. Holleran WM, Man MQ, Gao WN, *et al.* Sphingolipids are required for mammalian epidermal barrier function. Inhibition of sphingolipid synthesis delays barrier recovery after acute perturbation. *Journal of Clinical Investigation* 1991; **88**: 1338–1345.
10. Coderch L, Lopez O, de la Maza A, *et al.* Ceramides and skin function. *American Journal of Clinical Dermatology* 2003; **4**: 107–129.
11. Mizutani Y, Mitsutake S, Tsuji K, *et al.* Ceramide biosynthesis in keratinocyte and its role in skin function. *Biochimie* 2009; **91**: 784–790.
12. Uchida Y, Hara M, Nishio H, *et al.* Epidermal sphingomyelins are precursors for selected stratum corneum ceramides. *Journal of Lipid Research* 2000; **41**: 2071–2082.
13. Holleran WM, Takagi Y, Menon GK, *et al.* Processing of epidermal glucosylceramides is required for optimal mammalian cutaneous permeability barrier function. *Journal of Clinical Investigation* 1993; **91**: 1656–1664.
14. Holleran WM, Ginns EI, Menon GK, *et al.* Consequences of beta-glucocerebrosidase deficiency in epidermis. Ultrastructure and permeability barrier alterations in Gaucher disease. *Journal of Clinical Investigation* 1994; **93**: 1756–1764.

15. Hamanaka S, Hara M, Nishio H, *et al.* Human epidermal glucosylceramides are major precursors of stratum corneum ceramides. *Journal of Investigative Dermatology* 2002; **119**: 416–423.
16. Doering T, Proia RL, Sandhoff K. Accumulation of protein-bound epidermal glucosylceramides in beta-glucocerebrosidase deficient type 2 Gaucher mice. *FEBS Letters* 1999; **447**: 167–170.
17. Yanagi T, Akiyama M, Nishihara H, *et al.* Harlequin ichthyosis model mouse reveals alveolar collapse and severe fetal skin barrier defects. *Human Molecular Genetics* 2008; **17**: 3075–3083.
18. Finn LS, Zhang M, Chen SH, *et al.* Severe type II Gaucher disease with ichthyosis, arthrogryposis and neuronal apoptosis: molecular and pathological analyses. *American Journal of Medical Genetics* 2000; **91**: 222–226.
19. Akiyama M, Sugiyama Nakagiri Y, Sakai K, *et al.* Mutations in lipid transporter ABCA12 in harlequin ichthyosis and functional recovery by corrective gene transfer. *Journal of Clinical Investigation* 2005; **115**: 1777–1784.
20. Behne M, Uchida Y, Seki T, *et al.* Omega-hydroxyceramides are required for corneocyte lipid envelope (CLE) formation and normal epidermal permeability barrier function. *Journal of Investigative Dermatology* 2000; **114**: 185–192.
21. Herzinger T, Kleuser B, Schafer Korting M, *et al.* Sphingosine-1-phosphate signaling and the skin. *American Journal of Clinical Dermatology* 2007; **8**: 329–336.
22. Bäumer W, Rossbach K, Mischke R, *et al.* Decreased concentration and enhanced metabolism of sphingosine-1-phosphate in lesional skin of dogs with atopic dermatitis: disturbed sphingosine-1-phosphate homeostasis in atopic dermatitis. *Journal of Investigative Dermatology* 2011; **131**: 266–268.
23. Masukawa Y, Narita H, Sato H, *et al.* Comprehensive quantification of ceramide species in human stratum corneum. *Journal of Lipid Research* 2009; **50**: 1708–1719.
24. Yoon JS, Nishifuji K, Sasaki A, *et al.* Alteration of stratum corneum ceramide profiles in spontaneous canine model of atopic dermatitis. *Experimental Dermatology* 2011; **20**: 732–736.
25. Nishifuji K, Yoon JS. The stratum corneum: the rampart of the mammalian body. *Veterinary Dermatology* 2013; **24**: 60–72.
26. Uchida Y, Holleran WM. Omega-O-acylceramide, a lipid essential for mammalian survival. *Journal of Dermatological Science* 2008; **51**: 77–87.
27. Bouwstra JA, Gooris GS, Dubbelaar FE, *et al.* Role of ceramide 1 in the molecular organization of the stratum corneum lipids. *Journal of Lipid Research* 1998; **39**: 186–196.
28. de Jager M, Gooris G, Ponec M, *et al.* Acylceramide head group architecture affects lipid organization in synthetic ceramide mixtures. *Journal of Investigative Dermatology* 2004; **123**: 911–916.
29. Popa I, Thuy LH, Colsch B, *et al.* Analysis of free and protein-bound ceramides by tape stripping of stratum corneum from dogs. *Archives of Dermatological Research* 2010; **302**: 639–644.
30. Janssens M, van Smeden J, Gooris GS, *et al.* Lamellar lipid organization and ceramide composition in the stratum corneum of patients with atopic eczema. *Journal of Investigative Dermatology* 2011; **131**: 2136–2138.
31. Imokawa G, Abe A, Jin K, *et al.* Decreased level of ceramides in stratum corneum of atopic dermatitis: an etiologic factor in atopic dry skin? *Journal of Investigative Dermatology* 1991; **96**: 523–526.
32. Di Nardo A, Wertz P, Giannetti A, *et al.* Ceramide and cholesterol composition of the skin of patients with atopic dermatitis. *Acta Dermato-Venereologica* 1998; **78**: 27–30.
33. Ishikawa J, Narita H, Kondo N, *et al.* Changes in the ceramide profile of atopic dermatitis patients. *Journal of Investigative Dermatology* 2010; **130**: 2511–2514.
34. Macheleidt O, Kaiser HW, Sandhoff K. Deficiency of epidermal protein-bound omega-hydroxyceramides in atopic dermatitis. *Journal of Investigative Dermatology* 2002; **119**: 166–173.
35. Inman AO, Olivry T, Dunston SM, *et al.* Electron microscopic observations of stratum corneum intercellular lipids in normal and atopic dogs. *Veterinary Pathology* 2001; **38**: 720–723.
36. Piekutowska A, Pin D, Reme CA, *et al.* Effects of a topically applied preparation of epidermal lipids on the stratum corneum barrier of atopic dogs. *Journal of Comparative Pathology* 2008; **138**: 197–203.
37. Marsella R, Samuelson D, Doerr K. Transmission electron microscopy studies in an experimental model of canine atopic dermatitis. *Veterinary Dermatology* 2010; **21**: 81–88.
38. Reiter LV, Torres SM, Wertz PW. Characterization and quantification of ceramides in the nonlesional skin of canine patients with atopic dermatitis compared with controls. *Veterinary Dermatology* 2009; **20**: 260–266.
39. Popa I, Remoue N, Hoang LT, *et al.* Atopic dermatitis in dogs is associated with a high heterogeneity in the distribution of protein-bound lipids within the stratum corneum. *Archives of Dermatological Research* 2011; **303**: 433–440.
40. Wood SH, Clements DN, Ollier WE, *et al.* Gene expression in canine atopic dermatitis and correlation with clinical severity scores. *Journal of Dermatological Science* 2009; **55**: 27–33.
41. Steinert PM, Cantieri JS, Teller DC, *et al.* Characterization of a class of cationic proteins that specifically interact with intermediate filaments. *Proceedings of the National Academy of Sciences USA* 1981; **78**: 4097–4101.
42. Sandilands A, Sutherland C, Irvine AD, *et al.* Filaggrin in the frontline: role in skin barrier function and disease. *Journal of Cell Science* 2009; **122**: 1285–1294.
43. Dale BA, Resing KA, Lonsdale Eccles JD. Filaggrin: a keratin filament associated protein. *Annals of the New York Academy of Science* 1985; **455**: 330–342.
44. Gan SQ, McBride OW, Idler WW, *et al.* Organization, structure, and polymorphisms of the human profilaggrin gene. *Biochemistry* 1990; **29**: 9432–9440.
45. McKinley Grant LJ, Idler WW, Bernstein IA, *et al.* Characterization of a cDNA clone encoding human filaggrin and localization of the gene to chromosome region 1q21. *Proceedings of the National Academy of Sciences USA* 1989; **86**: 4848–4852.
46. Presland RB, Haydock PV, Fleckman P, *et al.* Characterization of the human epidermal profilaggrin gene. Genomic organization and identification of an S-100-like calcium binding domain at the amino terminus. *Journal of Biological Chemistry* 1992; **267**: 23772–23781.
47. Kanda S, Sasaki T, Shiohama A, *et al.* Characterization of canine filaggrin: gene structure and protein expression in dog skin. *Veterinary Dermatology* 2013; **24**: 25–31.
48. Kawasaki H, Kubo A, Sasaki T, *et al.* Loss-of-function mutations within the filaggrin gene and atopic dermatitis. *Current Problems in Dermatology* 2011; **41**: 35–46.
49. NemotoHasebe I, Akiyama M, Nomura T, *et al.* FLG mutation p.Lys4021X in the C-terminal imperfect filaggrin repeat in Japanese patients with atopic eczema. *British Journal of Dermatology* 2009; **161**: 1387–1390.
50. Sandilands A, Terron Kwiatkowski A, Hull PR, *et al.* Comprehensive analysis of the gene encoding filaggrin uncovers prevalent and rare mutations in ichthyosis vulgaris and atopic eczema. *Nature Genetics* 2007; **39**: 650–654.
51. Kawasaki H, Nagao K, Kubo A, *et al.* Altered stratum corneum barrier and enhanced percutaneous immune responses in filaggrin-null mice. *Journal of Allergy and Clinical Immunology* 2012; **129**: 1538–1546.

52. Palmer CN, Irvine AD, Terron Kwiatkowski A, *et al.* Common loss-of-function variants of the epidermal barrier protein filaggrin are a major predisposing factor for atopic dermatitis. *Nature Genetics* 2006; **38**: 441–446.
53. Carlsen BC, Johansen JD, Menne T, *et al.* Filaggrin null mutations and association with contact allergy and allergic contact dermatitis: results from a tertiary dermatology clinic. *Contact Dermatitis* 2010; **63**: 89–95.
54. Thyssen JP, Johansen JD, Linneberg A, *et al.* The association between null mutations in the filaggrin gene and contact sensitization to nickel and other chemicals in the general population. *British Journal of Dermatology* 2010; **162**: 1278–1285.
55. Novak N, Baurecht H, Schafer T, *et al.* Loss-of-function mutations in the filaggrin gene and allergic contact sensitization to nickel. *Journal of Investigative Dermatology* 2008; **128**: 1430–1435.
56. Fallon PG, Sasaki T, Sandilands A, *et al.* A homozygous frameshift mutation in the mouse *Flg* gene facilitates enhanced percutaneous allergen priming. *Nature Genetics* 2009; **41**: 602–608.
57. Hoste E, Kemperman P, Devos M, *et al.* Caspase-14 is required for filaggrin degradation to natural moisturizing factors in the skin. *Journal of Investigative Dermatology* 2011; **131**: 2233–2241.
58. Denecker G, Hoste E, Gilbert B, *et al.* Caspase-14 protects against epidermal UVB photodamage and water loss. *Nature Cell Biology* 2007; **9**: 666–674.
59. Marsella R, Samuelson D, Harrington L. Immunohistochemical evaluation of filaggrin polyclonal antibody in atopic and normal beagles. *Veterinary Dermatology* 2009; **20**: 547–554.
60. Chervet L, Galichet A, McLean WH, *et al.* Missing C-terminal filaggrin expression, NFkappaB activation and hyperproliferation identify the dog as a putative model to study epidermal dysfunction in atopic dermatitis. *Experimental Dermatology* 2010; **19**: e343–346.
61. Wood SH, Ollier WE, Nuttall T, *et al.* Despite identifying some shared gene associations with human atopic dermatitis the use of multiple dog breeds from various locations limits detection of gene associations in canine atopic dermatitis. *Veterinary Immunology and Immunopathology* 2010; **138**: 193–197.
62. Barros Roque J, O'Leary CA, Kyaw Tanner M, *et al.* Haplotype sharing excludes canine orthologous Filaggrin locus in atopy in West Highland White Terriers. *Animal Genetics* 2009; **40**: 793–794.
63. Salzmann CA, Olivry TJ, Nielsen DM, *et al.* Genome-wide linkage study of atopic dermatitis in West Highland White Terriers. *BMC Genetics* 2011; **12**: 37.
64. Vasilopoulos Y, Cork MJ, Murphy R, *et al.* Genetic association between an AACC insertion in the 3′UTR of the stratum corneumchymotryptic enzyme gene and atopic dermatitis. *Journal of Investigative Dermatology* 2004; **123**: 62–66.
65. Komatsu N, Saijoh K, Kuk C, *et al.* Human tissue kallikrein expression in the stratum corneum and serum of atopic dermatitis patients. *Experimental Dermatology* 2007; **16**: 513–519.
66. Voegeli R, Rawlings AV, Breternitz M, *et al.* Increased stratum corneum serine protease activity in acute eczematous atopic skin. *British Journal of Dermatology* 2009; **161**: 70–77.
67. De Benedetto A, Rafaels NM, McGirt LY, *et al.* Tight junction defects in patients with atopic dermatitis. *Journal of Allergy and Clinical Immunology* 2011; **127**: 773–786.
68. Stahl J, Paps J, Bäumer W, *et al.* *Dermatophagoides farinae* house dust mite allergen challenges reduce stratum corneum ceramides in an experimental dog model of acute atopic dermatitis. *Veterinary Dermatology* 2012; **23**: 497–e92.
69. Jensen JM, Folster Holst R, Baranowsky A, *et al.* Impaired sphingomyelinase activity and epidermal differentiation in atopic dermatitis. *Journal of Investigative Dermatology* 2004; **122**: 1423–1431.
70. Hara J, Higuchi K, Okamoto R, *et al.* High-expression of sphingomyelindeacylase is an important determinant of ceramide deficiency leading to barrier disruption in atopic dermatitis. *Journal of Investigative Dermatology* 2000; **115**: 406–413.
71. Imokawa G. A possible mechanism underlying the ceramide deficiency in atopic dermatitis: expression of a deacylase enzyme that cleaves the N-acyl linkage of sphingomyelin and glucosylceramide. *Journal of Dermatological Science* 2009; **55**: 1–9.
72. Murata Y, Ogata J, Higaki Y, *et al.* Abnormal expression of sphingomyelinacylase in atopic dermatitis: an etiologic factor for ceramide deficiency? *Journal of Investigative Dermatology* 1996; **106**: 1242–1249.
73. Ohnishi Y, Okino N, Ito M, *et al.* Ceramidase activity in bacterial skin flora as a possible cause of ceramide deficiency in atopic dermatitis. *Clinical and Diagnostic Laboratory Immunology* 1999; **6**: 101–104.

7

The role of bacterial agents in the pathogenesis of canine atopic dermatitis

David H. Lloyd

Department of Clinical Sciences and Services, Royal Veterinary College, Hatfield, UK

Conflict of interest: none declared.

Introduction

Earlier chapters have defined the nature of canine atopic dermatitis (CAD) and described the role of defects in the skin barrier (Chapter 6) and an aberrant immune system (Chapter 3) in its pathogenesis. Although it is recognised that genetic defects play an important role (Chapter 5), it is clear that the disease is substantially driven by environmental factors (Chapter 4), amongst which the influence of micro-organisms, and particularly bacteria, is increasingly apparent [1]. Although evidence of the involvement of bacteria in CAD is still fragmentary there is an increasing volume of data, from studies in experimental models and from the human field, which is helping us to build a picture of the range of microbial activities that may be involved in its pathogenesis.

Bacterial involvement in the pathogenesis of atopic dermatitis (AD) can be divided into two broad components. Firstly, there are effects associated with exposure of the immune system of young individuals to bacteria and their products within the environment. Secondly, there are effects associated with the micro-environment of the skin surface and colonisation and infection of the skin. Here, the bacteria are able to take advantage of barrier defects to promote their ability to persist and proliferate on skin; it is apparent that a vicious circle can be established where microbial activity promotes further degradation of the skin barrier and increases its susceptibility to bacterial proliferation and invasion. The predominant bacteria involved in this process are the pathogenic staphylococci: *Staphylococcus aureus* in humans and *S. pseudintermedius* in dogs. In this text, the name *S. pseudintermedius* will be used to refer to studies involving canine isolates of *S. intermedius* carried out before the new nomenclature for this species [2] was established. *S. aureus* and other staphylococci, including coagulase-variable species such as *S. schleiferi* and *S. hyicus*, and coagulase-negative species, may also be involved in infections associated with CAD but much less commonly than *S. pseudintermedius*.

This chapter will review knowledge of the involvement of bacteria in the pathogenesis of CAD, focusing on the pathogenic staphylococci, but will not extend to a description of cutaneous bacterial infection and bacterial overgrowth (see Chapter 26).

Environmental exposure

In humans, AD and other atopic conditions, such as asthma and IgE–mediated food allergy, have been increasing in prevalence and severity over the past three decades [3]. This increase has been attributed to reduced exposure to micro-organisms and their products, leading to an alteration in the balance of Th1 : Th2 and/or

Veterinary Allergy, First Edition. Edited by Chiara Noli, Aiden Foster, and Wayne Rosenkrantz.

reduced T-cell regulation of the immune response [3], a concept known as the 'hygiene hypothesis'. In a systematic review of research into this concept, there was convincing evidence to support an inverse relationship between the occurrence of AD and exposure to bacterial endotoxin/lipopolysaccharide, early day care, farm animals, and dogs. In addition, helminth infestation was considered at least partially protective [4]. A range of independent microbial signals, including those from both Gram-negative and Gram-positive bacteria, and moulds, seem to be involved [5]. In dogs, CAD is increasingly diagnosed and is perceived to be rising in prevalence, as in man, although reliable confirmatory data are lacking. There is also some evidence that hygiene may be involved in promoting the canine disease; an inverse relationship has been demonstrated between the occurrence of CAD and exposure to high indoor levels of endotoxin [6].

Response to probiotics

The concept that insufficient stimulation of the immune system is responsible, at least in part, for promotion of Th2 dominated responses and the development of AD is supported by increasing evidence from the human field, suggesting that the intestinal microbiota plays a critical role during early life [7]. This evidence includes responses to probiotics, in the form of ingested live cultures, principally of lactobacilli, with protection against atopic disease and amelioration of clinical signs in young children [8,9]. However, not all studies have yielded beneficial effects [10] and further work is required to define how probiotic use can be optimised in combating human atopic disease.

Evaluation of probiotics in dogs has been limited by confounding factors (differing diets, environments, and allergic sensitivities) but studies using a validated model of CAD have shown that early exposure to *Lactobacillus rhamnosus* can decrease allergen-specific IgE and partially prevent CAD when administered in the first 6 months of life [11]; follow-up of these dogs involving allergen challenge 3 years after discontinuation of the probiotic showed reduced clinical scores in probiotic-exposed dogs [12].

The defective skin barrier

Evidence for the role of a defective skin barrier in the pathogenesis of AD of humans is now quite extensive. Transepidermal water loss (TEWL) is elevated in AD lesions, pointing towards reduced stratum corneum function. Deficiencies of proteins and lipids, including filaggrin, involucrin, cholesterol, free fatty acids, and ceramides, have been demonstrated in the epidermis. Filaggrin gene mutations are involved but do not appear to be implicated in modification of the immune response and the importance of other environmental factors is increasingly recognised [1,13]. Down-regulation of filaggrin expression and other structural proteins and peptides by Th2 cytokines has been shown to occur in atopic skin [14].

In dogs, there is growing evidence of skin barrier impairment in CAD. Defective stratum corneum intracellular lamellae, evidence of decreased amounts of ceramides, and alteration of keratins, involucrin, and filaggrin gene expression have been demonstrated [15–17]. Micro-organisms, and particularly bacteria, are able to take advantage of such defects in the skin barrier in AD and this is demonstrated by bacterial colonisation, elevated populations and infection, particularly by pathogenic staphylococci, in affected individuals. These organisms can in turn exert a wide range of effects, which can protect them from host defences, promote the Th2 inflammatory environment, damage the skin, and facilitate cutaneous infection.

Staphylococcal colonisation/adherence

Bacteria need to adhere to host tissue in order to establish colonisation and proliferation, and for production of virulence factors. In AD, increased adherence has been demonstrated for *S. aureus* in humans and *S. pseudintermedius* in dogs, both to corneocytes [18,19] and to other substances within the epidermis, including fibronectin and fibrinogen [20,21]. Furthermore, in human immunocytochemical studies of AD, redistribution of fibronectin to the cornified layer of the epidermis has been demonstrated (an observation that was not seen in normal skin [22]), creating a situation likely to further enhance *S. aureus* colonisation and infection. Studies in mice sensitised with ovalbumin have also shown that a Th2 inflammatory environment can promote skin binding by *S. aureus* and that this binding is mediated by fibronectin and fibrinogen [22]. It is likely that such effects could also occur in CAD and further enhance the ability of *S. pseudintermedius* to colonise and infect the skin.

Antimicrobial peptides (AMPs)

AMPs are recognised as one of the important mechanisms of the epidermis controlling microbial colonisation and defending against infection. Reduced expression of the cathelicidin, LL-37, and of human beta-defensin-2 (hBD-2) has been demonstrated in lesional skin in AD, and it has been shown that exposure of keratinocytes in culture to Th2 cytokines (IL-4 and IL-13) reduces expression of hBD-2 [23]. Reduction of hBD-3 in AD lesions due to the presence of these cytokines has also been demonstrated [24,25]. Furthermore, defective killing of *S. aureus* associated with reduced mobilisation of hBD-3 has been reported in AD patients [26] indicating that AMPs of AD patients may not be sufficient to combat pathogenic skin infection even when up-regulated, or that that AMP function is disturbed in such patients [27]. One factor which is known to be capable of reducing activity of AMPs is the action of proteases, including those produced by coagulase-positive and coagulase-negative staphylococci [28,29]. In addition, staphylococci are able to promote their survival by induction of resistance mechanisms when exposed to AMPs via the *aps* AMP sensor/regulator system [30].

In CAD, canine beta defensin-1 (cBD-1) has been shown to be expressed at higher levels in both lesional and non-lesional skin compared with healthy skin, although cBD-103 was down-regulated in the skin of CAD dogs [31]. It is suggested that this down-regulation may be a factor predisposing dogs with atopic dermatitis to *S. pseudintermedius* infection [32].

Superantigens and related proteins

Bacterial superantigens are exotoxins exhibiting potent polyclonal T-lymphocyte-proliferating activity. Staphylococcal superantigens (SAGs) include the enterotoxins, named for their ability to cause vomiting and food poisoning, and toxic shock syndrome toxin [33,34]. These substances are involved in the pathogenesis of AD in a number of ways [35].

Superantigens are able to induce the skin homing receptor, cutaneous lymphocyte-associated antigen, on T cells to recruit these cells to the skin. It has been shown that such skin-homing phenotypically T regulatory ($CD4^+$ $FoxP3^+$) cells from AD patients actually exert a Th2 phenotype in skin in response to staphylococcal enterotoxin B stimulation [36]. There is also evidence supporting induction of T regulatory cells with functional suppressor activity by staphylococcal enterotoxin A [37]. Staphylococcal enterotoxin B has also been shown to be a potent inducer of IL-31 production by Th2 cells in the skin of patients with AD. IL-31 has been shown to cause severe pruritus in murine skin and there is increasing evidence that it is an important cause of pruritus in human AD [38,39]. Recent, as yet unpublished, studies presented at the Seventh World Congress of Veterinary Dermatology in July 2012 indicate that IL-31 is functionally active and can induce pruritus in dogs; it was detected in the skin of the majority of dogs with atopic dermatitis [40]. Self trauma as a consequence of such pruritus would cause further damage to the skin barrier.

SAGs are able to promote IgE production and the ability of AD patients to develop anti-SAG IgE antibodies, a recently recognised risk factor for human asthma, as well as IgE antibodies to other exotoxins, which may exacerbate the disease by promoting bacterial hypersensitivity [41–45]. A subgroup of AD patients has also been recognised with deficient ability to produce IgG2 antibodies to staphylococcal enterotoxin C1 [46]. In dogs, elevated levels of serum antistaphylococcal IgE have been demonstrated in idiopathic recurrent superficial pyoderma and in recurrent canine pyoderma secondary to atopic dermatitis, supporting the concept that bacterial hypersensitivity may be responsible for initiating or perpetuating skin lesions in these animals [47].

SAGs may also interfere with treatment of AD. In humans, they are known to induce glucocorticoid insensitivity and may render use of such drugs less effective in AD [48]. Interestingly, a study of staphylococcal isolates from steroid-resistant AD patients has shown that they contain more SAG genes than those from non-steroid-resistant patients, suggesting that use of glucocorticoids, a very common approach, may select for such resistant strains [49].

The staphylococcal superantigens-like proteins (SSLs) have structural similarity to superantigens but no superantigenic activity. Studies with murine and human inflammatory cells have shown that SSL3 is able to bind to Toll-like receptor 2 (TLR2) and inhibit stimulation of macrophages by TLR2 ligands, providing evidence of a novel mechanism for immune evasion by *S. aureus* by interfering with its recognition by innate immune cells [50,51].

Several studies have demonstrated production of SAGs by *S. pseudintermedius* from canine skin infections. Staphylococcal enterotoxins (SE) A, B, C, D, and E, and toxic shock syndrome toxin have been demonstrated, and stimulation of canine peripheral blood mononuclear cells *in vitro* and quantitative flow cytometry have revealed that SEA and SEB from canine isolates are potent stimulators of T cell blastogenesis [52,53].

Exfoliative toxins

Exfoliative toxins are virulence factors produced by pathogenic staphylococci, which can cause blister formation in the epidermis. In human *S. aureus* infections they are associated with bullous impetigo and staphylococcal scalded skin syndrome; in pigs, production of such toxins by *S. hyicus* is involved in the pathogenesis of porcine exudative epidermitis. Exfoliative toxin production has been demonstrated in *S. pseudintermedius*. The first toxin to be described (*Staphylococcus intermedius* exfoliative toxin; SIET) was shown to cause erythema, exfoliation, and crusting when injected into canine skin and the *siet* gene was shown to be present in a high proportion of isolates of *S. pseudintermedius* [53–55]. However, recent studies with recombinant SIET have failed to demonstrate lesion formation in canine skin

[56]. Two additional exfoliative toxins from *S. pseudintermedius* (EXI and ExpB) have now been described and shown to cause epidermal splitting in canine skin, an effect which appears to be mediated through degradation of desmoglein-1. Genes expressing these toxins have been shown to be present in 23% of *S. pseudintermedius* isolates from canine pyoderma [56,57]. It is very likely that the action of such toxins is responsible, at least in part, for the splitting of the epidermis and the formation of epidermal crusts and collarettes in canine pyoderma. Such damage to the skin barrier is likely to promote further invasion of the skin as well as atopic dermatitis in dogs with CAD.

Ceramidase

Ceramides are the dominant lipids in the human stratum corneum and play a crucial role in skin barrier function [58]. Studies also indicate that they are decreased in CAD [59] and reduced ceramide content within the stratum corneum of dogs with CAD has been correlated with transepidermal water loss, reflecting the situation observed in human AD [60]. High populations of bacteria are commonly found on the skin surface of individuals with AD and bacterial ceramidase is believed to be significant in further reducing the protective activity of ceramides. In studies of human AD, ceramidase secretion has been shown to be greater in bacterial flora, from both lesional and non-lesional skin, than from the skin of healthy subjects [61]. Ceramidase from *Pseudomonas aeruginosa* is inactivated in a dose-dependent way by citric acid and the use of citric acid has been shown to alleviate atopic dermatitis in an animal model [62], suggesting that ceramidase inhibitors may be useful in reducing damage to skin barrier function in AD caused by bacterial activity; further work is needed to demonstrate whether this approach may be effective in CAD and against ceramidase activity by other microbes.

Flagellin and thymic stromal lymphopoietin

Thymic stromal lymphopoietin (TSLP) is a cytokine that plays a crucial role in the development and progression of allergic diseases. It is thought to act as a driver of the Th2 environment and is highly expressed by keratinocytes in skin lesions of AD [63]. Flagellin, the major structural protein of the flagella of Gram-negative bacteria, is found in house dust and can promote allergic asthma by priming allergic responses to indoor allergens. Recent studies have shown that exposure of human keratinocytes to flagellin induces release of TSLP protein and up-regulation of gene expression for TSLP and other proinflammatory molecules [64]. This flagellin-induced release of TSLP was shown to be enhanced by Th2 cytokines and by transforming growth factor alpha, which is over-expressed in keratinocytes in atopic dermatitis, indicating that its effects in AD are likely to be amplified in patients' skin [65]. In CAD, TSLP expression is elevated in both lesional and non-lesional skin of affected dogs, and canine keratinocytes have been shown to have increased expression of TSLP when exposed to allergens or toll-like receptor ligands, including lipopolysaccharide, a major component of the outer membrane of Gram-negative bacteria [66]. Thus it seems likely that flagellin may play a role in the pathogenesis of CAD.

Bacterial virulence and the pathogenesis of canine pyoderma

Bacterial infection in skin is almost invariably a secondary event which occurs subsequent to reduction in the protective properties of the skin. Allergic dermatoses and particularly CAD are a common cause of this, largely for the reasons outlined above; reduced barrier function and impaired antimicrobial defences permit microbial colonisation and proliferation, and increased bacterial populations are then able to damage and invade the skin, causing superficial and deep pyoderma. Virulence factors are the mechanisms that enable bacteria to resist host defence mechanisms and damage host tissues, further promoting infection. Knowledge of virulence factors in *S. pseudintermedius* is quite limited but has been recently reviewed [67]. Like *S. aureus*, the virulence factors of *S. pseudintermedius* include a variety of substances capable of damaging host tissues, subverting host defence mechanisms, and promoting invasion. These include enzymes (coagulase, thermonuclease, proteases), surface proteins (clumping factor, protein A), a variety of toxins, and communication systems, such as the accessory gene regulator (Table 7.1). Of particular importance is the recognition of pathogen-associated molecular patterns, or PAMPs (e.g. lipoteichoic acid, peptidoglycan) by Toll-like receptors and other mechanisms, leading to the recruitment of granulocytes, the activation of mast cells, and the release of mediators promoting cutaneous inflammation and the clinical manifestations of canine pyoderma [73–75].

Conclusion

Data from human medicine, together with limited results from animals, indicate that exposure of young animals to microbes and their products, either through natural contact or by administration of probiotics, is likely to be of benefit in reducing the occurrence of CAD. It is clear that bacteria can also play an important part

Table 7.1 *Staphylococcus pseudintermedius* virulence factors and their activity*

Virulence factor	Recognised components	Activity
Cytotoxins	α- and β-haemolysin, leukotoxin Luk-I	Damage host cells including erythrocytes and leukocytes. Roles in pathogenesis are poorly understood. Luk-I is consistently found in the European MRSP clone ST71 [68].
Superantigens	Enterotoxins A, B, C, D and E, and toxic shock syndrome toxin	Enterotoxins can cause vomiting and food poisoning. Superantigens cause polyclonal T-lymphocyte proliferation (only demonstrated for SEA and SEB) [52].
Exfoliative toxins	SIET, EXI, ExpB	In canine skin: SIET can cause erythema, exfoliation and crusting [54,55]; EXI and ExpB cause epidermal splitting [56,57].
Cell-wall-anchored proteins	Protein A, clumping factor A, SpsD, SpsL, SpsO	Can act as MSCRAMMs. SpsD and SpsL adhere to fibrinogen, fibronectin, and cytokeratin 10 [69]. SpsD and SpsO mediate adherence to canine corneocytes [70].
Accessory gene regulatory (*agr*) system	Autoinducing peptide (AIP)	AIP activates the *agr* system in a population-dependent manner (quorum sensing) regulating the production of virulence factors and facilitating colonisation and infection [71].
Biofilm formation	Like most staphylococci, *S. pseudintermedius* has the capacity to form biofilms [72]	Composed principally of polysaccharide, biofilms bind and protect communities of cells giving increased resistance to host defence mechanisms and antimicrobials agents.

*Reviewed in more detail by Bannoehr and Guardabassi [67].
MSCRAMMs, microbial surface components recognising adhesive matrix molecules.

in the pathogenesis of AD and very probably CAD, in susceptible individuals, by promoting the allergic component of the disease and also by inducing conditions within the skin surface microenvironment that promote microbial survival, proliferation, and infection.

Whilst there is no convincing evidence yet in human medicine that antibacterial treatment is helpful in cases of atopic eczema that are not clinically infected [76], two studies indicate that shampooing is beneficial in dogs. In one of these, there was a reduction in pruritus in dogs with allergic or idiopathic pruritus treated with an antipruritic shampoo [77]. In the other study, a medicated shampoo was compared with the shampoo vehicle alone in dogs with mild to moderate allergic pruritus and both treatments gave reductions in pruritus [78]. Further studies are required to determine the nature of these beneficial effects in relation to microbial activity.

References

1. Ong PY, Leung DY. The infectious aspects of atopic dermatitis. *Immunology and Allergy Clinics of North America* 2010; **30**: 309–321.
2. Devriese LA, Vancanneyt M, Baele M, *et al. Staphylococcus pseudintermedius* sp. nov., a coagulase-positive species from animals. *International Journal of Systematic and Evolutionary Microbiology* 2005; **55**: 1569–1573.
3. Baker BS. The role of microorganisms in atopic dermatitis. *Clinical and Experimental Immunology* 2006; **144**: 1–9.
4. Flohr C, Yeo L. Atopic dermatitis and the hygiene hypothesis revisited. *Current Problems in Dermatology* 2011; **41**: 1–34.
5. Heederik D, von Mutius E. Does diversity of environmental microbial exposure matter for the occurrence of allergy and asthma? *Journal of Allergy and Clinical Immunology* 2012; **130**: 44–50.
6. Looringh van Beeck FA, Hoekstra H, Brunekreef B, *et al.* Inverse association between endotoxin exposure and canine atopic dermatitis. *Veterinary Journal* 2011; **190**: 215–219.
7. Russell SL, Finlay BB. The impact of gut microbes in allergic diseases. *Current Opinion in Gastroenterology* 2012; **28**: 563–569.
8. Ozdemir O. Various effects of different probiotic strains in allergic disorders: an update from laboratory and clinical data. *Clinical and Experimental Immunology* 2010; **160**: 295–304.
9. Sung-Il Woo, Ji-Yoon Kim, Yong-Ju Lee, *et al.* Effect of *Lactobacillus sakei* supplementation in children with atopic eczema–dermatitis syndrome. *Annals of Allergy, Asthma and Immunology* 2010; **104**: 343–348.
10. Brouwer ML, Wolt-Plompen SAA, Dubois AEJ, *et al.* No effects of probiotics on atopic dermatitis in infancy: a randomized placebo-controlled trial. *Clinical and Experimental Allergy* 2006; **36**: 899–906.
11. Marsella R. Evaluation of *Lactobacillus rhamnosus* strain GG for the prevention of atopic dermatitis in dogs. *American Journal of Veterinary Research* 2009; **70**: 735–740.
12. Marsella R, Santoro D, Ahrens K. Early exposure to probiotics in a canine model of atopic dermatitis has long-term clinical and immunological effects. *Veterinary Immunology and Immunopathology* 2012; **146**: 185–189.

13. Kubo A, Nagao K, Amagai M. Epidermal barrier dysfunction and cutaneous sensitization in atopic diseases. *Journal of Clinical Investigation* 2012; **122**: 440–447.
14. Ogg G. Role of T cells in the pathogenesis of atopic dermatitis. *Clinical and Experimental Allergy* 2009; **39**: 310–316.
15. Reiter LV, Torres SMF, Wertz PW. Characterization and quantification of ceramides in the nonlesional skin of canine patients with atopic dermatitis compared with controls. *Veterinary Dermatology* 2009; **20**: 260–266.
16. Roque JB, O'Leary CA, Kyaw-Tanner M, *et al.* Real-time PCR quantification of the canine filaggrin orthologue in the skin of atopic and non-atopic dogs: a pilot study. *BMC Research Notes* 2011; **4**: 554.
17. Theerawatanasirikul S, Sailasuta A, Thanawongnuwech R, *et al.* Alterations of keratins, involucrin and filaggrin gene expression in canine atopic dermatitis. *Research in Veterinary Science* 2012; **93**: 1287–1292.
18. Cole GW, Silverberg NL. The adherence of *Staphylococcus aureus* to human corneocytes. *Archives of Dermatology* 1986; **122**: 166–169.
19. McEwan NA. Adherence by *Staphylococcus intermedius* to canine keratinocytes in atopic dermatitis. *Research in Veterinary Science* 2000; **68**: 279–283.
20. Cho SH, Strickland I, Boguniewicz M, *et al.* Fibronectin and fibrinogen contribute to the enhanced binding of *Staphylococcus aureus* to atopic skin. *Journal of Allergy and Clinical Immunology* 2001; **108**: 269–274.
21. Schmidt V, Nuttall T, Fazakerley J, *et al. Staphylococcus intermedius* binding to immobilized fibrinogen, fibronectin and cytokeratin *in vitro*. *Veterinary Dermatology* 2009; **20**: 502–508.
22. Cho SH, Strickland I, Tomkinson A, *et al.* Preferential binding of *Staphylococcus aureus* to skin sites of Th2-mediated inflammation in a murine model. *Journal of Investigative Dermatology* 2001; **116**: 658–663.
23. Ong PY, Ohtake T, Brandt C, *et al.* Endogenous antimicrobial peptides and skin infections in atopic dermatitis. *New England Journal of Medicine* 2002; **347**: 1151–1160.
24. Nomura I, Goleva E, Howell MD, *et al.* Cytokine milieu of atopic dermatitis, as compared to psoriasis, skin prevents induction of innate immune response genes. *Journal of Immunology* 2003; **171**: 3262–3269.
25. Howell MD, Boguniewicz M, Pastore S, *et al.* Mechanism of HBD-3 deficiency in atopic dermatitis. *Clinical Immunology* 2006; **121**: 332–338.
26. Kisich KO, Carspecken CW, Fiéve S, *et al.* Defective killing of *Staphylococcus aureus* in atopic dermatitis is associated with reduced mobilization of human b-defensin-3. *Journal of Allergy and Clinical Immunology* 2008; **122**: 62–68.
27. Schittek B. The antimicrobial skin barrier in patients with atopic dermatitis. *Current Problems in Dermatology* 2011; **41**: 54–67.
28. Sieprawska-Lupa M, Mydel P, Krawczyk K, *et al.* Degradation of human antimicrobial peptide LL-37 by *Staphylococcus aureus*-derived proteinases. *Antimicrobial Agents and Chemotherapy* 2004; **48**: 4673–4679.
29. Lai Y, Villaruz AE, Li M, *et al.* The human anionic antimicrobial peptide dermcidin induces proteolytic defence mechanisms in staphylococci. *Molecular Microbiology* 2007; **63**: 497–506.
30. Li M, Cha DJ, Lai Y, *et al.* The antimicrobial peptide-sensing system aps of *Staphylococcus aureus*. *Molecular Microbiology* 2007; **66**: 1136–1147.
31. van Damme CMM, Willemse T, van Dijk A, *et al.* Altered cutaneous expression of β-defensins in dogs with atopic dermatitis. *Molecular Immunology* 2009; **46**; 2449–2455.
32. Leonard BC, Affolter VK, Bevins CL. Antimicrobial peptides: agents of border protection for companion animals. *Veterinary Dermatology* 2012; **23**: 177–e36.
33. Lina G, Bohach GA, Nair SP, *et al.* Standard nomenclature for the superantigens expressed by *Staphylococcus*. *Journal of infectious Diseases* 2004; **189**: 2334–2336.
34. Xu SX, McCormick JK. Staphylococcal superantigens in colonization and disease. *Frontiers in Cellular and Infection Microbiology* 2012; **2**: 52.
35. Schlievert PM, Strandberg KL, Lin YC, *et al.* Secreted virulence factor comparison between methicillin-resistant and methicillin-sensitive *Staphylococcus aureus*, and its relevance to atopic dermatitis. *Journal of Allergy and Clinical Immunology* 2010; **125**: 39–49.
36. Lin YT, Wang CT, Chao PS, *et al.* Skin-homing $CD4^+$ $Foxp3^+$ T cells exert Th2-like function after staphylococcal superantigen stimulation in atopic dermatitis patients. *Clinical and Experimental Allergy* 2011; **41**: 516–525.
37. Taylor AL, Llewelyn MJ. Superantigen-induced proliferation of human $CD4^+CD25^-$ T cells is followed by a switch to a functional regulatory phenotype. *Journal of Immunology* 2010; **185**: 6591–6598.
38. Sonkoly E, Muller A, Lauerma AI, *et al.* IL-31: a new link between T cells and pruritus in atopic skin inflammation. *Journal of Allergy and Clinical Immunology* 2006; **117**: 411–417.
39. Cornelissena C, Lüscher-Firzlaffa J, Malte Baronb J, *et al.* Signaling by IL-31 and functional consequences. *European Journal of Cell Biology* 2012; **91**: 552–566.
40. Gonzales A, Humphrey W, Teel J, *et al.* IL-31: Its role in canine pruritus and prevalence in naturally occurring canine atopic dermatitis. *Veterinary Dermatology* 2012; **23** (S1): 6.
41. Leung DY, Harbeck R, Bina P, *et al.* Presence of IgE antibodies to staphylococcal exotoxins on the skin of patients with atopic dermatitis. Evidence for a new group of allergens. *Journal of Clinical Investigation* 1993; **92**: 1374–1380.
42. Lin YT, Shau WY, Wang LF, *et al.* Comparison of serum specific IgE antibodies to staphylococcal enterotoxins between atopic children with and without atopic dermatitis. *Allergy* 2000; **55**: 641–646.
43. Cardona ID, Cho SH, Leung DY. Role of bacterial superantigens in atopic dermatitis: implications for future therapeutic strategies. *American Journal of Clinical Dermatology* 2006; **7**: 273–279.
44. Ong PY, Ferdman RM, Church JA. Late-onset of IgE sensitization to microbial allergens in young children with atopic dermatitis. *British Journal of Dermatology* 2010; **162**: 159–161.
45. Bachert C, van Steen K, Zhang N, *et al.* Specific IgE against *Staphylococcus aureus* enterotoxins: an independent risk factor for asthma. *Journal of Allergy and Clinical Immunology* 2012; **130**: 376–381.
46. Mrabet-Dahbi S, Breuer K, Klotz M, *et al.* Deficiency in immunoglobulin G2 antibodies against staphylococcal enterotoxin C1 defines a subgroup of patients with atopic dermatitis. *Clinical and Experimental Allergy* 2005; **35**: 274–281.
47. Morales CA, Schultz KT, DeBoer DJ. Antistaphylococcal antibodies in dogs with recurrent staphylococcal pyoderma. *Veterinary Immunology and Immunopathology* 1994; **42**: 137–147.
48. Hauk PJ, Hamid QA, Chrousos GP, *et al.* Induction of corticosteroid insensitivity in human PBMCs by microbial superantigens. *Journal of Allergy and Clinical Immunology* 2000; **105**: 782–787.
49. Schlievert PM, Case LC, Strandberg KL, *et al.* Superantigen profile of *Staphylococcus aureus* isolates from patients with steroid-resistant atopic dermatitis. *Clinical Infectious Diseases* 2008; **46**: 1562–1567.

50. Bardoel BW, Vos R, Bouman T, *et al.* Evasion of Toll-like receptor 2 activation by staphylococcal superantigen-like protein 3. *Journal of Molecular Medicine (Berlin)* 2012; **90**: 1109–1120.
51. Yokoyama R, Itoh S, Kamoshida G, *et al.* Staphylococcal superantigen-like protein 3 binds to the Toll-like receptor 2 extracellular domain and inhibits cytokine production induced by *Staphylococcus aureus*, cell wall component, or lipopeptides in murine macrophages. *Infection and Immunity* 2012; **80**: 2816–2825.
52. Hendricks A, Schuberth HJ, Schueler K, *et al.* Frequency of superantigen-producing *Staphylococcus intermedius* isolates from canine pyoderma and proliferation-inducing potential of superantigens in dogs. *Research in Veterinary Science* 2002; **73**: 273–277.
53. Yoon JW, Lee GJ, Lee SY, *et al.* Prevalence of genes for enterotoxins, toxic shock syndrome toxin 1 and exfoliative toxin among clinical isolates of *Staphylococcus pseudintermedius* from canine origin. *Veterinary Dermatology* 2010; **21**: 484–489.
54. Terauchi R, Sato H, Hasegawa T, *et al.* Isolation of exfoliative toxin from *Staphylococcus intermedius* and its local toxicity in dogs. *Veterinary Microbiology* 2003; **94**: 19–29.
55. Terauchi R, Sato H, Endo Y, *et al.* Cloning of the gene coding for *Staphylococcus intermedius* exfoliative toxin and its expression in *Escherichia coli*. *Veterinary Microbiology* 2003; **94**: 31–38.
56. Iyori K, Futagawa-Saito K, Hisatsune J, *et al.* *Staphylococcus pseudintermedius* exfoliative toxin EXI selectively digests canine desmoglein 1 and causes subcorneal clefts in canine epidermis. *Veterinary Dermatology* 2011; **22**: 319–326.
57. Iyori K, Hisatsune J, Kawakami T, *et al.* Identification of a novel *Staphylococcus pseudintermedius* exfoliative toxin gene and its prevalence in isolates from canines with pyoderma and healthy dogs. *FEMS Microbiology Letters* 2010; **312**: 169–175.
58. Choi MJ, Maibach HI. Role of ceramides in barrier function of healthy and diseased skin. *American Journal of Clinical Dermatology* 2005; **6**: 215–223.
59. Marsella R, Olivry T, Carlotti D-N. Current evidence of skin barrier dysfunction in human and canine atopic dermatitis. *Veterinary Dermatology* 2011; **22**: 239–248.
60. Shimada K, Yoon J-S, Yoshihara T, *et al.* Increased transepidermal water loss and decreased ceramide content in lesional and non-lesional skin of dogs with atopic dermatitis. *Veterinary Dermatology* 2009; **20**: 541–546.
61. Ohnishi Y, Okino N, Ito M, *et al.* Ceramidase activity in bacterial skin flora as a possible cause of ceramide deficiency in atopic dermatitis. *Clinical and Diagnostic Laboratory Immunology* 1999; **6**: 101–104.
62. Inoue H, Someno T, Kawada M, *et al.* Citric acid inhibits a bacterial ceramidase and alleviates atopic dermatitis in an animal model. *Journal of Antibiotics* 2010: **63**; 611–613.
63. Ziegler SF. Thymic stromal lymphopoietin and allergic disease. *Journal of Allergy and Clinical Immunology* 2012; **130**: 845–852.
64. Le TA, Takai T, Vu AT, *et al.* Flagellin induces the expression of thymic stromal lymphopoietin in human keratinocytes via Toll-like receptor 5. *International Archives of Allergy and Immunology* 2011; **155**: 31–37.
65. Wilson RH, Maruoka S, Whitehead GS, *et al.* 2012. The Toll-like receptor 5 ligand flagellin promotes asthma by priming allergic responses to indoor allergens. *Nature Medicine* 2012; **18**: 1705–1710.
66. Klukowska-Rotzler J, Chervett L, Muller EJ, *et al.* Expression of thymic stromal lymphopoietin in canine atopic dermatitis. *Veterinary Dermatology* 2013; **24**: 54–9.
67. Bannoehr J, Guardabassi L. *Staphylococcus pseudintermedius* in the dog: taxonomy, diagnostics, ecology, epidemiology and pathogenicity. *Veterinary Dermatology* 2012; **23**: 253–266.
68. Ruscher C, Lübke-Becker A, Wleklinski CG, *et al.* Prevalence of methicillin-resistant *Staphylococcus pseudintermedius* isolated from clinical samples of companion animals and equidae. *Veterinary Microbiology* 2009; **136**: 197–201.
69. Bannoehr J, Ben Zakour NL, Reglinski M, *et al.* Genomic and surface proteomic analysis of the canine pathogen *Staphylococcus pseudintermedius* reveals proteins that mediate adherence to the extracellular matrix. *Infection and Immunity* 2011; **79**: 3074–3086.
70. Bannoehr J, Brown JK, Shaw DJ, *et al.* *Staphylococcus pseudintermedius* surface proteins SpsD and SpsO mediate adherence to *ex vivo* canine corneocytes. *Veterinary Dermatology* 2012; **23**: 119–124.
71. Sung JM, Chantler PD, Lloyd DH. Accessory gene regulator locus of *Staphylococcus intermedius*. *Infection and Immunity* 2006; **74**: 2947–2956.
72. Futagawa-Saito K, Ba-Thein W, Sakurai N, *et al.* Prevalence of virulence factors in *Staphylococcus intermedius* isolates from dogs and pigeons. *BMC Veterinary Research* 2006; **2**: 4.
73. Sethi S, Chakraborty T. Role of TLR-/NLR-signaling and the associated cytokines involved in recruitment of neutrophils in murine models of *Staphylococcus aureus* infection. *Virulence* 2011; **2**: 316–328.
74. Feng BS, He SH, Zheng PY, *et al.* Mast cells play a crucial role in *Staphylococcus aureus* peptidoglycan-induced diarrhea. *American Journal of Pathology* 2007; **171**: 537–547.
75. Jawdat DM, Rowden G, Marshall JS. Mast cells have a pivotal role in TNF-independent lymph node hypertrophy and the mobilization of Langerhans cells in response to bacterial peptidoglycan. *Journal of Immunology* 2006; **177**: 1755–1762.
76. Bath-Hextall FJ, Birnie AJ, Ravenscroft JC, *et al.* Interventions to reduce *Staphylococcus aureus* in the management of atopic eczema: an updated Cochrane review. *British Journal of Dermatology* 2010; **163**: 12–26.
77. Löflath A, von Voigts-Rhetz A, Jaeger K, *et al.* The efficacy of a commercial shampoo and whirlpooling in the treatment of canine pruritus—a double-blinded, randomized, placebo-controlled study. *Veterinary Dermatology* 2007; **18**: 427–431.
78. Schilling J, Mueller RS. Double-blinded, placebo-controlled study to evaluate an antipruritic shampoo for dogs with allergic pruritus. *Veterinary Record* 2012; **171**: 97.

8

The role of fungal agents in atopic dermatitis

Ross Bond

Department of Clinical Sciences and Services, Royal Veterinary College, Hatfield, UK

Conflict of interest: none declared.

Introduction

The kingdom Fungi comprises a vast and diverse array of eukaryotic, uni- or multicellular, nutritionally-absorptive organisms that reproduce sexually or asexually, and whose cell walls contain chitin and β-glucans. The number of species in the fungal kingdom is unknown but may exceed 1.5 million [1]. Fungi play vital roles in agriculture, biotechnology, basic biological research, and medicine/veterinary medicine. Fungal pathogens of animals can be divided into **obligate** pathogens, which are able to infect even healthy individuals, and a larger group of **opportunistic** fungi, where host immunity must be compromised for infection to develop. Some species also express allergenic molecules that drive host hypersensitivity responses, which may induce disease without fungal invasion of the host. This chapter presents a comparative review of the role of fungi in the pathogenesis of human and canine atopic dermatitis (AD); similarities and differences, where known, between the two host species are emphasized.

Overview of fungi in human and canine atopic dermatitis

Atopic dermatitis (atopic eczema) is a chronic relapsing, inflammatory skin disease whose prevalence has increased markedly over the last 30 years with reports of 2–10% of adults and 15–30% of children now being affected in industrialized regions [2–4]. The majority of adult patients have the 'extrinsic' form of AD where the immediate skin reactivity to environmental allergens is believed to be involved in induction and maintenance of the disease. A smaller subset of patients have an 'intrinsic' form of AD wherein IgE-mediated allergen reactivity cannot be demonstrated; the analogous disorder in dogs is termed 'atopic-like dermatitis' [5].

The potential roles of fungi in the pathogenesis of human and canine AD are summarized here, schematically represented in Figure 8.1, and discussed in more detail in the following sections. Whilst pollens, house-dust mites, and animal dander account for a high percentage of cases, environmental moulds are commonly implicated as aeroallergens in humans [6] and in dogs, although there are important geographical differences. *Malassezia* spp. yeasts predominate amongst the resident skin mycobiota of both hosts and these yeasts may proliferate and trigger clinically relevant immediate hypersensitivity responses, although dogs are colonized by *M. pachydermatis* whereas humans are not. Cross-reactivity between *Malassezia*-derived antigens and self-antigens may result in a T-cell mediated autoimmunity in a subset of human patients based on molecular mimicry, but this is not described in dogs to the author's knowledge. Skin infections caused by dermatophytes may be more prevalent in humans with AD, but this association also does not appear to have been reported in dogs.

Veterinary Allergy, First Edition. Edited by Chiara Noli, Aiden Foster, and Wayne Rosenkrantz.

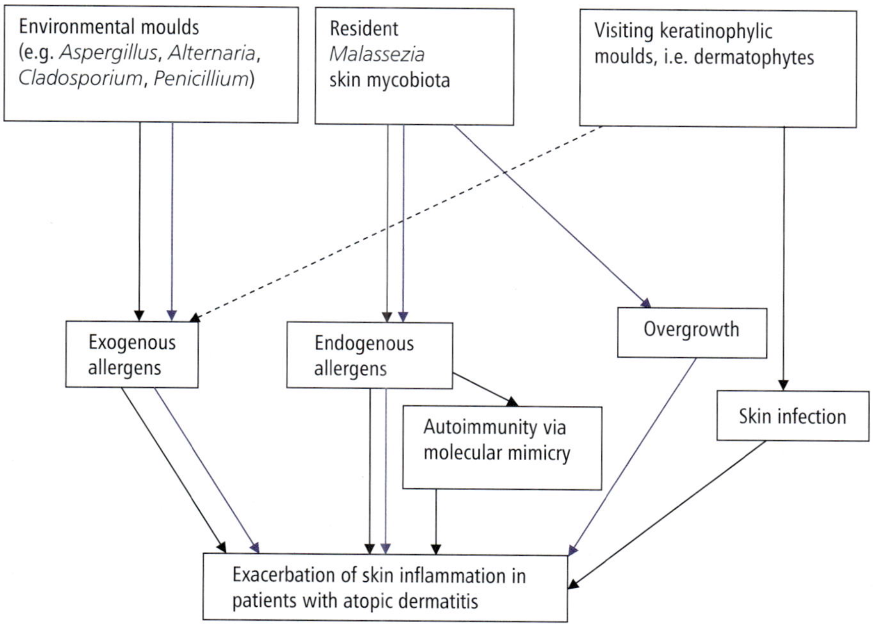

Figure 8.1 The role of fungi in the pathogenesis of human and canine atopic dermatitis is represented in this schematic diagram. The black lines indicate associations reported in human disease whereas the blue lines represent the canine situation. The dotted line reflects conflicting data.

Environmental fungal allergens in human atopic dermatitis

Sensitization to allergens from environmental fungi may be associated with allergic respiratory diseases or AD; fungi of the genera *Aspergillus*, *Cladosporium*, *Alternaria*, and *Penicillium* are commonly implicated [6,7]. In a review of the medical records of 133 atopic patients in Taiwan that were sensitive to at least one of the common fungi, the sensitization rates to *Aspergillus* and *Penicillium* were 69.2% and 63.2%, respectively; titres were highest in patients with AD, suggesting that fungal sensitization was more closely associated with AD than respiratory diseases in those patients [8]. By contrast, sensitization rates to *Alternaria alternata* determined by detection of IgE antibodies by western immunoblotting were comparable amongst 50 patients with AD (32%) and 50 patients with asthma (38%) [9]. Closely comparable sensitization rates to mixed mould allergens on skin testing (10–12%) were observed amongst a group of 1496 Puerto Rican patients with either AD, allergic rhinitis, or asthma [10]. In a US study of 73 patients with moderate to severe AD, 49% had IgE antibodies to *A. alternata* [11]. In a study of 6840 Italian children, only 213 (3.3%) were positive to *Alternaria alternata* on skin-prick or serological testing and only 1.3% had monosensitization to this mould [12]. Most of these patients had either asthma or allergic rhinitis, and only six had asthma associated with AD. Low rates (<2.8%) of fungal sensitization to *Cladosporium herbarum* and *A. alternata* were also observed in a large population of Finnish patients, whereas sensitization rates to animal dander or pollens ranged from 75 to 80% [13]. These data demonstrate the marked variation in sensitization rates observed amongst human patients in different geographical locations.

Work based on high-throughput cloning of fungal allergens revealed that fungi are able to produce extremely complex repertoires of species-specific and cross-reactive allergens [14]. Interestingly, studies of sensitization to *Aspergillus* and *Alternaria* that compared crude and recombinant allergens have shown that patients with AD recognize different recombinant allergens when compared with asthmatics [15,16], indicating that use of recombinant fungal allergens may provide more specific and standardized assessment of sensitization to fungi.

Environmental fungal allergens in canine atopic dermatitis

In a review of the role of environmental allergens in the pathogenesis of canine atopy, Hill and DeBoer concluded that the lack of standardization of extracts and techniques prevented current accurate definition of major or minor allergens for dogs [17]. Batch variations in crude mixtures, varied potency in allergens from different companies, irritant components, and use of different allergen concentrations in the tests were highlighted as likely factors in conflicting observations between studies. Nevertheless, these authors conducted a detailed review of studies completed prior to 1999, and several studies have been published subsequently.

In three studies of intradermal test reactivity in North American dogs [18,19], reactivity to individual mould allergens was usually seen in 33 to 48% of cases, although an earlier study reported reactivity in 79 to 84% of dogs [20]. In more recent studies of intradermal test reactivity to mould allergens in Korea and California, between 60 and 67% of dogs showed positive tests to at least one mould [21], with *Rhizopus* reactivity being reported in almost one-half of the Korean dogs [22]. By contrast, multiple European studies [23–26] have indicated that mould reactivity is much less frequently seen when compared with North American dogs; typically reactivity to moulds is seen in less than 7% of dogs, although 14% of Norwegian dogs were reactive to *Penicillium* [27]. Similarly, intradermal test data from Thailand [28], Japan [29], and a notably large study of 1000 Australian dogs [30] also indicated that mould reactivity can be expected in less than 10% of cases.

A similar relationship between geographical location and serological test results for IgE reactivity to moulds has been reported. For example, very frequent positive test results, commonly involving more than 80% of 35 dogs, were observed in a North American study [31]. By contrast, serological reactivity to moulds was not detected in any of 95 Japanese dogs with canine atopic dermatitis (CAD) [29]. Mould reactivity was seen in less than 5.0% of 265 British dogs [26], and less than 11% of 28 Norwegian dogs [27]. Overall, the more recent studies substantiate the previous conclusions of Hill and DeBoer [17] that mould antigens appear to be of major importance in the USA but of minor importance in Europe. The basis for these discrepancies merits further investigation.

Whilst recombinant flea [32,33], birch pollen [34], and grass pollen [35] allergens have been used in experimental studies, the author is not aware of reports of the use of recombinant fungal allergens in dogs, either experimentally or in the field.

Dermatophytosis in human and canine atopic dermatitis

The majority of humans with dermatophytosis are healthy and have no obvious predisposing factors, although there is a high incidence of AD (over 40% in some surveys) in patients with chronic infections [36,37]. Tinea pedis caused by *T. rubrum* also appears to be more frequent in atopic children and young adults [38], potentially reflecting dry skin, altered skin barrier function, immune dysregulation, or defective skin innate immunity [39,40]. The frequency of immediate reactivity to trichophytin determined by skin-prick test in atopic patients with chronic dermatophytosis significantly exceeded those of healthy patients without dermatophytosis in one study [41] but not in another [42]. Serum IgE antibodies to *T. mentagrophytes* were detected by enzyme-linked immunosorbent assay (ELISA) in 50% of patients with acute infections and 66% of patients with chronic dermatophytosis, whereas antibodies were not detected in atopic patients without dermatophytosis [41]. These hypersensitivity responses to fungal allergens could exacerbate the clinical signs of dermatophytosis in patients with AD.

Whilst dogs with CAD are known to be susceptible to staphylococcal pyoderma and *Malassezia* dermatitis, the author is unaware of any data establishing a relationship between dermatophytosis and CAD in dogs. At the time of writing, electronic literature searches did not yield any relevant publications in this area. Detailed reviews on CAD and dermatophytosis presented in the standard textbook of small animal dermatology mention no such association, other than to acknowledge that the administration of immunosuppressive drugs such as glucocorticoids (commonly used in the treatment of AD) might impair host immunity to dermatophytes [43]. Furthermore, this association is not recognized amongst the canine caseload in the author's institution, which sees large numbers of dogs with CAD, but relatively few dogs with dermatophytosis.

Malassezia yeasts in human atopic dermatitis

The genus *Malassezia* comprises a group of lipophilic and lipid-dependent yeasts that belong to the normal cutaneous mycobiota of a variety of mammals and birds [44]. The first report of an association between human AD and *Malassezia* spp. is attributed to Clemmensen and Hjort who reported in 1983 that patients with the 'head–neck' form of AD and positive skin-prick tests to *Malassezia* extract improved when treated with ketoconazole [45]. Subsequent studies on the role of these yeasts, particularly M. *sympodialis*, have supported the original report, and it is currently considered that *M. sympodialis* or other species may be involved in the perpetuation of an itch/scratch cycle in humans with AD [46]. Evidence to support this view includes the observations that: (1) IgE-mediated reactivity against a variety of *Malassezia* allergens frequently occurs in patients with AD but very rarely in patients with respiratory or contact allergy; (2) atopy patch tests responses show that direct contact with the yeast induces skin inflammation; (3) sensitization occurs to an array of recombinant allergens; (4) AD patients have Th2 cells specific to *Malassezia*; and (5) antifungal treatment results in a clinical improvement [46,47]. Sensitization to *M. sympodialis* has also been demonstrated in a small number of human patients with the so-called 'intrinsic form' of AD; these patients did not have elevated IgE titres to environmental or food allergens, but showed positive skin-prick or patch-test reactivity to *Malassezia* or peripheral blood mononuclear cell proliferative responses to crude or recombinant allergens [47].

The use of crude extracts of fungi such as *Malassezia* is potentially associated with difficulties relating to instability and variability, as previously discussed in relation to environmental moulds. The characterization and expression of *Malassezia*-derived recombinant proteins has led to recognition of sequence homology with human proteins; some of these host proteins have been shown to induce skin-prick test reactions and specific T-cell proliferation in patients sensitized to the corresponding fungal allergens, indicating that autoreactive skin-homing T cells might be relevant for cutaneous inflammation in patients with AD sensitized to *Malassezia* species based on molecular mimicry [48]. Mala s 11, a 22-kDa allergen cloned from *M. sympodialis*, has sequence homology with manganese superoxide dismutase [49]. Superoxide dismutase enzymes exist in eukaryotic cells to neutralize toxic reactive oxygen species generated in mitochondria by the process of oxidative phosphorylation [50]. In pathogenic fungi, superoxide dismutase enzymes may act as a virulence factor by providing resistance against reactive oxygen species generated within phagocytic cells [50]. Evidence has been presented that suggests IgE-mediated sensitization to *Malassezia*-derived manganese superoxide dismutase in humans might lead to cross-reaction and autoimmunity to manganese superoxide dismutase derived from host cells [51].

Similar issues of cross reactivity have been proposed in relation to Mala s 6, a cyclophilin [52] and Mala s 13, a thioredoxin (Trx). Mala s 13 T-cell clones generated from peripheral blood and skin biopsy specimens of positive patch-test reactions in patients with AD sensitized to Mala s 13 and human Trx were fully cross reactive with human Trx [53].

Whilst the allergens of *M. sympodialis* have been investigated in detail, much less is known about the allergens of *M. globosa*. A 40–45-kDa protein from *M. globosa* termed MG 42, shown to be highly reactive to IgE by western immunoblotting using sera from human AD patients, has been cloned and sequenced [54]. The sequence showed similarity to members of the heat shock protein 70 (hsp70) family, although no IgE cross-reactivity between MGp42 and human HSP70 was detected by immunoblot inhibition assays in this case.

It has been reported that *M. sympodialis* releases extracellular nanovesicles from the endosome of the cell containing allergens that induce IL-4 and TNF-α from human peripheral blood mononuclear cells; cytokine production from cells derived from patients with AD exceeded that of healthy controls [55]. These novel observations raise new possibilities in host–pathogen interaction and intercellular communication between *Malassezia* and host cells in the pathogenesis of AD.

Malassezia yeasts in canine atopic dermatitis

Malassezia pachydermatis is the predominant organism amongst the skin mycobiota of dogs [56]; the lipid-dependent *Malassezia* spp. associated with human diseases are only very rarely encountered [57–59]. An association between *Malassezia* dermatitis and CAD was recognized in one of the original case series describing *M. pachydermatis* as a skin pathogen in dogs; Mason and Evans diagnosed concurrent CAD in 2 out of 11 cases [60]. CAD tends to be the most frequently diagnosed concurrent disease in dogs with *Malassezia* dermatitis [61,62].

Studies of *Malassezia* colonization in dogs with CAD have consistently shown that, as a group, atopic dogs have higher skin populations of *M. pachydermatis* than healthy control dogs, particularly in the axilla, groin, interdigital skin, and beneath the tail [63,64]. More recently, Nardoni *et al.* [65] also showed that *M. pachydermatis* could be frequently isolated from the interdigital skin (71%) and ears (63%) in a group of 41 atopic dogs. Interestingly, a genetic subtype (3D) of *M. pachydermatis*, identified by sequencing of the intergenic spacer 1 (IGS-1) region of the ribosomal DNA, was found to be particularly prevalent in Japanese dogs with CAD [66]. Phospholipase activity from subtype 3D *in vitro* was higher when compared with subtypes isolated from healthy dogs [66]; phospholipase activity has recently been identified as a candidate virulence factor in *M. pachydermatis* infection in dogs [67], in parallel with reports of the potential role of lipases in the pathogenesis of *Malassezia*-associated skin diseases in humans [68,69].

The increased colonization of canine atopic skin by *M. pachydermatis* is associated with strong serum IgG responses that are not protective [70–73]. The role of IgE and immediate hypersensitivity is of particular interest in atopic dogs, particularly in view of the dramatic clinical response of some severely affected atopic dogs to antifungal therapy [74], and its role in human AD. Immediate intradermal test reactivity to *M. pachydermatis* allergens has been observed in atopic dogs using concentrations that cause no reaction in healthy dogs [75–77]. Reaginic antibody responses to the yeast have been further demonstrated by ELISA [77,78], western immunoblotting [79], and passive cutaneous anaphylaxis [80]. These observations are analogous to the suggestion that IgE-mediated hypersensitivity to *Malassezia*-derived allergens may be important in the pathogenesis of AD in humans [46,81]. Some dermatologists now include *Malassezia* allergens in allergen-specific immunotherapy courses for atopic dogs because induction of tolerance could be of clinical benefit, but the therapeutic benefit of this approach requires further assessment as most immunotherapy courses comprise multiple allergens and not just yeast allergens alone [74,82]. Because *Malassezia* dermatitis can exist in the absence of immediate hypersensitivity to the yeast [83,84], immunotherapy alone is unlikely to replace the need for antifungal therapy in dogs with high yeast counts in lesional skin. By contrast, immediate hypersensitivity to the yeast is infrequent amongst basset hounds with *Malassezia* dermatitis, in parallel with the low prevalence of CAD in this breed, whereas delayed responses on intradermal or patch testing are more common in this breed, which is predisposed to *Malassezia* colonization and infection [83,84].

Conclusion

A variety of yeasts and moulds is able to initiate or exacerbate skin inflammation in both humans and dogs with AD via diverse mechanisms. Molecular studies, particularly in human medicine, have highlighted the complexities of the interactions between fungi and their metabolites and the skin immune systems of the different hosts. A greater understanding of these processes is likely to lead to novel methods for preventing and controlling fungal exacerbation of these debilitating diseases.

References

1. Berbee ML, Taylor JW. Fungal phylogeny. In: Oliver RP, Schweizer M, eds. *Molecular Fungal Biology*. Cambridge: Cambridge University Press, 1999: 21–77.
2. Williams HC. Is the prevalence of atopic dermatitis increasing? *Clinical and Experimental Dermatology* 1992; **17**: 385–391.
3. Schmitz R, Atzpodien K, Schlaud M. Prevalence and risk factors of atopic diseases in German children and adolescents. *Pediatric Allergy and Immunology* 2012; **23**: 716–723.
4. Hong S, Son DK, Lim WR, *et al*. The prevalence of atopic dermatitis, asthma, and allergic rhinitis and the comorbidity of allergic diseases in children. *Environmental Health and Toxicology* 2012; **27**: e2012006.
5. Halliwell R. Revised nomenclature for veterinary allergy. *Veterinary Immunology and Immunopathology* 2006; **114**: 207–208.
6. Nolles G, Hoekstra MO, Schouten JP, *et al*. Prevalence of immunoglobulin E for fungi in atopic children. *Clinical and Experimental Allergy* 2001; **31**: 1564–1570.
7. Prester L. Indoor exposure to mould allergens. *Arhiv Za Higijenu Rada i Toksikologiju* 2011; **62**: 371–380.
8. Chang FY, Lee JH, Yang YH, *et al*. Analysis of the serum levels of fungi-specific immunoglobulin E in patients with allergic diseases. *International Archives of Allergy and Immunology* 2011; **154**: 49–56.
9. Hedayati MT, Arabzadehmoghadam A, Hajheydari Z. Specific IgE against *Alternaria alternata* in atopic dermatitis and asthma patients. *European Review for Medical and Pharmacological Sciences* 2009; **13**: 187–191.
10. Montealegre F, Meyer B, Chardon D, *et al*. Comparative prevalence of sensitization to common animal, plant and mould allergens in subjects with asthma, or atopic dermatitis and/or allergic rhinitis living in a tropical environment. *Clinical and Experimental Allergy* 2004; **34**: 51–58.
11. Scalabrin DM, Bavbek S, Perzanowski MS, *et al*. Use of specific IgE in assessing the relevance of fungal and dust mite allergens to atopic dermatitis: a comparison with asthmatic and nonasthmatic control subjects. *Journal of Allergy and Clinical Immunology* 1999; **104**: 1273–1279.
12. Cantani A, Ciaschi V. Epidemiology of *Alternaria alternata* allergy: a prospective study in 6840 Italian asthmatic children. *European Review for Medical and Pharmacological Sciences* 2004; **8**: 289–294.
13. Reijula K, Leino M, Mussalo-Rauhamaa H, *et al*. IgE-mediated allergy to fungal allergens in Finland with special reference to *Alternaria alternata* and *Cladosporium herbarum*. *Annals of Allergy, Asthma, and Immunology* 2003; **91**: 280–287.
14. Crameri R, Weichel M, Fluckiger S, *et al*. Fungal allergies: a yet unsolved problem. *Chemical Immunology and Allergy* 2006; **91**: 121–133.
15. Vailes LD, Perzanowski MS, Wheatley LM, *et al*. IgE and IgG antibody responses to recombinant Alt a 1 as a marker of sensitization to *Alternaria* in asthma and atopic dermatitis. *Clinical and Experimental Allergy* 2001; **31**: 1891–1895.
16. Disch R, Menz G, Blaser K, *et al*. Different reactivity to recombinant *Aspergillus fumigatus* allergen I/a in patients with atopic dermatitis or allergic asthma sensitised to *Aspergillus fumigatus*. *International Archives of Allergy and Immunology* 1995; **108**: 89–94.
17. Hill PB, DeBoer DJ. The ACVD task force on canine atopic dermatitis (IV): environmental allergens. *Veterinary Immunology and Immunopathology* 2001; **81**: 169–186.
18. Scott DW. Observations on canine atopy. *Journal of the American Animal Hospital Association* 1981; **17**: 91–100.
19. Nesbitt GH, Kedan GS, Cacciolo P. Canine atopy. 1. Etiology and diagnosis. *Compendium of Continuing Education for the Practising Veterinarian* 1984; **6**: 73–84.
20. Nesbitt GH. Canine allergic inhalant dermatitis. *Journal of the American Veterinary Medical Association* 1978; **172**: 55–60.
21. Zur G, Ihrke PJ, White SD, *et al*. Canine atopic dermatitis: a retrospective study of 266 cases examined at the University of California, Davis, 1992–1998. Part I. Clinical features and allergy testing results. *Veterinary Dermatology* 2002; **13**: 89–102.
22. Kim HJ, Kang MH, Park HM. Common allergens of atopic dermatitis in dogs: comparative findings based on intradermal tests. *Journal of Veterinary Science* 2011; **12**: 287–290.
23. Vollset I. Atopic dermatitis in Norwegian dogs. *Nordisk Veterinaermedicin* 1985; **35**: 97–106.
24. Bond R, Thorogood SC, Lloyd DH. Evaluation of two enzyme-linked immunosorbent assays for the diagnosis of canine atopy. *Veterinary Record* 1994; **135**: 130–133.

25. Sture GH, Halliwell RE, Thoday KL, *et al.* Canine atopic disease: the prevalence of positive intradermal skin tests at two sites in the north and south of Great Britain. *Veterinary Immunology and Immunopathology* 1995; **44**: 293–308.
26. Foster AP, Littlewood JD, Webb P, *et al.* Comparison of intradermal and serum testing for allergen-specific IgE using a Fcepsilon RIalpha-based assay in atopic dogs in the UK. *Veterinary Immunology and Immunopathology* 2003; **93**: 51–60.
27. Saevik BK, Ulstein TL, Larsen HJ. Evaluation of a commercially available enzyme-linked immunosorbent assay for the detection of allergen-specific IgE antibodies in dogs. *Research in Veterinary Science* 2003; **74**: 37–45.
28. Chanthick C, Anaman S, Buathet K. The prevalence of positive intradermal allergy tests in 114 dogs with atopic dermatitis in the Bangkok metropolis, Thailand. *Veterinary Immunology and Immunopathology* 2008; **126**: 256–262.
29. Park S, Ohya F, Yamashita K, *et al.* Comparison of response to immunotherapy by intradermal skin test and antigen-specific IgE in canine atopy. *Journal of Veterinary Medical Science* 2000; **62**: 983–988.
30. Mueller RS, Bettenay SV, Tideman L. Aero-allergens in canine atopic dermatitis in southeastern Australia based on 1000 intradermal skin tests. *Australian Veterinary Journal* 2000; **78**: 392–399.
31. Kleinbeck ML, Hites MJ, Loker JL, *et al.* Enzyme-linked immunosorbent assay for measurement of allergen-specific IgE antibodies in canine serum. *American Journal of Veterinary Research* 1989; **50**: 1831–1839.
32. McDermott MJ, Weber E, Hunter S, *et al.* Identification, cloning, and characterization of a major cat flea salivary allergen (Cte f 1). *Molecular Immunology* 2000; **37**: 361–375.
33. Jin J, Ding Z, Meng F, *et al.* An immunotherapeutic treatment against flea allergy dermatitis in cats by co-immunization of DNA and protein vaccines. *Vaccine* 2010; **28**: 1997–2004.
34. Egli KS, Schiessl B, Roosje PJ, *et al.* Evaluation of the usefulness of sensitization to aeroallergens as a model for canine atopic dermatitis in genetically predisposed Beagles. *American Journal of Veterinary Research* 2002; **63**: 1329–1336.
35. Schiessl B, Zemann B, Hodgin-Pickart LA, *et al.* Importance of early allergen contact for the development of a sustained immunoglobulin E response in a dog model. *International Archives of Allergy and Immunology* 2003; **130**: 125–134.
36. Jones HE, Reinhardt JH, Rinaldi MG. A clinical, mycological, and immunological survey for dermatophytosis. *Archives of Dermatology* 1973; **108**: 61–65.
37. Al Hasan M, Fitzgerald SM, Saoudian M, *et al.* Dermatology for the practicing allergist: Tinea pedis and its complications. *Clinical and Molecular Allergy* 2004; **2**: 5.
38. Svejgaard E, Faergeman J, Jemec G, *et al.* Recent investigations on the relationship between fungal skin diseases and atopic dermatitis. *Acta Dermato-Venereologica. Supplementum* 1989; **144**: 140–142.
39. Schittek B. The antimicrobial skin barrier in patients with atopic dermatitis. *Current Problems in Dermatology* 2011; **41**: 54–67.
40. Mrabet-Dahbi S, Maurer M. Innate immunity in atopic dermatitis. *Current Problems in Dermatology* 2011; **41**: 104–111.
41. Khosravi AR, Shokri H, Mansouri P. Immediate hypersensitivity and serum IgE antibody responses in patients with dermatophytosis. *Asian Pacific Journal of Allergy and Immunology* 2012; **30**: 40–47.
42. Escalante MT, Sanchez-Borges M, Capriles-Hulett A, *et al.* *Trichophyton*-specific IgE in patients with dermatophytosis is not associated with aeroallergen sensitivity. *Journal of Allergy and Clinical Immunology* 2000; **105**: 547–551.
43. Scott DW, Miller WH, Griffin CE. *Muller and Kirk's Small Animal Dermatology*, 6th edn. Philadelphia: W.B. Saunders, 2001: 339–361, 574–601.
44. Midgley G. The diversity of *Pityrosporum* (*Malassezia*) yeasts *in vivo* and *in vitro*. *Mycopathologia* 1989; **106**: 143–153.
45. Clemmensen OJ, Hjort N. Treatment of dermatitis of the head and neck with ketoconazole in patients with type 1 hypersensitivity to *Pityrosporum orbiculare*. *Seminars in Dermatology* 1983; **2**: 26–29.
46. Ashbee HR. Recent developments in the immunology and biology of *Malassezia* species. *FEMS Immunology and Medical Microbiology* 2006; **47**: 14–23.
47. Fischer Casagrande B, Fluckiger S, Linder MT, *et al.* Sensitization to the yeast *Malassezia sympodialis* is specific for extrinsic and intrinsic atopic eczema. *Journal of Investigative Dermatology* 2006; **126**: 2414–2421.
48. Zeller S, Glaser AG, Vilhelmsson M, *et al.* Immunoglobulin-E-mediated reactivity to self antigens: a controversial issue. *International Archives of Allergy and Immunology* 2008; **145**: 87–93.
49. Andersson A, Rasool O, Schmidt M, *et al.* Cloning, expression and characterization of two new IgE-binding proteins from the yeast *Malassezia sympodialis* with sequence similarities to heat shock proteins and manganese superoxide dismutase. *European Journal of Biochemistry* 2004; **271**: 1885–1894.
50. Frealle E, Noel C, Viscogliosi E, *et al.* Manganese superoxide dismutase in pathogenic fungi: an issue with pathophysiological and phylogenetic involvements. *FEMS Immunology and Medical Microbiology* 2005; **45**: 411–422.
51. Schmid-Grendelmeier P, Fluckiger S, Disch R, *et al.* IgE-mediated and T cell-mediated autoimmunity against manganese superoxide dismutase in atopic dermatitis. *Journal of Allergy and Clinical Immunology* 2005; **115**: 1068–1075.
52. Glaser AG, Limacher A, Fluckiger S, *et al.* Analysis of the cross-reactivity and of the 1.5 A crystal structure of the *Malassezia sympodialis* Mala s 6 allergen, a member of the cyclophilin pan-allergen family. *Biochemical Journal* 2006; **396**: 41–49.
53. Balaji H, Heratizadeh A, Wichmann K, *et al. Malassezia sympodialis* thioredoxin-specific T cells are highly cross-reactive to human thioredoxin in atopic dermatitis. *Journal of Allergy and Clinical Immunology* 2011; **128**: 92–99.
54. Ishibashi Y, Kato H, Asahi Y, *et al.* Identification of the major allergen of *Malassezia globosa* relevant for atopic dermatitis. *Journal of Dermatological Science* 2009; **55**: 185–192.
55. Gehrmann U, Qazi KR, Johansson C, *et al.* Nanovesicles from *Malassezia sympodialis* and host exosomes induce cytokine responses—novel mechanisms for host-microbe interactions in atopic eczema. *PLoS One* 2011; **6**: e21480.
56. Guillot J, Bond R. *Malassezia pachydermatis*: a review. *Medical Mycology* 1999; **37**: 295–306.
57. Yurayart C, Chindamporn A, Suradhat S, *et al.* Comparative analysis of the frequency, distribution and population sizes of yeasts associated with canine seborrheic dermatitis and healthy skin. *Veterinary Microbiology* 2011; **148**: 356–362.
58. Machado ML, Ferreiro L, Ferreira RR, *et al. Malassezia* dermatitis in dogs in Brazil: diagnosis, evaluation of clinical signs and molecular identification. *Veterinary Dermatology* 2011; **22**: 46–52.
59. Cafarchia C, Latrofa MS, Figueredo LA, *et al.* Physiological and molecular characterization of atypical lipid-dependent *Malassezia* yeasts from a dog with skin lesions: adaptation to a new host? *Medical Mycology* 2011; **49**: 365–374.
60. Mason KV, Evans AG. Dermatitis associated with *Malassezia pachydermatis* in 11 dogs. *Journal of the American Animal Hospital Association* 1991; **27**: 13–20.

61. Guaguère E, Prélaud P. A retrospective study of 54 dogs with *Malassezia pachydermatis* dermatitis: epidemiological, clinical, cytological, and histopathological results. *Practique Médicale et Chirurgicale de l'Animal de Compagnie* 1996; **31**: 309–323.
62. Bond R, Ferguson EA, Curtis CF, *et al.* Factors associated with elevated cutaneous *Malassezia pachydermatis* populations in dogs with pruritic skin disease. *Journal of Small Animal Practice* 1996; **37**: 103–107.
63. Bond R, Collin NS, Lloyd DH. Use of contact plates for the quantitative culture of *Malassezia pachydermatis* from canine skin. *Journal of Small Animal Practice* 1994; **35**: 68–72.
64. White SD, Bourdeau P, Blumstein P, *et al.*, Comparison via cytology and culture of carriage of *Malassezia pachydermatis* in atopic and healthy dogs. In: Kwochka KW, Willemse T, von Tscharner C, eds. *Advances in Veterinary Dermatology, Volume 3.* Oxford: Butterworth Heinemann, 1998: 291–298.
65. Nardoni S, Dini M, Taccini F, *et al.* Occurrence, distribution and population size of *Malassezia pachydermatis* on skin and mucosae of atopic dogs. *Veterinary Microbiology* 2007; **122**: 172–177.
66. Kobayashi T, Kano R, Nagata M, *et al.* Genotyping of *Malassezia pachydermatis* isolates from canine healthy skin and atopic dermatitis by internal spacer 1 (IGS1) region analysis. *Veterinary Dermatology* 2011; **22**: 401–405.
67. Cafarchia C, Dell'Aquila ME, Traversa D, *et al.* Expression of the micro-opioid receptor on *Malassezia pachydermatis* and its effect in modulating phospholipase production. *Medical Mycology* 2010; **48**: 73–78.
68. Vlachos C, Gaitanis G, Alexopoulos EC, *et al.* Phospholipase activity after beta-endorphin exposure discriminates *Malassezia* strains isolated from healthy and seborrhoeic dermatitis skin. *Journal of the European Academy of Dermatology and Venereology* 2012, in press.
69. Patino-Uzcategui A, Amado Y, Cepero de Garcia M, *et al.* Virulence gene expression in *Malassezia* spp from individuals with seborrheic dermatitis. *Journal of Investigative Dermatology* 2011; **131**: 2134–2136.
70. Chen TA, Halliwell REW, Hill PB. IgG responses to *Malassezia pachydermatis* antigens in atopic and normal dogs. *Veterinary Dermatology* 2000; **11** (Suppl 1): 13.
71. Chen TA, Halliwell REW, Hill PB. Immunoglobulin G responses to *Malassezia pachydermatis* antigens in atopic and normal dogs, In: Thoday KL, Foil CS, Bond R, eds. *Advances in Veterinary Dermatology, Volume 4.* Oxford: Blackwell Science, 2002: 202–209.
72. Chen TA, Hill PB. The biology of *Malassezia* organisms and their ability to induce immune responses and skin disease. *Veterinary Dermatology* 2005; **16**: 4–26.
73. Kim HJ, Kim ET, Lim CY, *et al.* The immunoglobulin G response to *Malassezia pachydermatis* extracts in atopic and non-atopic dogs. *Canadian Veterinary Journal* 2010; **51**: 869–872.
74. Nett CS, Reichler I, Grest P, *et al.* Epidermal dysplasia and *Malassezia* infection in two West Highland White Terrier siblings: an inherited skin disorder or reaction to severe Malassezia infection? *Veterinary Dermatology* 2001; **12**: 285–290.
75. Bond R, Curtis CF, Hendricks A, *et al.* Intradermal test reactivity to *Malassezia pachydermatis* in atopic dogs. *Veterinary Record* 2002; **150**: 448–449.
76. Morris DO, Olivier NB, Rosser EJ. Type-1 hypersensitivity reactions to *Malassezia pachydermatis* extracts in atopic dogs. *American Journal of Veterinary Research* 1998; **59**: 836–841.
77. Farver K, Morris DO, Shofer F, *et al.* Humoral measurement of type-1 hypersensitivity reactions to a commercial *Malassezia* allergen. *Veterinary Dermatology* 2005; **16**: 261–268.
78. Nuttall T, Halliwell REW. Serum antibodies to *Malassezia pachydermatis* extracts in atopic dermatitis. *Veterinary Dermatology* 2001; **12**: 327–332.
79. Chen TA, Halliwell RE, Pemberton AD, *et al.* Identification of major allergens of *Malassezia pachydermatis* in dogs with atopic dermatitis and *Malassezia* overgrowth. *Veterinary Dermatology* 2002; **13**: 141–150.
80. Morris DO, DeBoer DJ. Evaluation of serum obtained from atopic dogs with dermatitis attributable to *Malassezia pachydermatis* for passive transfer of immediate hypersensitivity to that organism. *American Journal of Veterinary Research* 2003; **64**: 262–266.
81. Kieffer M, Bergbrant IM, Faergemann J, *et al.* Immune reactions to *Pityrosporum ovale* in adult patients with atopic and seborrheic dermatitis. *Journal of the American Academy of Dermatology* 1990; **22**: 739–742.
82. Robson DC. Update on Malassezia—allergy, immunotherapy, therapy and resistance. In: *Proceedings of the Continuing Education Programme, 7th World Congress of Veterinary Dermatology*, 2012, Vancouver: World Congress of Veterinary Dermatology and the World Association for Veterinary Dermatology, 2012: 249–256.
83. Bond R, Patterson-Kane JC, Lloyd DH. Intradermal test reactivity to *Malassezia pachydermatis* in healthy basset hounds and bassets with *Malassezia* dermatitis. *Veterinary Record* 2002; **151**: 105–109.
84. Bond R, Perrins N, Patterson-Kane JC, *et al.* Patch test responses to *Malassezia pachydermatis* in healthy basset hounds and in basset hounds with *Malassezia* dermatitis. *Medical Mycology* 2006; **44**: 419–427.

9

Clinical signs of canine atopic dermatitis

Claude Favrot

Vetsuisse Faculty, University of Zurich, Zurich, Switzerland

Conflict of interest: none declared.

In veterinary dermatology, cutaneous adverse food reaction (CAFR) and canine atopic dermatitis (CAD) have been historically considered as two different conditions [1]. In fact, CAFR includes both immune-mediated and non-immune-mediated food intolerances and may be associated with a wide range of clinical signs such as gastrointestinal disturbances, urticaria, angioedema, and signs mimicking those of atopic dermatitis (see Chapter 16). This latter point led the International Task Force on Canine Atopic Dermatitis to suggest that some cases of CAFR may trigger flares of atopic dermatitis [2]. The clinical signs of CAD may thus be associated with sensitization to environmental (CAD *sensu stricto*) or food allergens (CAFR with clinical signs of CAD: food-induced atopic dermatitis: FIAD), or with atopic-like dermatitis (ALD). The present chapter will describe the clinical features of dogs affected by CAD from whatever cause. The clinical signs of food allergy without signs of CAD are described in Chapters 17 and 18.

Signalment of CAD dogs

The definition of CAD suggests a strong breed and/or familial predisposition. Reliable evaluation of breed predispositions for veterinary diseases is complicated by the fact that the population at risk is often unknown. Several studies have, however, addressed the question of breed predisposition for CAD [3]. Some studies only mentioned the most frequently represented breeds, while some others have been based on a comparison between atopic dogs and the hospital or insurance population [4–12]. The former do not present any statistical analysis and the latter may be biased by the absence or the under-representation of healthy dogs. One study was based on a large population of insured dogs but contained another potential bias—the authors did not make the diagnosis of CAD themselves but referred to the diagnosis of general practitioners, who may have used variable inclusion criteria [5]. To further complicate the analysis, predisposed breeds may vary by geographical areas [13,14]. Another study was based on the comparison of a population of atopic dogs and a validated population of healthy dogs [15]. This study was however limited to Switzerland. Some breeds, such as the West Highland white terrier (WHWT), boxers, and bulldogs, are, however, mentioned in virtually all these studies. Some others, such as German shepherd dogs (GSH), golden retrievers, and Labrador retrievers, seem to be predisposed for CAD only in some geographical regions.

Reports of sex predisposition in CAD are inconsistent. Studies have reported predisposition for male, female, or for neither sex [13]. In a study of a large population of 843 CAD dogs there was no sex predilection detected, when the whole population was taken into account [16]. However, some sex predisposition was detected in some breeds, such as golden or Labrador retrievers (more female) or boxer (more male).

The typical age at onset of CAD is reported to be between 6 months and 3 years [13]. We have shown that about 78% of dogs with CAD present with clinical signs

Veterinary Allergy, First Edition. Edited by Chiara Noli, Aiden Foster, and Wayne Rosenkrantz.

Table 9.1 Frequency of clinical features of CAD in dogs

Criterion	Frequency
Age at onset less than 2 years	0.52
Age at onset less than 3 years	0.68
Mostly indoor	0.84
Seasonality	0.24
Corticosteroid-responsive pruritus	0.78
Pruritus "with no skin changes"	0.61
Chronic or recurrent bacterial infections	0.66
Chronic or recurrent yeast infections	0.33
Chronic or recurrent otitis externa	0.5
Otitis externa, first episode before other signs	0.43
Affected front feet	0.79
Affected hind feet	0.75
Affected axillae	0.62
Affected abdomen/inguinal areas	0.66
Affected ear pinnae	0.58
Affected lips	0.42
Affected eyelids	0.32
Affected face (other sites)	0.31
Affected genitalia/ventral tail	0.43
Affected chest	0.32

before 3 years of age [16]. This means that every fifth atopic dog develops the first clinical signs later in life.

History of canine atopic dermatitis dogs

Clinical signs of CAD may be seasonal or not; seasonality is often present at onset (42–75%) [13]. Approximately 80% of dogs with seasonal signs are symptomatic in spring or summer while the others exhibit signs in winter or autumn [17]. It should be mentioned that some dogs with non-seasonal disease can exhibit worsening of clinical signs during one specific season (Table 9.1).

Pruritus must be present and its absence rules out a diagnosis of CAD. In fact, some CAD dogs do initially exhibit 'pruritus with no skin changes'. This feature was recorded in 61% of affected dogs in our study [16]. In 43% of atopic dogs the initial presentation was with an episode of otitis externa. CAD dogs are often treated with glucocorticoids and responses to such therapy should be evaluated carefully. In the same study, we found that 78% of CAD dogs responded adequately to such treatment. In the first stages of the disease, pruritus responds well and readily to the administration of glucocorticoids (i.e. 0.3–0.5 mg/kg prednisolone daily).

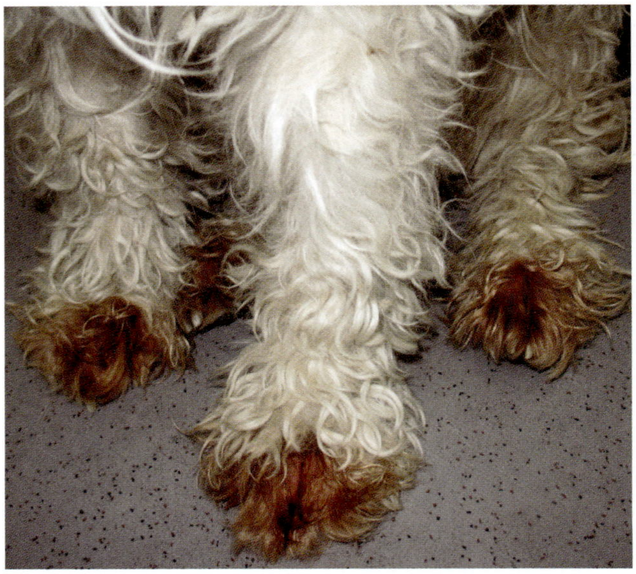

Figure 9.1 Saliva-coloured hairs is one of the first sign of chronic pruritus in dogs.

In chronic cases, however, the development of secondary bacterial or yeast infections is usually associated with a poorer response to such treatment.

We also found that 82% of atopic dogs spend most of their time indoors. This suggests that prolonged exposure to house dust mites may trigger or worsen CAD clinical signs.

Clinical signs of canine atopic dermatitis

Although common, CAD may be difficult to diagnose owing to the lack of pathognomonic signs and the protean clinical signs. Erythema and pruritus are virtually always present and often represent the first clinical signs. However, mild pruritus may remain unrecognized by the owner and the veterinarian may sometimes rely on indirect evidence of pruritus, such as excoriations and broken or saliva-coloured hairs (Figure 9.1).

Most of the signs are actually due to self-trauma and/or secondary infections. Small erythematous papules (Figure 9.2), which are considered the primary lesion of CAD, are rarely observed in atopic dogs [13]. The practitioner will usually observe the consequences of the inflammation and pruritus, namely excoriations and self-induced alopecia (Figure 9.3) and/or the signs of the secondary infections. These infections are caused by bacteria, resulting in papules, pustules, crusts, erosions, and epidermal collarettes (Figure 9.4), and/or by yeasts, which are mostly associated with epidermal hyperplasia, hyperpigmentation, and lichenification (Figure 9.5). Recurrent or chronic skin or ear infections (Figure 9.6)

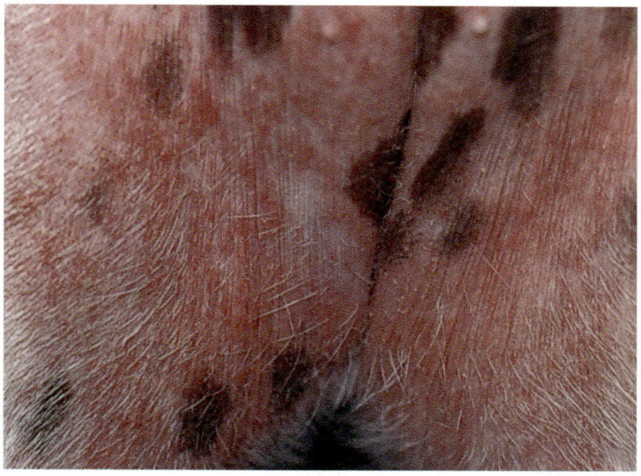

Figure 9.2 Some dogs with atopic dermatitis present with acute papulosis affecting mostly the abdomen.

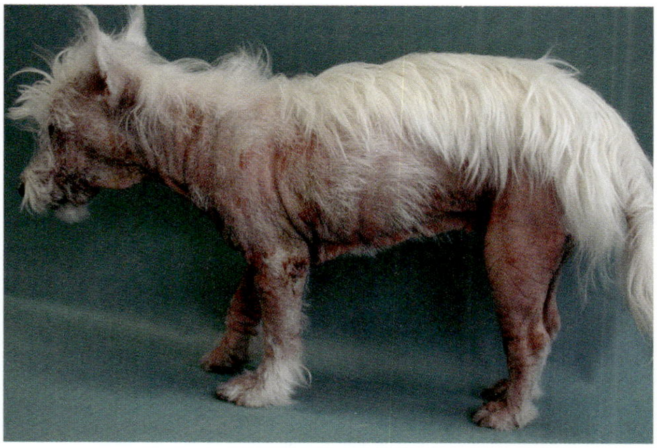

Figure 9.3 Self-induced alopecia, skin hyperplasia, and excoriations are the main signs of intense pruritus in chronic atopic dermatitis.

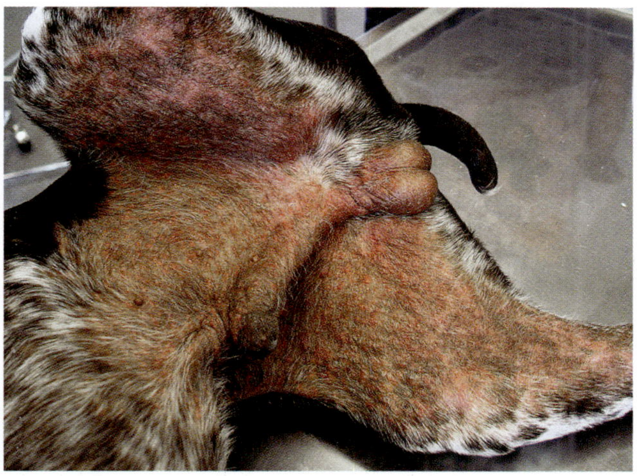

Figure 9.4 Pyoderma is a frequent cause of secondary infection in CAD dogs and often affects the abdomen, presenting with numerous pustules and papules.

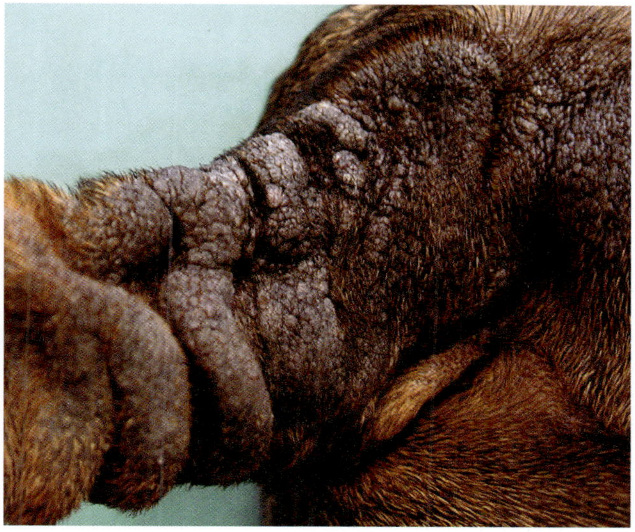

Figure 9.5 Malassezia dermatitis is often associated with lichenification, skin hyperplasia. and hyperpigmentation. Lesions from the hindlimb of a shar pei dog.

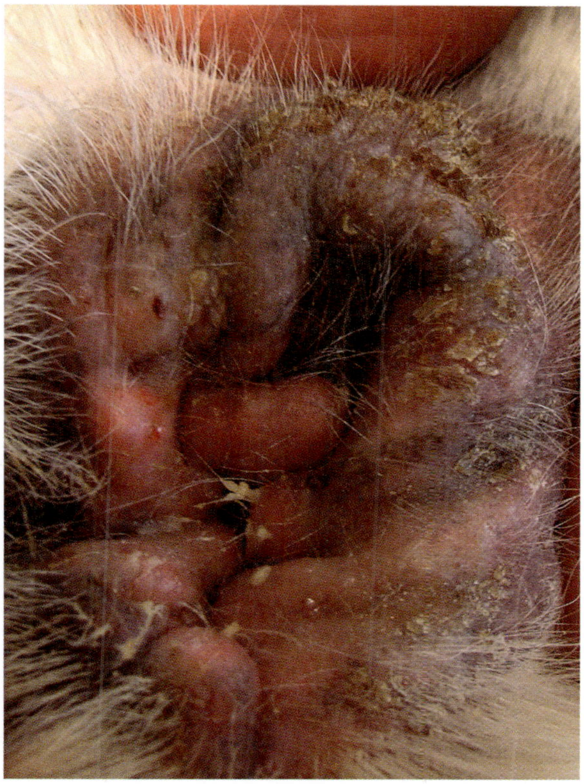

Figure 9.6 Otitis externa and lesions of the pinna are frequently observed in dogs with CAD.

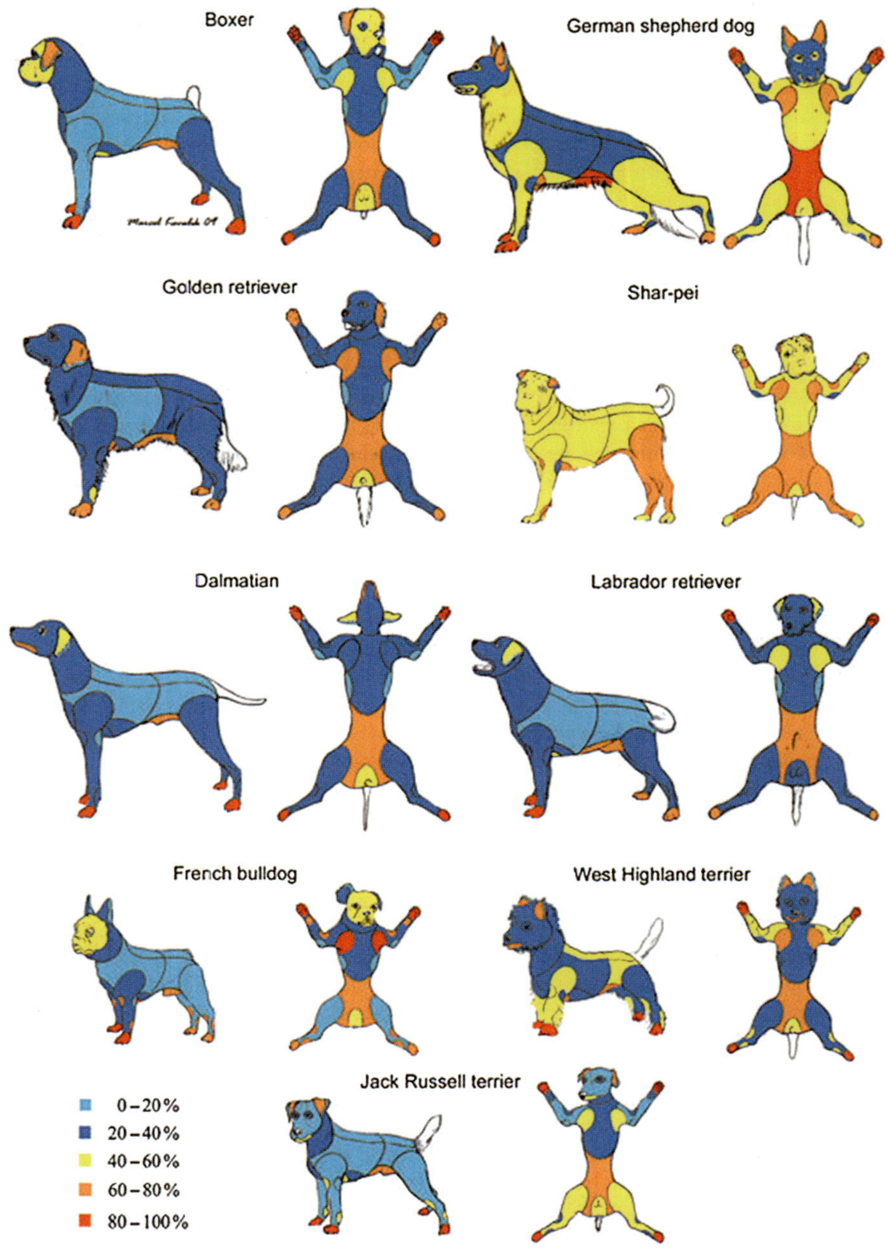

Figure 9.7 Silhouettes of atopic boxers, German shepherds, golden retrievers, shar peis, Dalmatians, Labrador retrievers, French bulldogs, West Highland white terriers, and Jack Russell terriers (in this order). Each colour corresponds to the percentage of affected animals. (Reprinted from [18]. © 2010, with the permission of John Wiley & Sons, Inc.)

are very frequently observed in CAD; in our study bacterial infections were observed in 66% of the cases while *Malassezia* dermatitis and otitis externa were present in 33% and 50% of all affected dogs, respectively [16].

Most of these signs are not specific and the distribution of these lesions is consequently more helpful (see Table 9.1). The most often affected areas are the pinnae (58%), the axillae (62%), the abdomen (66%), the front (79%) and hind feet (75%), the lips (42%), and the perineal area (43%). Unfortunately, all these areas are rarely simultaneously affected in the same individual, except in chronic cases (Figure 9.3).

Other dermatological (pyotraumatic dermatitis, interdigital fistulae) and non-dermatological signs are sometimes associated with CAD and their presence should reinforce the suspicion; spring/summer conjunctivitis, for example, is presented in approximately 20% of dogs.

Breed-associated phenotypes

Breed-associated phenotypic variability of CAD has been addressed in detail [18] (Figure 9.7). This study demonstrated that French bulldogs and shar peis are affected earlier than other breeds (i.e. 53.3% of French bulldogs and 66.7% of shar peis were affected during the first year of life, in comparison with 28.5% in the whole population). Some breeds, such as the GSH, Dalmatian, or shar pei, frequently present with pruritus without lesions while some other breeds frequently develop secondary infections, for example boxers (otitis), WHWT (*Malassezia* dermatitis), or seborrhoeic changes (WHWT, GSH). The GSH and WHWT are more often affected with widespread lesions of CAD compared with some other breeds that present with a rather localized phenotype. Some breeds may commonly present with signs in areas that are less frequently or rarely affected in others, for example in WHWT and shar peis lesions may occur on the dorsal aspect of the body and in GSH on elbows and hindlimbs.

References

1. Hillier A, Griffin CE. The ACVD task force on canine atopic dermatitis (X): is there a relationship between canine atopic dermatitis and cutaneous adverse food reactions? *Veterinary Immunology Immunopathology* 2001; **81**: 219–226.
2. Olivry T, Deboer DJ, Prélaud P, *et al.* Food for thought: pondering the relationship between canine atopic dermatitis and cutaneous adverse food reactions. *Veterinary Dermatology* 2007; **18**: 390–391.
3. Sousa CA, Marsella R. The ACVD task force on canine atopic dermatitis (II): genetic factors. *Veterinary Immunology Immunopathology* 2001; **81**: 153–158.
4. Koch HJ, Peters S. 207 intrakutantests bei hunden mit verdacht auf atopische dermatitis. *Kleintierpraxis* 1994; **39**: 25–36.
5. Nodtvedt A, Bergvall K, Emanuelson U, *et al.* Canine atopic dermatitis: validation of recorded diagnosis against practice records in 335 insured Swedish dogs. *Acta Veterinaria Scandinavia* 2006; **48**: 8.
6. Nodtvedt A, Egenvall A, Bergvall K, *et al.* Incidence of and risk factors for atopic dermatitis in a Swedish population of insured dogs. *Veterinary Record* 2006; **159**: 241–246.
7. Saridomichelakis MN, Koutinas AF, Gioulekas D, *et al.* Canine atopic dermatitis in Greece: clinical observations and the prevalence of positive intradermal test reactions in 91 spontaneous cases. *Veterinary Immunology Immunopathology* 1999; **69**: 61–73.
8. Sture GH, Halliwell RE, Thoday KL, *et al.* Canine atopic disease: the prevalence of positive intradermal skin tests at two sites in the north and south of Great Britain. *Veterinary Immunology Immunopathology* 1995; **44**: 293–308.
9. Tarpataki N, Papa K, Reiczigel J, *et al.* Prevalence and features of canine atopic dermatitis in Hungary. *Acta Veterinaria Hungaria* 2006; **54**: 353–366.
10. Willemse A, van den Brom WE. Investigations of the symptomatology and the significance of immediate skin test reactivity in canine atopic dermatitis. *Research in Veterinary Sciences* 1983; **34**: 261–265.
11. Willemse TA. Atopic dermatitis: a review and reconsideration of diagnostic criteria. *Journal of Small Animal Practice* 1986; **27**: 771–778.
12. Carlotti D, Costargent F. Analysis of positive skin tests in 449 dogs with allergic dermatitis. *European Journal of Companion Animal Practice* 1994; **4**: 42–59.
13. Griffin CE, Deboer DJ. The ACVD task force on canine atopic dermatitis (XIV): clinical manifestations of canine atopic dermatitis. *Veterinary Immunology Immunopathology* 2001; **81**: 255–269.
14. Nodtvedt A, Guitian J, Egenvall A, *et al.* The spatial distribution of atopic dermatitis cases in a population of insured Swedish dogs. *Preventive Veterinary Medicine* 2007; **78**: 210–222.
15. Picco F, Zini E, Nett C, *et al.* A prospective study on canine atopic dermatitis and food-induced allergic dermatitis in Switzerland. *Veterinary Dermatology* 2008; **19**: 150–155.
16. Favrot C, Steffan J, Seewald W. A prospective study on the clinical features of chronic canine atopic dermatitis and its diagnosis. *Veterinary Dermatology* 2010; **21**: 23–31
17. Scott DW. Observations on canine atopic dermatitis. *Journal of the American Animal Hospital Association* 1981; **17**: 89–102.
18. Wilhem S, Kovalik M, Favrot C. Breed-associated phenotypes in canine atopic dermatitis. *Veterinary Dermatology* 2010; **22**: 143–149.

10

Diagnosis of canine atopic dermatitis

Craig E. Griffin

Animal Dermatology Clinic, San Diego, CA, USA

Conflict of interest: Has served as a consultant to, serves or has served on advisory board, has received gifts and honoraria from, or has received research support from the following companies: Bayer, Dechra, Elanco, Greer, Merck, Novartis, Pinnaclife, Purina, Sogeval, VARL, Zoetis.

The approach to the chronic pruritic dog

Pruritus, the defining feature of canine atopic dermatitis (CAD), is a common presenting problem for veterinarians. Pruritus is a sensation in the skin that occurs with numerous skin diseases. However, the list of differential diagnoses for common causes of chronic pruritus, that appear clinically similar to CAD, is relatively small (Table 10.1). Causes of pruritus are often classified into **primary diseases**, able to cause pruritus directly, or **secondary causes**, which are diseases (usually infections, see Chapters 26 and 27) that occur as a consequence of the damage to the skin caused by a primary disease. The secondary causes of pruritus can occur with many different primary diseases, even ones not usually associated with pruritus, such as endocrinopathies. Thus, a major aspect and often the first step in making a diagnosis in cases of chronic pruritus is to determine if the primary disease is pruritic or not. This is only definitively done when any secondary cause of pruritus, such as infections, has been identified and eliminated.

Furthermore, there are **modulating factors** that occur in the skin or brain and that alter the pruritic threshold, such as stress, anxiety, dry environment, etc. (Table 10.1).

The diagnosis of chronic pruritus in dogs can be further complicated by the common occurrence of multiple causes of pruritus being present in the same dog. The possibility of several coexisting primary and/or secondary pruritic diseases should thus be considered. In particular, for the diagnosis of CAD it is important to determine if the pruritus and erythema observed are the result of environmental CAD, and/or presence of hypersensitivity to fleas, and/or adverse reaction to food, and/or of infections. Often a variety of therapeutic or diagnostic trials are indicated to really determine the causes of the clinical signs in dogs with pruritus (Table 10.2).

The main differential diagnosis of atopic dermatitis is **adverse food reaction**. However, many dermatologists now consider atopic dermatitis as a clinical presentation of both environmental and food allergens (see also Chapter 16). This has resulted in CAD being considered as food-induced (FIAD) and non-food-induced (thus environmentally induced or NFIAD) atopic dermatitis [1]. In fact, it is estimated that up to 40% of dogs with perennial signs are diet responsive and half of these have concurrent CAD and adverse food reactions (AFR) [2–4]. Other authors have found a lower but still significant incidence of dogs with these two diseases at the same time [5, 6]. It is essential for the best long-term control to determine how much of the dog's signs are due to food allergens. This can only be done by performing good elimination diet trials and provocative exposure testing (see Chapter 18).

Flea allergy dermatitis can also mimic and/or coexist with CAD, it is estimated that up to 79% of CAD dogs are also flea allergic in some areas of the world [7]. (Please refer to Chapters 20–25 for information on flea bite allergy, its diagnosis and its therapy.)

Veterinary Allergy, First Edition. Edited by Chiara Noli, Aiden Foster, and Wayne Rosenkrantz.

Table 10.1 Differential diagnoses for causes of chronic pruritus

Primary diseases	Secondary diseases	Modulating factors
Adverse food reaction	Pyoderma	Anxiety/stress
Atopic dermatitis	Malassezia dermatitis	Environment (dry warm air, UV radiation of skin)
Flea allergy dermatitis	Bacterial overgrowth	Heat
Contact allergy	Calcinosis cutis	Xerosis
Demodicosis		
Dermatophytosis		
Drug eruption		
Sarcoptic mange		
Other ectoparasites		
Neoplasia (epitheliotropic lymphoma)		
Pemphigus foliaceus		
Vasculitis		

Table 10.2 Trials for CAD dogs

Trial	Assesses
Aggressive flea control	To determine if fleas are the cause of disease or how much they aggravate CAD
Bathing trial	To help determine if there are environmental allergies
Diet trial	To determine if foods induce signs of CAD
Environmental restriction	To determine environmental, some parasitic and contact allergies
Antiparasitic drugs	To rule out the presence of scabies and some other internal and external parasites
Antibacterial therapy	To determine the role of bacteria in pruritus
Yeast therapy	To determine the role of yeast in pruritus and possibly allergy

Scabies can mimic CAD because it causes pruritus in a similar pattern to CAD, albeit with some subtle differences. In general, scabies presents with a papular rash, and pruritus without lesions is not seen. Trial therapy for scabies is advised in dogs that have a positive pinnal pedal reflex, and lesions on the ear margins or caudal and lateral elbow. The pinnal pedal reflex is positive in 82% of dogs with scabies and only 6.2% of 533 allergic and pruritic dogs with other diseases [8]. Trial therapy with selamectin or moxidectin/imidacloprid topically or milbemicine orally are the treatments of choice because they are approved or are licensed in many countries. Some clinicians use oral or subcutaneous ivermectin 250–300 µg/kg once weekly for three to five treatments, though this is an extra-label use in some countries and highly contraindicated in certain breeds [9]. There is a report of scabies failing to respond to both oral and subcutaneous ivermectin at 300 µg/kg [10].

Cytology is the most important test used to determine the presence of **bacterial pyoderma, bacterial overgrowth,** and ***Malassezia* dermatitis.** Once these infections are identified they should be treated and eliminated (please refer to Chapter 26 on bacterial and yeast infections in the atopic dog). After the treatment course, it is critical to evaluate the dog for changes in the level and pattern of pruritus as well as for residual presence of lesions. At this follow-up examination a new cytology is recommended because the therapy may have been ineffective in eliminating the microbes, particularly if meticillin-resistant *Staphylococcus pseudintermedius* is present and in some cases of bacterial rod overgrowth or pyoderma. The key to successfully using cytology in the diagnosis of CAD is to take multiple samples that reflect different aspects of the dog's disease, such as from lesions suggestive of pyoderma and *Malassezia* dermatitis as well as from pruritic areas with erythroderma or scaling. Essentially, if there are visible lesions at sites of pruritus then cytology is the only way to determine if the pruritus likely reflects the primary CAD or a microbial infection.

Establishing the diagnosis of CAD

A thorough diagnostic approach is needed to determine the presence of CAD and of secondary and modulating factors that may contribute to the dog's signs. This requires a systematic process to a work up that will invariably take some time to complete. Even when it is determined at an initial consultation that there is a likely diagnosis of CAD, it will still take more visits and generally one to several months to determine what role food, fleas, and micro-organisms play in the dog's signs and response to therapy.

No test has been developed to accurately diagnose CAD directly. Over the years, authors have reported a variety of different methods, combining clinical findings and trial therapies, for making a diagnosis of CAD. In 1986, Willemse proposed a set of major and minor diagnostic criteria that were used to make a compatible diagnosis [11]. These criteria were not validated and in 1998 Prélaud *et al.*, utilizing a relatively small number of cases, evaluated and modified these criteria [12]. Ten years after, a study by Favrot *et al.* on over 1000 dogs with chronic pruritus was performed by 34 veterinary dermatologist in 15 countries [5]. Canine atopic dermatitis was diagnosed in 843 dogs while 253 had either fleas, scabies, or other parasites causing pruritus. This study evaluated approximately 50 clinical findings and identified nine key observations that could be used in one of two sets of diagnostic criteria, which have differing sensitivity and specificity for the diagnosis of CAD. For the diagnosis of CAD, the highest sensitivity of 85.4% is reached by having any five of eight criteria in set 1 present (Table 10.3). The drawback is that approximately 20% of the cases may not have CAD. If the goal is to accurately diagnose CAD, which is preferred when deciding how a dog will be treated, likely for the remainder of its life, then set 2 is most useful. In set 2 there are seven criteria and if six are present then 93.7% of the dogs have CAD (Table 10.4). Unfortunately, requiring six of these seven criteria will not identify 58% of the cases (high specificity and low sensitivity). This study also did not evaluate dogs presenting for chronic or recurrent otitis externa, which often is associated with CAD.

There are some problems encountered when trying to use the nine criteria used in the diagnostic sets. In set 1 two criteria require that the case be presented on multiple occasions as the dog must have chronic or recurrent yeast infections or be corticosteroid responsive. What doses and types of corticosteroid the dog must respond to are not adequately known. In addition, this observation should only be made in cases that do not have concurrent pyoderma or yeast infections at the time of corticosteroid therapy. It is not uncommon for owners to report poor response to glucocorticoids due to the concurrent presence of skin infections. In these cases the CAD usually responds extremely well after the pyoderma, *Malassezia* dermatitis, or both, are eliminated. In addition, two studies that evaluated jointly 754 non-food-induced CAD dogs and 237 food-induced CAD dogs showed that 84.9% and 66.7% were corticosteroid responsive, respectively [5, 6]. In the larger study the difference was significant, showing that food-induced CAD does not respond as well as non-food-induced CAD to corticosteroid therapy. Another question relies on the owner to recall that the dog was lesion free at the onset of pruritus. Certainly in chronic cases the recollection of this finding can be difficult. Even in recent-onset cases the author has seen many cases where

Table 10.3 Diagnostic criteria set 1

Criteria
1. Age at onset <3 years
2. Mostly indoor
3. Corticosteroid-responsive pruritus
4. Chronic or recurrent yeast infections
5. Affected front feet
6. Affected ear pinnae
7. Non-affected ear margins
8. Non-affected dorsolumbar area

If 5 of 8 criteria are present the sensitivity for CAD is 0.854 and specificity is 0.791; however, this includes food-induced atopic dermatitis. The questions in bold differ from set 2.

Table 10.4 Diagnostic criteria set 2

Criteria
1. Age at onset <3 years
2. Mostly indoor
3. Pruritus with no visible lesions at onset
4. Affected front feet
5. Affected ear pinnae
6. Non-affected ear margins
7. Non-affected dorsolumbar area

If 6 of 7 criteria are present the sensitivity is 0.42 and the specificity is 0.937; however, this includes food-induced atopic dermatitis. The question in bold is different from set 1.

owners are not aware of lesions but they are present, particularly involving the paws. In spite of these drawbacks the criteria developed by Favrot *et al.* [5] are now routinely used in most studies evaluating CAD cases, even if practitioners on occasion see CAD cases that do not meet these criteria.

For those cases that do not have six criteria in set 2, a help to making a diagnosis is given by three key observations:

1 The pattern of pruritus, when no microbial disease is present, includes at least one body area that is typically affected in CAD (Box 10.1) (Figures 10.1 and 10.2).
2 Lesions (normal-appearing pruritic skin, erythema, very small papules) are typical for CAD and not for other causes of pruritus (Figure 10.3). A very helpful finding is to have owners carefully observe where their dog is scratching or licking. At follow-up examinations if dogs are itchy on the paws, forelegs, groin, and ears, with no lesions present, then that is very suggestive of atopic dermatitis. This finding is not the same as historical criteria of pruritus without lesions at onset, which is the reporting by the owner that when the dog initially was noted as being pruritic, the owners did not observe skin lesions.

Box 10.1 Typical sites for pruritus in canine atopic dermatitis

Paws, especially ventral interdigital
Concave base pinna
External orifice ears
Flexor surface metacarpal or metatarsal
Flexure of the elbow
Axilla
Abdomen/inguinal
Periocular
Perioral

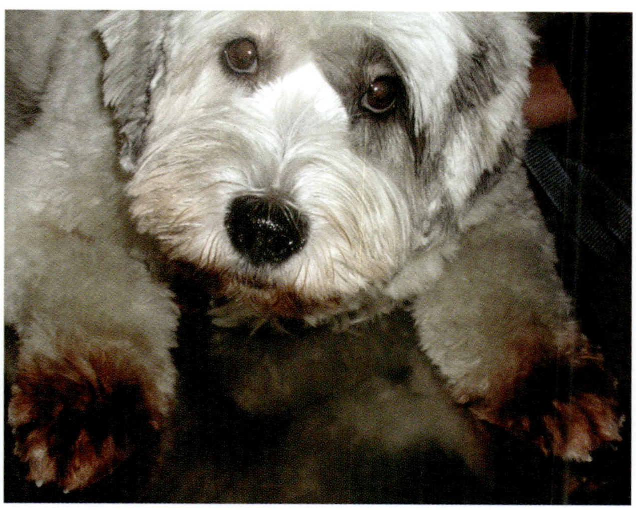

Figure 10.1 Front view of a dog with CAD. Areas of red-stained hair and some alopecia show typical sites where many CAD cases are pruritic. Note muzzle, perioral, and paws.

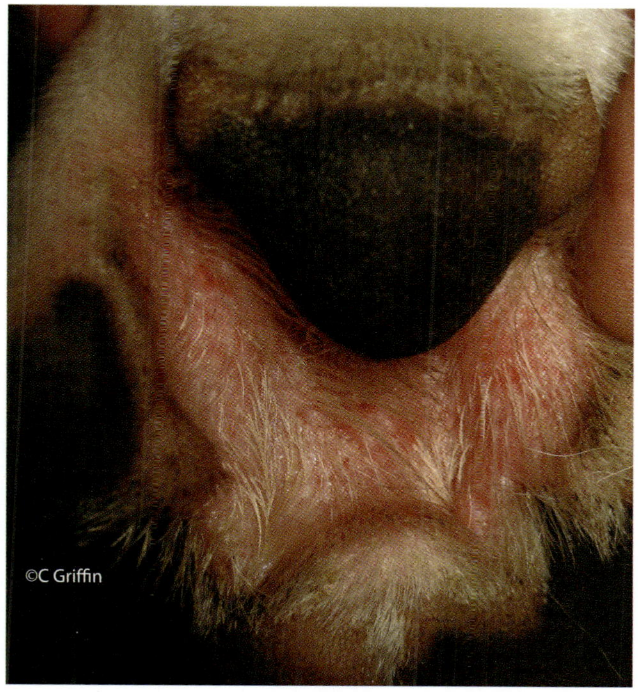

Figure 10.2 Palmar surface of the paw. This is a common site for erythema and pruritus in CAD cases, and in some that do not meet the Favrot *et al.* criteria as this may be the only site affected.

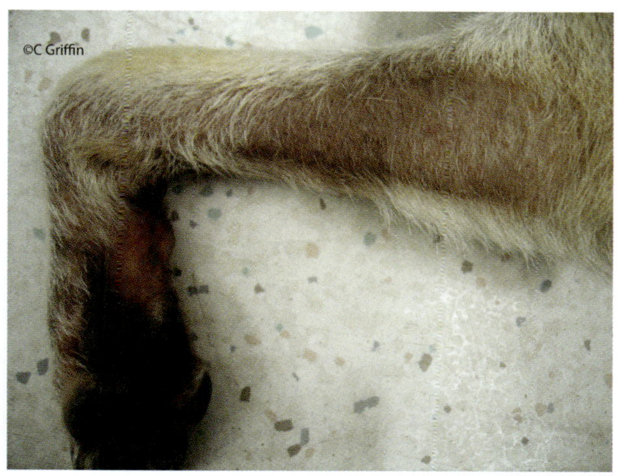

Figure 10.3 Close up of the lateral front leg and palmar aspect of a paw of a dog with CAD. Note alopecia, absence of skin lesions in some areas, and small papules or mild erythema in others.

3 Pruritus is correlated with environmental exposure to an allergen. The correlation may be based on seasonal exacerbation of signs or relapses following exposure to specific environments. If this is not possible then other causes of pruritus and lesions similar to those caused by CAD, particularly foods and parasites, should be ruled out. Seasonal exacerbation is typically seen in flea bite allergy or CAD. When seasonality is associated with otitis and pruritus in areas other than the dorsal lumbar region (typical of flea bite allergy), then CAD is likely to be present. Initial signs may be seasonal in 42–75% of the dogs in some areas of the world.

Other historical features help to support the diagnosis of CAD such as sneezing, reverse sneezing, and conjunctivitis. A lack of gastrointestinal signs in a dog with pruritus compatible with CAD also helps by decreasing, but not eliminating, food as a cause of the signs.

The role of 'allergy' testing in diagnosing CAD

Testing is *not* generally considered a major tool in the diagnosis of CAD [13]. Once the diagnosis of CAD is obtained clinically, it is mainly used to determine significant allergens. The diagnostic accuracy for CAD of a comprehensive intradermal and serum *in vitro* test is low, because there are multiple allergens that can give positive results in normal dogs [14–16]. However, intradermal testing can be very accurate in confirming CAD in some cases. The vast majority of pollen extracts that have been evaluated do not give positive results in normal dogs [17–19]. Based on those studies, it can be stated that positive intradermal test reactions to multiple pollens may in fact confirm a diagnosis of environmentally induced CAD. Unfortunately, a negative test does not rule out CAD; false negatives are a significant problem and were 40% in one study [20].

Identifying the role of the environment in the diagnosis of CAD

One study showed that confining dogs with CAD to an isolation room of a veterinary hospital for 2 weeks resulted in significant improvement in 63% of those that had not responded to diet trials [20]. The clinical improvement of hospitalized dogs maintained on the same diet strongly supports the diagnosis of environmentally induced CAD.

Another therapeutic trial is frequent bathing, as dogs with CAD that are bathed daily generally improve significantly. This has been supported by some studies in pruritic dogs [21,22]. It is not known if the benefit from bathing is due to antipruritic effects of moisturizing the skin, or to an antimicrobial effect, or to removal of environmental allergens from the skin. Though no controlled trial has been performed, it is the author's impression that dogs with adverse reactions to food do not respond to bathing as well as dogs with CAD. This could be explained by removal of allergen being an important mechanism, because the antimicrobial and antipruritic effects would likely be similar.

Determining environmental allergens for CAD

In general, allergen-specific IgE testing is indicated when a clinical diagnosis of atopic dermatitis has been made and it is considered desirable to know what allergens the dog is sensitive to. If the sensitivities are known, then this information may be used to attempt to avoid offending allergens or for the selection of allergens for allergen-specific immunotherapy (ASIT). There are two main methods for testing CAD dogs, *in vivo* and *in vitro* testing. Though both are used to determine significant allergens, the two types of test detect different things.

In vivo *testing*

In vivo testing may include patch or intradermal testing. Patch testing is when allergens are applied to the skin, generally under occlusion and left to react for 24–48 hours. Pruritus at the site has to be prevented throughout the testing time. To date, patch testing has been used more in research settings and not clinical practice [23–25].

Intradermal testing is the oldest, most studied method [17–19,26]. Intradermal testing is performed by administering injections of small amounts of allergen solutions directly into the dog's dermis. This is usually done with small-gauge (27 gauge) needles and injections of 0.05 to 0.1 mL at each site. The allergens will bind to mast cells that are coated with IgE to the specific allergen. The mast cells with bound allergen will degranulate, releasing mediators, including histamine, which will result in the formation of a wheal (Figure 10.4). This generally occurs within a few to 30 minutes. Most allergens have been tested at 1000 protein nitrogen units (PNU)/mL though some are tested at lower concentrations. Most notable are house dust mites, which are tested at 250 PNU/mL and flea which is tested at 500 PNU/mL [19]. Two studies have suggested that for most pollens this traditional testing concentration may not be appropriate and is likely too low in dogs [18,19]. Another factor is that there are several sources for allergens and they may not all be the same. One study reported that two different allergen sources of *Alternaria* used in the same dogs caused 1.9% versus 48% positive

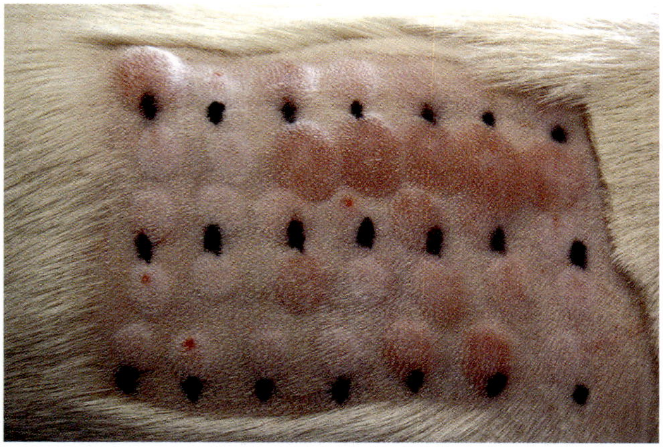

Figure 10.4 Lateral thorax of a dog after completing an intradermal skin test. Note numerous positive reactions. On the upper row left there are the positive control (erythematous wheal, histamine) and the negative control (no wheal, saline).

reactions [27]. These results indicate that each source needs to be evaluated for what is the most effective testing concentration. The positive reactions are arbitrarily interpreted by the presence of erythema, turgidity, height, and size of the wheal. One study compared an objective method for scoring reactions to one subjective method and found moderate agreement [28]. The authors concluded that the objective method may be sufficient while one is learning to use a subjective method. Controlled blinded studies comparing differences between different subjective training methods and intra- and interobserver variation have not been done. Additionally, late and delayed reactions may occur from hours to a day later [29,30]. The importance of late and delayed reactions for incorporation into ASIT formulations has not been evaluated. Even considering these problems the value of intradermal testing has been supported by the favourable response to ASIT [31,32]. The training required, variations in testing protocols, and the subjective interpretation of the results are the main reasons why most general practitioners refer their cases to those trained in intradermal testing, such as board certified veterinary dermatologists, or use serum *in vitro* testing.

In vitro *testing*

In vitro testing is more commonly used, compared to skin testing. Serum *in vitro* testing (SIVT), as previously discussed, is not to be used to diagnose atopic dermatitis because it is possible to have false-positive and -negative reactions [22,26,33]. The results may identify potential allergens that may be included in ASIT or avoided by the owner. Studies comparing intradermal test results to SIVT have also shown differences, though these vary from study to study [16,33–38]. The response to ASIT in dogs clinically diagnosed with atopic dermatitis is the most relevant criterion to compare SIVT versus IDT. In the few studies that have done this the results are similar [39–42].

A number of different commercial companies offer tests that detect IgE to a variety of environmental allergens and then formulate ASIT solutions. Though all the companies are essentially detecting canine allergen-specific IgE, they do use different methodologies, such as radioallergosorbent assay (RAST), enzyme linked assay (ELISA), or a liquid-phase allergen assay [33]. The techniques also vary in how they bind to canine IgE, with some using polyclonal, monoclonal, or mixed monoclonal anti-IgE antibodies, and others the FcEpsilon receptor (high affinity IgE receptor) [43,44]. All claim to be specific and reliable though only a little has been published in refereed journals.

One study evaluated three different companies that utilize an FcEpsilon receptor technology for detecting IgE. Blinded samples were submitted in duplicate. The evaluation of just positive versus negative results showed intralaboratory differences of 3.14% and interlaboratory differences for 4.76% of samples [44]. Another study evaluated a mixed monoclonal IgE-based test and showed an intra-assay coefficient of variation of 9.7% while the interassay concordance ranged from 91% to 94%, depending on the cut-off used for a positive value [45]. This study also compared its results to a FeEpsilon receptor test, and when evaluating just positive and negative it showed a 92% concordance.

The differences between serum and intradermal testing have been valuable in some cases that do not respond to ASIT based on one test but will respond if the results of the other test are used. Some veterinary specialists use both tests combined to determine the ASIT therapy and it has been suggested that this may improve ASIT results, though controlled studies showing this have not been published. Key features regarding the two tests are presented in Table 10.5.

Conclusion

The classic case of CAD is diagnosed when the history and physical examination meet Favrot's criteria. However, those criteria will fail to diagnose some cases. If the pruritus is associated with an environmental factor then atopic dermatitis is most likely. Therefore a complete diagnosis involves identifying and treating complicating infections and other factors and determining what signs reflect the uncomplicated case of CAD. Diet trials, aggressive flea control, cytology and appropriate antibiotic or antiyeast agents, used alone or in combination, are

Table 10.5 Comparison of tests to detect allergen-specific IgE

Intradermal test	*In vitro* serum test
Detects skin reactivity to intradermal injection of allergen extracts	Detects serum IgE (IgG_4) to specific allergens in laboratory situation
Positive test result determined subjectively by each investigator	Positive, negative and borderline values established by laboratory based on their individual controls and arbitrary cut offs
Generally can test more items, some up to 80 items	Testing often limited to 30–40 items
Drugs such as steroids, antihistamines effect test	Less sensitive to drugs though high dose steroids may effect test results
Training required to perform effectively	Interpretation offered by laboratory
Inventory and maintenance of testing solutions required	Only serum sample required then mailed to laboratory
Sedation and shaving hair at test site required	No shaving or sedation required
Very rare but risk of anaphylaxis during test	No risk of anaphylaxis from testing
Immediate results	Results take 1 to 2 weeks to return

often required to really determine how CAD manifests in a given patient. The diagnosis of CAD still remains the ultimate example of the art of practice in veterinary dermatology, as no two cases are the same.

References

1. Olivry T, DeBoer DJ, Prélaud P, *et al.* Food for thought: pondering the relationship between canine atopic dermatitis and cutaneous adverse food reactions. *Veterinary Dermatology* 2007; **18**: 390–391.
2. Biourge VC, Fontaine J, Vroom MW. Diagnosis of adverse reactions to food in dogs: efficacy of a soy-isolate hydrolyzate-based diet. *Journal of Nutrition* 2004;**134**: 2062S–2064S.
3. Loeffler A, Soares-Magalhaes R, Bond R, *et al.* A retrospective analysis of case series using home-prepared and chicken hydrolysate diets in the diagnosis of adverse food reactions in 181 pruritic dogs. *Veterinary Dermatology* 2006; **17**: 273–279.
4. Chesney C. Food sensitivity in the dog: a quantitative study. *Journal of Small Animal Practice* 2002; **43**: 203–207.
5. Favrot C, Steffan J, Seewald W, *et al.* A prospective study on the clinical features of chronic canine atopic dermatitis and its diagnoatsis. *Veterinary Dermatology* 2010; **21**: 23–31.
6. Proverbio D, Perego R, Spada E, *et al.* Prevalence of adverse food reactions in 130 dogs in Italy with dermatological signs: a retrospective study. *Journal of Small Animal Practice* 2010; **51**: 370–374.
7. Sousa CA, Halliwell REW. The ACVD task force on canine atopic dermatitis (XI): the relationship between arthropod hypersensitivity and atopic dermatitis in the dog. *Veterinary Immunology and Immunopathology* 2001; **81**: 233–237.
8. Mueller RS, Bettenay SV, Shipstone M. Value of the pinnal-pedal reflex in the diagnosis of canine scabies. *Vet Rec* 2001; **148**: 621–623.
9. Mealey KL. Therapeutic implications of the MDR-1 gene. *Journal of Veterinary Pharmoacological Therapy* 2004; **27**: 257–264.
10. Terada Y, Murayama N, Ikemura H, *et al.* Sarcoptes scabiei var. canis refractory to ivermectin treatment in two dogs. *Veterinary Dermatology* 2010; **21**: 608–612.
11. Willemse T. Atopic skin disease: a review and reconsideration of diagnostic criteria. *Journal of Small Animal Practice* 1986; **27**: 771–778.
12. Prélaud P, Guaguère E, Alhaidari Z, *et al.* Reevaluation of diagnostic criteria of canine atopic dermatitis. *Revue Veterinaire Medicale* 1998; **149**: 1057–1064.
13. DeBoer D, Hillier A. The ACVD task force on canine atopic dermatitis (XV): fundamental concepts in clinical diagnosis. *Veterinary Immunology and Immunopathology* 2001; **81**: 271–276.
14. Ginel PJ, Riaño C, Lucena R. Evaluation of a commercial ELISA test for the detection of allergen-specific IgE antibodies in atopic dogs. *Zentralblatt Veterinaermedizin B* 1998; **45**: 421–425.
15. Griffin CE, Moriello KA, DeBoer DJ. The effect of serum IgE on an in vitro ELISA test in the normal canine. In: von Tscharner C, Halliwell REW, eds. *Advances in Veterinary Dermatology I.* Philadelphia: Bailliere-Tindall, 1990: 137–144.
16. Codner EC, Lessard P. Comparison of intradermal allergy test and enzyme-linked immunosorbent assay in dogs with allergic skin disease. *Journal of the American Veterinary Medical Association* 1993; **202**: 739–743.
17. August J. The reaction of canine skin to the intradermal injection of allergenic extracts. *Journal of the American Animal Hospital Association* 1982; **18**: 157–163.
18. Bauer CL, Hensel P, Austel M, *et al.* Determination of irritant threshold concentrations to weeds, trees and grasses through serial dilutions in intradermal testing on healthy clinically nonallergic dogs. *Veterinary Dermatology* 2010; **21**: 192–197.
19. Hensel P, Austel M, Medleau L, *et al.* Determination of threshold concentrations of allergens and evaluation of two different histamine concentrations in canine intradermal testing. *Veterinary Dermatology* 2004; **15**: 304–308.
20. Fujimura M. The study of canine atopic dermatitis involving the isolation of dogs. *Polish Journal of Veterinary Science* 2011; **14**: 273–277.
21. Loflath A, von Voigts-Rhetz A, Jaeger K, *et al.* The efficacy of a commercial shampoo and whirlpooling in the treatment of canine pruritus—a double-blinded, randomized, placebo-controlled study. *Veterinary Dermatology* 2007; **18**: 427–431.
22. Olivry T, DeBoer DJ, Favrot C, *et al.* Treatment of canine atopic dermatitis: 2010 clinical practice guidelines from the International Task Force on Canine Atopic Dermatitis. *Veterinary Dermatology* 2010; **21**: 233–248.
23. Nogueira S, Torres SMF, Horne K, *et al.* Patch test reactions to house dust mites in dogs with atopic dermatitis. In: Hillier A, Foster AP, Kwocka KW, eds. *Advances in Veterinary Dermatology*, Vol. 4. Oxford: Blackwell Publishing, 2005: 49–59.
24. Olivry T, Deangelo KB, Dunston SM, *et al.* Patch testing of experimentally sensitized beagle dogs: development of a model

for skin lesions of atopic dermatitis. *Veterinary Dermatology* 2006; **17**: 95–102.
25. Pucheu-Haston CM, Jackson HA, Olivry T, *et al.* Epicutaneous sensitization with Dermatophagoides farinae induces generalized allergic dermatitis and elevated mite-specific immunoglobulin E levels in a canine model of atopic dermatitis. *Clinical and Experimental Allergy* 2008; **38**: 667–679.
26. Hillier A, DeBoer DJ. The ACVD task force on canine atopic dermatitis (XVII): intradermal testing. *Veterinary Immunology and Immunopathology* 2001; **81**: 289–304.
27. Hammerling R, de Weck AL. Comparison of two diagnostic tests for canine atopy using monoclonal anti-IgE antibodies. *Veterinary Dermatology* 1998; **9**: 191–199.
28. Hubbard TL, White PD. Comparison of subjective and objective intradermal allergy test scoring methods in dogs with atopic dermatitis. *Journal of the American Animal Hospital Association* 2011; **47**: 399–405.
29. Hillier A, Kwochka KW, Pinchbeck LRl. Reactivity to intradermal injection of extracts of *Dermatophagoides farinae, Dermatophagoides pteronyssinus*, house dust mite mix, and house dust in dogs suspected to have atopic dermatitis: 115 cases (1996–1998). *Journal of the American Veterinary Medical Association* 2000; **217**: 536–540.
30. Lorenz MD. Environmental allergens in small animal hypersensitivity disorders. *Veterinary Clinics of North America* 1974; **4**: 41–46.
31. Willemse A, Van den Brom WE, Rijnberk A. Effect of hyposensitization on atopic dermatitis in dogs. *Journal of the American Veterinary Medical Association* 1984; **184**: 1277–1280.
32. Loewenstein C, Mueller RS. A review of allergen-specific immunotherapy in human and veterinary medicine. *Veterinary Dermatology* 2009; **20**: 84–98.
33. Deboer DJ, Hillier A. The ACVD task force on canine atopic dermatitis (XVI): laboratory evaluation of dogs with atopic dermatitis with serum-based 'allergy' tests. *Veterinary Immunology and Immunopathology* 2001; **81**: 277–287.
34. Mueller RS, Burrows A, Tsohalis J. Comparison of intradermal testing and serum testing for allergen-specific IgE using monoclonal IgE antibodies in 84 atopic dogs. *Australian Veterinary Journal* 1999; **77**: 290–294.
35. Rosser E. Comparison of the results of intradermal testing and aeroallergen-specific IgE serum testing in dogs with warm weather, seasonal atopic dermatitis. *Veterinary Dermatology* 2004; **15** (Suppl. 1): 3 (abstract).
36. Olivry T, Jackson HA, Murphy KM, *et al.* Evaluation of a point-of-care immunodot assay for predicting results of allergen-specific intradermal and immunoglobulin E serological tests. *Veterinary Dermatology* 2005; **16**: 117–120.
37. Zunic M. Comparison between IMMUNODOT tests and the intradermal skin test in atopic dogs. *Veterinary Dermatology* 1998; **9**: 201–205.
38. Tarpataki N, Bigler B, Vajdovich P, *et al.* Comparison between an intradermal skin test and allergen-specific IgE-ELISA for canine atopic dermatitis. *Schweizer Archiv fuer Tierheilkunde* 2008; **150**: 117–122.
39. Zur G, White SD, Ihrke PJ, *et al.* Canine atopic dermatitis: a retrospective study of 169 cases examined at the University of California, Davis, 1992–1998. Part II. Response to hyposensitization. *Veterinary Dermatology* 2002; **13**: 103–111.
40. Scott K, White SD, Rosychuk RAW. A retrospective study of hyposensitization in atopic dogs in a flea-scarce environment. In Ihrke P, Mason I, White S, eds. *Advances in Veterinary Dermatology*, Vol 2. New York: Pergamon Press, 1993: 79–87.
41. Schnabl B, Bettenay SV, Dow K, *et al.* Results of allergen-specific immunotherapy in 117 dogs with atopic dermatitis. *Veterinary Record* 2006: **156**: 81–85.
42. Park S, Ohya F, Yamashita K, *et al.* Comparison of response to immunotherapy by intradermal skin test and antigen-specific IgE in canine atopy. *Journal of Veteterinary Medical Science* 2000; **62**: 983–988.
43. Derer M, Morrison-Smith G, De Weck ALl. Monoclonal anti-IgE antibodies in the diagnosis of dog allergy. *Veterinary Dermatology* 1998; **9**: 185–190.
44. Wassom D, Grieve R. In vitro measurement of canine and feline IgE: a review of FceR1a-based assays for detection of allergen-reactive IgE. *Veterinary Dermatology* 1998; **9**: 173–178
45. Lee KW, Blankenship KD, McCurry ZM, *et al.* Performance characteristics of a monoclonal antibody cocktail-based ELISA for detection of allergen-specific IgE in dogs and comparison with a high affinity IgE receptor-based ELISA. *Veterinary Dermatology* 2009; **20**: 157–164.

11

Allergen avoidance

Daniel O. Morris

School of Veterinary Medicine, University of Pennsylvania, Philadelphia, PA, USA

Conflict of interest: none declared.

Allergen avoidance is often said to be an important component of a comprehensive strategy for the symptomatic control of allergy in animals. While this is certainly true for dietary allergens and biting or sucking insects, complete avoidance of the ubiquitous aeroallergens that contaminate our natural and built environments is simply not achievable. In addition, very little evidence-based data are available regarding the clinical effects of aeroallergen remediation on allergic animals. Therefore, veterinarians often look to the scientific literature regarding human allergic diseases for information on useful targets and mechanisms for the remediation of environmental allergens. The bulk of this body of knowledge focuses on human respiratory allergies associated with indoor allergens such as pet danders and house dust mites [1,2]. Even so, it seems reasonable to expect that lessons learned from experiments and clinical trials in the human medical literature can be successfully extrapolated to our animal patients. Most aeroallergens segregate into groups that share similar properties in regards to molecular weight, dispersal by air and mechanical vectors, and susceptibility to destruction by chemical and physical means. Therefore, this chapter focuses on mitigation strategies gleaned from both the human and veterinary medical experiences (Table 11.1).

The role of indoor allergens

Improvements in indoor climate control and increased use of upholstered furnishings and carpets have occurred concurrently with an increased incidence of allergic diseases of people living in industrialized nations over recent decades [3,4]. This may be true for animals as well, although epidemiologic studies to support such a supposition are lacking [5]. Efficient indoor climate control reduces air exchange with the outdoor environment (reducing dilution of indoor allergens), while upholstery and carpeting trap moisture and indoor allergens, and complicate cleaning regimens [6]. The net effect has been enhanced ambient exposure to allergens in homes and public places. The aeroallergens with the most potential for avoidance or remediation originate from indoor sources such as dust mites, pet danders, cockroaches, and moulds [7]. However, the clinical relevance of these allergens to veterinary patients is variably understood at this time.

Environmental mites

The putative roles of dust mites and storage mites in canine atopic dermatitis have been described [8–10] and it is known that dust mite allergens are ubiquitous in the environments of pets, such as carpeting, upholstered furniture, mattresses, pet bedding, and pet toys [11–14]. There is also extensive cross-reactivity of the canine immune response to dust mites and storage mites, meaning that sensitization and exposure may occur independently of the specific mite species present at any given time [15]. Contamination of dry pet foods by dust and storage mites may occur [16–18], but is of low concern compared to environmental exposure [18]. However, opened pet food can be sealed in plastic containers to minimize contamination [18].

Veterinary Allergy, First Edition. Edited by Chiara Noli, Aiden Foster, and Wayne Rosenkrantz.

Table 11.1 Strategies for remediation of environmental allergens

Strategies	Goals
Home directed	
Maintain relative humidity <50%	Kill dust mites and reduce mould growth
Maintain temperature <18°C/65°F	Slow dust mite reproduction
Minimize/replace carpets, draperies, upholstery	Reduce dust mite habitat and allergen trapping
Encase pillows, box springs, and mattresses	Exclude dust mites and allergens
Vacuum weekly (minimum); HEPA filtered	Reduce reservoir dust and allergen trapping
Remove indoor plants	Reduce mould growth
Remediate damp basements, kitchens, baths	Reduce mould growth
Treat home/upholstery with benzyl benzoate	Kill dust mites
Professional extermination	Elimination of cockroaches
Keep kitchens clean/free of food particles	Reduce food sources for cockroaches
Pet directed	
Use commercial flea/tick control products	Reduce dust mites numbers
Rinsing/wiping feet when returning from outdoors	Remove pollens and mould spores
Bathing (whole-body) with shampoo products	Remove allergen from hair coat
Personal and pet items	
Seal dry pet foods in plastic containers	Avoid contamination by dust and storage mites
Freeze small pets toys, beds, and pillows (24 hours)	Kill dust mites
Launder clothing and bedding in hot water (55°C/130°F)	Kill dust mites and denature/remove allergen

To date, only a single report has addressed the effects of dust mite remediation efforts on the clinical signs of CAD in dogs with dust mite sensitivity. In that study, the acaricide benzyl benzoate was used for environmental treatment until a test for dust mite excretion products became negative, indicating destruction of live mites. Of the dust mite-sensitive dogs evaluated in these homes, 48% achieved an excellent clinical response while 36% were moderate responders, although there was no untreated (control) group [19]. In double-blind, placebo-controlled trials of acaricidal treatment of homes in which human patients with AD reside, results have been mixed. One trial showed significant benefit while another revealed none [20,21]. A Cochrane review of clinical trials for dust mite remediation has failed to prove benefit for people with asthma [22].

Perhaps the most effective intervention to reduce environmental mite burden is the maintenance of indoor relative humidity (RH) below 50% because mites must extract a sufficient amount of water from room air in order to survive [23]. Carpets, draperies, and other fabrics can retain moisture and provide an ideal habitat for mite reproduction. The use of high-efficiency dehumidifiers and air conditioners has been shown to be effective for RH control. Once live mites are destroyed, regular vacuuming and cleaning regimens should reduce the allergen pool in the home [24]. In especially humid climates, removal of carpets (in favour of hard surfaces) and replacement of curtains (with blinds or shades) can also be useful [23].

For small pet items, such as soft toys, beds, and pillows, freezing for at least 24 hours in a conventional freezer is an effective ways to kill mites, although their shed allergens may persist unless the items are properly laundered (see section "Laundering of textiles") [23].

Interestingly, the use of insecticidal flea control products on pets has been associated with decreased dust mite allergen levels in the homes of both cats and dogs, suggesting some lateral acaricidal effect [12,13].

Pet dander allergens

It is known that some degree of cross-reactivity occurs between canine and feline dander allergens (Can f 1 and Fel d 1, respectively), as recognized by the immune systems of pet-allergic people [25]. By comparison, very little is known about allergy of dogs, cats, and horses to one another. Although crude extracts of animal danders are used by many veterinary allergists when evaluating companion animals for aeroallergen sensitization [26], only one study has examined the role of a pet dander allergen that may be involved in sensitization. That report suggested that cats may autosensitize to their own Fel d 1 as part of the pathogenesis of eosinophilic skin lesions [27]. Regardless, it is clear that pet allergens are ubiquitous in homes and public places, including homes that do not house a pet [28]. Concepts relevant to pet dander allergen remediation are summarized in the section "General strategies for indoor allergen remediation".

Mould spores

In temperate climates, outdoor fungal spores appear in late winter when snow cover begins to dissipate and spore counts increase as the weather warms. Peak counts occur in the months of late summer and early autumn [29]. In tropical and subtropical climates, fungal spore counts may not vary greatly throughout the year. There is a direct relationship between indoor spore counts and outdoor conditions [30]. Spore infiltration from outdoors can be reduced by keeping doors and windows closed and using central air conditioning. Many of the strategies that are effective for dust mite mitigation are also useful for reducing fungal spore loads, such as maintenance of a low RH (≤50%) and removal of carpets and fabrics that trap moisture [29]. Providing for drier basements and better bathroom and kitchen ventilation will also reduce humidity and mould growth in the home. Live indoor plants that require irrigation are also a potential source of moulds and their spores, and should be removed from the home [29].

Cockroach allergens

Although there are no evidence-based data available regarding allergy to cockroaches in the veterinary literature, many veterinary allergists include crude cockroach extracts in their testing batteries for pruritic animals. Cockroach allergens are a common and well-documented source of asthma in people; they may also play a role in human urticaria and atopic dermatitis [31].

Although the kitchen is the primary site for cockroach infestation, allergen levels can often be detected in dust samples from furniture, bedding, and other rooms [32,33]. Approximately 20–48% of homes without visible cockroaches contain detectable cockroach allergen in dust samples [33,34].

Cockroach mitigation requires extermination and the important first step is home inspection by an experienced professional. An important adjunct for preventative maintenance is elimination of water and food sources [35], including scattered bits of pet food. However, detectable concentrations of cockroach allergen will persist in settled dust for several months even with repeated cleaning efforts [36].

General strategies for indoor allergen remediation

Despite a paucity of veterinary studies that have examined the utility of indoor allergen remediation, a significant body of evidence exists in the medical literature. The evidence suggests several strategies for consideration by veterinary allergists when planning general household allergen avoidance interventions.

Vacuuming and room air filtration

Perhaps the most significant factor that has contributed to the rise in allergic burden within human populations is the expanding prevalence of wall-to-wall fixed carpeting, which traps allergens but cannot be removed for laundering [37–39]. This factor has been exacerbated by the advent of vacuum cleaners of variable efficacy for allergen removal from carpeting. Allergen leakage from the machine and the vacuum bag is of major concern and vacuuming using older models may actually increase air-borne allergen concentrations [38]. In the past decade, improvements such as two- and three-layer microfiltration vacuum bags and high efficiency particulate arresting (HEPA) filters in both vacuum machines and room air cleaners (which claim to capture 99.9% of particles 0.3 μm diameter or larger) have improved allergen uptake and reduced leakage [40–42]. The use of such units has been correlated with decreased pet dander allergen in reservoir dust and improvements in asthmatic people [40], so it may be considered by pet owners when developing household allergen remediation strategies. Although there is a temporary increase in aerosolized allergen levels due to disturbance by the air exhaust flow and movements of the machine [41], one would expect reduced levels of allergen in reservoir dust to be the most important factor in mitigating the clinical signs of CAD, since the route of exposure is now presumed to be epicutaneous contact [43].

With regard to dust mites, vacuuming can remove dead mites and allergens at the surface but does not remove deeply imbedded allergens or reduce the number of live mites. Steam cleaning can kill mites at the surface if an adequate temperature is reached but it typically does not penetrate deeply enough into carpet or furniture fibre for significant effects. It may also be counterproductive if water residue is left behind that is capable of supporting mite population growth [23].

Trials utilizing HEPA-filtered air cleaners have produced mixed results. Some studies suggest excellent utility in reducing air-borne allergen levels [44–46], although not in reservoir dust [46], and not to a degree where they are likely to be effective alone [47,48]. Similar trials have not been reported in veterinary medicine, although the author has received many anecdotal reports from clients that the use of HEPA-filtered air cleaning units has failed to improve clinical signs in their pets with aeroallergen sensitivities. The effect of furniture dusting has been evaluated in simulation studies and, as might be expected, dry-dusting of wood surfaces releases allergens, whereas application of a spray polish to the dusting cloth or wood surface significantly reduces aerosolization of allergens [49,50].

Impermeable bedding covers

Because many pets have access to human bedding, encasement of mattresses and pillows in protective coverings manufactured for this purpose may be an effective way to reduce exposure to mites and their allergens, although the efficiency of allergen exclusion by such materials varies widely [51]. Mattresses are a known reservoir for dust mite and pet allergens and the quantity of trapped allergen increases with the advancing age of the mattress [52]. Also of interest is the finding that pillows stuffed with synthetic fibres harbour significantly more allergen than do feather pillows. This effect is likely due to the tighter weave used in pillow covers that prevent extrusion of feathers [53].

Laundering of textiles

In addition to house-keeping regimens, laundering of clothing plays an important role in allergen reduction. Clothing is often the point-source for indoor contamination with allergens. For example, levels of Fel d 1 in the homes of non-cat owners have correlated with the level of exposure experienced by their children in school, with the vehicle being the children's clothing [54]. Washing cotton fabrics in water is a simple and highly effective method for Fel d 1 removal [55]. Mechanical washing machines are highly effective for removal of pet allergens from cotton sheets at any water temperature but it was significantly better at the highest temperatures tested (60°C/140°F and steam) [56]. Detergents are superior to soap or water alone for removal of Fel d 1 [56], and two rinse cycles are the most beneficial with additional rinse cycles providing no additional gain [57]. For dust mites, weekly laundering in hot water (55°C/130°F or higher) kills mites and removes most allergen, while warm or cold water does not kill mites effectively (although it likely removes most mite allergens as they are water soluble) [23]. Mites are also killed by tumble driers if a temperature greater than 55°C (130°F) is maintained for 10 minutes [58]. Dry cleaning of woollens kills dust mites [59] and, while significantly reducing Fel d 1 allergen concentrations, does not abolish them entirely [60]. Allergen-free items can also become contaminated during the dry-cleaning process [60].

The role of outdoor allergens

The outdoor allergens of greatest relevance to allergic patients are pollens and mould spores. Veterinary allergists routinely utilize extensive panels of crude pollen and mould extracts to evaluate animal patients with pruritus or respiratory symptoms. The composition of these allergen panels are typically informed by human allergy clinics, regional pollen/mould spore maps, and local allergen counts.

General strategies for outdoor allergen avoidance

Monitoring pollen and mould spore counts

Avoidance of ubiquitous outdoor aeroallergens is virtually impossible but the public has become accustomed to monitoring the local pollen and mould spore counts, which are provided by various media outlets. Allergy sufferers may alter their outdoor activities during periods of moderate to high pollen and mould spore counts, in hopes of mitigating symptoms. The same may be true for owners of allergic pets. From a practical perspective however, there are several factors that limit the effectiveness of this approach to outdoor aeroallergen avoidance. Firstly, pollen and spore counts reported to the public often lag by 24 to 48 hours due to the collection and counting methods used and rapid changes in weather conditions can result in extreme daily variability. Counts may also exhibit significant geographical variation, even within a metropolitan area and these also fluctuate on a diurnal basis [61]. Additionally, dose–response relationships between pollen or spore exposure and symptoms are best characterized for nasal ('hay fever') and asthma symptoms in people, rather than with atopic dermatitis. For respiratory disease, dose–response relationships appear to often represent a threshold phenomenon (rather than linear relationship) [62]. These and other factors have led one author to question 'whether pollen and spore counts can be interpreted in a manner that can lead to reasonable recommendations for the lay public' [61].

Allergen removal from pets

Perhaps the most common (and reasonable) recommendation made to pet owners in regards to remediation of outdoor allergen exposure is bathing/ rinsing. This makes the most sense in view of an epicutaneous route of allergen exposure in the pathogenesis of CAD. Human hair is a well-known vehicle for Fel d 1 dispersal [63,64], and dust mite allergens can be extracted from the coats of dogs [65]. Therefore, it makes sense that the hair coat of animals could also be a significant reservoir for trapping of outdoor aeroallergens.

Studies have been performed to assess the utility of pet bathing for the reduction of their own dander allergen burdens. For both dogs and cats, bathing removes significant amounts of allergen from the pet but must be performed at least twice weekly to maintain a reduction relevant to pet-allergic people [66,67]. For dogs, this regimen achieved only a modest reduction of Can f 1 in room air [67]. Commercial products Allerpet/C® (for cats) and Allerpet/D® (for dogs) (Allerpet Inc., New York, NY, USA), available as shampoos (and as moistened wipes for cats), claim to substantially reduce the quantity of pet-related allergens in the home. However, an evaluation study showed that Allerpet/C® solution removed significantly less allergen than submersion in water and no more allergen than application of damp towels [68].

Anecdotal (owner-generated) reports of pets exhibiting increased levels of pedal pruritus after walking on damp grass (where pollens from plants may be concentrated) or generalized pruritus after swimming in ponds with a visible pollen film floating on the surface are not uncommon in the author's practice population. Many owners will also report some degree of relief after rinsing or bathing these pets when outdoor activities are completed. The results of a double-blind, randomized, placebo-controlled, cross-over study which evaluated the effects of weekly bathing on pruritus of dogs supports these anecdotal observations [69]. Although allergen loads within the hair coat were not evaluated in this study, dogs experienced better short-term relief of pruritus after bathing with a commercial emollient shampoo, in either a whirlpool tub or by conventional means, than after simple rinsing in a whirlpool tub without shampoo. However, multiple factors beyond mechanical removal of allergens could have correlated with clinical improvement including pharmacological and antimicrobial effects of the shampoo product [69].

The on-pet use of a putative allergen denaturing agent has been investigated in an experimental trial which utilized six dust mite-sensitized laboratory dogs. The product, which was marketed in pump spray and shampoo formats (Allerase®; Aveho Biosciences, Monterey, TN), claimed to denature protein allergens of all types therefore mitigating the clinical signs of CAD. When the product was compared to application of a saline control in a blinded cross-over design, clinical lesion scores were significantly higher for the test product. The authors speculated that it made allergens more soluble and available for absorption when wet [70]. This product is currently not marketed.

Conclusion

In conclusion, the balance of the evidence currently available regarding aeroallergen avoidance suggests that some clinical benefits can be gained from rigorous allergen remediation efforts. In general, removal of carpeting and upholstered furniture, extensive home-cleaning regimens, and encasement of mattresses and pillows with impermeable membranes can be quite costly and burdensome to sustain. For these reasons such measures are unlikely to be accepted by any but the most motivated of pet owners. Therefore, remediation efforts may best be focused on maintenance of a low indoor RH, as the simplest approach for reducing dust mite and mould spore burdens, and on pet bathing or rinsing for removal of outdoor allergens from the hair coat.

References

1. Morris DO. Human allergy to environmental pet danders: a public health perspective. *Veterinary Dermatology* 2010; **21**: 441–449.
2. Tovey ER, Marks GB. It's time to rethink mite allergen avoidance. *Journal of Allergy and Clinical Immunology* 2011; **128**: 723–727.
3. Matricardi PM. Prevalence of atopy and asthma in eastern versus western Europe: why the difference? *Annals of Allergy and Asthma Immunology* 2001; **87** (Suppl.): 24–27.
4. Sly RM. Changing prevalence of allergic rhinitis and asthma. Annals of Allergy and Asthma Immunology 1999; **82**: 233–252.
5. Hillier A. The ACVD task force on canine atopic dermatitis (I): incidence and prevalence. *Veterinary Immunology and Immunopathology* 2001; **81**: 147–151.
6. Liccardi G, D'Amato G, Russo M, *et al.* Focus on cat allergen (Fel d 1): immunological and aerodynamic characteristics, modality of airway sensitization and avoidance strategies. *International Archives of Allergy and Immunology* 2003; **132**: 1–12.
7. Peyton A, Eggleston PA, Bush RK. Environmental allergen avoidance: An overview. *Journal of Allergy and Clinical Immunology* 2001; **107**: S403–405.
8. Marsella R, Samuelson D. Unravelling the skin barrier: a new paradigm for atopic dermatitis and house dust mites. *Veterinary Dermatology* 2009; **20**: 533–540.
9. Nuttall TJ, Hill PB, Bensignor E, *et al.* House dust and forage mite allergens and their role in human and canine atopic dermatitis. *Veterinary Dermatology* 2006; **17**; 223–235.
10. Arlian LG, Schumann RJ, Morgan S, *et al.* Serum immunoglobulin E against storage mite allergens in dogs with atopic dermatitis. *American Journal of Veterinary Research* 2003; **64**: 32–36.
11. Randall A, Hillier A, Cole LK, *et al.* Quantitation of house dust mites and house dust mite allergens in the microenvironment of dogs. *American Journal of Veterinary Research* 2003; **64**: 1580–1588.
12. Raffan E, Lawrence H, Henderson T, *et al.* Prevalence of the group 1 Dermatophagoides allergens Der p 1 and Der f 1 in homes with

no dogs, healthy dogs and Dermatophagoides-sensitized atopic dogs in Liverpool. *Veterinary Dermatology* 2005; **16**: 253–260.
13. Loft KE, Rosser EJ. Group 1 and 2 Dermatophagoides house dust mite allergens in the microenvironment of cats. *Veterinary Dermatology* 2009; **21**: 152–158.
14. Wallace JC, Vogelnest LJ. Evaluation of the presence of house dust mites in horse rugs. *Veterinary Dermatology* 2010; **21**: 602–607.
15. Saridomichelakis MN, Marsella R, Lee KW, *et al.* Assessment of cross-reactivity among five species of house dust and storage mites. *Veterinary Dermatology* 2008; **19**: 67–76.
16. DeBoer DJ, Schreiner TA. Commercial dry dog food in the north central United States is not contaminated by *Dermatophagoides* house dust mites. *Veterinary Dermatology* 2001; **12**: 183–187.
17. Pilar Brazis P, Serra M, Sellés A, *et al.* Evaluation of storage mite contamination of commercial dry dog food. *Veterinary Dermatology* 2008; **19**: 209–214
18. Gill C, McEwan N, McGarry J, *et al.* House dust and storage mite contamination of dry dog food stored in open bags and sealed boxes in 10 domestic households. *Veterinary Dermatology* 2010; **22**: 162–172.
19. Swinnen C, Vroom M. The clinical effect of environmental control of house dust mites in 60 house dust mite-sensitive dogs. *Veterinary Dermatology* 2004; **15**: 31–36.
20. Boon B Tan BB, Weald D, Strickland I, *et al.* Double-blind controlled trial of effect of housedust-mite allergen avoidance on atopic dermatitis. *Lancet* 1996; **347**: 15–18.
21. Gutgesell C, Heise S, Seubert S, *et al.* Double-blind placebo-controlled house dust mite control measures in adult patients with atopic dermatitis. *British Journal of Dermatology* 2001; **145**: 70–74.
22. Gotzsche PC, Johansen HK. House dust mite control measures for asthma: systematic review. *Allergy* 2008; **63**: 646–659.
23. Arlian LG, Platts-Mills TAE. The biology of dust mites and the remediation of mite allergens in allergic disease. *Journal of Allergy and Clinical Immunology* 2001; **107**: S406–413.
24. Arlian LG, Neal JS, Morgan MS, *et al.* Reducing relative humidity is a practical way to control dust mites and their allergens in homes in temperate climates. *Journal of Allergy and Clinical Immunology* 2001; **107**: 99–104.
25. Reininger R, Varga EM, Zach M, *et al.* Detection of an allergen in dog dander that cross-reacts with the major cat allergen, Fel d 1. *Clinical and Experimental Allergy* 2007; **37**: 116–214.
26. Hill PB, DeBoer DJ. The ACVD task force on canine atopic dermatitis (IV): environmental allergens. *Veterinary Immunology and Immunopathology* 2001; **81**: 169–186.
27. Wisselink MA, van Ree R, Willemse T. Evaluation of Felis domesticus allergen I as a possible autoallergen in cats with eosinophilic granuloma complex. *American Journal of Veterinary Research* 2002; **63**: 338–341.
28. Arbes SJ, Cohn RD, Yin M, *et al.* Dog allergen (Can f 1) and cat allergen (Fel d 1) in US homes: results from the National Survey of Lead and Allergens in Homes. *Journal of Allergy and Clinical Immunology* 2004; **114**: 111–117.
29. Bush RK, Portnoy JM. The role and abatement of fungal allergens in allergic diseases. *Journal of Allergy and Clinical Immunology* 2001; **107**: S430–440.
30. Platts-Mills TA, Hayden ML, Chapman MD, *et al.* Seasonal variation in dust mite and grass-pollen allergens in dust from the houses of patients with asthma. *Journal of Allergy and Clinical Immunology* 1987; **79**: 781–791.
31. Peruzzi M, de Luca M, Novembre E, *et al.* Incidence of cockroach allergy in atopic Italian children. *Annals of Allergy* 1999; **83**: 167–171.
32. De Blay F, Sanchez J, Hedelin G, *et al.* Dust and airborne exposure to allergens derived from cockroach (Blattella germanica) in low-cost public housing in Strasbourg (France). *Journal of Allergy and Clinical Immunology* 1997; **99**: 107–112.
33. Gelber LE, Seltzer LH, Bouzoukis JK, *et al.* Sensitization and exposure to indoor allergens as risk factors for asthma among patients presenting to the hospital. *American Reviews of Respiratory Disease* 1993; **147**: 573–578.
34. Chew GL, Burge HA, Dockery DW, *et al.* Limitations of a home characteristic questionnaire as a predictor of indoor allergen levels. *American Journal of Respiratory Critical Care Medicine* 1998; **157**: 1526–1541.
35. Peyton A. Eggleston PA, Arruda LK. Ecology and elimination of cockroaches and allergens in the home. *Journal of Allergy and Clinical Immunology* 2001; **107**: S422–429.
36. Eggleston PA, Wood RA, Rand C, *et al.* Removal of cockroach allergen from inner city homes. *Journal of Allergy and Clinical Immunology* 1999; **104**: 842–846.
37. Erwin EA, Woodfolk JA, Custis N, *et al.* Animal danders. *Immunology and Allergy Clinics of North America* 2003; **23**: 469–481.
38. Torrent M, Sunyer J, Garcia R, *et al.* Early-life exposure and atopy, asthma, and wheeze up to 6 years of age. *American Journal of Respiratory Critical Care Medicine* 2007; **176**: 446–453.
39. Popplewell EJ, Innes VA, Lloyd-Hughes S, *et al.* The effect of high-efficiency and standard vacuum cleaners on mite, cat and dog allergen levels and clinical progress. *Pediatric Allergy and Immunology* 2000; **11**: 142–148.
40. Gore RB, Durrell B, Bishop S, *et al.* High-efficiency particulate arrest-filter vacuum cleaners increase personal cat allergen exposure in homes with cats. *Journal of Allergy and Clinical Immunology* 2003; **111**: 784–787.
41. Vaughan JW, Woodfolk JA, Platts-Mills TA. Assessment of vacuum cleaners and vacuum cleaner bags recommended for allergic subjects. *Journal of Allergy and Clinical Immunology* 1999; **104**: 1079–1083.
42. Green R, Simpson A, Custovic A, *et al.* The effect of air filtration on airborne dog allergen. *Allergy* 1999; **54**: 484–488.
43. Olivry T, Hill PB. The ACVD task force on canine atopic dermatitis (IX): the controversy surrounding the route of allergen challenge in canine atopic dermatitis. *Veterinary Immunology and Immunopathology* 2001; **81**: 219–225.
44. Gore RB, Bishop S, Durrell B, *et al.* Air filtration units in homes with cats: can they reduce personal exposure to cat allergen? *Clinical and Experimental Allergy* 2003; **33**: 765–769.
45. van der Heide S, van Aalderen WM, Kauffman HF, *et al.* Clinical effects of air cleaners in homes of asthmatic children sensitized to pet allergens. *Journal of Allergy and Clinical Immunology* 1999; **104**: 447–451.
46. Sulser C, Schulz G, Wagner P, *et al.* Can the use of HEPA cleaners in homes of asthmatic children and adolescents sensitized to cat and dog allergens decrease bronchial hyper-responsiveness and allergen contents in solid dust? *International Archives of Allergy and Immunology* 2009; **148**: 23–30.
47. van der Heide S, Kauffman JF, Dubois AE, *et al.* Allergen reduction measures in houses of allergic asthma patients: effects of air-cleaners and allergen-impermeable mattress covers. *European Respiratory Journal* 1997; **10**: 1217–1223.
48. Jerrim KL, Whitmore LF, Hughes JF, *et al.* Airborne dust and allergen generation during dusting with and without spray polish. *Journal of Allergy and Clinical Immunology* 2002; **109**: 63–67.
49. Ko G, Burge HA. Effects of furniture polish on release of cat allergen-laden dust from wood surfaces. *Indoor Air* 2004; **14**: 434–438.
50. Liccardi G, Russo M, Barber D, *et al.* Washing the clothes of cat owners is a simple method to prevent cat allergen dispersal. *Journal of Allergy and Clinical Immunology* 1998; **102**: 143–144.

51. Perry TT, Wood RA, Matsui EC, *et al.* Room-specific characteristics of suburban homes as predictors of indoor allergen concentrations. *Annals of Allergy and Asthma Immunology* 2006; **7**: 628–635.
52. Almqvist C, Wickman M, Perfetti L, *et al.* Worsening of asthma in children allergic to cats, after indirect exposure to cats at school. *American Journal of Respiratory Critical Care Medicine* 2001; **163**: 694–698.
53. Peroni DG, Ress M, Pigozzi R, *et al.* Efficacy in allergen control and air permeability of different materials used for bed encasement. *Allergy* 2004; **59**: 969–972.
54. Instanes C, Hetland G, Berntsen S, *et al.* Allergens and endotoxin in settled dust from day-care centers and schools in Oslo, Norway. *Indoor Air* 2005; **15**: 356–362.
55. Liccardi G, Russo M, Barber D, *et al.* Efficacy of dry-cleaning in removing Fel d 1 allergen from wool fabric exposed to cats. *Annals of Allergy and Asthma Immunology* 2002; **88**: 301–305.
56. Reininger R, Varga EM, Zach M, *et al.* Detection of an allergen in dog dander that cross-reacts with the major cat allergen, Fel d 1. *Clinical and Experimental Allergy* 2007; **37**: 116–124.
57. Choi SY, Lee IY, Sohn JH, *et al.* Optimal conditions for the removal of house dust mite, dog dander, and pollen allergens using mechanical laundry. *Annals of Allergy and Asthma Immunology* 2008; **100**: 583–588.
58. Miller JD, Miller A. Ten minutes in a clothes dryer kills all mites in blankets. *Journal of Allergy and Clinical Immunology* 1996; **97**: 423.
59. Vandehove T, Soler M, Birnbaum J, *et al.* Effect of dry cleaning on the mite allergen levels in blankets. *Allergy* 1993; **48**: 264–266.
60. Tovey ER, Taylor DJ, Mitakakis TZ, *et al.* Effectiveness of laundry washing agents and conditions in the removal of cat and dust mite allergen from bedding dust. *Journal of Allergy and Clinical Immunology* 2001; **108**: 369–374.
61. Portnoy J, Barnes C. Clinical relevance of spore and pollen counts. *Immunology and Allergy Clinics of North America* 2003; **23**: 389–410.
62. Lebel B, Bousquet J, Morel A, *et al.* Correlation between symptoms and the threshold for release of mediators in nasal secretions during nasal challenge with grass pollen grains. *Journal of Allergy and Clinical Immunology* 1988; **82**: 869–877.
63. D'Amato G, Liccardi G, Russo M, *et al.* Clothing is a carrier of cat allergens. *Journal of Allergy and Clinical Immunology* 1997; **99**: 577–578.
64. Karlsson AS, Renstrom A. Human hair is a potential source of cat allergen contamination of ambient air. *Allergy* 2005; **60**: 961–964.
65. Jackson AP, Foster AP, Hart, BJ, *et al.* Prevalence of house dust mites and dermatophagoides group 1 antigens collected from bedding, skin and hair coat of dogs in south-west England. *Veterinary Dermatology* 2005; **16**: 32–38.
66. Avner DB, Perzanowski MS, Platts-Mills TAE, *et al.* Evaluation of different techniques for washing cats: quantitation of allergen removal from the cat and the effect on airborne Fel d 1. *Journal of Allergy and Clinical Immunology* 1997; **100**: 307–312.
67. Hodson T, Custovic A, Simpson A, *et al.* Washing the dog reduces dog allergen levels but the dog needs to be washed twice a week. *Journal of Allergy and Clinical Immunology* 1999; **103**: 581–585.
68. Perzanowski MS, Wheatley LM, Avner DB, *et al.* The effectiveness of Allerpet/c in reducing the cat allergen Fel d 1. *Journal of Allergy and Clinical Immunology* 1997; **100**: 428–430.
69. Löflath A, von Voigts-Rhetz A, Jaeger K, *et al.* The efficacy of a commercial shampoo and whirlpooling in the treatment of canine pruritus—a double-blinded, randomized, placebo-controlled study. *Veterinary Dermatology* 2007; **18**: 427–431.
70. Marsalla R, Nicklin C, Lopez J. Evaluation of the effects of Allerase® spray on clinical signs in house dust mite allergic high IgE Beagle dogs using a randomized, double blinded, placebo controlled design. *Veterinary Dermatology* 2005; **16**: 202.

12

Allergen-specific immunotherapy

Ralf S. Mueller

Centre for Clinical Veterinary Medicine, Ludwig Maximilian University, Munich, Germany

Conflict of interest: in the last 5 years, Ralf Mueller has obtained funding, lectured, or consulted for Almapharm, Dermcare, Bayer Animal Health, Boehringer Ingelheim, Dechra Veterinary Products, Intervet, Merial, Novartis Animal Health, Pfizer Animal Health, Procter and Gamble, Royal Canin, Selectavet, and Virbac.

Introduction

Atopic disease in humans was rare, when it was first reported more than a century ago. Allergen-specific immunotherapy (ASIT) in humans was reported as early as 1911 by Noon [1]. With the dramatic increase of the prevalence of allergic diseases in the last 50 years, this treatment modality became a topic of major research interest because it is the only specific therapy for atopy. With the advent of veterinary specialization in the last four decades, ASIT has also become a topic of interest for veterinarians and is now available widely in the developed world. However, there is still a marked paucity of published scientific information about ASIT. Although there are a number of case reports and retrospective case cohort studies [2], the literature contains only a few prospective and blinded studies [3–5]. In 2009, a non-systematic review attempted to summarize the most current information and concluded that there was a great need for further studies in veterinary medicine on this treatment modality [2].

Most of the research has been undertaken on dogs, although there are some publications about ASIT in cats and horses and individual case reports in other species. In this chapter the focus is on canine atopic dermatitis (CAD). A short summary of the mechanism of action of ASIT is followed by some information about the selection of allergens for the extract, the efficacy and protocol of conventional immunotherapy, factors possibly influencing treatment outcome, and adverse effects. Special subsets of ASIT, such as rush, intralymphatic, and sublingual immunotherapy, are discussed briefly, although not much information is available in the veterinary literature about those routes at this point.

Mechanism of action

Allergen-specific immunotherapy in dogs has been associated with an increase of allergen-specific serum IgG within the first 6 months of treatment [6,7]. These so-called 'blocking antibodies' are thought to decrease availability of antigen for mast cell-bound allergen-specific IgE in humans [8]. In the two studies in dogs, the increase of IgG was not correlated with the clinical response [6,7]. Allergen-specific serum IgE did not decrease with clinical signs, but rather increased initially, although this increase was less pronounced in those dogs that responded clinically. Despite this initial difference between the species, after 1 year, successful immunotherapy led to a decrease in allergen-specific IgE in dogs [9].

More recently, T cells have been the focus of research in atopic dermatitis, in both humans and dogs. An

Veterinary Allergy, First Edition. Edited by Chiara Noli, Aiden Foster, and Wayne Rosenkrantz.

imbalance between T helper 1 and T helper 2 cells was identified in atopic dermatitis of humans and dogs [10–12]. In humans an increase in regulatory T cells with ASIT was identified [11]. Similar changes have been noted in dogs. In a study of ten dogs with atopic dermatitis the IFN-gamma/IL-4 ratio significantly increased with ASIT [13]. In a more recent study evaluating dogs with atopic dermatitis before and 12 months after ASIT, regulatory T cell numbers more than doubled and serum concentrations of IL-10 significantly increased compared to a healthy control group. Numbers of regulatory T cells as well as concentrations of serum IL-10 were higher in those dogs that responded to therapy than in the non-responders [9].

Based on these limited studies, successful ASIT for CAD seems to be associated with an increased regulatory T-cell response, which is similar to observations in human medicine.

Selection of allergens

'Allergy' testing must be undertaken in order to identify clinically significant allergens for inclusion in the ASIT. Intradermal testing was considered the gold standard for years when many of the early serum tests were not very accurate [14]. With the validated tests developed in recent years, serum testing has become far more reliable [15]. Independent of the test, it is essential that allergens for the treatment extract are selected based on a careful correlation between the test results and clinical history. Positive reactions with intradermal testing to house dust mite and storage mite antigens have been reported in normal dogs [16,17]. Similarly, tests for dust mite-specific serum IgE were positive in normal dogs [16]. If an allergen is included in the extract that is not involved in the clinical disease then improvement seems an unlikely outcome and, more importantly, there is a risk of sensitization of the dog. Thus, in a dog living in a temperate climate, exhibiting pruritus exclusively in autumn and winter and showing test reactions to birch pollens (which pollinate in early spring), ASIT with birch pollens will probably not lead to a satisfactory treatment outcome and may even be contraindicated.

Conventional allergen-specific immunotherapy

Protocol of conventional allergen-specific immunotherapy

In conventional ASIT the allergen extract is administered subcutaneously in steadily increasing volumes and concentrations during an induction period of several weeks to months [2]. The concentration of an allergen extract is measured differently in different studies and with allergens from different companies, and may be stated for example in protein nitrogen units (PNU), biological activity, reactive indices, or molecular weight. These measures are not directly translatable, consequently comparison of the various published studies is difficult. However, they generally have shown a similar approximate success rate in larger case cohorts (see section 'Efficacy of ASIT') [5,18–23]. Allergens in the induction period are typically first injected at a dilution of 1 : 10 to 1 : 100 of the allergen extract and then gradually increased to the final concentration.

In many dogs the dose and frequency of allergen injections need to be tailored based on the individual response in the induction and/or the maintenance therapy phases [20]. Two common scenarios may be encountered and a general rule can be applied. Some dogs repeatedly show increased pruritus following the ASIT injection, which gradually resolves over the next few days. A repeat treatment produces a repeat 'post injection flare'. In this case the dose should be decreased. Another pattern is when dogs tolerate injections well but the pruritus increases with time until the next injection leads to a reduction/resolution of the pruritus. In this circumstance (preinjection flare) the injections should be administered more often. This adjustment requires experience, patience, and excellent client communications, and without them an optimal outcome is impossible.

Efficacy of allergen-specific immunotherapy

It is difficult to compare different studies due to the different protocols, definitions of treatment success, and different follow-up periods [2]. Evaluation is further complicated by the fact that only one placebo-controlled, randomized study has been published [5]. A few other studies have compared different ASIT protocols in a randomized, blinded fashion [3,4], but most reports are retrospective case series, albeit with larger numbers of dogs [18–23]. Even so, when evaluating all those reports a common picture emerges. Approximately 20% of the dogs respond excellently with no further need for medications. In a larger number of dogs (40–50%), the outcome is satisfactory, clinical signs improve, and the need for concurrent medication decreases. The residual 30–40% of the dogs either show unsatisfactory response or do not improve at all. The time until response to treatment is highly variable. Improvement is reported after 2 to 9 months in most dogs [2].

Factors potentially influencing treatment outcome

In contrast to humans, the age of the dog or duration of the disease does not seem to influence the success rate of ASIT [2]. Similarly, at this point, there is no consistent evidence that either gender or breed of the dog, type and number of the allergens or the seasonality of the disease, or signs influence the treatment outcome [2].

It has been reported that mould proteases degrade pollen allergens when stored in the same vial [24,25]. It has been questioned whether this degradation has real immunologic consequences. However, in one study evaluating ASIT in dogs with atopic dermatitis, the success rate was much lower with allergen treatment sets which contained both moulds and pollens than with those which contained no mould antigens [18]. Subsequently, mould and pollen antigens were dispensed in separate vials and the success rate of ASIT containing mould antigens increased and was comparable to that of ASIT containing pollens alone [21]. All of those studies were conducted with aqueous allergens. Further studies evaluating the influence of moulds on pollen antigens in ASIT are urgently needed.

Some studies compare high- or low-dose immunotherapy protocols with conventional doses. An increased response rate of 85% versus 68% was noted when using an increased maintenance concentration of allergen (40 000 PNU/mL) versus the conventional concentration of 20 000 PNU/mL and defining a response as symptom improvement of more than 50% [26]. However, low-dose protocols have also been reported as efficacious [27]. In the light of published results and the differences in allergen requirements of individual dogs, no consistent trend emerges and the allergen concentration is best determined on the basis of the individual dog's response.

Adverse effects of allergen-specific immunotherapy

The most common adverse effect reported is increased pruritus after the injection, which is seen in up to 50% of the dogs [20]. Usually a decrease in the amount of allergen injected will resolve this reaction pattern. Premedication with an antihistamine has also been advocated and is recommended by some veterinary dermatologists as a routine treatment on the morning of the "allergy shot". Localized reactions such as small nodules at the site of injection are rare and do not require treatment. Systemic adverse effects occur in approximately 1% of the dogs and include diarrhoea, vomiting, anxiety, depression, weakness, urticaria/angioedema, and anaphylaxis [2]. Their severity will determine symptomatic treatment; subsequent allergen injections should be modified and administered after premedication of the dog with antihistamines or even low-dose glucocorticoids. In the event of an anaphylactic/anaphylactoid reaction, adrenaline is the initial treatment of choice; antihistamines and/or glucocorticoids may be additionally administered. Subsequently, injections must be administered under direct medical supervision. There are anecdotal reports of dogs that have exhibited an anaphylactic reaction once, but have gone on to complete their ASIT with no further adverse effects (under direct medical supervision and preinjection antihistamine administration) but many owners will choose not to continue with such therapy.

Rush immunotherapy

In humans rush protocols abbreviating the induction period to one or a few days have been reported. These protocols lead to a faster response rate although half the patients have been reported to show adverse effects and thus rush immunotherapy in humans is usually conducted in hospitalized patients. Rush immunotherapy has also been reported in dogs [4,28–30]. Dogs are hospitalized for a day and premedicated with an antihistamine. Injections are administered every 30 minutes and the dogs are discharged on the maintenance dose [29]. In a double-blind, randomized trial rush immunotherapy was as effective as conventional immunotherapy for the treatment of CAD [4]. The time to maximal resolution was shorter than with conventional ASIT (6.8 versus 9.2 months) but this difference was not statistically significant. The only adverse effect seen was increased pruritus in some dogs toward the end of the first day. One advantage of rush immunotherapy unique to veterinary medicine, where owners frequently administer the allergen injections themselves, is the decreased likelihood of confusion about how much to inject out of which of the (up to three) different vials. With the rush therapy owners and dogs go home with one maintenance vial and a specific dose given at specific intervals, which of course may also be altered to suit the individual. Rush immunotherapy has been routinely used in the author's clinic for almost a decade.

Intralymphatic immunotherapy

Intralymphatic immunotherapy in 14 dogs that failed conventional ASIT was reported in a short abstract [31]. Eight of the dogs showed complete remission after therapy. This concept was further evaluated in a mouse model where an increased IgG and T-cell response was seen in sensitized mice after intralymphatic ASIT when compared to subcutaneous ASIT [32]. In humans with rhinoconjunctivitis, three intralymphatic injections with allergens increased tolerance to intranasal provocation, caused fewer adverse effects than 3 years of subcutaneous ASIT, and were less painful than venipuncture [33]. A double-blind, randomized study compared intralymphatic ASIT using aqueous allergens with subcutaneous ASIT in dogs [34]. A small amount of allergen extract (0.08 mL) was injected under ultrasound guidance into the submandibular lymph node four times within a 2-month period. After 2 months of therapy there was a more prominent decrease in pruritus and lesion scores in the intralymphatic treatment group, although the difference was not significant. Based on these data, intralymphatic therapy is as effective short term as conventional immunotherapy although long-term data are lacking.

Sublingual immunotherapy

A number of studies evaluating sublingual immunotherapy in humans have been published over more than two decades. It has been shown that there are distinct immunologic changes with this therapy, induced by a sophisticated immunological network in the oral mucosa [35]. In veterinary medicine such sublingual immunotherapy has been conducted in individual cases but evidence has been largely anecdotal. A pilot trial of sublingual immunotherapy was reported in ten dogs allergic to house dust mites [36]. After 6 months, eight dogs had improved on average by 72% in relation to the pruritus. Median CADESI scores and mean methylprednisolone use also declined significantly [36]. This improvement was associated with a significant decrease in dust mite-specific serum IgE [37]. Although the number of dogs evaluated was small, sublingual immunotherapy could become an interesting treatment alternative in years to come.

Allergen-specific immunotherapy and concurrent drug therapy

Atopic animals often require concurrent medical therapy. However, many of these immunomodulatory drugs could possibly influence the T-cell response to ASIT. In humans, montelukast treatment significantly impaired the induction of regulatory T cells [38]. Similarly, oral prednisolone led to a decreased efficacy of ASIT in asthmatic children [39]. H1 antihistamines reduced adverse effects during ASIT with honeybee venom without affecting the efficacy [40]. This was in contrast to mice, where the efficacy of bee venom immunotherapy was reduced by the H1-receptor antagonist clemastine [41]. To the author's knowledge, no such studies have been conducted in dogs, cats, or horses. It seems logical that drugs suppressing T-cell response may also suppress the induction of regulatory T cells associated with successful therapy. However, studies are urgently needed to assess if, and at what dose, this inhibition is decreasing response to ASIT in a clinically relevant fashion.

References

1. Noon L. Prophylactic inoculation against hay fever. *Lancet* 1911; **177**: 1572–1573.
2. Löewenstein C, Mueller RS. A review of allergen-specific immunotherapy in human and veterinary medicine. *Veterinary Dermatology* 2009; **20**: 84–98.
3. Colombo S, Hill PB, Shaw DJ, *et al.* Effectiveness of low dose immunotherapy in the treatment of canine atopic dermatitis: a prospective, double-blinded, clinical study. *Veterinary Dermatology* 2005; **16**: 162–170.
4. Mueller RS, Fieseler KV, Zabel S, *et al.* Conventional and rush immunotherapy in the treatment of canine atopic dermatitis. In: Hillier A, Foster AP, Kwochka KW, eds. *Advances in Veterinary Dermatology*, Vol. 5. Oxford: Blackwell Publishing, 2005: 61–69.
5. Willemse A, Van den Brom WE, Rijnberk A. Effect of hyposensitization on atopic dermatitis in dogs. *Journal of the American Veterinary Medical Association* 1984; **184**: 1277–1280.
6. Fraser MA, McNeil PE, Gettinby G. Examination of serum total IgG1 concentration in atopic and non-atopic dogs. *Journal of Small Animal Practice* 2004; **45**: 186–190.
7. Hites MJ, Kleinbeck ML, Loker JL, *et al.* Effect of immunotherapy on the serum concentrations of allergen-specific IgG antibodies in dog sera. *Veterinary Immunology and Immunopathology* 1989; **22**: 39–51.
8. Mothes N, Heinzkill M, Drachenberg KJ, *et al.* Allergen-specific immunotherapy with a monophosphoryl lipid A-adjuvanted vaccine: reduced seasonally boosted immunoglobulin E production and inhibition of basophil histamine release by therapy-induced blocking antibodies. *Clinical and Experimental Allergy* 2003; **33**: 1198–1208.
9. Keppel KE, Campbell KL, Zuckermann FA, *et al.* Quantitation of canine regulatory T cell populations, serum interleukin-10 and allergen-specific IgE concentrations in healthy control dogs and canine atopic dermatitis patients receiving allergen-specific immunotherapy. *Veterinary Immunology and Immunopathology* 2008; **123**: 337–344.
10. Varney VA, Hamid QA, Gaga M, *et al.* Influence of grass pollen immunotherapy on cellular infiltration and cytokine mRNA expression during allergen-induced late-phase cutaneous responses. *Journal of Clinical Investigation* 1993; **92**: 644–651.
11. Jutel M, Akdis M, Budak F, *et al.* IL-10 and TGF-beta cooperate in the regulatory T cell response to mucosal allergens in normal immunity and specific immunotherapy. *European Journal of Immunology* 2003; **33**: 1205–1214.
12. Nuttall TJ, Knight PA, McAleese SM, *et al.* Expression of Th1, Th2 and immunosuppressive cytokine gene transcripts in canine atopic dermatitis. *Clinical and Experimental Allergy* 2002; **32**: 789–795.
13. Shida M, Kadoya M, Park SJ, *et al.* Allergen-specific immunotherapy induces Th1 shift in dogs with atopic dermatitis. *Veterinary Immunology and Immunopathology* 2004; **102**: 19–31.
14. Plant J. The reproducibility of three in-vitro canine allergy tests: a pilot study. In: *Proceedings of the 10th Annual Meeting of the American Academy of Veterinary Dermatology and the American College of Veterinary Dermatology*, 1994: 16–18.
15. Thom N, Favrot C, Failing K, *et al.* Intra- and interlaboratory variability of allergen-specific IgE levels in atopic dogs in three different laboratories using the Fc-epsilon receptor testing.

Veterinary Immunology and Immunopathology 2010; **133**: 183–189.
16. Lian TM, Halliwell RE. Allergen-specific IgE and IgGd antibodies in atopic and normal dogs. *Veterinary Immunology and Immunopathology* 1998; **66**: 203–223.
17. Mueller RS, Fieseler KV, Rosychuk RA, *et al.* Intradermal testing with the storage mite *Tyrophagus putrescentiae* in normal dogs and dogs with atopic dermatitis in Colorado. *Veterinary Dermatology* 2005; **16**: 27–31.
18. Mueller RS, Bettenay SV. Long-term immunotherapy of 146 dogs with atopic dermatitis—a retrospective study. *Australian Veterinary Practitioner* 1996; **26**: 128–132.
19. Nuttall TJ, Thoday KL, van den Broek AH, *et al.* Retrospective survey of allergen immunotherapy in canine atopy. *Veterinary Record* 1998; **143**: 139–142.
20. Rosser EJ. Aqueous hyposensitization in the treatment of canine atopic dermatitis: a retrospective and prospective study of 100 cases. In: Kwochka KW, Willemse T, von Tscharner C, eds. *Advances in Veterinary Dermatology*, Vol. 3. Oxford: Butterworth Heinemann, 1998: 169–176.
21. Schnabl B, Bettenay SV, Dow K, *et al.* Results of allergen-specific immunotherapy in 117 dogs with atopic dermatitis. *Veterinary Record* 2006; **158**: 81–85.
22. Scott KV, White SD, Rosychuk RAW. A retrospective study of hyposensitization in atopic dogs in a flea-scarce environment. In: Ihrke PJ, Mason IS, White SD, eds. *Advances in Veterinary Dermatology*, Vol. 2. Oxford: Pergamon Press, 1992: 79–87.
23. Zur G, White SD, Ihrke PJ, *et al.* Canine atopic dermatitis: a retrospective study of 169 cases examined at the University of California, Davis, 1992–1998. Part II. Response to hyposensitization. *Veterinary Dermatology* 2002; **13**: 103–111.
24. Esch B. Role of proteases on the stability of allergenic extracts. Arbeiten aus dem Paul Ehrlich Institut (Bundesamt für Sera und Impfstoffe) zu Frankfurt am Main 1992; **85**: 171–177.
25. Rosenbaum MR, Esch RE, Schwartzman RM. Effects of mold proteases on the biological activity of allergenic pollen extracts. *American Journal of Veterinary Research* 1996; **57**: 1447–1452.
26. Garfield RA. Injection immunotherapy in the treatment of canine atopic dermatitis: a comparison of three hyposensitization protocols. In: *Proceedings of the 8th Annual conference of the American Academy of Veterinary Dermatology and American College of Veterinary Dermatology*, 1992: 7–8.
27. Wagner R. A retrospective study of hyposensitization using low concentrations of alum-precipitated allergens. In: *Proceedings of the 15th Annual Congress of the European Society of Veterinary Dermatology and the European College of Veterinary Dermatology*, 1998: 167.
28. McDonald JM. Rush hyposensitization in the treatment of canine atopy. In: *Proceedings of the 15th Annual Meeting of the American Academy of Veterinary Dermatology and the American College of Veterinary Dermatology*, 1999: 95–97.
29. Mueller RS, Bettenay SV. Evaluation of the safety of an abbreviated course of injections of allergen extracts (rush immunotherapy) for the treatment of dogs with atopic dermatitis. *American Journal of Veterinary Research* 2001; **62**: 307–310.
30. Paterson R, Harris KE. Rush immunotherapy in a dog with severe ragweed and grass pollen allergy. *Annals of Asthma, Allergy and Immunology* 1999; **83**: 213–216.
31. Juillard GJ, Bubbers JE. Experimental intralymphatic immunotherapy of canine allergic disease. *Federation Proceedings of the 67th Annual Meeting of the American Societies for Experimental Biology* 1983; **42**: 441.
32. Martinez-Gomez JM, Johansen P, Erdmann I, *et al.* Intralymphatic injections as a new administration route for allergen-specific immunotherapy. *International Archives of Allergy and Immunology* 2009; **150**: 59–65.
33. Senti G, Prinz Vavricka BM, Erdmann I, *et al.* Intralymphatic allergen administration renders specific immunotherapy faster and safer: a randomized controlled trial. *Proceedings of the National Academy of Sciences of the United States of America* 2008; **105**: 17908–17912.
34. Hatzmann K, Mueller RS. Practicability and safety of intralymphatic allergen-specific immunotherapy in dogs with atopic dermatitis. *Veterinary Dermatology* 2011; **22**: 463–464.
35. Novak N, Bieber T, Allam JP. Immunological mechanisms of sublingual allergen-specific immunotherapy. *Allergy* 2011; **66**: 733–739.
36. DeBoer DJ, Verbrugge M, Morris M. Pilot trial of sublingual immunotherapy (SLIT) in mite-sensitive atopic dogs. *Veterinary Dermatology* 2010; **21**: 325.
37. DeBoer DJ, Verbrugge M, Morris M. Changes in mite-specific IgE and IgG levels during sublingual immunotherapy (SLIT) in dust-mite sensitive dogs with atopic dermatitis. *Veterinary Dermatology* 2010; **21**: 531–532.
38. Majak P, Rychlik B, Pulaski L, *et al.* Montelukast treatment may alter the early efficacy of immunotherapy in children with asthma. *Journal of Allergy and Clinical Immunology* 2010; **125**: 1220–1227.
39. Majak P, Rychlik B, Stelmach I. The effect of oral steroids with and without vitamin D3 on early efficacy of immunotherapy in asthmatic children. *Clinical and Experimental Allergy* 2009; **39**: 1830–1841.
40. Müller UR, Jutel M, ReimersA, *et al.* Clinical and immunologic effects of H1 antihistamine preventive medication during honeybee venom immunotherapy. *Journal of Allergy and Clinical Immunology* 2008; **122**: 1001–1007.
41. Johansen P, Senti G, Gomez MM, *et al.* Medication with antihistamines impairs allergen-specific immunotherapy in mice. *Clinical and Experimental Allergy* 2008; **38**: 512–519.

13

Guidelines for symptomatic medical treatment of canine atopic dermatitis

Douglas J. DeBoer

Department of Medical Sciences, School of Veterinary Medicine, University of Wisconsin–Madison, Madison, WI, USA

Conflict of interest: consultant for Zoetis, Inc.

With recognition of the complexity of the pathogenesis of canine atopic dermatitis (CAD), we now also recognize that treatment approaches must be individualized and flexible, must combine several modes of therapy, and must be aimed at both the primary disease and at secondary complications. Within this integrated approach, we see each of the potential treatment elements as 'tools'. Our goal with each dog is to find just the right combination of tools that will provide lifelong therapy that is effective, affordable, convenient, and with as few adverse effects as possible. This combination will vary with both individual patient characteristics and with owner preferences. This chapter will discuss the elements of successful treatment plans and how these elements are best combined for different clinical situations. The focus will be on conventional medical management, though with recognition that drug treatment is only part of a successful therapy. Information on other elements such as avoidance, allergen-specific immunotherapy, and unconventional drug treatments can be found in other chapters of this volume.

An integrated approach to treatment

Historically, management of CAD has been aimed at the end process of the disease, in other words focused on anti-inflammatory therapies. 'Managing inflammation' was the first goal of therapy. This traditional approach was a rather blunt instrument, often consisting principally of oral corticosteroids, with antihistamines or fatty acids as possible adjuncts. As our understanding grew, we gained additional tools to manage the inflammation, for example the calcineurin inhibitors such as ciclosporin and effective topical corticosteroid products that could manage inflammation with less systemic effect. We also gained a renewed understanding of the importance of treating secondary complications such as bacterial and yeast infections. All of these approaches, even as they evolved, were still completely *reactive*—reacting to the inflammatory process, after it had already become well established in the skin.

A newer approach to treating CAD encompasses a broader, whole-patient view, stressing a multifaceted approach, based on a multifaceted pathogenesis and multifaceted clinical signs, which are likely different in each patient. In addition, where possible we now stress a *proactive* approach to treatment—in other words, correcting the underlying pathogenesis of the disease where possible, preventing acute flares where we can, and forestalling the development of chronic inflammatory changes in the skin that become much more difficult to reverse. Important elements of this new approach include:

- identification and elimination of relevant allergens (avoidance) where possible, especially any food or parasite allergens;

Veterinary Allergy, First Edition. Edited by Chiara Noli, Aiden Foster, and Wayne Rosenkrantz.

- control of secondary infections, which contribute to discomfort and augment the allergic and inflammatory responses;
- restoration of the epidermal barrier, to reduce entry of allergens and irritants and reduce colonization by micro-organisms;
- modification of the aberrant immunologic response through allergen-specific immunotherapy;
- careful use of medications to manage of any remaining inflammatory and pruritic response that persists despite the above measures.

This new approach also requires renewed efforts at educating clients about treatment of CAD. Therapies such as improvement of epidermal barrier function and modification of the immune response are 'proactive treatments', which will not work instantly as do the 'reactive treatments' such as anti-inflammatory drugs. They are not expected to produce immediate results but rather, gradual, prolonged improvement over a longer time period. Owners must be educated that this preventive approach represents our best chance of controlling this lifelong disease with minimal use of drugs that may be detrimental over the long term.

Evidence-based guidelines for treatment of canine atopic dermatitis

Published systematic reviews on drug treatment of CAD [1–3] provide evidence-based, rational information on successful therapy. In addition, the development of 'Practice Guidelines' is a newer concept that applies principles of evidence-based medicine to treatment of the most common clinical patient presentations, providing practical recommendations to assist clinicians in choosing effective treatment protocols. The International Task Force on Canine Atopic Dermatitis, an independent group of clinicians and researchers in veterinary allergy, published a set of Practice Guidelines for CAD, which can be downloaded free of cost [4] in many different languages. These guidelines stress that one approach or set of therapies is appropriate for short-term or immediate management of sudden flares of clinical signs. A second approach is used in parallel, in an attempt to gain longer-term control of the disease. These evidence-based guidelines will form the basis of the treatment recommendations made in this chapter.

Managing acute flares of canine atopic dermatitis

The most common clinical situation faced by a veterinarian in treating CAD is an acute flare, i.e. the dog whose clinical signs have gone out of control. This may be a first-time visit by an owner of a dog with mild, perhaps even longstanding, disease that has finally reached the point where additional intervention is necessary. Alternatively, it may be a sudden flare in a dog previously well-controlled on a steady management plan. The patient may have erupted with lesions, may be so pruritic as to be causing extensive self-trauma, and may be dramatically affecting the owner's own quality of life through frustration and lack of sleep. In any clinic visit with these characteristics, treating acute flares should focus on three important elements of the clinical situation: (1) identification and elimination of flare factors; (2) improvement of skin and coat hygiene and care; and (3) reducing pruritus and lesions with short-term medication.

Identification and elimination of flare factors

Flare factors are short-term alterations in the pet's environment or clinical status that have caused an immediate worsening of clinical signs. Such factors as varying environmental exposure (pollen counts, etc.) may be responsible for the flare, as might things as simple as development of flea infestation, or dietary indiscretion in a dog with a food-hypersensitivity component to their disease. These factors need to be considered, and eliminated where possible. *Perhaps the most common factor in an acute flare—and one of the most commonly overlooked—is the development of a staphylococcal or yeast infection.* Identification and treatment of such infections are paramount; both as a short-term consideration and in a longer-term preventive approach, and should be a primary question in the clinician's mind when examining a dog in acute flare. Examination and diagnostic evaluations such as cytology should be followed by appropriate systemic and/or topical antimicrobial treatment, based upon culture and susceptibility if necessary. Experienced dermatologists frequently find that merely identifying and treating secondary skin infections produces rapid and substantial remission of overall clinical signs without the necessity of resorting to administration of corticosteroids.

Improving skin and coat hygiene and care

A number of studies have demonstrated the benefit of frequent bathing in CAD [5,6]. Bathing provides multiple beneficial actions, including providing temporary relief from pruritus, removal of microbial and environmental allergens from the skin and hair coat, and limiting further microbial colonization of the skin. Much of the benefit may come merely from the action of mechanical washing with any non-irritating cleansing shampoo and twice-weekly bathing for at least the first month is recommended. From an evidence-based standpoint, there is no demonstrated consistent superiority of any specific shampoo product and no evidence for increased efficacy of shampoos containing ingredients such as oatmeal, local anaesthetics, or antihistamines. Clinicians should therefore select a shampoo based on other details of the specific case. For example dogs with active infections (or those prone to development of such infections) are best treated with a shampoo containing antimicrobial ingredients such as chlorhexidine and/or an azole antifungal; dogs with a strong tendency to develop secondary seborrhoea may best be served by bathing in an antiseborrhoeic formulation containing ingredients such as sulphur, salicylic acid, or phytosphingosine.

Reducing pruritus and lesions with short-term medications: What works and what doesn't?

In the situation of an acute flare, after infections have been considered and treated, a brief course of oral corticosteroids is a frequent treatment of choice if the pruritus is widespread. Systemic corticosteroids generally provide rapid and effective control of pruritus in CAD (Box 13.1) and are a useful and important 'rescue treatment' for acute flares, though much less satisfactory for long-term use due to the potential for development of adverse effects.

Box 13.1 Therapy capsule: Oral corticosteroids

Effectiveness: Typically very effective, and safe short-term (up to 3–4 months per year) or intermittently. With longer-term use, effectiveness may decline substantially due to corticosteroid 'resistance' or tachyphylaxis and adverse effects become limiting.

Adverse effects: Short-term — olyuria, polydypsia, polyphagia, possible behavioural changes, panting. With long-term use, signs of iatrogenic hyperadrenocorticism common, including alopecia, thin skin, pendulous abdomen, etc. Less commonly, calcinosis cutis, steroid hepatopathy, and/or diabetes mellitus possible with long-term treatment.

Dosing: Prednisone or prednisolone, induction dose of 0.5–1 mg/kg per day (as a single daily dose or divided) until remission, typically 5–7 days, then gradual tapering to maintenance dose of 0.25–0.5 mg/kg or less, every other day. Concurrent administration of fatty acid supplements or antihistamines may help to lower required dosage over the long term.

Patient monitoring: Not necessary if short-term; with long-term use monitor for silent urinary tract infection with urine culture 1–2 times annually. Monitor liver enzymes annually. Corticosteroids induce alkaline phosphatase and elevations are expected; ALT/AST elevations indicate development of steroid hepatopathy and may require discontinuation of therapy.

A pet with more localized signs can often be rapidly controlled with a topically applied corticosteroid product, several of which provide equivalent therapeutic response without the systemic effects of an oral glucocorticoid [7,8] (Box 13.2).

Although not available for review at the time the Practice Guidelines were first published, new non-steroidal drugs have the potential to rapidly reduce the pruritus and inflammatory changes of CAD without glucocorticoid adverse effects. In particular, the Janus Kinase (JAK) inhibitor drug oclacitinib has shown great promise of effectiveness in both canine models of pruritus and in early clinical trials of atopic dogs [9,10]. The JAK enzymes are a family of molecules that associate with various cell-surface receptors, and function in cellular signaling. They are important in many different processes including those related to immune function, inflammation, and hematopoiesis. Oclacitinib targets JAK-1, resulting in inhibition of inflammation and pruritus mediated by cytokines including interleukin-31 and others, while preserving other critical JAK functions. It represents a new and important therapeutic option for acute control of CAD and other pruritic, allergic skin conditions (Box 13.3).

Considering specifically the case of an acute flare of CAD where rapid relief is desired, interventions of little or no benefit in this clinical situation include antihistamines, fatty acid supplements, and calcineurin inhibitors such as ciclosporin. Fatty acid supplements may be beneficial in the long term (see discussion in section 'Improvement of skin condition and epidermal barrier function'), but their slow onset of action (typically occurring over months of time) makes them inappropriate for acute use. Likewise, though ciclosporin is often an extremely effective treatment over time, it may take several weeks to have a substantial effect, thus limiting its usefulness as an acute rescue medication.

Box 13.2 Therapy capsule: Topical corticosteroids

Effectiveness: Approved products (see 'Dosing' in this box) often at least as effective as oral corticosteroids, but best suited for regional inflammation rather than generalized due to mechanics of application. Weaker steroid preparations such as 1% hydrocortisone are of unproven efficacy.

Adverse effects: Alopecia and thinning of skin reported with chronic use in some dogs; generally no systemic effects.

Dosing: Triamcinolone 0.015% or hydrocortisone aceponate 0.054% per label instructions. Daily application is necessary until remission; taper to every 2–3 days for maintenance if possible.

Patient monitoring: No specific monitoring necessary.

Box 13.3 Therapy capsule: Oclacitinib

Effectiveness: Clear evidence for effectiveness in CAD and other pruritic allergic skin diseases, with approximately 49–67% of patients showing benefit. Rapid onset of efficacy makes drug appropriate for acute as well as chronic use.

Adverse effects: Short-term gastrointestinal upset in 3–5% of dogs; typically mild and self-limiting.

Dosing: Starting dose of 0.4–0.6 mg/kg twice daily for up to 14 days, then reduce to same dose once daily if used longer. Not for use in dogs under 12 months of age, or in dogs with serious infections, demodicosis, or neoplastic conditions.

Patient monitoring: Monitor patient for development of infections, demodicosis, or neoplasia with appropriate examinations and testing. At present no specific monitoring interval is recommended, but prudence would dictate at least once annually until we gain more long-term experience with this newly-approved drug.

From a strictly evidence-based point of view, there is no convincing evidence that conventional antihistamines are beneficial in treating CAD, especially in an acute and severe flare. In fact, the majority of studies of antihistamines in CAD provide either poor-quality evidence of effectiveness, or else conclude that antihistamines are no more effective than placebo [1,3]. Despite this gap, many owners and clinicians do perceive that antihistamines provide some benefit to their atopic dogs [11] and current evidence may be overridden by future studies of use in different clinical situations. It may be, for example, that antihistamines provide such a small level of improvement that it is not apparent in placebo-controlled studies of patients with moderately severe disease, but that very mildly affected dogs may benefit more; or, as some have suggested, that antihistamines may be useful as synergistic medications when combined with corticosteroids or other drugs [12,13]. These clinical situations have not been studied adequately. The current uncertainty regarding antihistamine use has led many clinicians to conclude that, especially considering their low cost and safety, it is reasonable to propose them, especially in dogs with mild signs (Box 13.4).

Box 13.4 Therapy capsule: Antihistamines

Effectiveness: Limited study to date provides insufficient evidence for effectiveness. Popular perception suggests limited effectiveness in mild cases, or when combined with other drugs. Thus, even in the face of limited rationale, antihistamines are often tried as part of therapy. No evidence for greater effectiveness of newer, non-sedating antihistamines as used for human allergy (e.g. loratidine, cetirizine, fexofenadine).

Adverse effects: Drugs appear safe for longer-term use without adverse effects. Some owners report mild sedative effects, but this has not been strictly documented in dogs.

Dosing: Diphenhydramine or hydroxyzine, 2 mg/kg 2–3 times daily as needed; cetirizine, 0.5–1 mg/kg q 24 hr.

Patient monitoring: No specific monitoring necessary.

Long-term management of chronic atopic dermatitis

After the inflammation of an acute flare is extinguished, the clinician and owner must focus on a management plan consisting of treatments that will provide safe, effective, long-term relief. Again, client communication is important here: owners must be told explicitly that CAD is a lifelong, controllable, but not curable disease. Owners should expect that treatment will not go perfectly—there will be relapses and secondary problems, and they should plan on higher-than-normal medical care costs over the pet's life. The owner must be made aware of the 'integrated approach' concepts and accept that maximum clinical benefit occurs only over time. For the owner and dog presented with a goal of developing a long-term management plan, the following treatment elements should be especially considered and discussed with the owner: (1) identification and *avoidance* of flare factors; (2) long-term improvement of skin condition, including consideration of epidermal barrier function; (3) options for long-term treatment with medications; and (4) modifying the underlying disease pathogenesis where possible.

Identification and avoidance of flare factors

Many clinicians have observed that the factors responsible for flare in individual patients tend to be repeated over time. Thus, in long-term treatment emphasis must be given to identifying which flare factors are historically and typically important for the particular dog and instituting measures to prevent additional flares. For example, if fleas have been a periodic or recurring factor, monthly parasite preventive treatment should be instituted. If flares typically occur during a certain time of year due to increases in pollen count, it may be helpful to prospectively and temporarily institute (or increase the dose of) medications during this season for best control.

Because infections are so commonly implicated as flare factors, consideration should be given to reducing skin colonization longer term with regular application of topical products containing such ingredients as chlorhexidine, phytosphingosine, azole antifungal drugs, nisin, or hypochlorite ions. Such preventive therapy must be made easy for the owner to comply with long term. For example, through periodic bathing will still be helpful, use of convenient disinfectant wipes, sprays, or foam mousse formulations allow more frequent application of these ingredients with greater ease.

Improvement of skin condition and epidermal barrier function

In addition to bathing and prevention of infection with topical products, therapies aimed at enhancing epidermal barrier function should be considered as part of long-term treatment. From an evidence-based standpoint, it should be noted that, at the time of this writing, there is only moderate evidence for altered barrier function as part of the pathogenesis of CAD [14], and limited and insufficient evidence for effectiveness of such measures exist in dogs, in spite of their widespread and effective use in human atopic dermatitis. Despite this, products promising to improve or enhance barrier function have appeared on the veterinary market and as they are studied further, evidence may accumulate. The measures being considered and which may become useful include dietary approaches, for example supplementation with oral fatty acids [15] or barrier-enhancing micronutrients [16]. Topical approaches with spray-on or spot-on products containing fatty acids, ceramides, and/or phytosphingosine are the subject of considerable investigation and may be useful in certain cases [17,18]. Our knowledge of this area of therapy is likely to expand greatly over the coming years.

There may be two reasons why fatty acid supplementation may be of benefit in CAD. First, there is evidence that they may have some anti-inflammatory action in skin, though the effect is mild and may be reflected mostly as synergism with other medications. For example, administration of oral fatty acids along with oral corticosteroids allows a lower total dosage of corticosteroid to be used [19]. Second, there is emerging evidence that fatty acid administration influences the composition of epidermal lipids [15]. In theory, this may augment epidermal barrier function, though critical studies to demonstrate this benefit are lacking. It is also clear that any of these effects take months to reach maximum effect. There is currently insufficient evidence of the superiority of any particular form or ratio of omega-3 to omega-6 fatty acids in the supplement (Box 13.5).

Long-term medical treatment options

Conventional drugs that have proven effective for long-term control of pruritus and lesions of chronic CAD include oral or topical glucocorticoids and oral ciclosporin.

Box 13.5 Therapy capsule: Fatty acid supplementation

Effectiveness: Moderate evidence of effectiveness, though effects are mild and may be mostly reflected in lower required doses of other concurrent medications.
Adverse effects: None reported.
Dosing: General recommendation of at least 25 mg/kg/day of the anti-inflammatory fatty acids; consult label for details. Requires 1–2 months of treatment to observe effects. Some prescription diets may be supplemented at or above this level, making capsule or liquid supplementation unnecessary, though this may be difficult to discern from label.
Patient monitoring: None required.

Box 13.6 Therapy capsule: Ciclosporin modified

Effectiveness: Strong, clear evidence for effectiveness in CAD, with approximately 75% of dogs showing benefit. Efficacy appears to persist over time and does not wane with long-term use.
Adverse effects: Short-term, gastrointestinal upset common (inappetance, vomiting, or diarrhoea) but often resolves within a few weeks. If vomiting is a problem initially, maropitant may be given concurrently for a few weeks. Longer term, an important but uncommon effect is gingival hyperplasia, occurring in perhaps 1% of dogs.
Dosing: Starting dose of 5 mg/kg/day for induction; response may not occur at lower initial doses. If response occurs, dose may be tapered in many dogs to 25–50% of initial dose for long-term maintenance.
Patient monitoring: No specific laboratory monitoring typically necessary. Measuring plasma levels of CsA is generally unnecessary because they are uncorrelated to clinical efficacy.

The prospect of treating a patient continuously with corticosteroids over a period of years is quite different than short-term or intermittent use, and should be considered only as a last resort if other treatments are not effective or affordable to the owner. Efficacy often declines with time, and the chances of serious adverse effects (e.g. steroid hepatopathy, diabetes mellitus) are much greater with long-term use (Boxes 13.1 and 13.2).

Ciclosporin has proven both effective and safe for long-term use in CAD [20,21]. Though expensive, it has strong advantages of minimal adverse effects and no specific toxicity over time (Box 13.6).

Oclacitinib has received regulatory approval for chronic use in treatment of canine AD, and as of this writing, a few dogs have been treated for as long as 2 years with the drug without adverse effect; see Box 13.3.

Additional 'non-traditional' medication options, such as topical tacrolimus and injectable interferon products, are less studied but have demonstrated efficacy in CAD [22–24]. Cost and availability vary and these products will be discussed in Chapter 14 of this volume. All of these medications must be individually targeted for patient use, considering not only variation in efficacy but their costs and individual longer-term adverse effect profiles.

Modifying underlying disease pathogenesis

Allergen-specific immunotherapy (ASIT) remains one of the single most valuable and proven long-term treatments for CAD. It is one of the very few treatments currently available that is aimed at actually reversing an important part of the underlying pathogenesis of the disease, has an excellent safety profile, and is the only treatment that in some cases can effect a virtual cure of the disease. For needle-shy owners, there is initial evidence that a new sublingual 'allergy drop' formulation is effective, and may even work via different mechanisms as it may benefit dogs that have failed conventional 'allergy shots'. Further information on ASIT can be found in Chapter 12 of this volume.

References

1. Olivry T, Mueller RS. International Task Force on Canine Atopic Dermatitis. Evidence-based veterinary dermatology: a systematic review of the pharmacotherapy of canine atopic dermatitis. *Veterinary Dermatology* 2003; **14**: 121–146.
2. Steffan J, Favrot C, Mueller R. A systematic review and meta-analysis of the efficacy and safety of cyclosporine for the treatment of atopic dermatitis in dogs. *Veterinary Dermatology* 2006; **17**: 3–16.
3. Olivry T, Foster AP, Mueller RS, *et al.* Interventions for atopic dermatitis in dogs: a systematic review of randomized controlled trials. *Veterinary Dermatology* 2010; **21**: 4–22.
4. Olivry T, DeBoer DJ, Favrot C, *et al.* Treatment of canine atopic dermatitis: 2010 clinical practice guidelines from the International Task Force on Canine Atopic Dermatitis. *Veterinary Dermatology* 2010; **21**: 233–248.
5. Loeflath A, von Voigts-Rhetz A, Jaeger K, *et al.* The efficacy of a commercial shampoo and whirlpooling in the treatment of canine pruritus—a double-blinded, randomized, placebo-controlled study. *Veterinary Dermatology* 2007; **18**: 427–431.
6. Schilling J, Mueller RS. Double-blinded, placebo-controlled study to evaluate an antipruritic shampoo for dogs with allergic pruritus. *Veterinary Record* 2012; **171**: 97.
7. Nuttall T, Mueller R, Bensignor E, *et al.* Efficacy of a 0.0584% hydrocortisone aceponate spray in the management of canine atopic dermatitis: a randomised, double blind, placebo-controlled trial. *Veterinary Dermatology* 2009; **20**: 191–198.
8. DeBoer DJ, Schafer JH, Salsbury CS, *et al.* Multiple-center study of reduced-concentration triamcinolone topical solution for the treatment of dogs with known or suspected allergic pruritus. *American Journal of Veterinary Research* 2002; **63**: 408–413.
9. Cosgrove S, Wren J, King V, *et al.* A multicenter clinical trial to evaluate the efficacy and field safety of oclacitinib. *Veterinary Dermatology* 2012; **23** (Suppl. 1): 38.
10. Fleck T, Humphrey W, Coscarelli E, *et al.* Comparison of the janus kinase (JAK) inhibitor, oclacitinib, and prednisolone in canine models of pruritus. *Veterinary Dermatology* 2012; **23** (Suppl. 1): 38.
11. Dell DL, Griffin CE, Thompson LA, *et al.* Owner assessment of therapeutic interventions for canine atopic dermatitis: a long-term retrospective analysis. *Veterinary Dermatology* 2012; **23**: 228–e47.
12. Paterson S. Additive benefits of EFAs in dogs with atopic dermatitis after partial response to antihistamine therapy. *Journal of Small Animal Practice* 1995; **36**: 389–394.
13. DeBoer DJ, Griffin CE. The ACVD task force on canine atopic dermatitis (XXI): antihistamine pharmacotherapy. *Veterinary Immunology and Immunopathology* 2001; **81**: 323–329.
14. Marsella R, Olivry T, Carlotti DN, *et al.* Current evidence of skin barrier dysfunction in human and canine atopic dermatitis. *Veterinary Dermatology* 2011; **22**: 239–248.
15. Popa I, Pin D, Remoue N, *et al.* Analysis of epidermal lipids in normal and atopic dogs, before and after administration of an oral omega-6/omega-3 fatty acid feed supplement. A pilot study. *Veterinary Research Communications* 2011; **35**: 501–509.
16. Watson AL, Fray TR, Bailey J, *et al.* Dietary constituents are able to play a beneficial role in canine epidermal barrier function. *Experimental Dermatology* 2006; **15**: 74–81.
17. Popa I, Remoue N, Osta B, *et al.* The lipid alterations in the stratum corneum of dogs with atopic dermatitis are alleviated by topical application of a sphingolipid-containing emulsion. *Clinical and Experimental Dermatology* 2012; **37**: 665–671.
18. Tretter S, Mueller RS. The influence of topical unsaturated fatty acids and essential oils on normal and atopic dogs. *Journal of the American Animal Hospital Association* 2011; **47**: 236–240.
19. Saevik BK, Bergvall K, Holm BR, *et al.* A randomized, controlled study to evaluate the steroid sparing effect of essential fatty acid supplementation in the treatment of canine atopic dermatitis. *Veterinary Dermatology* 2004; **15**: 137–145.
20. Olivry T, Rivierre C, Jackson HA, *et al.* Cyclosporine decreases skin lesions and pruritus in dogs with atopic dermatitis: a blinded randomized prednisolone-controlled trial. *Veterinary Dermatology* 2002; **13**: 77–87.
21. Radowicz SN, Power HT. Long-term use of cyclosporine in the treatment of canine atopic dermatitis. *Veterinary Dermatology* 2005; **16**: 81–86.
22. Yasukawa K, Saito S, Kubo T, *et al.* Low-dose recombinant canine interferon-gamma for treatment of canine atopic dermatitis: an open randomized comparative trial of two doses. *Veterinary Dermatology* 2012; **21**: 42–49.
23. Carlotti DN, Boulet M, Ducret J, *et al.* The use of recombinant omega interferon therapy in canine atopic dermatitis: a double-blind controlled study. *Veterinary Dermatology* 2009; **20**: 405–411.
24. Bensignor E, Olivry T. Treatment of localized lesions of canine atopic dermatitis with tacrolimus ointment: a blinded randomized controlled trial. *Veterinary Dermatology* 2005; **16**: 52–60.

14

Non-conventional treatments

Ralf S. Mueller

Centre for Clinical Veterinary Medicine, Ludwig Maximilian University, Munich, Germany

Conflicts of interest: in the last 5 years Ralf Mueller has obtained funding, lectured, or consulted for Almapharm, Dermcare, Bayer Animal Health, Boehringer Ingelheim, Dechra Veterinary Products, Intervet, Merial, Novartis Animal Health, Pfizer Animal Health, Procter and Gamble, Royal Canin, Selectavet, and Virbac.

Introduction

Atopic dermatitis is a common disease in veterinary medicine and the treatment of the disease is not always straightforward. Two recent publications have succinctly summarized available evidence for the various therapies in the dog [1,2]. Two main treatment options exist in principle, symptomatic antipruritic therapy and allergen-specific immunotherapy. The latter is discussed in Chapter 12. The former can be grouped in treatments commonly used in small animal practice, which are summarized in Chapter 13, and therapies that are not commonly used. This may be due to their hitherto questionable efficacy, or because they are not widely available, or not practical in many cases, or a combination of these factors. This chapter will focus on such treatments and summarize published evidence as well as advantages and disadvantages of some of these therapies.

Pentoxifylline

The methylxanthine and phosphodiesterase inhibitor pentoxifylline has been used in human medicine for many years as a rheological agent. It has effects on leukocyte deformability and decreases platelet activation; it decreases endothelial leukocyte adhesion, neutrophil degranulation, production of a number of cytokines such as tumour necrosis factor, and inhibits T- and B-cell activation [3]. The drug is metabolized by the liver and by red blood cells; there is extensive enterohepatic recycling of metabolites.

Pentoxifylline is administered to dogs orally at an empirical dose of 10–20 mg/kg, two to three times daily. In humans adverse effects are rare and are dose related; these may include vomiting, diarrhoea, nausea, dizziness, and headaches. Adverse effects in dogs are not reported; the author has rarely seen vomiting.

Pentoxifylline was administered for 4 weeks in a placebo-controlled, double-blinded, cross-over trial and was shown to significantly decrease pruritus and erythema by approximately 30% [4]. In another study both pentoxifylline and a combination of pentoxifylline and polyunsaturated fatty acids led to a significant improvement (up to 90%) for lesions and pruritus after 2 months compared to placebo; the combination therapy was more efficacious than pentoxifylline alone [5]. In the author's experience improvement of more than 50% in lesions or pruritus is not common. Based on available evidence pentoxifylline can be recommended for the treatment of canine atopic dermatitis [2].

Tacrolimus

Tacrolimus is a macrolide lactone and a calcineurin inhibitor like ciclosporin. It inhibits cytokine production (predominantly IL-2, but also IL-3, IL-4, IFN-gamma, and tumour necrosis factor-α) and thus activation of T

Veterinary Allergy, First Edition. Edited by Chiara Noli, Aiden Foster, and Wayne Rosenkrantz.

cells; it also down-regulates cytokine production in other cells involved in allergic inflammation, such as mast cells, eosinophils, keratinocytes, and Langerhans cells [6].

Tacrolimus is available as an ointment that is only minimally absorbed and thus very safe. However, due to this formulation it is best suited for small localized lesions of atopic dermatitis. It is administered twice daily and may be tapered to once daily or every other day after clinical signs have improved. A burning or stinging sensation can be associated with its administration in some dogs; other adverse effects are not reported to the author's knowledge.

In the first study published, tacrolimus at 0.3% constituted by a pharmacy, significantly improved clinician-judged erythema, but not owner-judged pruritus scores, in a double-blinded, placebo-controlled, cross-over study in a small number of dogs [7]. Two further studies used the commercial 0.1% tacrolimus ointment [8,9]. In both studies, pruritus and lesion scores improved significantly compared to placebo. Thus, there is good evidence for the use of topical tacrolimus ointment at 0.1% for localized lesions of canine atopic dermatitis.

Misoprostol

Misoprostol is a synthetic prostaglandin E1 analogue with antiallergic action [10]. In an open study 20 dogs with atopic dermatitis were given 3–6 µg/kg misoprostol three times daily for a month [11]. Pruritus and skin lesions decreased by >50% in more than half of the dogs. Some dogs showed vomiting and diarrhoea when given the drug. In a subsequent placebo-controlled trial 12 dogs with atopic dermatitis were treated with misoprostol at 5 µg/kg three times a day and eight dogs with placebo [12]. In contrast to placebo therapy, misoprostol treatment was associated with a significant improvement in pruritus and skin lesions after 3 weeks, the median improvement of both pruritus and lesions was 30%. Thus, there is evidence for the use of misoprostol in canine atopic dermatitis. Unfortunately, availability and cost of this drug varies greatly from country to country.

Chinese herbal medicine

Chinese herbal medicine is increasingly popular with a subgroup of dog owners preferring alternative medicine to classical established therapies. P07P is a product derived from traditional Chinese herbal medicine, containing the herbs *Glycyrizzha uralensis*, *Paeonia lactiflora*, and *Rehmannia glutinosa* (Phytopica, Intervet-Schering-Plough Animal Health). It was first evaluated in 2001 in a randomized, double-blinded, placebo-controlled study with 50 dogs [13]. P07P was administered at 200 mg/kg once daily. Adverse effects noted were soft stool, diarrhoea, and flatulence in a small number of dogs. Although there was a significantly higher withdrawal rate due to deterioration in the placebo group compared to treated dogs (13/23 versus 7/24) and nine treated dogs improved versus three dogs in the placebo group, there was no statistically significant difference in clinical outcome between the two groups [13]. In a subsequent study, it was shown that this preparation has a glucocorticoid-sparing effect in atopic dogs [14]. There is currently insufficient evidence to recommend this product generally for the treatment of atopic dermatitis in the dog and further studies are recommended. It seems, however, that individual dogs may benefit from this treatment option. However, at the time of writing this product was not available anymore in some countries.

Capsaicin

Capsaicin is an alkaloid, the active component of chilli peppers, that binds to a receptor on neurons and leads to neuronal depletion of substance P, a neurotransmitter involved in pain and neurogenic inflammation [6]. In a double-blinded, placebo-controlled, cross-over study 12 dogs with atopic dermatitis were treated with 0.025% capsaicin or vehicle lotion twice daily for 6 weeks [15]. Investigator evaluation showed no significant change, although all but one dogs improved on treatment and the improvement in owner scores was significant. However, cutaneous concentrations of substance P did not change significantly with time and treatment and did not correlate with pruritus. These findings point to a possible role for capsaicin as adjunctive treatment for atopic dermatitis, although further studies are needed.

Leukotriene inhibitors

Leukotrienes are important inflammatory mediators in humans and animals. There is a report documenting excellent bioavailability of a leukotriene inhibitor and nearly complete suppression of leukotriene production in dogs [16]. Furthermore, two reports in the literature evaluate products for dogs that are available in human medicine [17, 18]. In one placebo-controlled, cross-over trial, nine dogs were treated with zileuton at 2 mg/kg three times daily for 4 weeks and showed a significant decrease in erythema, but not pruritus. Three of them showed a decrease of >50% in lesion scores and pruritus [17]. Clinical adverse effects were not seen; one dog showed a mild elevation of liver enzymes. In another trial, 18 dogs were treated with zafirlukast for 2–4 weeks and two of those dogs showed a sustained effect with

>50% improvement in pruritus [18]. Two dogs vomited during treatment. Based on those reports, the efficacy of leukotriene inhibitors is limited, although they may be moderately beneficial in individual cases. More randomized clinical trials would be needed for a final recommendation.

Serotonin uptake inhibitors and tricyclic antidepressants

Serotonin is one of the preformed inflammatory mediators released with mast cell degranulation. There are a number of reports about drugs that act as serotonin uptake inhibitors and tricyclic antidepressants, often in addition to their antihistaminic action. In a pilot study, six dogs with allergic dermatitis and five dogs with acral lick dermatitis were treated with fluoxetine at a dose of 1 mg/kg daily. Two of the six atopic dogs and two of the dogs with acral lick dermatitis showed a marked, and one of the atopic dogs a moderate, improvement. Adverse effects seen were lethargy and wheals in four dogs [19]. In a second presentation good results with similar treatment were reported, but exact modes of evaluation and numbers of dogs were unclear [20].

Cyproheptadine has been administered orally at a dose of 0.1–0.2 mg/kg daily to 16 dogs with allergic pruritus and no improvement was seen in any of the dogs [21]. Four of the dogs showed polyphagia with cyproheptadine administration. Amitriptyline was evaluated in 31 pruritic dogs and led to elimination of the pruritus in five and reduction by half in another five dogs [22]. Hydroxyzine (2 mg/kg three times daily) and doxepin (1–2 mg/kg twice daily) are further tricyclic antidepressants that were cited as being efficacious in 30% of the dogs in one study, without further details [23]. In summary, there are individual allergic dogs reported to respond to a number of different serotonin uptake inhibitors/tricyclic antidepressants, but randomized, double-blinded studies are lacking and are urgently needed to allow any evidence-based recommendation.

Probiotics

Probiotic organisms are live micro-organisms that are thought to be beneficial to the host. They have been evaluated in many studies in human atopy after a promising Finnish study showed decreased development of atopy in babies supplemented with lactobacilli [24,25]. After more than a decade of research in the field probiotics are still controversial; however, a recent review found evidence to recommend probiotics as a preventative measure in pregnant mothers and infants [26].

In veterinary medicine a clinical pilot study showed that mRNA expression of filaggrin, a molecule essential for the epidermal barrier, was increased in atopic beagles after probiotic therapy [27]. After this therapy, lesion scores of atopic beagles were lower than those of the siblings that were not treated. In addition, IL-10 concentrations were much higher in dogs not treated [28]. In these studies, laboratory beagles were used. *Lactobacillus rhamnosus* strain GG was administered at a dose of 100–200×10^9 CFU, because this is one of the best studied strains in human medicine and was shown to also be a probiotic in dogs [29]. Further studies with larger numbers of dogs with naturally occurring atopic dermatitis are needed to determine the optimal therapeutic dose and organism; the evidence for efficacy in canine atopic dermatitis is too limited at this point.

Therapy with helminths

In recent years, the 'hygiene hypothesis' has been developed. It assumes that children with an increased risk of infection are at a lesser risk of suffering from atopic dermatitis. A negative correlation between the occurrence of helminth infections and atopic diseases has been reported [30]. Therefore it seems feasible that an infection with an intestinal parasite may decrease clinical signs of atopy by interaction with the immune system. In a pilot study, 12 dogs with atopic dermatitis were treated with *Trichuris vulpis* eggs or larvae of *Uncinaria stenocephala* orally for 12 weeks [31]. Lesion scores improved in all dogs and pruritus in 9/12. A subsequent placebo-controlled, double-blinded study treating dogs with 2500 *T. vulpis* eggs every month did not show any statistically significant difference between placebo and the helminth eggs [31]. However, dogs in the blinded trial had mostly mild to moderate CAD, while dogs in the pilot study were almost all severely atopic. None of the dogs receiving placebo improved, but four dogs in the treatment group improved by more than 50% and those were dogs with more severe disease. Further studies are needed to evaluate if helminth treatment is only suitable for dogs with severe atopic dermatitis.

Interferon-γ

Interferons are cytokines belonging to a family of proteins with three subtypes. They play an important role in innate and adapted immunity. In atopic humans, IL-4 (a cytokine produced by Th2 cells) is expressed in abundance whereas IFN-γ (a type II IFN produced by Th1 cells) expression is suppressed in comparison to healthy individuals. In several Japanese studies, canine atopic dermatitis was treated successfully with recombinant canine interferon-γ (rCaIFN-γ) (Interdog, Toray, Japan) administered subcutaneously with no adverse effects [32,33]. Unfortunately, rCaIFN-γ is not widely available. Carlotti *et al.* reported treating CAD using recombinant feline interferon-ω (rFeIFN-ω) (Virbagen Omega, Virbac, France) for 6 months [34]. In this double-blinded, controlled study, rFeIFN-ω was as efficacious as orally administered ciclosporin [34]. In a more recent study, rFeIFN-ω was administered subcutaneously to dogs with atopic dermatitis in a protocol similar to that of Carlotti *et al.*, while another group of atopic dogs received the drug orally. Comparison of pruritus scores, CADESI and total scores between days 0 and 120 showed improvement in both groups; however, significant improvement could only be detected in the oral group with CADESI and total scores [35]. Antibody production against rFeIFN-ω could not be detected. More studies are needed to evaluate rFeIFN-ω in CAD, whereas rCaIFN-γ seems to be an efficacious therapy for this disease.

Hardy kiwi preparation

A multicentre, randomized, double-blinded, placebo-controlled study tested the efficacy of *Actinidia arguta* (hardy kiwi) (EFF1001) in dogs with mild/moderate CAD [36]. Dogs received prednisolone for 2 weeks, responders then continued to receive either the kiwi preparation or placebo. Although dogs on the kiwi preparation showed an improved response (in regard to pruritus and CADESI) compared to the dogs on placebo, this was not significant.

Heat-killed *Mycobacterium vaccae*

A single intradermal injection of heat-killed *M. vaccae* was evaluated in dogs with atopic dermatitis in a multicentre, placebo-controlled, double-blinded study [37]. Three months after the injection, there was improvement in both groups; a significant difference between groups could only be noted in pruritus. However, when dogs with mild atopic dermatitis were analysed separately, there was a more pronounced improvement of CADESI and pruritus with the treated dogs compared to the dogs receiving a placebo injection. More studies are needed to evaluate the effects of heat-killed *M. vaccae* on canine atopic dermatitis.

Conclusion

There are a number of interesting therapies for atopic dermatitis but at this point many of them cannot be recommended for routine use without further studies. However, there is evidence for a moderate efficacy of systemic pentoxifylline and misoprostol, good efficacy for topical tacrolimus and rCaIFN-γ, and moderate efficacy for capsaicin.

References

1. Olivry T, DeBoer DJ, Favrot C, *et al.* Treatment of canine atopic dermatitis: 2010 clinical practice guidelines from the International Task Force on Canine Atopic Dermatitis. *Veterinary Dermatology* 2010; **21**: 233–248.
2. Olivry T, Foster AP, Mueller RS, *et al.* Interventions for atopic dermatitis in dogs: a systematic review of randomized controlled trials. *Veterinary Dermatology* 2010; **21**: 4–22.
3. Samlaska CP, Winfield EA. Pentoxifylline. *Journal of the American Academy of Dermatology* 1994; **30**: 603–621.
4. Marsella R, Nicklin CF. Double-blinded, placebo-controlled crossover study on the effects of pentoxifylline in canine atopy. *Veterinary Dermatology* 2000; **11**: 255–260.
5. Singh SK, Dimri U, Saxena SK, *et al.* Therapeutic management of canine atopic dermatitis by combination of pentoxifylline and PUFAs. *Journal of Veterinary Pharmacology and Therapeutics* 2010; **33**: 495–498.
6. Marsella R, Olivry T. The ACVD task force on canine atopic dermatitis (XXII): nonsteroidal anti-inflammatory pharmacotherapy. *Veterinary Immunology and Immunopathology* 2001; **81**: 331–345.
7. Marsella R, Nicklin CF. Investigation on the use of 0.3% tacrolimus lotion for canine atopic dermatitis: a pilot study. *Veterinary Dermatology* 2002; **13**: 203–210.
8. Bensignor E, Olivry T. Treatment of localized lesions of canine atopic dermatitis with tacrolimus ointment: a blinded randomized controlled trial. *Veterinary Dermatology* 2005; **16**: 52–60.
9. Marsella R, Nicklin CF, Saglio S, *et al.* Investigation on the clinical efficacy and safety of 0.1% tacrolimus ointment (Protopic) in canine atopic dermatitis: a randomized, double-blinded, placebo-controlled, cross-over study. *Veterinary Dermatology* 2004; **15**: 294–303.
10. Smith WG, Thompson JM, Kowalski DL, *et al.* Inhaled misoprostol blocks guinea pig antigen-induced bronchoconstriction and airway inflammation. *American Journal of Respiratory Critical Care Medicine* 1996; **154**: 295–299.
11. Olivry T, Guaguère E, Héripret D. Treatment of atopic dermatitis with misoprostol, a prostaglandin E1 analogue—an open study. *Journal of Dermatological Treatment* 1997; **8**: 243–247.
12. Olivry T, Dunston SM, Rivierre C, *et al.* A randomized controlled trial of misoprostol monotherapy for canine atopic dermatitis: effects on dermal cellularity and cutaneous tumour necrosis factor-alpha. *Veterinary Dermatology* 2003; **14**: 37–46.
13. Nagle TM, Torres SM, Horne KL, *et al.* A randomized, double-blind, placebo-controlled trial to investigate the efficacy and safety of a Chinese herbal product (P07P) for the treatment of canine atopic dermatitis. *Veterinary Dermatology* 2001; **12**: 265–274.
14. Schmidt V, McEwan N, Volk A, *et al.* The glucocorticoid sparing efficacy of Phytopica in the management of canine atopic dermatitis. *Veterinary Dermatology* 2010; **21**: 96–105.
15. Marsella R, Nicklin CF, Melloy C. The effects of capsaicin topical therapy in dogs with atopic dermatitis: a randomized, double-blinded, placebo-controlled, cross-over clinical trial. *Veterinary Dermatology* 2002; **13**: 131–139.
16. Bell RL, Bouska J, Young PR, *et al.* The properties of A-69412: a small hydrophilic 5-lipoxygenase inhibitor. *Agents Actions* 1993; **38**: 178–187.

17. Crow DW, Marsella R, Nicklin CF. Double-blinded, placebo-controlled, cross-over pilot study on the efficacy of zileuton for canine atopic dermatitis. *Veterinary Dermatology* 2001; **12**: 189–195.
18. Senter DA, Scott DW, Miller WH, Jr. Treatment of canine atopic dermatitis with zafirlukast, a leukotriene-receptor antagonist: a single-blinded, placebo-controlled study. *Canadian Veterinary Journal* 2002; **43**: 203–206.
19. Shoulberg N. The efficacy of fluoxetime (Prozac) in the treatment of acral lick and allergic inhalant dermatitis in canines. In: *Proceedings of the Annual Meeting of the American Academy of Veterinary Dermatology and American College of Veterinary Dermatology*, 1990: 31–32.
20. Melman S. Prozac (fluoxatime), Zoloft (sertraline) and Anafranil (clomipramine) use in animals for selected dermatological and behavioral conditions. In: *Proceedings of the 11th Annual Congress of the American Academy of Veterinary Dermatology and American College of Veterinary Dermatology*, 1995: 82.
21. Scott DW, Miller WH, Jr., Decker GA, *et al.* Failure of cyproheptadine hydrochloride as an antipruritic agent in allergic dogs: results of a double-blinded, placebo-controlled study. *Cornell Veterinarian* 1992; **82**: 247–251.
22. Miller WH, Jr., Scott DW, Wellington JR. Nonsteroidal management of canine pruritus with amitriptyline. *Cornell Veterinarian* 1992; **82**: 53–57.
23. Scott DW, Miller WH, Jr. Antihistamines in the management of allergic pruritus in dogs and cats. *Journal of Small Animal Practice* 1999; **40**: 359–364.
24. Kalliomaki M, Salminen S, Arvilommi H, *et al.* Probiotics in primary prevention of atopic disease: a randomised placebo-controlled trial. *Lancet* 2001; **357**: 1076–1079.
25. Kalliomaki M, Salminen S, Poussa T, *et al.* Probiotics and prevention of atopic disease: 4-year follow-up of a randomised placebo-controlled trial. *Lancet* 2003; **361**: 1869–1871.
26. Pelucchi C, Chatenoud L, Turati F, *et al.* Probiotics supplementation during pregnancy or infancy for the prevention of atopic dermatitis: a meta-analysis. *Epidemiology* 2012; **23**: 402–414.
27. Santoro D, Marsella R, Bunicke D, *et al.* Longterm effect of probiotics on filaggrin mRNA and protein expression in atopic beagles. *Veterinary Dermatology* 2010; **21**: 322.
28. Marsella R, Santoro D, Ahrens K. Early exposure to probiotics in a canine model of atopic dermatitis has long-term clinical and immunological effects. *Veterinary Immunology and Immunopathology* 2012; **146**: 185–189.
29. Weese JS, Anderson ME. Preliminary evaluation of *Lactobacillus rhamnosus* strain GG, a potential probiotic in dogs. *Canadian Veterinary Journal* 2002; **43**: 771–774.
30. Cooper PJ, Chico ME, Rodrigues LC, *et al.* Reduced risk of atopy among school-age children infected with geohelminth parasites in a rural area of the tropics. *Journal of Allergy and Clinical Immunology* 2003; **111**: 995–1000.
31. Mueller RS, Specht L, Helmer M, *et al.* The effect of nematode administration on canine atopic dermatitis. *Veterinary Parasitology* 2011; **181**: 203–209.
32. Iwasaki T, Hasegawa A. A randomized comparative clinical trial of recombinant canine interferon-gamma (KT-100) in atopic dogs using antihistamine as control. *Veterinary Dermatology* 2006; **17**: 195–200.
33. Yasukawa K, Saito S, Kubo T, *et al.* Low-dose recombinant canine interferon-gamma for treatment of canine atopic dermatitis: an open randomized comparative trial of two doses. *Veterinary Dermatology* 2010; **21**: 42–49.
34. Carlotti DN, Boulet M, Ducret J, *et al.* The use of recombinant omega interferon therapy in canine atopic dermatitis: a double-blind controlled study. *Veterinary Dermatology* 2009; **20**: 405–411.
35. Litzlbauer P, Weber K, Mueller RS. Recombinant feline interferon-omega as oral or subcutaneous treatment of canine atopic dermatitis. *Veterinary Dermatology* 2012; **23** (Suppl. 1): 39.
36. Marsella R, Messinger L, Zabel S, *et al.* A randomized, double-blind, placebo-controlled study to evaluate the effect of EFF1001, an Actinidia arguta (hardy kiwi) preparation on CADESI score and pruritus in dogs with mild to moderate atopic dermatitis. *Veterinary Dermatology* 2010; **21**: 50–57.
37. Ricklin Gutzwiler ME, Reist M, Peel JE, *et al.* Intradermal injection of heat-killed *Mycobacterium vaccae* in dogs with atopic dermatitis: a multicentre pilot study. *Veterinary Dermatology* 2007; **18**: 87–93.

Section 2

Food Hypersensitivity

15

The pathogenesis of food allergy

Hilary A. Jackson

Dermatology Referral Service Ltd, Glasgow, UK

Conflict of interest: none declared.

Introduction: lessons from human food allergy

As defined in the 2010 US National Institutes of Allergy and Infectious Diseases (NIAID) sponsored guidelines, **food allergy** is an 'adverse health effect arising from a specific immune response that occurs reproducibly on exposure to a given food' [1]. This covers both IgE and non-IgE-mediated reactions and combinations of both.

Food intolerances include lactose intolerance, responses to pharmacologically active food components such as histamines, and reactions to toxins produced by bacterial contamination (Table 15.1).

Natural development of oral tolerance

Oral tolerance develops with repeated low-dose exposure to antigen and is mediated by regulatory T cells, such as $CD8^+$ cells, Th3 cells, Tr1 cells, $CD4^+$ $CD25^+$ cells, and $NK1.1^+$ T cells. These cells migrate to the local lymph nodes and stimulate the production of suppressive cytokines such as IL-10 and TGF-beta. High-dose antigen exposure can also induce tolerance if T-cell receptors engage in the absence of co-stimulation. In practice, a combination of these effects probably occurs during weaning [2,3].

Mechanism of development of food allergy

In humans, sensitization is complex and thought to arise from a breakdown of normal tolerance and immune regulation. Immaturity of the gastrointestinal tract may account for the increased incidence of food allergies in children. Additional factors, such as increased intestinal permeability due to disease, administration of immunosuppressive drugs, or protracted use of antacids, may also play a part. Environmental factors also play a significant role, and the timing, route, and method of allergen exposure appear to be important to the genetically susceptible individual [4].

In the majority of cases in humans, food allergy is IgE mediated [2], but cell-mediated and mixed reactions can occur. Mechanisms were reviewed by Burks *et al.* in 2012 [5]. After primary exposure to and processing of the antigen, antigen-presenting cells present peptide fragments (epitopes) in conjunction with MHC class II molecules to T cells. The ensuing T-cell proliferation and generation of Th2-type cytokines stimulate the production of food-specific IgE from B cells. Immunoglobulin E binds to tissue mast cells. On re-exposure to antigen, adjacent antigen-specific IgE molecules are cross-linked and cellular degranulation is induced, resulting in the release of inflammatory mediators such as histamine and eicosanoids.

Clinically, IgE reactions are characterized by an acute onset, usually within 2 hours of exposure to the allergenic food, and can involve the skin, gastrointestinal, and respiratory systems. Cell-mediated reactions are less common. Food-induced atopic dermatitis is considered to be a mixed reaction and clinical signs generally occur within 2 days of allergen exposure.

Avoidance of food allergens during pregnancy, lactation, and early infancy has not consistently been shown to reduce the incidence of IgE-mediated food

Veterinary Allergy, First Edition. Edited by Chiara Noli, Aiden Foster, and Wayne Rosenkrantz.

Table 15.1 Definitions

Adverse food reaction	Any clinically abnormal response attributable to the ingestion of food or food additive
Food intolerance	Abnormal physiological response to food with no immunological basis
Food allergy	Immunologically mediated adverse food reaction

Table 15.2 Major food allergens in man

Allergen	Food source
Animal proteins	
Caseins	Milk
Tropomyosin	Fish
EF-hand proteins (i.e. parvalbumin)	Crustaceans and molluscs
Plant proteins	
Bet v 1 superfamily	Fruit, soy, vegetables
Cupin superfamily	Nuts, legumes, seeds
Prolamin superfamily	Cereals, fruits, vegetables
Cysteine protease C1 family	Soy, kiwi
Profilins	Fruits, vegetables, legumes

allergy in at-risk infants [6] and this recommendation has been withdrawn by both the American Academy of Pediatrics and the similar organization in Europe. Furthermore, there is increasing evidence that sensitization to food allergens may occur also by the epicutaneous route and atopic patients with impaired barrier function are at increased risk [4].

Allergens

Food allergens are usually proteins, although carbohydrates have been recognized to be allergenic in some cases [7]. In man, relatively few protein families account for the majority of reactions (Table 15.2). The allergenic portion of the protein (epitope) may be linear or conformational. In the latter case, the protein is more likely to be denatured by digestion or cooking processes. For example milk- or egg-allergic children can often tolerate baked products containing these ingredients [8,9].

A significant geographic variation in the allergens involved in food allergy is recognized and depends on local dietary practices; thus birds nest soup allergy is recognized in Singapore [10] and mustard seed allergy in France [11].

Clinical and immunological differences are also noted between patients with allergy to the same food in different locations. American patients with peanut allergy have more severe clinical signs and higher sensitization to the major peanut allergens Ara h 1, Ara h 2, and Ara h 3; Spanish patients recognize more commonly the lipid transfer protein Ara h 9; and Swedish patients react to the Bet v 1 homolog Ara h 8 [12]. These differences have been attributed to environmental influences, genetic variability, and differences in the preparation of foods.

The natural evolution of food allergy

Food allergy is more common in infants. In 85% of children allergic to antigens such as cow's milk, soy, egg, wheat, and cereal grains tolerance to the allergen will develop spontaneously with age, whereas in the case of nut and shellfish allergies only 15–20% will develop spontaneous tolerance [13] and the allergy will persist. Adults may develop food allergy after primary sensitization to aeroallergens such as birch pollen. This arises from protein cross-reactivity. There are similar epitopes on fruits such as melon and kiwi; ingestion of these fruits result in acute oral inflammation—the so-called 'oral allergy syndrome' [4].

Increasing knowledge of the pathogenesis of food allergy in people has led to the development of new treatment strategies and, although strict avoidance of known allergens is generally recommended, studies looking at controlled introduction of allergen at certain ages may induce tolerance [13].

What do we know about canine food allergy?

The majority of dogs reported in the veterinary literature with 'food allergy' have been identified by feeding a limited antigen diet containing novel or hydrolysed proteins, which has been selected after detailed review of the individual's dietary history. A challenge with previously fed foods is performed after a period of 6–10 weeks on the new diet and clinical deterioration demonstrated [14]. However, on the basis of these clinical observations we can only describe these animals as having adverse food reactions (AFR).

Epidemiology

Populations of dogs with variable clinical presentations and age of onset of clinical signs appear to exist. Whether this is a reflection of differences in disease pathogenesis is unclear. In a Swiss study in which the allergic population was compared with all registered dogs, West Highland white terriers, Rhodesian ridgebacks, and pugs were predisposed to AFR, supporting a genetic predisposition to the disease. It should be noted, however, that these breeds are also affected with canine atopic dermatitis (CAD). In the same study, gastrointestinal signs were more common in the population with AFR and clinical signs tended to develop earlier: 48% <1 year as compared with 16% of dogs with CAD [15]. These findings are similar to a study carried out by the author on client-owned dogs in North Carolina (38% <1 year) [16].

Immunological investigations

Positive intradermal test reactivity to food antigens and serum food allergen-specific IgE can be measured in dogs with suspected food allergies, although at this time these tests are unreliable both in the diagnosis of food allergy or as an aid to the selection of a novel protein diet. Whether this relates to the test methodology, allergens employed, or the lack of IgE involvement in canine AFR is unclear [17,18]. Food allergen-specific serum IgE tends to be more positive in dogs with AFR and dogs with CAD as compared with normal dogs but could not be used to distinguish between the two groups [18,19]. No change in the concentration of food allergen-specific IgE or IgG could be demonstrated in dogs with AFR after a period on an elimination diet [20]. Serum food-specific IgG can also be elevated in dogs with AFR and CAD [21], although another study found allergen-specific IgG to be higher in normal dogs as compared with CAD and dogs with gastrointestinal disease [22]. Detection of allergen-specific IgG may either indicate exposure or cross-reacting antigens, and a role for IgG in the pathogenesis of AFR has not been demonstrated.

Antigen-specific lymphocyte proliferation has also been investigated in dogs with AFR and CAD. Again, positive reactions are more frequent in both groups than in the normal dog population but could not be used to distinguish between the two groups. The lymphocyte proliferation response to antigens was shown to reduce after more than 6 weeks on an elimination diet. A correlation with clinically relevant allergens, however, was not made in this study and the number of dogs investigated was small [19]. Antigen-specific lymphocyte activation might occur in both humoral and cell-mediated reactions. Increased histamine release after food antigen-specific stimulation of peripheral blood leukocytes harvested from affected dogs supports a role for IgE [23].

Patch testing with food allergens in dogs with AFR has also been a subject of investigation. Positive reactions are more common in dogs with AFR than in normal dogs, again suggesting a cell-mediated component to canine AFR. A lack of allergen specificity, however, precludes the use of this methodology as a diagnostic test [24].

Allergen specificity

Increased IgE specific to bovine serum albumin was identified in dogs with clinical hypersensitivity to beef but not in normal dogs [25]. Additional studies have looked at dogs with clinical signs of AFR and suggest that muscle phosphoglucomutase and bovine and ovine IgG might be significant allergens [26]. Since muscle phosphoglucomutase is a ubiquitous mammalian protein and ovine and bovine IgG share structural homology, sensitization to these proteins may account for clinical intolerance of both beef and lamb.

One dog was described with clinical signs similar to the oral allergy syndrome. Primary sensitization was thought to arise through exposure to Japanese cedar (CJ; *Cryptomeria japonica*) and subsequent hypersensitivity to the ingestion of tomato developed. Cross reactivity between CJ and tomato was demonstrated [27].

A small number of dogs have been reported in which a home-cooked diet was tolerated but when the equivalent commercial diet was fed clinical signs developed [28,29]. Whether this related to conformational changes in allergen or other ingredients in the commercial diets is not known.

Other immunological findings

Gastrointestinal immune function may vary with age. Foxp3, a marker for T regulatory cell expression, was found to be reduced in juvenile and older animals when compared with healthy middle-aged dogs. This might support reduced oral tolerance in these age groups. Expression was also reduced in dogs with inflammatory bowel disease (IBD). Subject numbers in this study were small and whether reduced expression in dogs with IBD was due to cause or effect was not determined [30].

Using a population of client-owned dogs with AFR, the duodenal gene expression of Th1, Th2, and Treg-related cytokines was investigated before and after dietary provocation and compared with normal dogs. Gene expression was similar in both groups and did not change with dietary provocation in the dogs with AFR [31]. The same investigators looked at T-cell phenotypes and gene expression in the lesional skin of client-owned dogs with AFR before (with active lesions) and after amelioration with an elimination diet. Whilst clinical signs resolved on the elimination diet, the predominantly CD8 T-cell phenotype persisted. Interferon gamma gene expression was also increased in lesional skin [32]. These novel studies provide a snapshot of the immunological processes occurring in canine AFR but further work is required to determine the precise pathogenesis.

Canine models

Canine models have been used to investigate sensitization and treatment of food allergy. The Maltese×beagle dog colony at North Carolina State University, USA, manifests spontaneous food allergy. This colony was originally established to express an autosomal recessive glycogen storage disease. Dogs fed on a regular canine diet from weaning developed signs of allergic disease to components of that diet, notably corn, soy, milk, and pork. The allergic response was manifest as pruritus of the feet, limbs, face, ears, and ventrum as early as 4 months of age and within hours of ingesting specific proteins. An allergen-specific IgE response was measured in these dogs during sensitization and after oral challenge; this led to the conclusion that, at least in this group of dogs, IgE may play a role in the pathogenesis of the disease [33,34]. Furthermore, treatment with oral ciclosporin failed to ameliorate the acute response to oral challenge with food allergen, supporting a role for an immediate humoral reaction [35].

Non-physiological sensitization of colonies of high IgE responder dogs to food antigens has facilitated by-pass of normal immune tolerance. The timing of sensitization has been shown to be critical to the subsequent development of a robust IgE response. Predictable outcome measures, both clinical and immunological, have allowed for the testing of novel therapeutic strategies such as testing the immunogenicity of genetically modified foods, or treatment strategies for nut allergies in man [36,37]. This technique has also been exploited in the pet food industry for evaluation of hydrolysed diets. Dogs sensitized to chicken protein developed antibodies to a 68–70-kDa protein, thought to be chicken serum albumin, and *in vitro* tests showed that these antibodies did not recognize epitopes in the same protein after hydrolysis [38]. Similarly, dogs experimentally sensitized to soy proteins had reduced immune-reactivity to the native protein after hydrolysis [39]. Extrapolation of data from these canine models to the client-owned dog population, however, should be undertaken with care and it is quite likely that the dogs diagnosed with 'food allergy' represent a highly heterogeneous group, which include immunological and non-immunological aetiologies.

Conclusion

Over the past decade, our understanding of the pathogenesis of food allergy in man has significantly improved and this is leading to revision in the management recommendations for the potentially atopic infant and food-allergic individual. Unfortunately, the current status of our appreciation of the pathogenesis of adverse food reactions and food allergy in companion animals is minimal. Investigations to date in client-owned dogs suggest that various arms of the immune system may be activated and it is an over-simplification to consider canine food allergy to be IgE mediated. It should be remembered, however, that study populations to date probably include dogs with non-immunological food intolerance, making it difficult to draw accurate conclusions from published data.

References

1. Boyce J, Assa'ad A, Burks A, *et al.* Guidelines for the diagnosis and management of food allergy in the United States: report of the NIAID-sponsored expert panel. *Journal of Allergy and Clinical Immunology* 2010; **126** (Suppl.): S1–58.
2. Wang J, Sampson H. food allergy. *Journal of Clinical Investigation* 2011; **121**: 827–835.
3. Chehade M, Mayer L. Oral tolerance and its relation to food hypersensitivities. *Journal of Allergy Clinical Immunology* 2005; **115**: 3–12.
4. Lack G. Update on risk factors for food allergy. *Journal of Allergy and Clinical Immunology* 2012; **129**: 1187–1197.
5. Burks AW, Tang M, Sicherer S, *et al.* ICON: Food Allergy 2012. *Journal of Allergy and Clinical Immunology* **194**: 900–920.
6. Greer FR, Sicherer SH, Burks AW. Effects of early nutritional interventions on the development of atopic disease in infants and children: the role of maternal dietary restriction, breastfeeding, timing of introduction of complementary foods, and hydrolyzed formulas. *Pediatrics* 2008; **121**: 183–191.
7. Commins SP, Satinover SM, Hosen J, *et al.* Delayed anaphylaxis, angio-edema, or urticaria after consumption of red meat in patients with IgE antibodies specific for galactose-alpha-1,3-galactose. *Journal of Allergy and Clinical Immunology* 2009; **123**: 426–433.
8. Lemon-Mule H, Sampson HA, Sicherer SH, *et al.* Immunologic changes in children with egg allergy ingesting extensively heated egg. *Journal of Allergy and Clinical Immunology* 2008; **122**: 977–983.
9. Nowak-Wegrzyn A, Bloom KA, Sicherer SH, *et al.* Tolerance to extensively heated milk in children with cow's milk allergy. *Journal of Allergy and Clinical Immunology* 2008; **122**: 342–347.
10. Goh D, Lau Y, Chew F, *et al.* Pattern of food-induced anaphylaxis in children of an Asian community. *Allergy* 1999; **54**: 84–86.
11. Rance F, Dutau G, Abbal M. Mustard allergy in children. *Allergy* 2000; **55**: 496–500.
12. Vereda A, Hage Mv, Ahlstedt S, *et al.* Peanut allergy: clinical and immunological differences among patients from 3 different geographical regions. *Journal of Allergy and Clinical Immunology* 2011; **127**: 603–607.
13. Nowak-Wegrzyn A, Sampson HA. Future therapies for food allergies. *Journal of Allergy and Clinical Immunology* 2011; **127**: 558–573.
14. Verlinden A, Hesta M, Millet S, *et al.* Food allergy in dogs and cats: a review. *Critical Reviews Food Science Nutrition* 2006; **46**: 259–273.
15. Picco F, Zini E, Nett C, *et al.* A prospective study on canine atopic dermatitis and food induced allergic dermatitis in Switzerland. *Veterinary Dermatology* 2008; **19**: 150–155.
16. Jackson H, Murphy KM, Tater KC, *et al.* The pattern of allergen hypersensitivity (dietary or environmental) of dogs with non-

seasonal atopic dermatitis cannot be differentiated on the basis of historical or clinical information: a prospective evaluation 2003–2004. *Veterinary Dermatology* 2005; **16**: 200.
17. Mueller R, Tsohalis J. Evaluation of serum allergen specific IgE for the diagnosis of adverse food reactions in dogs. *Veterinary Dermatology* 1998; **9**: 167–171.
18. Kunkle G, Horner S. Validity of skin testing for diagnosis of food allergy in dogs. *Journal of the American Veterinary Medical Association* 1992; **200**: 677–680.
19. Fujimura M, Masuda K, Hayashiya M, *et al.* Flow cytometric analysis of lymphocyte proliferative responses to food allergens in dogs with food allergy. *Journal of Veterinary Medicine and Science* 2011; **73**: 1309–1317.
20. Zimmer A, Bexley J, Halliwell REW, *et al.* Food allergen-specific serum IgG and IgE before and after elimination diets in allergic dogs. *Veterinary Immunology and Immunopathology* 2011; **144**: 442–447.
21. Halliwell REW, Gordon CM, Horvath C. IgE and IgG antibodies to food antigens in sera from normal dogs, dogs with atopic dermatitis and dogs with adverse food reactions. In: Hillier A, Foster AP, Kwochka KW, eds. *Advances in Veterinary Dermatology*. Oxford: Blackwell Publishing, 2005: 28–35.
22. Foster AP, Knowles TG, Moore AH, *et al.* Serum IgE and IgG responses to food antigens in normal and atopic dogs, and dogs with gastrointestinal disease. *Veterinary Immunology and Immunopathology* 2003; **92**: 113–124
23. Ishida R, Masuda K, Kurata K. Lymphocyte blastogenic responses to inciting food allergens in dogs with food hypersensitivity. *Journal of Veterinary Internal Medicine* 2004; **18**: 25–30.
24. Bethlehem S, Bexley J, Mueller RS. Patch testing and allergen-specific serum IgE and IgG antibodies in the diagnosis of canine adverse food reactions. *Veterinary Immunology and Immunopathology* 2012; **145**: 582–589.
25. Ohmori K, Masuda K, Ohno K, *et al.* Bovine serum albumin is one of the common allergens in dogs with spontaneous beef allergy. *Journal of Allergy and Clinical Immunology* 2005; **115**: S243.
26. Martín AU, Sierra MA, González JL, *et al.* Identification of allergens responsible for canine cutaneous adverse food reactions to lamb, beef and cow's milk. *Veterinary Dermatology* 2004; **15**: 349–356.
27. Fujimura M, Ohmori K, Masuda K, *et al.* Oral allergy syndrome induced in a dog with Japanese cedar (*Cryptomeria japonica*) pollinosis. *Journal of Veterinary Medical Science* 2002; **64**: 1069–1070.
28. White SD. Food hypersensitivity in 30 dogs. *Journal of the American Veterinary Medical Association* 1986; **188**: 695–698.
29. Jeffers EJ, Meyer EK Sosis EJ. Responses of dogs with food allergies to single ingredient dietary provocation. *Journal of the American Veterinary Medical Association* 1996; **209**: 608–611.
30. Junginger J, Schwittlick U, Lemensieck F, *et al.* Immunohistochemical investigation of Foxp3 expression in the intestine in healthy and diseased dogs. *Veterinary Research* 2012; **43**: 1–14.
31. Veenhof EZ, Rutten VP, Noort RV, *et al.* Evaluation of T-cell activation in the duodenum of dogs with cutaneous food hypersensitivity. *American Journal of Veterinary Research* 2010; **71**: 441–446.
32. Veenhof E, Knol E, Schlotter Y, *et al.* Characterisation of T cell phenotypes, cytokines and transcription factors in the skin of dogs with cutaneous adverse food reactions. *Veterinary Journal* 2011; **187**: 320–324.
33. Jackson H, Jackson MW, Coblentz L, *et al.* Evaluation of the clinical and allergen specific serum IgE responses to oral challenge with cornstarch, corn, soy and a soy hydrolysate in dogs with spontaneous food allergy. *Veterinary Dermatology* 2003; **14**: 181–187.
34. Hammerburg B, Jackson H, Paps J, *et al.* Spontaneous IgE associated food allergy in dogs as a model of human peanut allergy. *Journal of Allergy and Clinical Immunology* 2005; **115**: S34.
35. Jackson H, Olivry T, Hammerberg B, *et al.* The effect of cyclosporine therapy on acute oral challenge in a spontaneous canine model of food allergy. *Veterinary Dermatology* 2006; **17**: 358.
36. Day MJ. The canine model of dietary hypersensitivity. *Proceedings of the Nutrition Society* 2005; **64**: 458–464.
37. Kimber I, Dearman RJ, Andre H. Penninks, *et al.* Assessment of protein allergenicity on the basis of immune reactivity: animal models. *Environmental Health Perspectives* 2003; **111**: 1125–1130.
38. Cave NJ, Guilford WG. A method for in vitro evaluation of protein hydrolysates for potential inclusion in veterinary diets. *Research in Veterinary Science* 2004; **77**: 231–238.
39. Serra M, Brazís P, Fondati A, *et al.* Assessment of IgE binding to native and hydrolyzed soy protein in serum obtained from dogs with experimentally induced soy protein hypersensitivity. *American Journal of Veterinary Research* 2006; **67**: 1895–1900.

16

Cutaneous manifestations of food hypersensitivity

Didier N. Carlotti

Service de Dermatologie, Aquivet Clinique Vétérinaire, Eysines, Bordeaux, France

Conflict of interest: none declared.

Historical perspective

Food allergies in humans have been known for nearly a century. In 1923, Dr. Prausnitz injected himself intradermally with serum from a fish-allergic individual (Mr. Küstner), and the allergy was confirmed by a positive skin test with Prausnitz reacting to the intradermal injection of fish extract on the same site 24 hours later. This was the first passive transfer test, indicating that a reaginic substance was present in the serum of a food-allergic patient.

In the veterinary literature, hypersensitivity reactions to various foods have been reported in dogs, cats, cattle, pigs, horses, rabbits, and even pandas and walruses [1–12]. The first cases of skin disorders in dogs were described in 1934 by Pomeroy (allergy to salmon) [1] and subsequently in dogs and cats in 1967 by Walton [2].

Epidemiology

Until the end of the last century, 1 to 6% of all dermatological diseases and 5 to 20% of all allergic dermatitides were thought to be attributable to food allergy [4–8,10,13]. These percentages are somewhat variable, possibly because the offending food items had still not been identified and reintroduced [13]. More recently, some authors have observed that 20 to 35% of cases of non-seasonal canine pruritus were due to a food reaction [14–20]. It could be argued that about 10% of canine dermatology cases and about 25% of cases of allergic skin disease are attributable to food reactions. Food hypersensitivity is thus a common skin disease in dogs. In fact, in a recent study the diagnosis of food hypersensitivity in dogs with dermatological signs was made in 48% of dogs subjected to dietary trial [18]. In humans, the incidence of food allergy is increasing in developed countries, with one-third of anaphylactic shock flares attributable to food allergy [12].

Sex, age (at onset), and breed predilection

No sex predilection has been recognized [10,11,18,20,21]. It has been observed that the age of food hypersensitivity onset can range from a few months to over 10 years of age in dogs [6,10,11,18–21]. Picco *et al.* showed that initial clinical symptoms occur before 3 years of age in 83% of cases [20]. It should be emphasized that in some studies, young dogs (aged less than 1 year) were commonly affected as opposed to the situation for canine atopic dermatitis (CAD) *sensu stricto*, i.e. due to aeroallergens [11,13,18,20,21]. The percentage of affected dogs aged younger than 1 year was as high as 48% in one study [20]. Moreover, unlike CAD *sensu stricto*, no breed predilection was recognized in most of the studies of food hypersensitivity, although some canine breeds such as boxer, cocker and springer spaniel, collie, Dalmatian, German shepherd, Lhasa apso, miniature schnauzer, dachshund, West Highland white terrier, shar pei, and

Veterinary Allergy, First Edition. Edited by Chiara Noli, Aiden Foster, and Wayne Rosenkrantz.

Labrador retriever were suspected to be predisposed [10,11,13,22]. In fact, Labradors were predisposed in one study [14] and another study showed a predisposition of pug, boxer, Rhodesian ridgeback, and German shepherd to a lesser extent [20].

Pruritus

Non-seasonal pruritus, mostly widespread and generalized, is the most common manifestation of food hypersensitivity [1–13,18–28]. Pruritus can be *sine materia* (47% in one study [28]) but this is probably the case only at the beginning of the disease. The period between ingestion and the onset of signs may depend on the predominant type of hypersensitivity and the specific antigens involved, but most dogs presenting with food hypersensitivity have permanent pruritus that is not obviously related to the time of ingestion of food. Pruritus is usually severe, relatively constant from the onset, and oral or parenteral glucocorticoids provide variable efficacy, ranging from poor (particularly in longstanding cases) [5,10] to good [11,20,28] (e.g. in 75% of the cases [20]), which makes this response a poor diagnostic criterion [26]. In some cases a poor response to long-term glucocorticoid therapy may lead to iatrogenic Cushing's syndrome [5].

Lesions and pattern of distribution

In dogs, erythema and a papular eruption represent the most common primary lesions. However, in most cases, secondary lesions predominate and develop rapidly. These include alopecia, excoriations, crusting, lichenification, and hyperpigmentation [9,10,12,29]. A rare primary lesion, hyperhidrosis, has been noticed in 15% of the cases in one study [28].

Dogs with food allergy can present clinical primary and secondary lesions with a pattern identical to that CAD *sensu stricto*, or with a completely different pattern. In fact, there are clinical presentations without the classical pattern of CAD, which respond to an elimination diet, such as pruritus, with or without lesions, limited principally to the face and pinnae, or paws [30] (Figure 16.1), perianal area [17,18], and dorsolumbar area [17,18]. Six of eight dogs in which pruritus and erythema were recorded as mainly in the perianal region were diagnosed with food hypersensitivity or concurrent food hypersensitivity [17]. In less than 20% of cases, dry skin (xerosis) or seborrhoea oleosa may occur [28]. Particular clinical presentations can also occur, such as urticaria and angioedema [9,10,12,29], pyotraumatic dermatitis [20,28], otitis externa (see section 'Otitis externa'), and perianal fistulae [11,17,18].

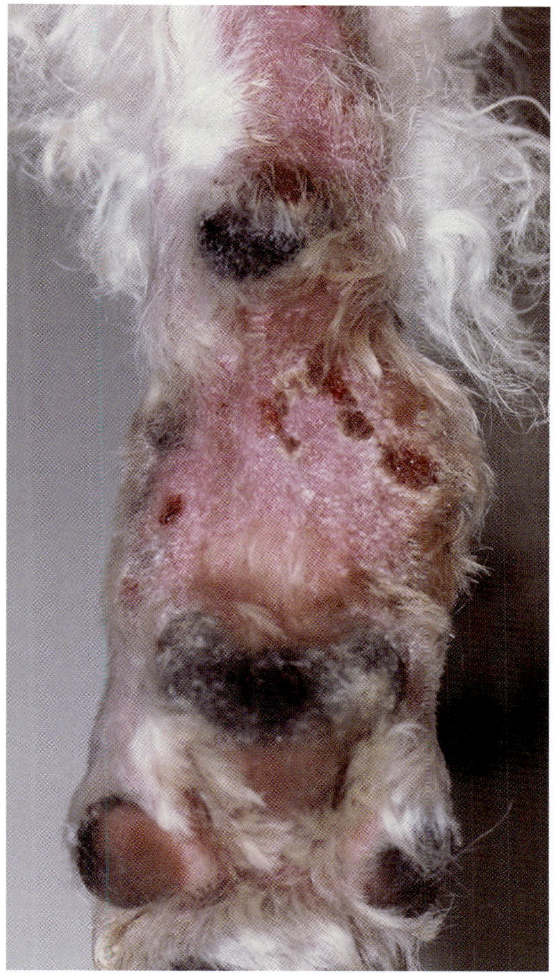

Figure 16.1 Close up of one forefoot in a wire-haired fox terrier with an exclusive pododermatitis of the four feet due to food allergy to chicken meat (no other lesions elsewhere, pedal pruritus was intense).

On the other hand, some cases with the classical pattern of CAD will respond to an elimination diet and it has been reported since the 1960s that food-allergic dogs can present with signs typical of atopic dermatitis [2,3,6,10,11,17,20,21]. These dogs present with facial lesions and rubbing of the face, pododermatitis accompanied by biting the extremities, bilateral otitis externa, and frequently with pinnal and axillary/inguinal involvement [14,18,20,26,28] (Figures 16.2 and 16.3). In the past, clinicians used to say that food hypersensitivity can mimic CAD *sensu stricto*, but it is preferable to consider today that food hypersensitivity can be a cause of CAD *sensu lato*. Furthermore , the International Task Force on Canine Atopic Dermatitis supports the concept that cutaneous adverse food reactions (food allergies) might manifest as atopic dermatitis in some canine patients, or, in other words, that food components might

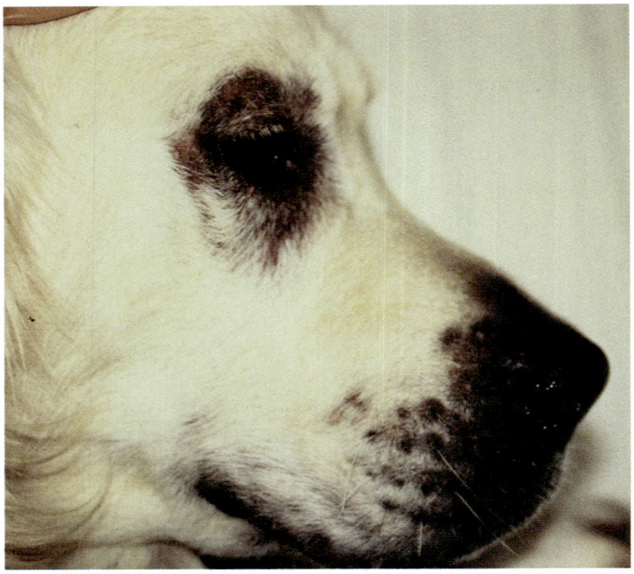

Figure 16.2 Food allergy to beef meat in a golden retriever, with a clinical pattern of atopic dermatitis (food-induced atopic dermatitis). Aspect of the face.

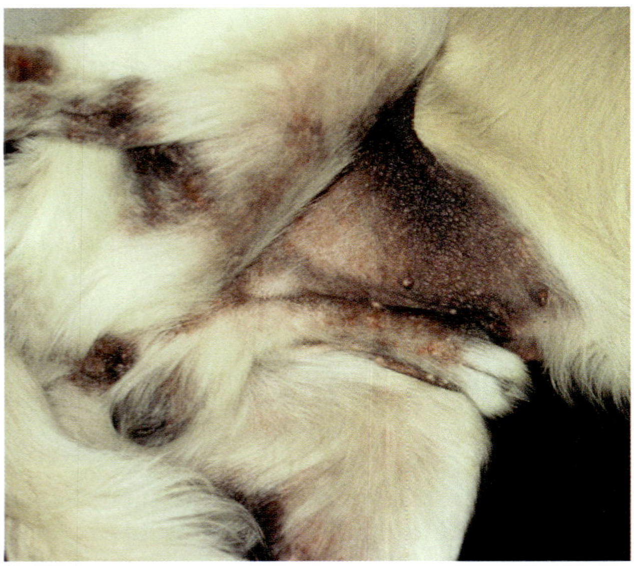

Figure 16.3 Food allergy to beef meat in a golden retriever, with a clinical pattern of atopic dermatitis (food-induced atopic dermatitis). Aspect of the ventrum.

trigger flares of atopic dermatitis in dogs hypersensitive to such allergens [31]. In other words, CAD being a clinical diagnosis (CAD *sensu lato*), there are cases of food-induced CAD and cases of non-food-induced CAD, which include CAD *sensu stricto* and atopic-like dermatitis [28]. In clinical practice every dog diagnosed with non-seasonal (i.e. perennial) atopic dermatitis should undergo one or more dietary restriction–provocation challenges (i.e. 'elimination diets') [31].

Many studies have explored the similarities between food- and non-food-induced CAD (including a large-scale worldwide study of 1096 dogs [28]). Findings from these studies are summarized as follows.

- Percentage of food-allergic dogs exhibiting a CAD pattern:
  - Loeffler *et al.* reported that 40% of food hypersensitivity cases have a CAD pattern [17].
- Percentage of atopic dogs with CAD due to food hypersensitivity:
  - Chesney found that one-third (33%) of CAD cases were food-induced [14].
  - Favrot *et al.* found that 23% of CAD cases were food-induced [28].
- Percentage of dogs with food hypersensitivity affected simultaneously with CAD *sensu stricto*:
  - Jackson *et al.* reported that 10% of dogs with food hypersensitivity were also suffering from CAD *sensu stricto* [19].
- Percentages of dogs with CAD *sensu stricto* suffering simultaneously from food hypersensitivity:
  - Carlotti *et al.* found that only 2% of dogs with CAD *sensu stricto* were also suffering from food hypersensitivity [32].
  - Griffin and DeBoer report that up to 30% of dogs with CAD *sensu stricto* have concurrent food hypersensitivity and they stated that combining food-allergic patients with those with CAD may have led to inaccurate descriptions of clinical signs of CAD *sensu stricto* [29].
  - Zur *et al.* report that 7% of dogs with CAD *sensu stricto* were also affected by food hypersensitivity [33].
  - Jackson *et al.* reported that 33% of dogs with CAD *sensu stricto* were also affected by food hypersensitivity [19].
- Percentages of dogs with allergic skin disease due to CAD *sensu stricto*, due to food hypersensitivity, or both:
  - Jackson *et al.* reported that amongst cases of allergic skin diseases, 48% had CAD *sensu stricto*, 27% food hypersensitivity, and 24% both diseases [19].
  - Proverbio *et al.* reported that amongst cases of allergic skin diseases 26% had food hypersensitivity [18].
  - Picco *et al.* reported that amongst cases of allergic skin disease, 71% had CAD *sensu stricto*, 25% had adverse food reactions, and 4% are complex cases [20].

All these data are difficult to compare because of different study designs or study group size. In summary:

- 40% of food-allergic dogs have a CAD disease pattern;
- one-quarter to one-third of dogs with a CAD pattern are in fact food-allergic dogs;
- 10% of food-allergic dogs also have CAD *sensu stricto*;
- up to one-third of dogs with CAD *sensu stricto* also have food hypersensitivity (very variable);
- allergic skin disease can be roughly divided into: 50–75% CAD *sensu stricto*, 25% food hypersensitivity, and 5–25% with both CAD *sensu stricto* and food hypersensitivity.

These studies did not take into account simultaneous flea allergy dermatitis, which may have influenced the clinical outcome (see Section 'Particular and rare dermatological signs') [18,19,33].

Most of the above studies suggest that only some minor differences exist in the clinical presentation of dogs suffering from CAD due to food hypersensitivity and CAD *sensu stricto* and that the 'two diseases' are clinically indistinguishable with a similar phenotype [14,19,20,28,34]. The few differences noted include:

- Age at onset is rarely under 1 year for CAD *sensu stricto* whereas about half of the dogs with CAD due to food hypersensitivity have initial clinical symptoms before 1 year (16% versus 48%, respectively, in one study [20]); an earlier onset of clinical signs in food-induced CAD being suspected in other reports [14,28]. A possible late onset of food-induced CAD has also been mentioned [14,28].
- Seasonality is mostly seen in CAD *sensu stricto*, as would be expected [20,28].
- Pruritus *sine materia* was more common in CAD *sensu stricto* than in food-induced CAD (63% versus 47%, respectively) in one study [28].
- Pruritus was more corticosteroid responsive in CAD *sensu stricto* than in food-induced CAD (85% versus 64%, respectively) in one study [28].
- Interdigital involvement was more common in CAD *sensu stricto* in one study [19].
- In one study, perianal pruritus was more frequent in food-allergic dogs than in the atopic cases *sensu stricto* (six vs. two) [17].
- *Malassezia* dermatitis was two times more common in food-induced CAD in comparison with CAD *sensu stricto* (43% versus 20%, respectively) in one study [20].
- Gastrointestinal signs are more common in cases of CAD due to food hypersensitivity as compared to CAD *sensu stricto*, according to various studies: 65% versus 25% [17], 31% versus none [20], and 26% versus 11% [28]).

Otitis externa

It is important to appreciate the role of chronic otitis as a presenting sign of canine food hypersensitivity (Figures 16.4 and 16.5). This was confirmed in a study in which there was a significant association between adverse food reactions and otitis externa in dogs [18], with three times more dogs with otitis in a food-allergic canine population than in a non-affected population. In other studies, otitis externa has been observed in 26 [14], 53 [28], 55 [20], 63 [18], and 80% [17] of cases of food hypersensitivity. Otitis externa was the principal sign of food hypersensitivity in one of these studies in 26% of 19

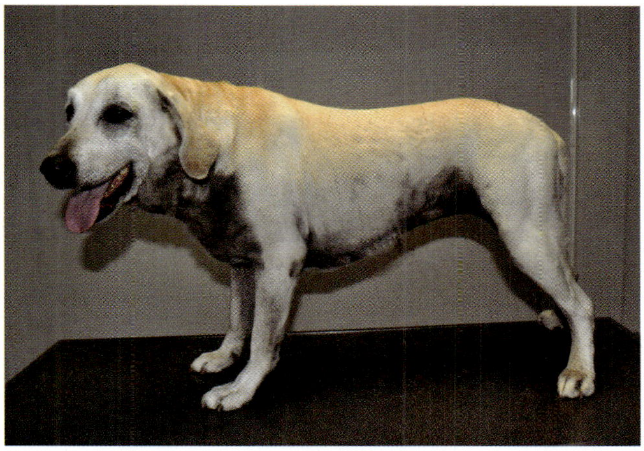

Figure 16.4 Chronic generalized skin disease in an atopic dog, with both food and environmental allergens involved.

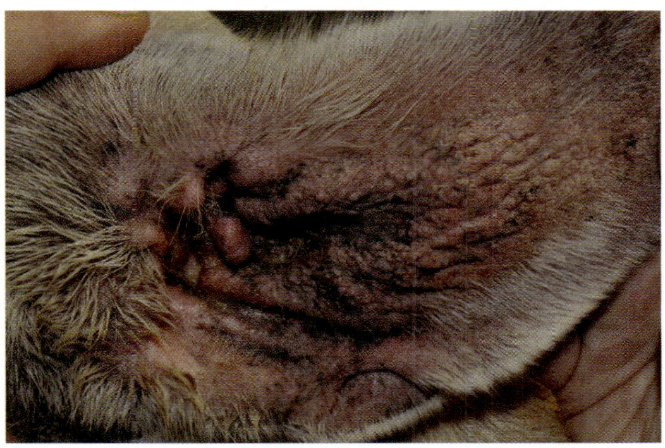

Figure 16.5 Close up of the ear pinna from the dog illustrated in Figure 16.4. Note erythema, lichenification, and hyperpigmentation.

cases [14]. It is the impression of the author that chronic otitis externa is often the main clinical presentation for food hypersensitivity. Otitis externa linked to food hypersensitivity appeared to occur with approximately the same frequency as otitis externa due to atopic dermatitis *sensu stricto* in two studies (food hypersensitivity 53% versus CAD *sensu stricto* 49% [28] and food hypersensitivity 55% versus CAD *sensu stricto* 44% [20]). Otitis media is a mid to long-term consequence of poorly managed otitis externa. Otitis externa (and media) can also occur in man in cases of food hypersensitivity [35].

Secondary skin diseases

Pyotraumatic dermatitis, superficial bacterial pyoderma (folliculitis), *Malassezia* dermatitis, infectious otitis externa (possibly chronic and severe), bacterial pododermatitis, perianal furunculosis, and secondary keratoseborrhoeic disorders are common complications [6,9–11,13,14,17,18,20,28]. In one study, secondary pyoderma and *Malassezia* dermatitis were diagnosed in 32 and 24% of the cases, respectively [17]. In another study, these percentages were similar (44 and 25%, respectively) [18]. In a large-scale study, bacterial infection and yeast infection were diagnosed in 70 and 38% of the cases, respectively, with no statistical difference with CAD *sensu stricto* [28]. In another study, bacterial infection was diagnosed in 69% of cases with no difference with CAD *sensu stricto* (66%) and yeast infection was diagnosed in 43% of cases but in contrast this was higher than in CAD *sensu stricto* (20%), as mentioned above [20]. Overall, it would seem that secondary bacterial infection occurs in one-third to two-thirds of cases of food hypersensitivity whereas secondary *Malassezia* dermatitis occurs in about 25 to 40% of cases, which could be higher than in CAD *sensu stricto* for *Malassezia*. A few cases of recurrent superficial pyoderma have been attributed to a food reaction, in spite of the absence of pruritus [14,21], and recurrent pyoderma can be the principal clinical sign of food hypersensitivity (11% in a study [14]).

Particular and rare dermatological signs

A variety of uncommon to rare cases with unusual clinical presentations of food hypersensitivity have been reported and these include one case with clinical signs mimicking flea allergy dermatitis [17]. A case of granulomatous sebaceous adenitis and one case of dermatosis mimicking mycosis fungoides resulting from a food hypersensitivity have been reported [36,37]. A case of erythema multiforme was reported in 1999 (beef and soy), and another in 2006 (commercially available foods) [38,39]. In a prospective study involving 24 dogs with claw disease, Mueller *et al.* observed a partial remission in two dogs and complete remission in two others after an elimination diet; the complete remission patients relapsed 2 days following reintroduction of their old food. One proved to be allergic to beef by sequential rechallenges, which were not performed in the other three dogs. Curiously, in three of these four dogs, apoptosis was not demonstrated on histological examination of the claws. Mueller *et al.* recommended setting up an elimination diet in cases of exclusive claw disease [40].

Gastrointestinal signs in dogs with skin disease

Some authors reported the gastrointestinal signs usually described in humans, such as vomiting and diarrhoea, in only 10 to 15% of cases in dogs with skin disease [2,6,10,13,41]. In another study, Jackson reported observing intermittent vomiting, diarrhoea, signs of colitis, or borborygmus in 50 to 60% of canine cases [26]. Loeffler *et al.* reported that 65% of food-allergic canine patients presented with gastrointestinal signs [17], Picco *et al.* reported this in 31% [20], and Favrot reported this in 26% [28] of cases, with a significant difference with CAD *sensu stricto* in all studies (see section 'Lesions and pattern of distribution'). In Leoffler's study, the elimination diet resulted in their disappearance in two-thirds of cases [17]. In a more recent study, the prevalence of associated gastrointestinal signs was only 6% [18]. In summary, gastrointestinal signs seem to vary from less than 10% to more than 50% of cases. Paterson reported 20 cases of colitis-associated cutaneous food hypersensitivity [42]. The colitis associated with perianal fistulae can respond to high-dose prednisone and diet therapy [43]. As mentioned in Section "Lesions and pattern of distribution", perianal fistulae can indeed be associated with food hypersensitivity [11,17,18]. Details about gastrointestinal adverse reactions can be found in Chapter 17.

Other non-dermatological signs associated with skin disease

Neurological signs (convulsions) are rarely observed in dogs [2,9,11]. The study by Loeffler *et al.* reported behavioural changes in three dogs (two dogs became lethargic and one dog overexcited) [17]. Many owners report that their dogs appear to improve after an elimination diet is started [22]. Although food allergy-induced canine asthma is very uncommon, its presence has been mentioned [2].

References

1. Pomeroy BS. Allergy and allergic reactions in the dog. *Cornell Vet* 1934; **24**: 335–341.
2. Walton GS. Skin responses in the dog and cat to ingested allergens. Observations on one hundred confirmed cases. *Veterinary Record* 1967; **81**: 709–713.
3. Baker E. Food allergy. *Veterinary Clinics of North America* 1974; **4**: 79–89.
4. Walton GS. Allergic responses to ingested allergens. In: Kirk RW, ed. *Current Veterinary Therapy VI*. Philadelphia: WB Saunders, 1977: 576–579.
5. August JE. Dietary hypersensitivity in dogs: Cutaneous manifestations, diagnosis and management. *Compendium* 1985; **7**: 469–477.
6. White SD. Food hypersensitivity in 30 dogs. *Journal of the American Veterinary Medical Association* 1986; **18**: 695–698.
7. Sousa CA. Nutritional dermatoses. In: Nesbitt GH, ed. *Contemporary Issues in Small Animal Practice*, Vol. 8, Dermatology. New York: Churchill Livingstone, 1987: 189–208.
8. Ackerman L. Food hypersensitivity: A rare but manageable disorder. *Veterinary Medicine* 1988; **83**: 1142–1148.
9. White SD. Food hypersensitivity. *Veterinary Clinics of North America: Small Animal Practice* 1988; **18**: 1043–1048.
10. Carlotti DN, Remy I, Prost C. Food allergy in dogs and cats: a review and report of 43 cases. *Veterinary Dermatology* 1990; **1**: 55–62.
11. Rosser Jr EJ. Diagnosis of food allergy in dogs. *Journal of the American Veterinary Medical Association* 1993; **209**: 259–262.
12. Guaguère E, Prélaud P. Les intolérances alimentaires. *Pratique Médicale et Chirurgicale de l'Animal de Compagnie* 1998; **33** (Suppl. 3): 389–407.
13. Denis S, Paradis M. L'allergie alimentaire chez le chien et le chat. Etude rétrospective. *Le Médecin Vétérinaire du Québec* 1994; **24**: 15–20.
14. Chesney CJ. Food sensitivity in the dog: a quantitative study. *Journal of Small Animal Practice* 2002; **43**: 203–207.
15. Biourge VC, Fontaine J, Vroom MW. Diagnosis of adverse reactions to food in dogs: efficacy of a soy-isolate hydrolysate-based diet. *Journal of Nutrition* 2004; **134**: 2064S–2062S.
16. Loeffler A, Lloyd DH, Bond R, *et al.* Dietary trials with a commercial chicken hydrolysate diet in 63 pruritic dogs. *Veterinary Record* 2004; **154**: 519–522.
17. Loeffler A, Soares-Magalhaes R, Bond R, *et al.* A retrospective analysis of case series using home-prepared and chicken hydrolysate diets in the diagnosis of adverse food reactions in 181 pruritic dogs. *Veterinary Dermatology* 2006; **17**; 273–279.
18. Proverbio D, Perego R, Spada E, *et al.* Prevalence of adverse food reactions in 130 dogs in Italy with dermatological signs: a retrospective study. *Journal of Small Animal Practice* 2010; **51**: 370–374.
19. Jackson HA, Murphy KM, Tater KC, *et al.* The pattern of allergen hypersensitivity (dietary or environmental) of dogs with non-seasonal atopic dermatitis cannot be differentiated on the basis of historical or clinical information: a prospective evaluation 2003–2004. *Veterinary Dermatology* 2005; **16**: 200.
20. Picco F, Zini E, Net C, *et al.* A prospective study on canine atopic dermatitis and food-induced allergic dermatitis in Switzerland. *Veterinary Dermatology* 2008; **19**: 150–155.
21. Harvey RG. Food allergy and dietary intolerance in dogs: A report of 25 cases. *Journal of Small Animal Practice* 1993; **34**: 175–179.
22. White SD. Food allergy in dogs. *Compendium on Continuing Education for the Practicing Veterinarian* 1997; **20**: 261–268.
23. Ferguson E, Scheidt VJ. Hypoallergenic diets and skin disease. In: Ihrke PJ, Mason I, White SD, eds. *Advances in Veterinary Dermatology*, Vol. 2. Oxford: Pergamon Press, 1993: 459–461.
24. Jeffers JG, Meyer EK, Sosi EJ. Responses of dogs with food allergies to single ingredient dietary provocation. *Journal of the American Veterinary Medical Association* 1996; **209**: 608–611.
25. Roudebush P, Cowell CS. Results of hypoallergenic diet survey of veterinarians in North America with a nutritional evaluation of homemade diet prescriptions. *Veterinary Dermatology* 1992; **3**: 23–28.
26. Jackson HA. Dermatological manifestations and nutritional management of adverse food reactions. *Veterinary Medicine* 2007; **1**: 51–64.
27. Rosser EJ. Food allergy in dogs and cats: a review. *Journal of Veterinary Allergy and Clinical Immunology* 1998; **6**: 21–24.
28. Favrot C, Steffan J, Seewald W, *et al.* A prospective study on the clinical features of chronic atopic dermatitis and its diagnosis. *Veterinary Dermatology* 2010; **21**: 23–31.
29. Griffin CE, Deboer DJ. The ACVD task force on canine atopic dermatitis (XIV): clinical manifestations of canine atopic dermatitis. *Veterinary Immunology and Immunopathology* 2001; **81**: 255–269.
30. White SD. Pododermatitis. *Veterinary Dermatology* 1989; **1**: 1–18.
31. Olivry T, DeBoer DJ, Bensignor E, *et al.* for the International Task Force on Canine Atopic Dermatitis. Food for thought: pondering the relationship between canine atopic dermatitis and cutaneous adverse food reactions. *Veterinary Dermatology* 2007; **18**: 390–391.
32. Carlotti DN, Costargent F. Analysis of positive skin tests in 449 dogs with allergic dermatitis. *European Journal of Companion Animal Practice* 1994; **4**: 42–59.
33. Zur G, Ihrke PJ, White SD, *et al.* Canine atopic dermatitis: a retrospective study of 266 cases examined at the University of California, Davis, 1992–1998. Part I: Clinical features and allergy testing results. *Veterinary Dermatology* 2002; **13**: 89–102.
34. Wilhem S, Kovalik M, Favrot C. Breed-associated phenotypes in canine atopic dermatitis. *Veterinary Dermatology* 2010; **22**: 143–149.
35. Yariktas M, Doner F, Dogru H, *et al.* Asymptomatic food hypersensitivity prevalence in patients with eczematous external otitis. *American Journal of Otolaryngology* 2004; **25**: 1–4.
36. Koutinas AF, Toutes D. Granulomatous sebaceous adenitis in the dog: a report of two clinical cases. *Bulletin of the Hellenic Veterinary Medical Association* 1994; **45**: 59–66.
37. Ghernatti I, Peyronnet L, Chabanne L, *et al.* A case of food allergy immunohistopathologically mimicking mycosis fungoides. In: Kwochka KW, Willemse T, von Tscharner C, eds. *Advances in Veterinary Dermatology*, Vol. 3. Oxford: Butterworth Heinamann, 1998: 432–433.
38. Scott DW, Miller WH. Erythema multiforme in dogs and cats: literature review and case material from the Cornell University College of Veterinary Medicine (1988–1996). *Veterinary Dermatology* 1999; **10**: 297–309.
39. Itoh T, Nibe K, Kojimoto A, *et al.* Erythema multiforme possibly triggered by food substances in a dog. *Journal of Veterinary Medical Science* 2006; **68**: 869–871.

40. Müller RS, Friend S, Shipstone MA, *et al.* Diagnosis of canine claw disease—a prospective study of 24 dogs. *Veterinary Dermatology* 2000; **11**: 133–141.
41. Rosser PJ, White SD. Workshop report: Diet and the skin in companion animals. In: Kwochka KW, Willemse T, von Tscharner C, eds. *Advances in Veterinary Dermatology*, Vol. 3. Oxford: Butterworth Heinemann, 1998: 401–405.
42. Paterson S. Food hypersensitivity in 20 dogs with skin and gastrointestinal signs. *Journal of Small Animal Practice* 1995; **36**: 529–534.
43. Harkin KR, Walsham R, Mullaney TP. Association of perianal fistula and colitis in the German Shepherd dog: response to high dose prednisone and dietary therapy. *Journal of the American Animal Hospital Association* 1996; **32**: 515–520.

17

Adverse reactions to food: a gastroenterologist's perspective

Paola Gianella

Dipartimento di Scienze Veterinarie, Università degli Studi di Torino, Grugliasco, Italy

Conflict of interest: none declared.

Adverse food reactions

Adverse food reactions (AFRs) are defined as reactions to an otherwise harmless dietary component, which are experienced by certain individuals on ingestion [1]. They can be divided into two categories based on their aetiology: immunological AFRs (food allergy (FA), also called dietary/food hypersensitivity) and non-immunological AFRs (food intolerance). Food allergy is defined as an aberrant immune response caused by exposure to a particular food substance, most often protein or glycoprotein [2]. In dogs the most common food allergens are beef, dairy products, wheat, eggs, and chicken; in cats they are beef, dairy products, fish, and lamb [3]. In addition, there is evidence that non-protein molecules can also function as allergens. For instance, certain carbohydrates have been implicated as protein-binding haptens (e.g. inulin), and as parts of antigenic glycoproteins [4–6]. They also have a role in causing cross-reactivity between plant allergens and are incriminated in false-positive IgE binding-assays, such as ELISA 'allergy' tests [6]. In contrast, food intolerance denotes non-immunological reactions to a food or a food additive. Food idiosyncrasy, food toxicity, food poisoning, anaphylactic, pharmacological, and metabolic food reactions are all forms of food intolerance.

In recent years, the importance of the diet in the management of dogs and cats with chronic idiopathic intestinal disorders has received much attention and the new term 'diet-responsive' or 'food-responsive chronic enteropathy' has been proposed by gastroenterologists [7]. This definition includes all types of AFRs as well as mild intestinal inflammatory conditions that benefit from the properties of a new diet. For these reasons, diet elimination trials are now recommended in most dogs and cats with chronic idiopathic enteric signs of gastrointestinal (GI) disease [8]. Dogs and cats that respond to an elimination trial but do not relapse after provocation with their original diet almost certainly do not have true AFR, such as food intolerance or FA. It is likely that they are affected by enteritis, colitis, or enterocolitis of different origin and benefit from the higher bioavailability of the nutrients, higher n3–n6 fatty acid ratio, and probiotics in the special diet.

Gluten sensitivity

A characteristic dietary hypersensitivity to gluten causing weight loss with or without small intestine diarrhoea has been reported in genetically related Irish setter dogs [9]. Vomiting and panhypoproteinaemia (low albumin and globulines) are also observed. Unfortunately, these clinical signs and the panhypoproteinaemia are not pathognomonic, but are similar to those observed in other chronic inflammatory enteropathies, such as idiopathic inflammatory bowel disease (IBD). Commonly reported histological alterations are reduced brush-border enzyme expression, villous atrophy, diffuse

Veterinary Allergy, First Edition. Edited by Chiara Noli, Aiden Foster, and Wayne Rosenkrantz.

infiltration of the lamina propria and epithelium with increased numbers of lymphocytes, and goblet cell hyperplasia [10]. Clinical signs and histopathological alterations are reversible when dogs are maintained on a gluten-free diet [9]. It has been hypothesized that an intestinal permeability abnormality may be involved in the pathogenesis of gluten-sensitive enteropathy [9]. This enteropathy in Irish setters has been shown to be inherited at a single autosomal recessive locus, but currently there is no DNA test available [11]. Although similar, the disease is not perfectly analogous to coeliac disease in humans; indeed, it differs because it does not correlate with MCH II haplotypes [12]. The true prevalence of gluten sensitivity among dogs is not available and a confirmed case of gluten sensitivity in any other canine breed (or in cats) has not yet been published. However, despite the lack of scientific evidence, gluten is perceived to be a common food allergen and, as a result, most formulated diets are now gluten free.

Epidemiology of adverse food reactions

Prevalence

The prevalence of dogs with cutaneous AFR showing signs of GI disease varies between studies from 10% to 31% [13–15]. In one of these studies [14], many dogs showed only mild GI signs, such as tendency to develop loose stool and flatulence, whereas few had overt diarrhoea and vomiting.

By comparison, the proportion of dogs with GI signs (vomiting, weight loss, small and large bowel diarrhoea, and decreased appetite) that responded completely to a 10-day elimination trial was 56% in a study conducted in Switzerland [7]. Surprisingly, 79% of these diet-responsive dogs could be switched back to their original diet after receiving a salmon, trout, and rice novel protein diet for 14 weeks. The remaining dogs (21%) relapsed when the novel protein diet was discontinued and improved again when it was resumed. These dogs were considered to have true AFR. One of these dogs with true AFR could not be successfully managed thereafter and was euthanized; this dog had initially presented with chronic signs of GI disease and pruritus.

In another study of dogs with small intestinal diarrhoea, a high percentage of them (90%) responded to either an exclusive highly digestible or a hydrolysed diet over 2–3 months. After performing a dietary challenge with the original food, 65% of dogs that responded to a novel diet (either hydrolysed or highly digestible), relapsed [16]. No difference in the relapse rate between dogs receiving the hydrolysed diet and dogs receiving the highly digestible control diet was found. Interestingly, the vast majority of dogs receiving the hydrolysed diet remained in remission for up to 3 years, compared to only 12% of those on the control diet.

Breed and age predisposition

To date, no definitive breed predisposition has been reported in dogs, with the exception of soft-coated wheaten terriers and a colony of Maltese beagle cross-bred dogs [17,18]. Based on a Swiss study [7], dogs with diet-responsive enteropathy (CE) are usually relatively young, with a median age of 3.4 years.

Clinical presentation

Adverse food reactions may manifest clinically with dermatologic and/or GI signs. It may be difficult to distinguish between food intolerance, FA, and idiopathic IBD in dogs with GI signs, unless cutaneous disease is seen. Indeed, the presence of cutaneous disease and pruritus should raise a suspicion of FA [8,19,20]. With regard to GI signs, AFRs can affect any part of the gastrointestinal tract; however, the most common presenting problems are vomiting, small and large intestinal diarrhoea, and abdominal pain/discomfort [3]. Excessive flatus/borborygmus and altered appetite or anorexia have also been reported. Serious clinical signs such as marked weight loss, depression, melena, haematemesis, and protracted vomiting are usually not observed, although some types of AFRs can be severe.

In a Swiss study, the vast majority of dogs with diet-responsive chronic enteropathy (71%) had exclusively mild to moderate large bowel diarrhoea with signs of tenesmus, frequent defecation, mucoid faeces, and/or haematochezia [7]. Mixed small and large bowel diarrhoea was present in 24% of dogs, whereas 5% had only small bowel diarrhoea. By comparison, most dogs having protein-losing enteropathy or requiring steroid treatment in addition to a diet for the remission of the clinical signs showed severe small bowel diarrhoea. Interestingly, all dogs included in the study were given a clinical score named Canine Chronic Enteropathy Activity Index (CCECAI), derived from the Canine IBD Activity Index (CIBDAI) established by Jergens *et al.* [21]. The CCECAI scoring system is based on the evaluation of six gastrointestinal variables (attitude and activity, appetite, vomiting, stool consistency, stool frequency, weight loss) in addition to serum albumin concentration, the subjective owner assessment of severity of pruritus, and the subjective scoring of peripheral oedema or ascites. After summation, the total composite score is determined to be clinically insignificant (score 0–3), mild (score 4–5), moderate (score 6–8), severe (score 9–11), or very severe (score ≥12). This scoring system was shown to be useful in predicting the response to therapy and a negative outcome in dogs with chronic enteropathy. Therefore the CCECAI may be valuable for all dogs with chronic intestinal disease, including ARFs, after exclusion of endoparasites and enteropathogens.

Differential diagnoses [22]

Dogs with AFRs may present with a wide range of clinical signs; therefore, AFRs should be considered in the differential diagnoses of any case of vomiting and/or diarrhoea, both acute and chronic, unless serious clinical signs or other obvious reasons (e.g. parasites) are present.

Some of the differential diagnoses for AFR are: parasites (nematodes and protozoa), antibiotic-responsive enteropathies, idiopathic IBD, granulomatous colitis, protein-losing enteropathy (i.e. intestinal lymphangectasia, enteropathy of soft-coated wheaten terriers), gluten-sensitive enteropathy of Irish setters, histoplasmosis, alimentary lymphoma, GI neoplasia, and chronic idiopathic large bowel diarrhoea.

In particular, parasite, diet-responsive enteropathies, granulomatous colitis, and IBD are often associated with large bowel diarrhoea, like in AFR.

Diagnosis

Dogs with AFRs do not usually present with pathognomonic clinical findings on physical examination, therefore it is impossible to differentiate dogs with AFR from dogs with other forms of chronic enteropathy by physical examination and routine laboratory tests alone. The combination of cutaneous and GI signs should raise a suspicion of AFR [20]. The index of suspicion is also increased when a temporal association between the ingestion of a specific ingredient and the development of clinical signs is observed. Unfortunately, this is not always the case, because reactions can occur hours or even days after ingestion, and because other GI disorders, such as acute gastritis, pancreatitis, or hepatic failure, may cause clinical signs shortly after feeding. The aim of the physical examination in a dog with suspected AFR is to detect abnormalities that might support other differential diagnoses, such as parasites, antibiotic-responsive enteropathy, idiopathic IBD, or GI neoplasia.

In animals with suspected ARF, a systematic elimination of all possible differential diagnoses is required. The first step is to rule out the presence of intestinal parasites with faecal examination and ELISA test for *Giardia*. A 3- to 5-day course of fenbendazole is generally empirically prescribed (50 mg/kg once daily per os). However, a food elimination trial is usually recommended very early in the diagnostic process, because of the high number of responders. An early dietary elimination trial is pivotal, because animals that improve with appropriate dietary manipulation alone do not require other invasive and expensive diagnostic tests such as an intestinal biopsy.

The clinical diagnosis of AFRs is often based on the response to therapy, that is the abatement of clinical signs while the animal is fed an appropriate diet (hydrolysed, restricted/novel protein diet, home-prepared) and the relapse of the clinical signs upon reintroduction of the previous diet (see Chapters 18 and 19). By feeding an appropriate diet the clinical signs of GI disease usually improve within 2 weeks.

The management of other chronic enteropathies, that do not respond to dietary manipulation and are not thought to be associated with an AFR can involve a variety of therapeutic options [23]. The reader should refer to other reference sources because these are not of allergic origin and are not discussed here.

References

1. Cianferoni A, Spergel JM. Food allergy: review, classification and diagnosis. *Allergology International* 2009; **58**: 457–466.
2. Ortolani C, Pastorello EA. Food allergies and food intolerances. *Best Practice and Research Clinical Gastroenterology* 2006; **20**: 467–483.
3. Verlinden A, Hesta M, Millet S, *et al.* Food allergy in dogs and cats: a review. *Critical Reviews in Food Science and Nutrition* 2006; **46**: 259–273.
4. van Ree R. Carbohydrate epitopes and their relevance for the diagnosis and treatment of allergic diseases. *International Archives of Allergy and Immunology* 2002; **129**: 189–197.
5. Frank P, Moneret-Vautrin DA, Morisset M, *et al.* Anaphylactic reaction to inulin: first identification of specific IgEs to an inulin protein compound. *International Archives of Allergy and Immunology* 2005; **136**: 155–158.
6. Foetisch K, Westphal S, Lauer I, *et al.* Biological activity of IgE specific for cross-reactive carbohydrate determinants. *Journal of Allergy and Clinical Immunology* 2003; **111**: 889–896.
7. Allenspach K, Wieland B, Grone A, *et al.* Chronic enteropathies in dogs: evaluation of risk factors for negative outcome. *Journal of Veterinary Internal Medicine* 2007; **21**: 700–708.
8. Guilford WG, Jones BR, Markwell PJ, *et al.* Food sensitivity in cats with chronic idiopathic gastrointestinal problems. *Journal of Veterinary Internal Medicine* 2001; **15**: 7–13.
9. Hall EJ, Batt RM. Dietary modulation of gluten sensitivity in a naturally occurring enteropathy of Irish Setter dogs. *Gut* 1992; **33**: 198–205.
10. Hall EJ, Batt RM. Development of wheat-sensitive enteropathy in Irish Setters: biochemical changes. *American Journal of Veterinary Research* 1990; **51**: 978–982.
11. Garden OA, Pidduck H, Lakhani KH, *et al.* Inheritance of gluten-sensitive enteropathy in Irish Setters. *American Journal of Veterinary Research* 2000; **61**: 462–468.
12. Polvi A, Garden OA, Houlstgon RS, *et al.* Genetic susceptibility to gluten sensitive enteropathy in Irish setters dogs is not linked to the major histocompatibility complex. *Tissue Antigens* 1998; **52**: 543–549.

13. Favrot C, Steffan J, Seewald W, *et al.* A prospective study on the clinical features of chronic canine atopic dermatitis and its diagnosis. *Veterinary Dermatology* 2010; **21**: 23–31.
14. Chesney CJ. Food sensitivity in the dog: a quantitative study. *Journal of Small Animal Practice* 2002; **43**: 203–207.
15. Picco F, Zini E, Nett C, *et al.* A prospective study on canine atopic dermatitis and food-induced allergic dermatitis in Switzerland. *Veterinary Dermatology* 2008; **19**: 150–155.
16. Mandigers PJ, Biourge V, van de Ingh TS, *et al.* A randomized, open-label, positively controlled field trial of a hydrolyzed protein diet in dogs with chronic small bowel enteropathy. *Journal of Veterinary Internal Medicine* 2010; **24**: 1350–1357.
17. Vaden SL, Hammemberg B, Davenport DJ, *et al.* Food hypersensitivity reactions in Soft Coated Wheaten Terriers with protein-losing enteropathy or protein-losing nephropathy or both: gastroscopic food sensitivity testing, dietary provocation, and fecal immunoglobulin E. *Journal of Veterinary Internal Medicine* 2000; **14**: 60–67.
18. Jackson HA, Hammemberg B. Evaluation of a spontaneous canine model of immunoglobulin E-mediated food hypersensitivity: dynamic changes in serum and fecal allergen-specific immunoglobulin E values relative to dietary change. *Comparative Medicine* 2002; **52**: 316–321.
19. Olivry T, DeBoer DJ, Prélaud P, *et al.* Food for thought: pondering the relationship between canine atopic dermatitis and cutaneous adverse food reaction. *Veterinary Dermatology* 2007; **18**: 390–391
20. Löeffler A, Soares-Magalhaes R, Bond R, *et al.* A retrospective analysis of case series using home-prepared and chicken hydrolysate diets in the diagnosis of adverse food reactions in 181 pruritic dogs. *Veterinary Dermatology* 2006; **17**: 273–279.
21. Jergens AE, Schreiner CA, Frank DE, *et al.* A scoring index for disease activity in canine inflammatory bowel disease. *Journal of Veterinary Internal Medicine* 2003; **17**: 291–297.
22. Gaschen FP, Merchant SR. Adverse food reactions in dogs and cats. *Veterinary Clinics of North America: Small Animal Practice* 2006; **41**: 361–379.
23. Washabau RJ, Day MJ. *Canine and Feline Gastroenterology*. St. Louis, MI: Elsevier Saunders, 2013: 445–537.

18

Diagnostic workup of food hypersensitivity

Edmund J. Rosser Jr

Department of Small Animal Clinical Sciences, College of Veterinary Medicine, Michigan State University, East Lansing, MI, USA

Conflict of interest: none declared.

Hypoallergenic diets

The diagnosis of food hypersensitivity in dogs and cats is first based on one's index of suspicion after considering several historical features and clinical signs [1–11] (see Chapters 16 and 17).

The most accurate method of diagnosing food hypersensitivity in dogs is the use of a *home-cooked* elimination diet. The author does not recommend the use of commercial diets because there are too many possibilities of the presence of some common ingredients or processing agents when changing from one brand of commercially prepared food to another. In addition, it has been documented that cross-contamination of commercial diets can occur in the processing plants. Therefore the animal may have been exposed to proteins and carbohydrates not even listed on the pet food label [12].

The protein source chosen for feeding during the elimination diet trial should be based on the known past exposure of the dog to various foods. If it can be documented that the animal has been exposed to a wide variety of dietary proteins, then each of these proteins must be avoided during the diet trial. Therefore a thorough and extensive review of the pet's dietary history is critical. This needs to include the pet's conventional diet, other dog or cat foods in multiple animal households, table foods, pet treats, dietary supplements, and chewable or flavoured heartworm preventative medications [13].

The protein sources most often found to be suitable, based on the previous dietary history include: lamb, venison, duck, rabbit, kangaroo, and ostrich. The meat should be prepared by boiling, baking, or broiling, with nothing added during the cooking process. The carbohydrate sources most often found to be suitable include: potatoes, sweet potatoes (yams), barley, oats, squash, green peas, or rutabagas (Swedish or yellow turnip (*Brassica napobrassica*)) and must be of the fresh variety because the instant or minute packaged cooking versions of these carbohydrates must be avoided. The carbohydrate is also prepared by boiling or baking, with nothing added during the cooking process.

For dogs, the diet is made by mixing the protein and carbohydrate sources together in equal cooked portions, feeding 2 cups (500 mL) of the cooked mixture per 10 kg of body weight. No supplements need to be added to the diet for the duration of the elimination diet trial. The use of lamb-based baby foods in small dogs should be avoided. Even these food items have been found to contain some offending allergen, which results in the appearance of pruritus after exposure to these foods in a confirmed food-allergic dog [5,14]. Therefore the only thing that 'passes the pet's lips' during the elimination diet trial, is the home-cooked diet and tap water.

When it is deemed appropriate to continue heartworm preventative medication during the elimination diet trial, a non-chewable and non-flavoured formula, or topically applied selamectin or imidacloprid plus moxidectin should be used. No chewable or flavoured versions of a heartworm preventative can be used because

Veterinary Allergy, First Edition. Edited by Chiara Noli, Aiden Foster, and Wayne Rosenkrantz.

it has been documented to have both clinical and immunological reactions to a flavoured monthly oral heartworm prophylactic in 12 dogs with spontaneous food allergy [13]. As these instructions can be overwhelming to most pet owners it is useful to provide a client handout when starting the elimination diet trial (Boxes 18.1 and 18.2).

The duration for feeding the elimination diet is the next most crucial aspect of establishing or ruling out the diagnosis of a food allergy in a dog or cat. Historically and empirically the recommendation was to feed the elimination diet for a 3-week period. It is known that dogs and cats may take as long as 9–10 weeks to show a significant clinical improvement while eating a restricted diet [4,5]. Therefore, the current recommendation is that the home-cooked elimination diet should be fed for a *minimum* duration of 9–10 weeks. In selected instances, dogs and cats may take as long as 12 weeks to show a

Box 18.1 Food allergy elimination diet for dogs

We believe that your pet may have a food allergy. Not an allergy to a particular brand of food, but to one of the individual ingredients. We therefore want to feed a diet that your pet has not eaten before. For this diet we will use a source of fresh protein and a fresh carbohydrate. The protein source can be lamb, venison, elk, moose, ostrich (emu), kangaroo, horse, rabbit, goat, fish (ocean perch, white fish), or duck. The carbohydrate source can be white or redskin potatoes, sweet potatoes (yams) rutabagas, squash, green beans, green peas, barley, or oats. It is very important that you adhere to the following guidelines:

1. The meat must be pure without any additives (spices, other meats such as beef). Be sure to mention to your butcher it **must** be PURE meat. If the meat is ground, make sure that if they grind the meat they use a clean meat grinder.
2. The meat should be trimmed of any excess fat and then boiled, broiled, microwaved, or baked. If using duck, either skin it before cooking, or poke large holes through the skin to allow the excessive fat to drain. If boiling meat the water and fat should be drained. You can skim the fat off the water and let it harden into lard. This can then be used to help give your pet a pill. Nothing should be added to it (seasoning etc.). Larger quantities may be prepared and then frozen for daily feeding. If boiling (poaching) fish it should be cooked until it is white and flakes easily.
3. The white or redskin potatoes, sweet potatoes (yams), rutabagas, barley, or oats must be FRESH—not pre-cooked or pre-seasoned. They should be boiled with nothing added to the water. Larger quantities may be prepared and then refrigerated for daily feeding.
4. Occasionally, we will use pinto or kidney beans as a fresh source of protein to decrease the amount of meat needed for the diet. To prepare them: soak beans in water over night. Throw out this water and put in fresh water. Boil till cooked—typically approximately one hour.
5. The proportion of food should be 50% meat and 50% carbohydrates by volume. Begin with 2 cups (500 mL) of the cooked mixture per 10 kg of body weight per day. Should the dog seem to still be hungry, you can add up to double the amount of the carbohydrate.
6. Some pets won't drink much water during this time because there is so much water in this diet. Don't worry.
7. Always make the diet change from your current diet to the home-cooked diet GRADUALLY, by feeding ¾ by volume of the old diet and ¼ by volume of the new diet on Day 1, then feeding ½ by volume of the old diet and ½ by volume of the new diet on Day 2, then feeding ¼ by volume of the old diet and ¾ by volume of the new diet on Day 3, and finally only the new diet on Day 4.
8. It is very important to emphasize that your animal should not be allowed to put anything in his/her mouth except the home cooked diet and water. This means NO vitamin or essential fatty acid supplement, chew toys, biscuits, rawhides, or table food. NOTHING! If your pet is receiving any MEDICATION please check with us **before** discontinuing it. If your pet is on a chewable form (i.e. beef flavoured biscuit) of heartworm medicine please have your referring veterinarian change it to a NON-chewable form.
9. Occasionally, a change in diet may cause a digestive upset—either vomiting or diarrhoea. Your pet may refuse to eat the above diet. If he/she does not eat for 2 days or a digestive upset occurs, please call us for instructions before giving up. Frequently, they will only have a bowel movement every other day because the food is so well digested. Please call if your pet goes more than 2–3 days without a bowel movement.
10. In order to determine if your pet has a food allergy this diet must be **strictly** maintained for 8–12 weeks. You may not see complete relief from itching, scratching, or licking, but you should see some improvement. It is very important that you keep a DAILY ITCH CALENDAR. Please contact us before you change your pet's diet, whether improvement is noted or not.
11. Your pet will **not** be on the elimination diet for the rest of its life. Once we have established that your pet has a food allergy we will then outline procedures to determine which foods cause an allergic response. When we know which pure foods cause a problem and which ones don't, we can then choose a commercial preparation that your pet will tolerate.

Box 18.2 Guidelines for determination of specific food allergies

Your animal has shown improvement on the home-made elimination diet. We must now continue with the next phase of the programme.

1. Start your pet back on ALL the SAME things he/she ate prior to the special homemade diet. We are doing this to establish that there is a definite food allergy and that the improvement was not due to other factors. If, after feeding the original diet for 14 days, the itching hasn't increased, please call us for the next step. However, if the itching increases, **immediately stop** the pet food and re-institute the homemade elimination diet. Continue this homemade diet trial until the itching has again reduced, then proceed to the next step. If after 14 days the itching doesn't decrease please call us.
2. Now we want to try ____________________ commercial pet food for 14 days. If your pet does not experience an increase of itching go to Step 3.
3. Now that we have established for CERTAIN that your pet has a food allergy we must determine what individual ingredients are causing the problem. Make a list with 2 columns. One column says 'safe' food and the other column says 'unsafe' food. Each week add a new ingredient to the above commercial pet food as directed below. If no increase in itching is noted after 1 week, list this food in the column labelled 'safe'. You may immediately start on the next food mixture on the list, following the same procedure. If your pet's itching increases, list the new food in the 'unsafe' column. Stop that food and resume feeding ________________ commercial pet food (only) until the animal is as itch-free as it was prior to adding the offending food. Once the itching has subsided, resume feeding as directed below. When you have completed the list, schedule a follow-up examination and evaluation (please bring your list of 'safe' and 'unsafe' foods).

USE __________AND ONE OF THE FOLLOWING (depending on the week):

Week #1 and 2 Ground beef
Week #3 and 4 Chicken
Week #5 and 6 Pork
Week #7 and 8 Cottage cheese
Week #9 and 10 Boiled eggs (1 egg/10 kg body weight)
Week #11 and 12 Ground whole-wheat flour
Week #13 and 14 Corn oil (half tablespoon per 10 kg body weight)
Week #15 and 16 Soybean
Week #17 and 18 Lamb
Week #19 and 20 Fish

noticeable clinical improvement. Interestingly, in one study of food hypersensitivity in humans, it was shown that it may require 4–6 months of an allergen-avoidance diet for the rate of basophil-derived histamine release to decline into the normal range [15]. This suggests that a given patient could manifest clinical signs of pruritus for as long as 6 months after avoiding an offending food allergen.

In cases where the pruritus is severe, during the onset of the elimination diet trial it may be necessary to treat the pet with a decreasing dosage of an anti-inflammatory corticosteroid for the first 3 weeks of the diet trial (e.g. oral prednisone or prednisolone at a dosage of 0.5 mg/kg twice daily for 7 days, 0.5 mg/kg once daily for 7 days, and 0.5 mg/kg every other day for 7 days). Additionally, any concurrent secondary problems identified, including a superficial pyoderma, *Malassezia* dermatitis, seborrhoeic dermatitis, or otitis externa/media, should be treated aggressively with the appropriate therapy during the initiation of the elimination diet trial.

When the owner absolutely refuses to feed a home-cooked diet one could use one of the commercially available hydrolysed diets. For dogs these diets include Hill's z/d Canine Ultra Allergen-Free, Purina HA Hypoallergenic Canine Formula, Royal Canin Hypoallergenic Hydrolyzed Protein Adult HP Canine, and Royal Canin Anallergenic. However, it is important to note that in the author's practice approximately 25% of dogs do not improve on any so-called 'hypoallergenic or allergen-free' commercial diet. Subsequently, approximately 25% of our dogs that do improve on only the home-cooked formula need to be maintained on a balanced, home-cooked diet as their long-term maintenance diet. Therefore, the client should be made aware that if one of these diets is chosen as the diagnostic elimination diet, there is a possible 25% failure rate and the dog's food allergy will not be completely ruled out during such a trial.

Once the dog has shown a complete remission of clinical signs, the animal should be challenged with the previously eaten foods for a 14-day observation period. A dog with a confirmed food allergy will exhibit a recurrence of its clinical signs at any time from 15 minutes to 14 days after eating the original offending food. The foods fed should include not only the commercial diet, but also any table foods, pet treats, dietary supplements, and chewable or flavoured heartworm preventative medication because these may be the primary source of allergen as well as the commercial diet. During this time period of dietary challenge, the pet needs to be observed closely because the return of pruritus can be marked, resulting in severely excoriated lesions (Box 18.2).

Each time the clinical signs recur and an offending dietary ingredient is established, the animal is then fed the original elimination diet until the clinical signs resolve. This process is then repeated until each of the major proteins and carbohydrates have been examined, based on the knowledge of the pet's previous dietary exposure. In some instances, the dog seems able to eat any source of home-cooked protein or carbohydrate without exhibiting any clinical signs. However, when these foods are fed in a commercially prepared form, the clinical signs return [1,16]. This has led to the belief that some cases with a food hypersensitivity may actually be reacting to a preservative, dye, or processing agent present in the food.

In some instances, the dog may only show a partial remission of clinical signs during the elimination diet trial, which remain constant for over a 2-week time period without exhibiting any further clinical improvement. This can occur when the animal has more than one cause for its pruritic skin disease, such as a concurrent flea allergy dermatitis or atopic dermatitis.

In vivo tests: intradermal testing and gastroscopy

All studies performed to date examining the potential usefulness of intradermal testing as an aid to the diagnosis of food hypersensitivity in dogs have indicated that these methods are unreliable [17,18]. In one study there were 28 dogs with positive intradermal test reactions to various foods that completed a home-cooked elimination diet trial. Of these dogs only three improved when fed a home-cooked elimination diet and had an exacerbation of clinical signs when re-exposed to their original diet, indicating a problem with false-positive reactions in a majority of the dogs [18]. In another study using 13 dogs with confirmed food hypersensitivity, the sensitivity value for intradermal testing with food allergens was only 10.3%, indicating a poor ability to detect true-positive reactions based on dietary provocation [17]. Lastly, in a study using 14 Maltese × beagle dogs from a breeding colony with a genetic predisposition for allergic disease that were sensitized to various dietary proteins, the dogs were evaluated for their clinical responses and intradermal test reactions upon exposure to corn or soy proteins [19]. When exposed to corn and soy the dogs showed a rapid increase in their cutaneous clinical scores (CCS) and a rapid decrease in their CCS when the food allergen was avoided. However, the positive and negative predictive values of the results of intradermal testing did not approach a level at which the authors would endorse this diagnostic test for specific food hypersensitivities in this or any other population of dogs.

There has been only one study evaluating the usefulness of gastroscopic food sensitivity testing (GFST) in dogs [20]. Several food extracts (corn, soy, wheat, beef, milk, and chicken) were dripped onto the dependent aspect of the stomach via plastic tubing passed through an endoscope in anaesthetized dogs. Six atopic dogs with a history of sensitivity to pollens and foods were evaluated. Of these, three dogs with a food-hypersensitivity component had mucosal reactions of swelling, erythema, and hyperperistalsis observed within 2–3 minutes of the application of food allergens. The dogs were then orally food challenged with the suspected dietary allergen and acute reactions were observed as follows: one dog reacted to milk proteins with acute eructation and vomiting, and one dog react to corn and one to wheat with acute, profuse watery diarrhoea. Based on these observations, it was suggested that some dogs' gastrointestinal food hypersensitivity may have an IgE-mediated disease process due to the acute reactions upon oral food challenge and the observation of the mucosal changes via endoscopy occurring with 2–3 minutes. The authors indicated that the diagnostic accuracy of GFST could not be precisely determined in this study because of the small number of food-hypersensitive dogs evaluated.

Patch testing with foods using a Finn chamber method while keeping the food antigen in contact with the skin for 48 hours has been examined and a negative reaction has a high probability that that food will be well tolerated [21,22]. However, false-positive reactions were observed.

In vitro tests

Similar to intradermal testing, all studies performed to date examining the potential usefulness of *in vitro* serological testing as an aid to the diagnosis of food hypersensitivity in dogs have indicated that these methods are unreliable. In the same study using 13 dogs with confirmed food hypersensitivity for the evaluation of intradermal testing, a food allergen-specific serum IgE ELISA test was evaluated and a sensitivity value of only 13.8% was reported, again indicating a poor ability to detect true-positive reactions based on dietary provocation [17]. Another study was unable to demonstrate food antigen-specific IgE antibodies in the serum of known food-allergic dogs using the Prausnitz–Kustner (PK) tests or the oral PK test [23]. Another study attempted to demonstrate the presence of food antigen-specific IgE from the serum of eight confirmed food-hypersensitive dogs, and the results were negative for all eight of the dogs tested [24]. In another study of 12 dogs with a know hypersensitivity to chicken, most of the dogs had undetectable levels of chicken allergen-specific IgE by the ELISA testing method [25]. Similarly, in the same study mentioned above using 14 Maltese × beagle dogs from a breeding colony with a genetic predisposition for allergic disease that were sensitized to various dietary proteins, the results of the levels of the soy and corn-specific serum IgE levels after oral challenge were not statistically significant and could not be used to predict clinical hypersensitivity [19].

References

1. White SD. Food hypersensitivity in 30 dogs. *Journal of the American Veterinary Medical Association* 1986; **188**: 695–698.
2. White SD, Sequoia D. Food hypersensitivity in cats: 14 cases (1982–1987). *Journal of the American Veterinary Medical Association* 1989; **194**: 692–695.
3. Carlotti DN, Remy I, Prost C. Food allergy in dogs and cats. A review and report of 43 cases. *Veterinary Dermatology* 1990; **1**: 55–62.
4. Rosser EJ. Diagnosis of food allergy in dogs. *Journal of the American Veterinary Medical Association* 1993; **203**: 259–262.
5. Rosser EJ. Food allergy in the cat: A prospective study of 13 cats. In: *Advances in Veterinary Dermatology*, Vol. 2. Ihrke PJ, Mason IS, White SD, eds. Oxford: Pergamon Press, 1993: 33–39.
6. Harvey RG. Food allergy and dietary intolerance in dogs: a report of 25 cases. *Journal of Small Animal Practice* 1993; **34**: 175–179.
7. Kennis RA. Food allergies: Update of pathogenesis, diagnosis, and management. *Veterinary Clinics of North America: Small Animal Practice* 2006; **36**: 175–184.
8. Verlinden A, Hesta M, Millet S, *et al.* Food allergy in dogs and cats: a review. *Critical Reviews in Food Science and Nutrition* 2006; **46**: 259–273.
9. Guaguère E, Prélaud P. Food hypersensitivity in the cat. *European Journal of Companion Animal Practice* 2009; **19**: 234–241.
10. Bryan J, Frank L. Food allergy in the cat: A diagnosis by elimination. *Journal of Feline Medicine and Surgery* 2010; **12**: 861–866.
11. Gaschen FP, Merchant SR. Adverse food reactions in dogs and cats. *Veterinary Clinics of North America: Small Animal Practice* 2006; **41**: 361–379.
12. Raditic DM Remillard RL, Tater KC. ELISA testing for common food antigens in four dry dog foods used in dietary elimination trials. *Journal of Animal Physiology and Animal Nutrition* 2011; **95**: 90–97.
13. Jackson HA, Hammerberg B. The clinical and immunological reaction to a flavoured monthly oral heartworm prophylactic in 12 dogs with spontaneous food allergy. *Veterinary Dermatology* 2002; **13**: 213.
14. Reedy LM. Food hypersensitivity to lamb in cat. *Journal of the American Veterinary Medical Association* 1994; **204**: 1039–1040.
15. Sampson HA Broadbent KR, Bernhisel-Broadbent J. Spontaneous release of histamine from basophils and histamine-releasing factor in patients with atopic dermatitis and food hypersensitivity. *New England Journal of Medicine* 1989; **321**: 228–232.
16. Jeffers JG Meyer EK, Sosis EJ. Responses of dogs with food allergies to single ingredient dietary provocation. *Journal of the American Veterinary Medical Association* 1996; **209**: 608–611.
17. Jeffers JG Shanley KJ, Meyer EK. Diagnostic testing of dogs for food hypersensitivity. *Journal of the American Veterinary Medical Association* 1991; **198**: 245–250.
18. Kunkle K, Horner S. Validity of skin testing for diagnosis of food allergy in dogs. *Journal of the American Veterinary Medical Association* 1992; **200**: 677–680.
19. Jackson HA, Jackson MW, Coblentz L, *et al.* Evaluation of the clinical and allergen specific serum immunoglobulin E responses to oral challenge with cornstarch, corn, soy, and a soy hydrolysate diet in dogs with spontaneous food allergy. *Veterinary Dermatology* 2003; **14**: 181–187.
20. Guilford WG, Strombeck DR, Rogers Q, *et al.* Development of gastroscopic food sensitivity testing in dogs. *Journal of Veterinary Internal Medicine* 1994; **8**: 414–422.
21. Bethlehem S, Bexley J, Mueller RS. Patch testing and allergen-specific serum IgE and IgG antibodies in the diagnosis of canine adverse food reactions. *Veterinary Immunology and Immunopathology* 2012; **145**: 582–589.
22. Johansen C, Mueller RS. Evaluation of canine adverse food reactions by patch testing. *Veterinary Dermatology* 2012; **23** (Suppl. 1): 49.
23. Hillier A, Kunkle G. Inability to demonstrate food antigen-specific IgE antibodies in the serum of food allergic dogs using the PK and oral PK tests. *10th Proceedings of the Annual Meeting of the American College of Veterinary Dermatology*, 1994.
24. Mueller R, Toshalis J. Evaluation of serum allergen-specific IgE for the diagnosis of food adverse reactions in the dogs. *Veterinary Dermatology* 2003; **9**: 167–171.
25. Ricci R, Hammerberg B, Paps J, *et al.* A comparison of the clinical manifestations of feeding whole and hydrolyzed chicken to dogs with hypersensitivity to the native protein. *Veterinary Dermatology* 2010; **21**: 358–366.

19

Long-term management of food hypersensitivity in the dog

Nick J. Cave

Institute of Veterinary, Animal and Biomedical Sciences, Massey University, Palmerston North, New Zealand

Conflict of interest: none declared.

Abbreviations

AAFCO	American Association of Feed Control Officials
CFH	Cutaneous food hypersensitivity
CLA	Cutaneous lymphocyte antigen
DHA	Docosahexanoic acid (C22:6 n-3)
EFA	Essential fatty acids
EPA	Eicosapentaenoic acid (C20:5 n-3)
FEDIAF	European Pet Food Industry Federation
GLA	γ-linolenic acid (C20:3 n-6)
HPD	Home-prepared diet
LA	Linoleic acid (C18:2 n-6)
PUFA	Polyunsaturated fatty acids
Th1, Th2	Type 1 and 2 T-helper lymphocytes

Introduction

Confirming a diagnosis of food hypersensitivity requires the satisfaction of four diagnostic criteria:

1. resolution or improvement of clinical signs on an elimination diet;
2. relapse on subsequent challenge with the original diet;
3. resolution on re-introduction of the elimination diet;
4. demonstration of an immunological basis (i.e. hypersensitivity) for the adverse response.

It is rare, even in academic institutions, that all four criteria are met, especially the demonstration of the immunological basis. Thus it is frequently more precise to diagnose an adverse reaction to food, rather than a hypersensitivity to food. In addition, it is reasonable for a client to be uninterested in subjecting their pet to a challenge trial when the clinical signs are well controlled on an elimination diet. Thus, the long-term management of dogs with suspected food hypersensitivity will be for dogs that range from those that have simply improved on an elimination diet, to those in which the specific allergen has been defined and an immunological basis has been demonstrated.

Despite this range of diagnostic certainty, the two primary concerns for the long-term management of cutaneous food hypersensitivity (CFH) are: avoidance of the known or suspected allergen(s) and meeting the nutritional requirements of the dog. Thus, the long-term management requires two questions to be answered:

- What should this animal be fed?
- For how long should the particular diet be complied with?

This chapter will attempt to address these questions.

Diets for food hypersensitivity

The term 'hypoallergenic' is not used in this chapter. The term is, at best, an ambiguous one, and has been widely misused. It should be reserved for diets that have, at the

Veterinary Allergy, First Edition. Edited by Chiara Noli, Aiden Foster, and Wayne Rosenkrantz.

very least, been demonstrated to possess a substantial reduction in antigenicity, and preferably been shown to be tolerated by the vast majority patients known to be hypersensitive to the intact source protein. However, any reduction in antigenicity or clinical reactivity at which point a diet could be considered 'hypoallergenic' is arbitrary, unless it is absolute. The only commercial diets for which this term would approach suitability would be extensively hydrolysed diets. This chapter includes discussion, and perhaps is largely devoted to, conventional intact protein diets. Although they are novel to the patient, and will not elicit an allergic response in a patient sensitized to another protein, they are in no way 'hypoallergenic'. Therefore, the term is not used in this chapter.

Nutritional considerations

Long-term feeding of a specific diet should only be recommended if the diet is known to be complete and balanced. There are three methods for determining if a diet is complete and balanced:

1 computerized analysis
2 chemical analysis
3 feeding trial.

A computerized analysis calculates the concentrations of individual nutrients in a diet by combining established analyses of the individual ingredients in the proportion they appear in the diet. This approach is used for the formulation of home-prepared recipes by nutritionists, and by some commercial manufacturers. Serious limitations to computerized analyses include:

- differences between the actual ingredients in the diet and those ingredient analyses used in the calculations;
- lack of information on nutrient digestibility or bioavailability;
- inability to identify nutrient interactions;
- absence of information on the presence of toxins;
- no guarantee of palatability.

A chemical analysis of a diet enables a definitive statement of the content of assayed nutrients and is thus more accurate than a computerized analysis. None-theless, similar limitations exist in regards to digestibility, bioavailability, nutrient interactions, safety, and palatability.

The best available information regarding a diet is derived from a feeding trial, whereby a diet is fed to a group of suitable animals for a sufficient length of time under controlled conditions, during which the animals are monitored for the presence of diet refusal, weight loss, or disease. Both the American Association of Feed Control Officials (AAFCO) and the European Pet Food Industry Federation (FEDIAF) have well-established protocols for conducting feeding trials and diets that have been subjected to these can be held to be truly complete and balanced (see http://www.fediaf.org/self-regulation/nutrition/and http://petfood.aafco.org/).

It is the author's opinion that veterinarians should recommend diets that have passed one of these feeding trials if a suitable diet exists. An acceptable alternative is a diet that is formulated to meet the requirements established by AAFCO or FEDIAF. If the pertinent clinical signs have been acceptably controlled on an AAFCO/FEDIAF tested diet, then the simplest approach is to maintain that elimination diet in the long term, whilst considering the points below.

Immunological considerations

The successful diagnosis of an adverse food reaction will have required the elimination of the offending ingredient from the diet. If challenge trials have been conducted, then it is possible to provide an owner with a list of commercial foods or recipes that exclude the ingredient. In the majority of cases, the incriminated ingredient will be an ingredient included as a primary source of protein. In some cases, ingredients typically described as carbohydrate or lipid sources may be incriminated. In cases where a dietary carbohydrate is implicated as a source of allergen, e.g. corn (maize), it is more likely that the dog is sensitized to proteins within the carbohydrate source than the dog having a true hypersensitivity to the carbohydrate molecules. Maize proteins ('zeins') have been identified as the allergenic component of corn starch for some humans [1]. Similarly, lipophilic protein allergens have been isolated in refined vegetable oils [2]. Thus the carbohydrate and lipid ingredients may be an important source of conventional protein allergens in commercial diets.

If the exact ingredient remains uncertain, then one must choose between three options:

1 Avoid all protein sources consumed within the period of clinical signs. It is frequently difficult to identify a completely accurate dietary history that would enable confidence. Additionally, many dogs have eaten so many ingredients that selecting a diet that excludes them all may preclude any commercial diet and force the creation of a home-prepared recipe using uncommon ingredients.
2 Avoidance of the most likely protein sources. In the majority of food allergic dogs, the allergen is within one of the major ingredients in the diet [3–5]. On that basis, the simple avoidance of the major protein and carbohydrate sources from the previous diet will usually be successful. A more rigorous exclusion would also consider the lipid source.

3 Long-term feeding of the elimination diet, or a balanced version of it. If the elimination diet is an incomplete home-prepared recipe, an attempt should be made to complete and balance it through the options discussed in Section Home-prepared diets. Alternatively, the dog can be weaned onto a commercial diet that includes the same protein source as the elimination diet and contains none of the known or suspected allergenic ingredients of the prior diet.

Whatever diet is selected for the immediate long term, it is frequently desirable, sometimes necessary, to consider if the original dietary hypersensitivity is transient or lifelong and if a new hypersensitivity to the new diet might develop.

Home-prepared diets

Home-prepared diets (HPDs) can, and should, be formulated to be the equal of commercial diets. However, a combination of inadequate recipes, owner (and veterinarian) ignorance, and the natural tendency for 'recipe drift' combine to produce a large proportion of inadequate diets.

In Europe, a survey of HPDs fed to dogs found that energy, fat, and protein were above AAFCO recommendations, whereas calcium, Ca:P ratio, and vitamins A and E and potassium, copper, and zinc concentrations were below recommendations [6]. Relative fatty acid contents of serum phospholipid fractions of HPD-fed dogs were significantly lower in 18:2(n-6) and 20:4(n-6) than those from a population of 37 normal dogs consuming commercial dry, USA-manufactured diets. In the USA, the great majority (>90%) of HPD recipes used by veterinarians and owners are nutritionally inadequate [7]. Unfortunately, even textbook and refereed publications may not contain adequate recipes. In one study of 49 maintenance and 36 growth diets published in six veterinary nutrition books, the majority had one or more significant nutrient deficiency [8]. The most common nutritional inadequacy was a deficiency of calcium and too low Ca:P ratio, which is an inevitable consequence of an unsupplemented meat-based diet. Other common deficiencies included vitamins B_{12}, E, D, and A, and copper, manganese, and iodine. Common excesses included total fat, 18:2(n-6), and B vitamins.

Proper formulation of HPD recipes can be performed by consulting a veterinary nutritionist through either the American College of Veterinary Nutrition or the European College of Veterinary Comparative Nutrition. Alternatively, recipes can be created using a web-based service created by a veterinary nutrition specialist (www.balanceit.com). Most properly formulated HPDs contain a minimum of six, and up to nine, separate ingredients. Although not studied, client compliance probably decreases with increased ingredient list. Formulating complete diets without using 'supplements' is perfectly possible, but requires many more ingredients.

Since most veterinarians prescribe HPDs for short periods of time (up to 10 weeks for the diagnosis of cutaneous food hypersensitivity), it is worth considering the significance of nutritional deficiencies encountered during that feeding period in an adult dog.

That dogs do not apparently become ill with short-term feeding of such diets is credit to several factors including:

- our inability to measure the effects of short-term nutritional inadequacy;
- the uncertainty of the absolute physiology requirements;
- the difference between long-term requirements averaged out as a daily requirement vs. a true short-term requirement;
- non-compliance and the pragmatic tendency for a varied diet to be more likely to be complete than a restricted one.

Although not properly surveyed, the most commonly reported deficiencies are calcium, phosphorus, protein, thiamine, taurine, and vitamins E, A, and D; the most common excesses are vitamin A and D. Most home-prepared elimination diets have a single protein source (usually a meat), often as the dominant ingredient. Such diets will be very high in protein, B vitamins, and phosphorus, but grossly deficient in calcium (see Tables 19.1 and 19.2). Thus the most commonly reported clinical effects from meat-based diets are due to osteopenia and fibrous osteodystrophy from inadequate calcium [10,11].

Table 19.1 Key nutrient deficiencies and excesses in a diet of lamb and rice, fed 50:50 by weight, for a dog

Nutrient	Percentage of NRC requirement[a]
Calcium	4%
Copper	27%
Iodine	0%
Potassium	30%
Iron	54%
Zinc	27%
Vitamin A	0%
Vitamin D_3	0%

[a] Nutrient requirements of dogs (and cats), National Research Council [9].

Table 19.2 The suitability of commonly used elimination diets for growth

Suitable for growth	Not suitable for growth
Royal Canin Hypoallergenic Canine	Hill's Canine z/d
Royal Canin Sensitivity Control Canine	Hill's Feline z/d
Royal Canin Sensitivity Control Feline	Hill's Canine Ultra z/d
Nestle-Purina HA Canine	Hill's Canine d/d
Nestle-Purina HA Feline	Hill's Feline d/d
Nestle-Purina DRM Dermatologic Management® Canine	Royal Canin Hypoallergenic Feline

Malnutrition is more likely to occur during growth than in an adult, and it is important to realize how quickly significant clinical disease can develop. It may be many months before a severely calcium-deficient diet causes clinical signs of osteopenia in an adult [12]. In contrast, severe signs of fibrous osteodystrophy can develop within 6–8 weeks in puppies when fed deficient diets during the first 3–6 months of life [13]. Not all commercial diets marketed for the diagnosis of food hypersensitivity are suitable for long-term feeding to growing animals. Examples of both suitable and unsuitable diets are presented in Table 19.2.

Hydrolysed protein diets

Dietary proteins can be hydrolysed into individual amino acids or peptides using acid or proteases [14]. The resulting hydrolysate can then be incorporated in a diet as the source of amino acids. If the parent proteins have been fragmented sufficiently then there will be no intact allergens and the diet can be fed to a patient sensitized to the parent protein without causing any clinical signs. In addition, if the proteins are sufficiently hydrolysed, an animal eating that diet cannot become sensitized to the parent protein.

It is not known what the limit is, under which the remaining peptide fragments are small enough to prevent clinical signs in all sensitized patients. Indeed, although there is an absolute limit for all proteins, the actual limit for individual proteins will vary according to the antigenic epitopes within that protein.

Ensuring that a hydrolysate has no peptides greater than 1 kDa would give the greatest chance of eliminating any residual allergens, although 3 kDa would be sufficient for the great majority of patients sensitized to the parent protein. However, hypersensitivity reactions have been identified in children fed even the most hydrolysed formulae [15]. It should also be realized that the presence of fragments of greater than 5 kDa or even greater than 10 kDa does not guarantee that they can act as allergens. Nor is there any useful information in citing an 'average' molecular weight of a product. The reduction of allergenic epitopes is dependent on the specificity for the proteolytic enzymes as to whether any given epitope is cleaved or disrupted and rendered non-allergenic.

Complete and balanced hydrolysed diets also contain lipid and carbohydrate sources, either of which can contain very small quantities of intact allergens, such as maize zeins in corn starch and lipophilic protein allergens in refined vegetable oils [16,17]. Thus the carbohydrate and lipid sources chosen for incorporation into hydrolysed protein diets may be a source of conventional protein allergens because they are not subjected to enzymic hydrolysis and should be considered when evaluating commercial diets. It is not sensible to use a hydrolysed protein diet that is made from protein sources that the patient may be allergic to when alternatives exist.

The palatability of a protein source changes significantly with hydrolysis, and although it is often reduced, that cannot be assumed. The taste of a hydrolysate is dependant on the mixtures of peptides and cannot be assumed to be any one flavour, or easily predicted from the protein source. In addition to changes in taste and digestibility, osmolarity increases significantly with increasing hydrolysis, and has been blamed for a high incidence of diarrhoea in infants fed extensively hydrolysed formulae [18]. Feeding high osmolarity enteral solutions has been associated with diarrhoea in humans [19,20]. Dogs that develop diarrhoea when a hydrolysed protein diet is introduced may not be tolerant to the higher osmolarity of that diet.

Pragmatic considerations about diets for food hypersensitivity

Hidden antigen sources

The same difficulties in conducting an elimination diet trial are present in successfully feeding a diet for long-term maintenance. There is great variation between manufacturers and products in the accuracy of the ingredient list. Ingredient lists on many diets can be incomplete or misleading. For instance, it is common for plant-derived ingredients to be included in diets in which only animal by-products are listed [21]. Ambiguity or inaccuracy of ingredient lists, proteins in non-protein ingredients, the feeding of treats and chews, and scavenging present constant challenges. The difficulty obtaining owner compliance with weight management plans is testament to how often diet recommendations are not kept to.

Recipe drift

An unpublished phone survey of clients of the Nutrition Consulting Service of the University of California, Davis, USA, found that within weeks of starting a prescribed HPD the great majority of clients modify, add commercial food to, or abandon the diet completely. Clinicians who prescribe HPDs should be aware of this long-term limitation and if relapse of clinical signs occurs, careful re-evaluation of what is actually being fed is warranted.

Non-allergen aspects of the diet associated with clinical improvement

Essential fatty acids

It is now well recognized that canine atopic dermatitis (CAD) is associated with impaired ceramide production within the stratum corneum, which leads to increased water loss, and likely increased allergen absorption [22,23]. The effect of the diet on ceramide production has not been carefully studied in dogs. However, in one study, enrichment of the diet with a mixture of fatty acids (including LA, GLA, EPA, and DHA) resulted in an increase in both free and protein bound ceramides, cholesterol, and free fatty acids in and on the dermis [24]. In another study, a commercial dry food based on potato, fish, and animal fat, was compared with a home-prepared diet of fish (cod or hake) and potato [25]. Disease severity scores improved within 4 weeks of being fed the commercial diet. Although the study design precluded conclusions as to the mechanism of improvement, the commercial diet contained more LA, EPA, and DHA than the home-prepared diet.

In addition to alterations in ceramide production in the dermis, atopic dogs appear to have altered fatty acid metabolism, presumably in the liver. Atopic dogs appear to have reduced fatty acid desaturase activity, suggesting an impaired ability to produce long-chain desaturated fatty acids [26]. This could indicate that extra benefits may be seen from feeding higher concentrations of longer-chain polyunsaturated fatty acids (20 to 24 carbon PUFA) than is required by normal animals. However, it is not known if these findings also apply to dogs with CFH.

Many, perhaps most, studies of the efficacy of PUFA supplementation on CAD are hampered by failure to consider the dietary fat content concurrently ingested by the trial subjects. In one of the few to evaluate supplementation of a controlled diet, an n-3 PUFA supplement enabled a significant reduction in the use of prednisone required to control pruritus after 8 weeks of supplementation [27].

In another study of atopic dermatitis, supplementation with flax seed or fish oil for 10 weeks resulted in clinical improvement without changing the total FA content in skin biopsies [28]. It may be that whole tissue change does not occur in 10 weeks, although the authors showed that the plasma concentration did, and perhaps superficial lipids of the stratum corneum do too.

Dietary influence on type 2 T-helper lymphocyte development

Several nutrients influence lymphocyte development and the commitment towards a specific T-helper immunophenotype. There may be specific concentrations of these nutrients that will assist resolution of clinical signs and the development of oral tolerance to dietary and other allergens. Vitamins D, A, and E can influence T-lymphocyte development and cytokine production and epidemiological studies in humans have implicated both low and high dietary concentrations of vitamin D as a risk factor for allergic disease [29,30]. In addition, vitamins A and D can affect lymphocyte homing to the dermis and dietary vitamin D can selectively decrease the expression of cutaneous lymphocyte antigen (CLA) without affecting homing to other tissues [31]. At present, it is unknown which, if any, nutrients are especially important in CFH and thus it is not possible to recommend one dietary approach over another. However, until the effective concentrations have been established, it is prudent to avoid deficiency or over-supplementation beyond normal dietary concentrations.

Alternative non-dietary treatments of food hypersensitivity

It has traditionally been assumed that sensitization to food allergens occurs through the intestinal tract. However, the difficulty in explaining CFH in the light of the conventional understanding of oral tolerance and lymphocyte migration suggests that we should question that assumption. Antigens absorbed through the epidermis are ingested by Langerhans cells, which migrate to regional lymph nodes and present antigens to T cells there. Activation of T cells in those nodes induces the expression of CLA and sequestration of antigen-specific T cells into regions of the dermis where local inflammation has resulted in up-regulation of E-selectin [32,33].

In humans and rodents, sensitization through the epidermis is easily demonstrated, and can lead to IgE production, resulting in allergen-primed mast cells in the dermis and other tissues [34]. Oral feeding of the allergen can then produce cutaneous signs or even systemic anaphylaxis [35]. A prerequisite for this to occur is the lack of oral exposure prior to epicutaneous sensitization, because this would induce oral tolerance, or even prevent dermal sensitization [36]. Likewise, small doses of food allergen applied to a disrupted or abnormally permeable epidermis can prevent the development of normal oral tolerance when that food is subsequently ingested in mice [36]. The increased permeability of a disrupted epidermis to proteins is well established in humans and suspected but not yet proven in dogs. Perturbation of the barrier function of the stratum corneum may stimulate inflammation, epidermal hyperplasia, entry of allergens, and serve as a natural sensitization pathway for food allergy.

These concepts support the idea that CFH is a cutaneous allergy and not an 'oral allergy', even though clinical signs are elicited following ingestion. If that is the case, it opens the intriguing possibility that strategies that employ the induction of oral tolerance, such as the gradual reintroduction of the offending allergen, might be successful therapeutic approaches.

A key difference in the management of CFH and atopic dermatitis is that control of the inflammatory component of the dermatopathy is presumed to occur by means of allergen avoidance. However, improvement of the epidermal barrier function may be important for prevention of sensitization and perhaps resolution of existing sensitization.

Thus, there may still be a benefit to promoting optimal cutaneous barrier function, minimizing Th2 lymphocyte development, and reducing inflammatory responses to future dietary indiscretions. At present, dietary approaches to these goals are limited to the avoidance of dietary deficiency and excess, and adequate concentrations of LA, EPA, and DHA.

Sensitization to novel proteins

In the majority of food-hypersensitive dogs, it is not possible at present to determine what was the underlying predisposition of the dog. That means it is also not possible to speculate about the risk of sensitization to the novel diet, with subsequent recrudescence of the clinical signs. Just as there is little information of the frequency of restoration of oral tolerance, there are very few reports of sensitization to the novel protein. Some authors have reported the development of new dietary sensitivities within 1 to 3 years [37]. Questions that remain to be answered include:

- Are there features of the dog at the time of initial diagnosis that predict the risk of neosensitization in the future?
- Is a strict adherence to one diet better than a varied diet with avoidance? There may be a difference in the risk of neosensitization between constant exposure to a single diet and exposure to a variety of dietary proteins.

In dogs that become sensitized to a new protein it may be that long-term maintenance on an extensively hydrolysed diet would significantly reduce the risk of further dietary sensitization.

Eventual restoration of tolerance to allergens

Hypersensitivity to dietary antigens is not necessarily a lifelong state. Although not clear, the expert opinion is that in humans food allergies that start in childhood are often outgrown, whereas food allergy that starts in adulthood often persists [38]. In people with IgE-mediated hypersensitivity to cow's milk it is predominantly a disease of early childhood, which resolves within a few years. In a recent study of cow's milk allergy in children, almost 60% were no longer clinically allergic by 5 years of age and the majority of those patients were no longer allergic within the first 2 years [39]. In another larger study the rate of resolution was less, with 19% resolved by age 4 years, 42% by age 8 years, 64% by age 12 years, and 79% by 16 years [40]. In a study of soy allergy in children, 25% had resolved by age 4 years, 45% by age 6 years, and 69% by age 10 years [41]. In contrast, only about 21% of children that acquire peanut hypersensitivity will become tolerant by age 20 and only 9% of a study of 278 children with tree nut allergy were tolerant at adulthood [42,43].

The resolution of confirmed food hypersensitivity in dogs has not been well described. In study of 55 cats with chronic vomiting and/or diarrhoea, 16 cats were diagnosed as having food sensitivity based on elimination–challenge trials [44]. However, a further 14 cats responded completely to an elimination diet, but did not recrudesce during a challenge with the staple diet. Whilst some of those cats may not have been challenged with the offending food allergen due to an incomplete dietary history, some cats may have rapidly re-established oral tolerance. It is possible that following a period of intestinal quiescence, those cats became clinically tolerant to the food protein, despite potentially still having sensitized antigen-specific lymphocytes. A similar study in feline or canine food allergic patients with CFH has not been published. Indeed, although the author has seen several cases in clinical practice where there has been an apparent resolution, there are no published cases of food hypersensitivity that were shown to have subsequently resolved.

Conclusions and recommendations

It is frequently difficult to find diets that are truly novel to a dog. For long-term feeding, after a diagnosis has been made, only diets that are complete and balanced and that are appropriate for that life-stage should be recommended. Although growing animals are more susceptible to malnutrition, clinical disease is still seen in adult animals on deficient diets. Clinically significant signs of nutritional deficiency can occur within a few weeks on some commonly used elimination diets. Home-prepared recipes offer flexibility and allow for the formulation of a truly novel diet; however, they need to be properly formulated, and owners frequently alter recipes in the long term. Multiple nutrients have the potential to affect short and long-term allergic disease but we do not know enough yet to make recommendations about supplementation or restriction beyond the normal ranges used by respectable manufacturers. Until more is known, the long-term management of food hypersensitivity should focus on a few basic tenets:

- Feed a proven commercial complete and balanced diet suitable for the life-stage if possible, to avoid excess or deficiency.
- If using a home-prepared recipe, ensure it is properly balanced and be aware of poor long-term compliance.
- Resolution of food hypersensitivity is possible, but it is not known how commonly or when it might occur.
- If there is recrudescence of clinical signs on a maintenance diet, consider lack of compliance, hidden antigens, or sensitization to the new diet.

References

1. Frisner H, Rosendal A, Barkholt V. Identification of immunogenic maize proteins in a casein hydrolysate formula. *Pediatric Allergy and Immunology* 2000; **11**: 106–110.
2. Zitouni N, Errahali Y, Metche M, *et al.* Influence of refining steps on trace allergenic protein content in sunflower oil. *Journal of Allergy and Clinical Immunology* 2000; **106**: 962–967.
3. Baker E. Food allergy. *Veterinary Clinics of North America* 1974; **4**: 79–89.
4. Jeffers JG, Meyer EK, Sosis EJ. Responses of dogs with food allergies to single-ingredient dietary provocation. *Journal of the American Veterinary Medical Association* 1996; **209**: 608–611.
5. Paterson S. Food hypersensitivity in 20 dogs with skin and gastrointestinal signs. *Journal of Small Animal Practice* 1995; **36**: 529–534.
6. Streiff EL, Zwischenberger B, Butterwick RF, *et al.* A comparison of the nutritional adequacy of home-prepared and commercial diets for dogs. *Journal of Nutrition* 2002; **132**: 1698S–1700S.
7. Roudebush P, Cowell CS. Results of a hypoallergenic diet survey of veterinarians in North America with a nutritional evaluation of homemade diet prescriptions. *Veterinary Dermatology* 1992; **3**: 23–28.
8. Lauten SD, Smith TM, Kirk CA, *et al.* Computer analysis of nutrient sufficiency of published home-cooked diets for dogs and cats. *Journal of Veterinary Internal Medicine* 2005; **19**: 476.
9. Beitz DC, Bauer JE, Behnke KC, *et al. Nutrient Requirements of Dogs and Cats*, revised edn. National Research Council. Washington: National Academies Press, 2006: 357–358.
10. Aithal HP, Singh GR, Amarpal, *et al.* Fractures secondary to nutritional bone disease in dogs: a review of 38 cases. *Zentralblatt fur Veterinarmedizin Reihe A* 1999; **46**: 483–487.
11. Tomsa K, Glaus T, Hauser B, *et al.* Nutritional secondary hyperparathyroidism in six cats. *Journal of Small Animal Practice* 1999; **40**: 533–539.
12. de Fornel-Thibaud P, Blanchard G, Escoffier-Chateau L, *et al.* Unusual case of osteopenia associated with nutritional calcium and vitamin D deficiency in an adult dog. *Journal of the American Animal Hospital Association* 2007; **43**: 52–60.
13. McMillan CJ, Griffon DJ, Marks SL, *et al.* Dietary-related skeletal changes in a Shetland sheepdog puppy. *Journal of the American Animal Hospital Association* 2006; **42**: 57–64.
14. Cave NJ. Hydrolyzed protein diets for dogs and cats. *Veterinary Clinics of North America Small Animal Practice* 2006; **36**: 1251–1268.
15. Ellis MH, Short JA, Heiner DC. Anaphylaxis after ingestion of a recently introduced hydrolyzed whey protein formula. *Journal of Pediatrics* 1991; **118**: 74–77.
16. Frisner H, Rosendal A, Barkholt V. Identification of immunogenic maize proteins in a casein hydrolysate formula. *Pediatric Allergy and Immunology* 2000; **11**: 106–110.
17. Zitouni N, Errahali Y, Metche M, *et al.* Influence of refining steps on trace allergenic protein content in sunflower oil. *Journal of Allergy and Clinical Immunology* 2000; **106**: 962–967.
18. Hyams JS, Treem WR, Etienne NL, *et al.* Effect of infant formula on stool characteristics of young infants. *Pediatrics* 1995; **95**: 50–54.
19. Ladas SD, Isaacs PE, Sladen GE. Post-prandial changes of osmolality and electrolyte concentration in the upper jejunum of normal man. *Digestion* 1983; **26**: 218–223.
20. Fruto LV. Current concepts: management of diarrhea in acute care. *Journal of Wound, Ostomy Continence Nursing* 1994; **21**: 199–205.
21. Bell KM, Rutherfurd SM, Hendriks WH. The isoflavone content of commercially-available feline diets in New Zealand. *New Zealand Veterinary Journal* 2006; **54**: 103–108.
22. Popa I, Remoue N, Hoang LT, *et al.* Atopic dermatitis in dogs is associated with a high heterogeneity in the distribution of protein-bound lipids within the stratum corneum. *Archives for Dermatological Research Archiv fur Dermatologische Forschung* 2011; **303**: 433–440.
23. Shimada K, Yoon JS, Yoshihara T, *et al.* Increased transepidermal water loss and decreased ceramide content in lesional and non-lesional skin of dogs with atopic dermatitis. *Veterinary Dermatology* 2009; **20**: 541–546.
24. Popa I, Pin D, Remoue N, *et al.* Analysis of epidermal lipids in normal and atopic dogs, before and after administration of an oral omega-6/omega-3 fatty acid feed supplement. A pilot study. *Veterinary Research Communications* 2011; **35**: 501–509.
25. Bensignor E, Morgan DM, Nuttall T. Efficacy of an essential fatty acid-enriched diet in managing canine atopic dermatitis: a randomized, single-blinded, cross-over study. *Veterinary Dermatology* 2008; **19**: 156–162.
26. Fuhrmann H, Zimmermann A, Guck T, *et al.* Erythrocyte and plasma fatty acid patterns in dogs with atopic dermatitis and healthy dogs in the same household. *Canadian Journal of Veterinary Research* 2006; **70**: 191–196.
27. Saevik BK, Bergvall K, Holm BR, *et al.* A randomized, controlled study to evaluate the steroid sparing effect of essential fatty acid supplementation in the treatment of canine atopic dermatitis. *Veterinary Dermatology* 2004; **15**: 137–145.

28. Mueller RS, Fettman MJ, Richardson K, *et al.* Plasma and skin concentrations of polyunsaturated fatty acids before and after supplementation with n-3 fatty acids in dogs with atopic dermatitis. *American Journal of Veterinary Research* 2005; **66**: 868–873.
29. Litonjua AA. Vitamin D deficiency as a risk factor for childhood allergic disease and asthma. *Current Opinion in Allergy and Clinical Immunology* 2012; **12**: 179–185.
30. Li-Weber M, Giaisi M, Treiber MK, *et al.* Vitamin E inhibits IL-4 gene expression in peripheral blood T cells. *European Journal of Immunology* 2002; **32**: 2401–2408.
31. Yamanaka K, Dimitroff CJ, Fuhlbrigge RC, *et al.* Vitamins A and D are potent inhibitors of cutaneous lymphocyte-associated antigen expression. *Journal of Allergy and Clinical Immunology* 2008; **121**: 148–157.
32. Eigenmann PA. T lymphocytes in food allergy: overview of an intricate network of circulating and organ-resident cells. *Pediatric Allergy and Immunology* 2002; **13**: 162–171.
33. Santamaria-Babi LF. CLA(+) T cells in cutaneous diseases. *European Journal of Dermatology* 2004; **14**: 13–18.
34. Beck LA, Leung DY. Allergen sensitization through the skin induces systemic allergic responses. *Journal of Allergy and Clinical Immunology* 2000; **106**: S258–263.
35. Hsieh KY, Tsai CC, Wu CH, *et al.* Epicutaneous exposure to protein antigen and food allergy. *Clinical and Experimental Allergy* 2003; **33**: 1067–1075.
36. Strid J, Hourihane J, Kimber I, *et al.* Epicutaneous exposure to peanut protein prevents oral tolerance and enhances allergic sensitization. *Clinical and Experimental Allergy* 2005; **35**: 757–766.
37. White SD. Food hypersensitivity. *Veterinary Clinics of North America Small Animal Practice* 1988; **18**: 1043–1048.
38. Burks AW, Tang M, Sicherer S, *et al.* ICON: Food allergy. *Journal of Allergy and Clinical Immunology* 2012; **129** 906–920.
39. Elizur A, Rajuan N, Goldberg MR, *et al.* Natural course and risk factors for persistence of IgE-mediated cow's milk allergy. *Journal of Pediatrics* 2012; **161**: 482–487.
40. Skripak JM, Matsui EC, Mudd K, *et al.* The natural history of IgE-mediated cow's milk allergy. *Journal of Allergy and Clinical Immunology* 2007; **120**: 1172–1177.
41. Savage JH, Kaeding AJ, Matsui EC, *et al.* The natural history of soy allergy. *Journal of Allergy and Clinical Immunology* 2010; **125**: 683–686.
42. Fleischer DM, Conover-Walker MK, Matsui EC, *et al.* The natural history of tree nut allergy. *Journal of Allergy and Clinical Immunology* 2005; **116**: 1087–1093.
43. Skolnick HS, Conover-Walker MK, Koerner CB, *et al.* The natural history of peanut allergy. *Journal of Allergy and Clinical Immunology* 2001; **107**: 367–374.
44. Guilford WG, Jones BR, Markwell PJ, *et al.* Food sensitivity in cats with chronic idiopathic gastrointestinal problems. *Journal of Veterinary Internal Medicine* 2001; **15**: 7–13.

Section 3

Flea Bite Allergy

20

Flea biology and ecology

Marie-Christine Cadiergues

Toulouse Veterinary School, Toulouse, France

Conflict of interest: none declared.

Introduction

Fleas represent the most important ectoparasites in companion animals. They have a history of about 60 million years and were already found on prehistoric mammals. More than 2000 species and subspecies are identified throughout the world. Nevertheless, very few species are encountered on dogs and cats and, amongst these, *Ctenocephalides felis felis* is by far the most common. Various aspects of flea biology and ecology may be useful in improving flea control and/or understanding failure or inadequacy of flea control programmes [1,2]. This chapter aims to review the biological and ecological features of flea infestations in dogs and cats, as essential background for following chapters on pathogenesis, clinical signs, diagnostic testing, and management of flea bite allergy.

Morphology

Fleas are wingless insects, belonging to the Order Siphonapterida. The genera *Ctenocephalides*, *Spilopsyllus*, *Pulex*, and *Archaeopsylla* belong to the Family Pulicidae. Their body is laterally compressed and measures about 1–8 mm. Anatomical peculiarities that are of biological importance are the mouth parts and legs [3].

The suctorial mouth parts are well adapted to piercing and sucking. The flea penetrates the epidermis with its maxillae. The epipharynx is inserted in the capillary vessel, allowing blood to be sucked by three pumps (one cibarian, two pharyngeal) through the feeding tube, formed by the maxillae together with the epipharynx. A salivary pump pushes saliva through the laciniae [4]. The sialotranscriptome of *C. felis* has been analysed. The sialomes of cat and rat fleas contain the enzyme families of phosphatases (inactive), CD-39-type apyrase, adenosine deaminases, and esterases, as well as antigen-5 members and defensins. Fleas, in contrast to mosquitoes or sand flies, have a sialome that is comprised of a good portion of small polypeptides, none of which have a known function but they may act as inhibitors of haemostasis or inflammation. They are also unique in terms of the expansion of a phosphatase family that appears to be deficient of enzyme activity and has an unknown function [5].

The third pair of legs is of particular use for jumping. Modifications of the hind leg include an enlarged, muscular femur and an elastic protein (called resilin) in the integument. Resilin is compressed during the flexion of the coxa in the metathorax, and then rapidly relaxed [6]. Jump performances of *C. canis* and *C. felis felis* have been measured and compared on unfed young imagos. The mean length of the *C. felis felis* jump was 19.9±9.1 cm; minimum jump was 2 cm, and the maximum was 48 cm. The *C. canis* jump was significantly longer (30.4±9.1 cm; from 3 to 50 cm). The mean height of the jump was 15.5 and 13.2 cm for *C. canis* and *C. felis*, respectively. The highest jump was 25 cm for *C. canis* and 17 cm for *C. felis* [7].

Veterinary Allergy, First Edition. Edited by Chiara Noli, Aiden Foster, and Wayne Rosenkrantz.

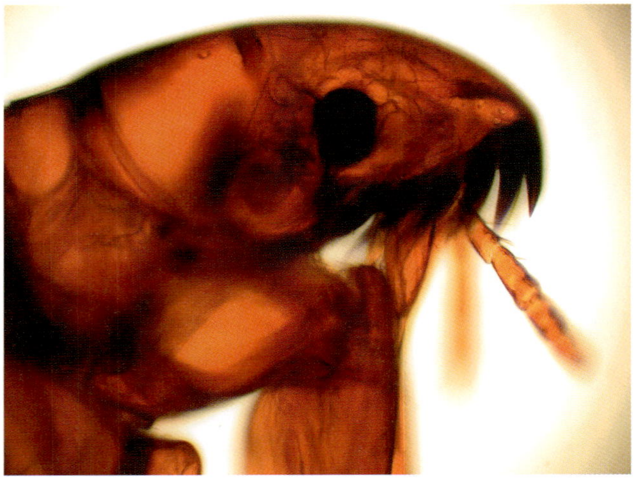

Figure 20.1 Cephalic capsule of *Ctenocephalides felis felis* (adult stage).

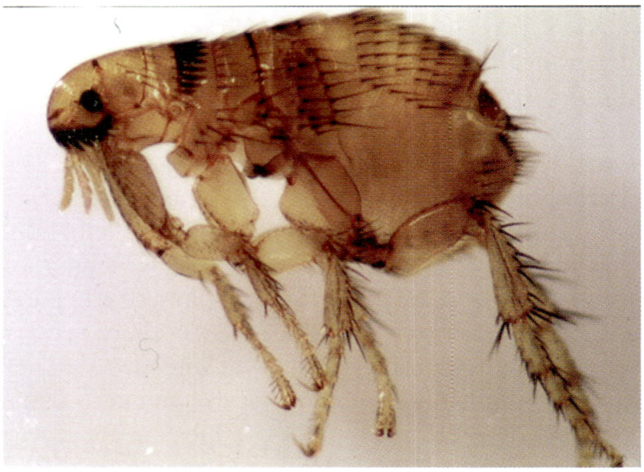

Figure 20.2 *Ctenocephalides canis* (adult stage).

Distribution

Fleas have a global distribution, being found on dogs and cats worldwide. More than 50 epidemiological studies have been conducted all over the world. In all world regions, *C. felis* (Figure 20.1), *C. canis* (Figure 20.2), and *P. irritans* have been identified on dogs. The most prevalent flea species found globally on dogs is the cat flea (*C. felis*). The dog flea (*C. canis*) also occurs globally, but at lower rates. *Archaeopsylla erinacei* (the hedgehog flea) has been found in Europe. Bird fleas (*Echidnophaga gallinacea*, *Ceratophyllus gallinae*) and rodent fleas (*Xenopsylla cheopis* and *Nosopsyllus fasciatus*) are also present [8,9].

Data about flea species encountered in wild canids are sparse. *Chaetopsylla* seems the most prevalent, followed by *P. irritans* and less commonly by *C. canis* and *C. felis* [8].

Life cycle

Various aspects of flea biology may be useful in improving flea control and/or understanding failure or inadequacy of flea control programmes.

Host phase

The adult stage of both *C. felis felis* and *C. canis* lives permanently in the hair coat of its host. Exchanges between animals are possible but limited and should not be considered the main source of infestation. In normal conditions, when fleas are in the hair of a dog or a cat, they walk. Fleas have a tendency to leave their host when the host's temperature decreases (e.g. death, anaesthesia), when the species is not well adapted to the host (e.g. *C. canis* in cats), or when the on-host population is extremely high [10]. Jumping is also used by young imagos catching the host.

Early onset of blood feeding

Once the adult (imago) has colonized a new host, it will take its first blood meal very rapidly. About 25% of cat fleas start to feed within 5 minutes of being free in the coat and about 97% have taken a blood meal within 1 hour [11]. Although *C. canis* takes its meal more slowly, 72.5% of fleas begin blood feeding within 1 hour [12]. The mean duration of the first blood meal, evaluated on individual fleas confined on animals, has been found to be 25±18 minutes in female *C. felis* and 11±8 minutes in male *C. felis* [11]. It was significantly shorter (5 and 6 minutes, respectively for *C. canis*) [12]. More recently, using PCR methods, Wang *et al.* showed that after 15 minutes on a dog, male and female *C. felis* had ingested low, but similar, amounts of approximately 1.1 nL blood. Saturation uptake of 118 and 100 nL blood per flea was found at 30 and 60 minutes on the dog, respectively [13].

These data demonstrate the difficulty, if not the impossibility, of preventing newly emerged fleas from taking a blood meal and hence injecting their saliva.

Blood feeding and lifespan

Although it is clearly established that blood-feeding is necessary for mating and laying viable eggs [10], the number of blood meals and their frequency remain unknown. It is thought that fleas will continue to bite and have blood meals until they die. The lifespan of *C. felis felis* is usually considered to be between 2 and 3 weeks. Under experimental conditions, mean survival of *C. canis* in the canine coat was 8.6 days [14]. Clearly, flea lifespan depends highly on the level of grooming (by the animal itself or the owner). In allergic animals, survival is likely to be shortened.

Survival of 250 unfed fleas of both species was evaluated in the environment at 19°C and 27°C (relative humidity 70%). Mean survival of 50% of *C. canis* was 15.9 days (19°C) and 9.0 days (27°C). Under similar conditions, mean survival of *C. felis* was 11.7 days (19°C) and 9.6 days (27°C). After 48 hours on a dog, mean survival of females was 7.9 days (19°C) and 4.8 days (27°C) for *C. canis* and 4.9 days (19°C) and 3 days (27°C) for *C. felis*. Survival of males was shorter [14].

First eggs

Female fleas lay their first eggs between 24 and 36 hours after colonizing a host. Eggs are pearly white, oval with rounded ends and approximately 0.5 mm long (Figure 20.3), they are laid in the coat and subsequently fall to the ground. They are then susceptible to insect development inhibitors applied on the coat or on the ground, as well as insecticidal products. Egg production reaches a peak (around 15–20 eggs per day) during the second and third week and then decreases, but a female will lay eggs until it dies. Cat flea egg production usually peaks during the night, coinciding with normal sleep periods for indoor pet dogs and cats [15], hence a higher density of immature stages in animal resting places, including bedrooms. Around areas such as sofas and beds, where pets jump and play, eggs and flea faeces will be more easily dislodged from the haircoat [15].

Environmental phase and factors affecting egg and larval development

Once on the ground, eggs require favourable environmental conditions (humidity and temperature) to develop further. Ideal conditions for the life cycle of the cat flea (relative humidity of 70% and a temperature of between 20 and 30°C) are provided by a modern home environment. The environmental phase has major implications in control because of the development of larval and pupal stages and because pupae remain dormant in the environment for an extended period of time.

Larval instars (Figure 20.4)

The first-instar larvae hatch from eggs in the pet's immediate environment. They then tend to move to the depth of the carpet, not travelling far from where they hatched. They search for suitable food, particularly dried blood flea faeces (Figure 20.5) [15] but also other debris including non-viable flea eggs [16]. The second-instar larvae tend to search more widely for food and darker areas where they are less likely to be disturbed. They tend to move away from carpets, making vacuuming a rather ineffective procedure, since it only removes 15–27% of the larvae. However, regular vacuuming of pet resting places can remove 90% or more of flea eggs as well as flea faeces [15].

Pupal stage

The third-instar larva becomes a pupa encased within a cocoon formed out of various bits of environmental

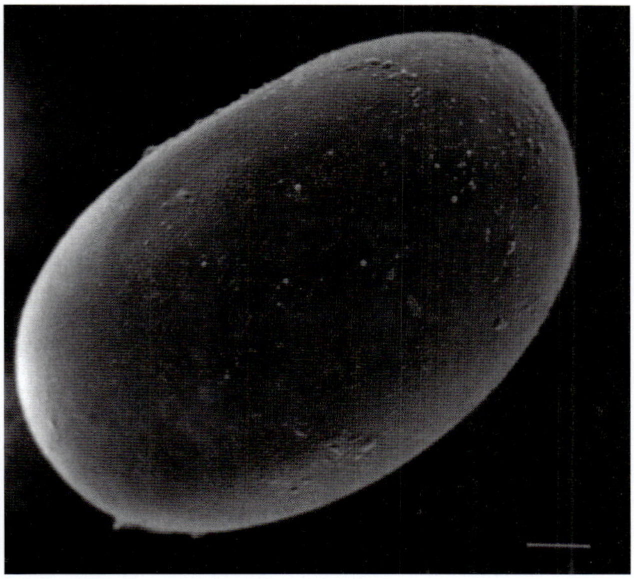

Figure 20.3 Dog flea egg (bar = 50 μm).

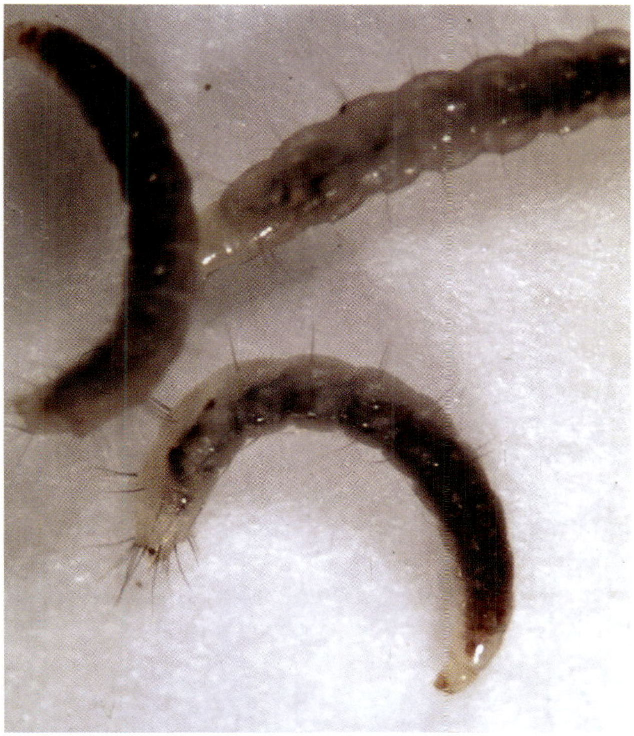

Figure 20.4 Cat flea larvae.

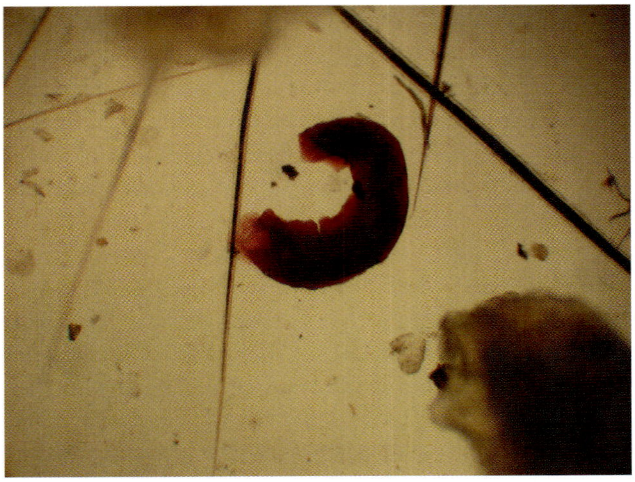

Figure 20.5 Typical curved flea faeces.

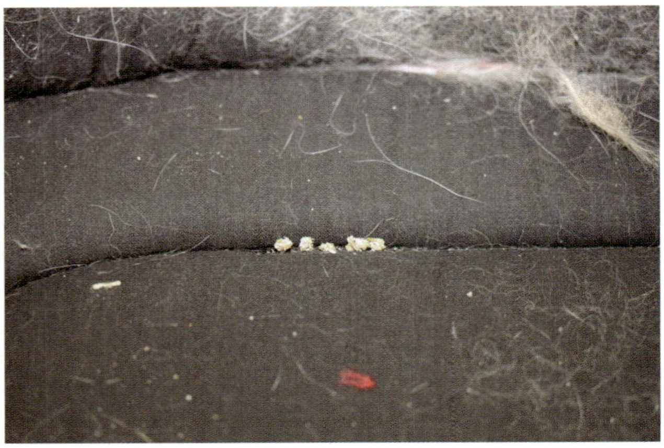

Figure 20.6 Cat flea cocoons with adherent debris on a cat basket.

debris stuck together. Pupae are often found in well-protected areas such as the back of carpets, skirting boards, and cushion seams (Figure 20.6). Inside, the future imagos remain dormant for several months (the so-called 'pupal window') until stimulated to hatch by triggers such as vibrations, increased carbon dioxide levels, and/or temperature changes. Pupae are resistant to freezing, desiccation, insecticides, and insect development inhibitors.

Imago

Once stimulated, the imago tears open the cocoon, probably as a consequence of its agitated movements, and jumps onto the first mobile, warm 'object', usually an animal. The young, unfed adult is susceptible to adulticides and insect development inhibitors. As stated earlier, the unfed flea survives longer in the environment than fed fleas.

The entire life cycle can be completed in 13 to 14 days under optimal conditions but can take up to 7–9 months.

Preventing a new life cycle would require killing all the adults in the first 24–36 hours of infestation and/or applying an insect development inhibitor either to the adult or to the immature stages before pupa formation. Vacuuming is not very effective due to the mobility and positive geotaxis of the larvae. Although immature stages concentrate in rooms or areas where animals spend most of their time, it is crucial to take into account places visited infrequently or visited by other animals, including wildlife.

Veterinary importance

Direct role

Fleas are primarily a nuisance for dogs and cats due to mechanical irritation and in heavily infested animals, possible anaemia. Dermatological signs become evident when animals develop flea bite allergy (see Chapters 22 and 39).

Transmission of pathogens

Fleas can carry specific infectious diseases and have played a historical role in human plague. Flea-borne infections are considered as emerging or re-emerging throughout the world. Fleas are vectors of *Bartonella* spp. including *B. henselae*, causing the cat-scratch disease. In addition to *Rickettsia typhi* (the pathogen of murine typhus), they can also transmit *R. felis*, the agent of the flea-borne spotted fever [8,17].

Intermediate host

Dipylidium caninum, the double-pored tapeworm, needs *C. felis* as an intermediate host. Fleas can also be intermediate hosts for *Rodentolepis nana* (syn. *Hymenolepis nana*, the dwarf tapeworm) and *H. diminuta*, the rodent tapeworm. Finally, fleas can transmit microfilaria stages of *Acanthocheilonema reconditum* [8,17].

Conclusion

Appropriate knowledge of the flea life cycle and flea-related biology is required to better control fleas, particularly when their presence becomes a nuisance, i.e. in allergic dogs. The veterinarian should ensure that the client understands these relevant basic principles of flea biology.

References

1. Rust MK. Advances in the control of *Ctenocephalides felis* (cat flea) on cats and dogs. *Trends in Parasitology* 2005; **21**: 232–236.
2. Blagburn BL, Dryden MW. Biology, treatment, and control of flea and tick infestations. *Veterinary Clinics of North America: Small Animal Practice* 2009; **39**: 1173–1200.

3. Soulsby EL. *Helminths, Arthropods and Protozoa of Domesticated Animals*. London: Bailliere Tindall, 1982: 475.
4. Matsuda R. Insect head. *Memoirs of the American Entomological Institute* 1965; **4**: 257–265.
5. Ribeiro JM, Assumpção TC, Ma D, *et al.* An insight into the sialotranscriptome of the cat flea, *Ctenocephalides felis*. *PLoS One* 2012; **7**: e44612.
6. Rothschild M, Schlein Y, Parker K, *et al.* The flying leap of the flea. *Scientific American* 1973; **229**: 92–100.
7. Cadiergues MC, Joubert C, Franc M. A comparison of jump performances of the dog flea, *Ctenocephalides canis* (Curtis, 1826) and the cat flea, *Ctenocephalides felis felis* (Bouche, 1835). *Veterinary Parasitology* 2000; **92**: 239–241.
8. Dobler G, Pfeffer M. Fleas as parasites of the family Canidae. *Parasites and Vectors* 2011; **4**: 139.
9. Cadiergues MC. *Ctenocephalides canis (Curtis, 1826) [Siphonaptera: Pulicidae]: Epidemiological and Biological Data*. PhD thesis. Toulouse: Polytechnic National Institute of Toulouse; 2000, no. 1749.
10. Hsu MH, Wu WJ. Off-host observations of mating and postmating behaviors in the cat flea (Siphonaptera: Pulicidae). *Journal of Medical Entomology* 2001; **38**: 352–360.
11. Cadiergues MC, Hourcq P, Cantaloube B, *et al.* First bloodmeal of Ctenocephalides felis felis (Siphonaptera: Pulicidae) on cats: time to initiation and duration of feeding. *Journal of Medical Entomology* 2000; **37**: 634–636.
12. Cadiergues MC, Santamarta D, Mallet X, *et al.* First blood meal of *Ctenocephalides canis* (Siphonaptera: Pulicidae) on dogs: time to initiation of feeding and duration. *Journal of Parasitology* 2001; **87**: 214–215.
13. Wang C, Mount J, Butler J, *et al.* Real-time PCR of the mammalian hydroxymethylbilane synthase (HMBS) gene for analysis of flea (*Ctenocephalides felis*) feeding patterns on dogs *Parasit Vectors* 2012; **5**: 4.
14. Cadiergues MC, Roques M, Franc M. Survival performances of the dog flea, *Ctenocephalides canis* and the cat flea, *Ctenocephalides felis felis*: a comparative study. *Veterinary Dermatology* 2003; **14**: 245.
15. Robinson WH. Distribution of cat flea larvae in the carpeted household environment. *Veterinary Dermatology* 1995; **6**: 145–150.
16. Hsu MH, Hsu YC, Wu WJ. Consumption of flea faeces and eggs by larvae of the cat flea, *Ctenocephalides felis*. *Medical and Veterinary Entomology* 2002; **16**: 445–447.
17. Bitam I, Dittmar K, Parola P, *et al.* Fleas and flea-borne diseases. *International Journal of Infectious Diseases* 2010; **14**: e667–676.

21

The pathogenesis of flea bite allergy in dogs

Richard E.W. Halliwell

Royal (Dick) School of Veterinary Studies, University of Edinburgh, Roslin, Midlothian, UK

Conflict of interest: none declared.

Introduction

Flea allergy dermatitis in dogs has a wide geographic distribution and is only absent from regions where climatic conditions are unfavourable for the survival of the cat flea *Ctenocephalides felis*, which is most commonly implicated as the causative agent. Although infestation with other flea species, whose natural hosts are wildlife, may occur in colder climates, allergic responses are infrequently reported and flea control is readily achieved. Thus all of the experimental work reported in this chapter has employed *Ct. felis*, or allergenic extracts derived there from. It is still a matter of controversy as to whether all dogs that show dermatitis when infested with fleas are in fact hypersensitive to them. However, in temperate climates dogs are not infrequently seen to harbour large populations of fleas for long periods and yet they may suffer no observable untoward effects [1,2]. This observation suggests that flea bite dermatitis is equivalent to flea allergic dermatitis (FAD).

The flea allergen

Studies in the 1960s by Benjamini *et al.* employed a guinea pig model [3]. They claimed that the flea allergen was present in a low-molecular-weight fraction of flea saliva, which was believed to act as a hapten. It remains unclear whether any relevant higher-molecular-weight protein allergens were present but not identified, or whether the pathogenesis in the guinea pig is different. However, since the 1980s, a number of studies have examined the IgE reactivity of sera from flea-allergic dogs against protein allergens derived from whole body extracts or flea saliva. In 1987, it was reported that such sera recognized a number of allergens ranging from 14.4 K to >67 K [4]. Although there were some dominant allergens that were recognized by most if not all sera, the patterns identified by the different sera were quite variable. Six years later, another study similarly identified at least 15 different protein components ranging from 14 to 150 K [5]. Again, the patterns recognized by each of 20 sera from dogs with FAD were highly variable. However, three components with molecular weights of 25, 40, and 58 K were recognized by >40% of the sera. Some years later, a further study used fractionated extracts of >2000 flea salivary glands for intradermal tests (IDTs) in dogs with FAD [6]. The major activity was attributed to two fractions of 40 K and 12–8 K, respectively.

Molecular techniques have also been used. Firstly, mRNA was isolated from a homogenate of adult fleas and showed that it encoded at least eight allergens recognized by sera from dogs with FAD, most of which had molecular weights of 14–45 K [7]. Secondly, a major allergen (Cte f 1) with a molecular weight of 18 K was identified, cloned, and characterized [8]. The recombinant allergen was recognized by sera from 100% of experimentally sensitized dogs, but interestingly by only 80% of sera from client-owned dogs suffering from FAD. Although when used to inhibit an enzyme-linked

Veterinary Allergy, First Edition. Edited by Chiara Noli, Aiden Foster, and Wayne Rosenkrantz.

immunosorbent assay (ELISA) it was able to block some 90% of the reactivity against a flea saliva antigen preparation, paradoxically when employed for IDTs in dogs with FAD, positive reactions resulted in only 40% of cases [1]. It is also difficult to reconcile the obvious importance of this allergen with previous work that showed reactivity, both *in vitro* and *in vivo*, against allergens of widely varying molecular weights. Cloning and expression of further allergens is a prerequisite for a greater understanding of this area.

Finally, mention must be made of a study investigating possible cross-reactivity of flea allergens with allergens of other insects [9]. Employing ELISA inhibition and a pool of sera highly reactive to flea allergen, binding to the solid phase was inhibited by black ant, black fly, and cockroach antigens. It is thus theoretically possible for dogs to become sensitized to flea allergen from prior sensitization to other insect allergens and even exhibit clinical signs upon first exposure to fleas. The practical implications of this observation are a matter of conjecture.

The immunopathogenesis of FAD

Immediate and delayed hypersensitivity

It is well known that FAD involves both immediate (IgE) and delayed (cell-mediated) hypersensitivity. In response to flea bites or an IDT, most allergic animals react with clearly demarcated erythematous wheals within 15 minutes. In the case of flea bites they range from 0.3 mm to >1 cm in diameter [10]. This reaction generally persists for 2–4 hours. It then may fade gradually over the next 12 hours to be replaced by smaller, firmer erythematous papules surrounded by a zone of oedema, which persist for 24–48 hours and in some cases for up to 96 hours. The presence of immediate hypersensitivity should be demonstrable by both IDT and serology. However, there is variation in the reliability of different commercially available allergen preparations [1] and such preparations are generally unsuitable for use in ELISAs unless they are enhanced for allergen content by chromatography. In one study of 20 dogs with FAD in which this procedure was followed, there was a significant correlation between the level of allergen-specific IgE and the dilution of allergen to which a positive IDT resulted [4]. The presence of delayed hypersensitivity is documented by the use of the IDT and observation of a positive reaction at 24–48 hours [10].

However, not all cases show both types of hypersensitivity [11]. Which is of the greater importance in the pathogenesis of FAD is not known. Most emphasis is usually placed on the role of IgE as this is more readily quantified, but in one extensive survey of flea-allergic dogs, 33% showed delayed reactions only [11]. It is also noteworthy that in a study in which dogs were experimentally sensitized, there was a rather poor correlation between flea antigen-specific IgE and clinical signs [12]. Thus 5/34 dogs showing a clinical response to flea exposure failed to develop significant IgE titres. Conversely, three dogs with demonstrable IgE showed no evidence of dermatitis upon flea exposure. Unfortunately, the presence or absence of delayed hypersensitivity was not assessed in this study.

The histopathology of FAD

The histopathology of skin affected by FAD

There is generally mild to moderate superficial oedema accompanied by a perivascular dermatitis comprising mast cells, eosinophils, and mononuclear cells [12]. Intraepidermal eosinophilic pustules may be seen [13]. However, the findings are quite variable, which is probably attributable to the magnitude and type of hypersensitivity shown in the individual case and the nature and extent of recent flea exposure. This variability implies that dermatopathology is not regarded as a diagnostic test of choice for FAD. Certainly, some biopsies may be highly suggestive of insect hypersensitivity, but others less so.

The sequential pathological changes

There is only one study in which biopsies taken from sensitized dogs at varying times after both IDT and natural flea exposure were examined [10]. Five dogs that showed both strong immediate and delayed reactions were chosen for the study. Biopsies were taken at 15 minutes, 2, 4, 24, and 48 hours. Following flea bites, an oedematous reaction manifested by separation of collagen fibres was evident. It peaked at 15 minutes and waned gradually over the ensuing 48 hours, but was still evident at that time. A superficial perivascular infiltrate was present throughout. Eosinophils were the predominant cell type up to 4 hours (Figure 21.1), gradually diminishing in numbers although always present over the ensuing 48 hours. Small numbers of neutrophils persisted throughout. Mononuclear cells were first evident at 4 hours, peaking at 24 hours and still abundant at 48 hours (Figure 21.2). Mast cells were present in small to moderate numbers in the majority of dogs at all stages except at 15 minutes, which was likely to reflect their prior degranulation in response to antigen and subsequent regranulation. The response to intradermal injection of allergen was similar, except that the oedema was more severe and the reaction was generally deeper in the dermis and most pronounced in the mid-dermis. In another study, which examined biopsies of IDT sites

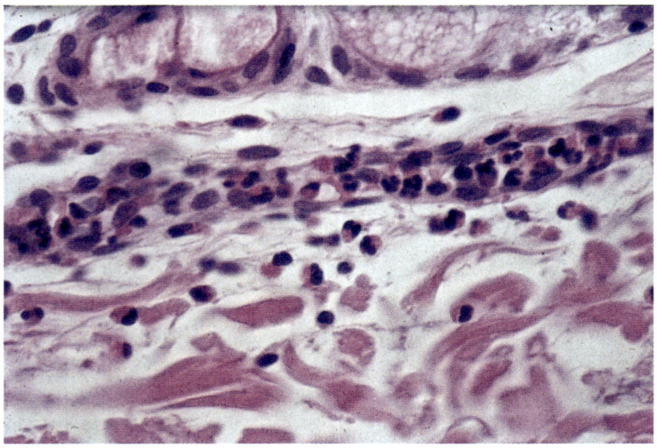

Figure 21.1 Immediate skin test reaction showing superficial dermal oedema and a blood vessel packed with eosinophils, some of which have reached the surrounding dermis. H&E × 40. Reprinted with permission from the *European Journal of Companion Animal Practice* 19(3).

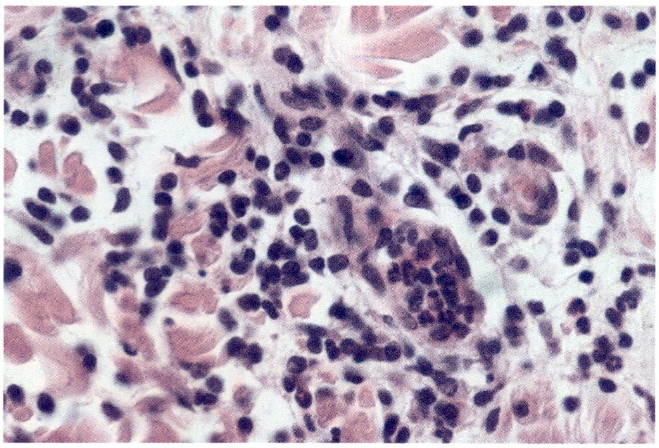

Figure 21.2 Delayed reaction at 48 hours. The infiltrate is still dense and predominantly mononuclear. H&E × 40. Reprinted with permission from the *European Journal of Companion Animal Practice* 19(3).

only, the proportion of eosinophils remained fairly constant at 1, 4, 8, 12, 18, 24, and 48 hours, whilst the proportion of mononuclear cells peaked at 48 hours [14].

Mast cells

Mast cells are increasingly recognized as being of major importance in FAD. In the dog, mast cells can be subdivided according to their protease content, i.e. those that contain tryptase, chymase, or both [15]. In a study comparing normal dogs previously sensitized to fleas with non-sensitized controls, there was no difference in the numbers of toluidine blue-staining mast cells prior to flea exposure [13]. However, the number of cells in the sensitized dogs that were positive for both chymase and tryptase was significantly greater than the numbers staining with toluidine blue, implying a selective up-regulation of proteases in the sensitized dogs and possibly lowered levels of glycosaminoglycans. When sensitized dogs were exposed to fleas, there was a significant increase in the proportion of chymase-staining cells, and a concomitant decrease in the number of tryptase-staining cells. Similar changes were evident in adjacent, non-exposed sites of the sensitized dogs following flea exposure. In a parallel manner, the percentage of cells that stained for both chymase and tryptase decreased significantly. This implies a selective release of tryptase in response to the antigen challenge. However, the question of mast cell numbers as revealed by toluidine blue staining in sensitized dogs not exposed to fleas remains controversial. A later study employed 10 dogs previously sensitized to fleas and who developed clinical signs upon exposure [16]. The controls comprised a further 10 dogs that had been similarly exposed to fleas without developing clinical signs. Two months after the last flea exposure the mast cells density was significantly higher in the sensitized dogs than in the non-allergic controls [16]. Following flea exposure, mast cell numbers in the allergic group, as assessed by toluidine blue staining, dropped significantly, reflecting degranulation. In contrast, there was no change in the apparent mast cell density in the non-allergic group in response to flea exposure.

The role of basophils

Basophils are not routinely observed in skin biopsies following formalin fixation and haematoxylin and eosin staining. Special preservatives, such as Karnovsky's fixative, followed by embedding in methacrylate and ultrathin sections are required. This technique was used to examine biopsies from IDT sites in 10 flea-allergic dogs, all of whom showed strong delayed reactions [13]. Basophils were prominent amongst the inflammatory infiltrate between 4 and 18 hours post injection (Figure 21.3). The proportion of this cell type exceeded 10% of the infiltrating cells in 7/10 dogs, with the highest percentage being 22.1%. This suggests a likely immunopathogenic role for basophils in FAD.

Factors involved in the development of clinical FAD

Th1 versus Th2 polarization

Wuersch *et al.* [16] examined mRNA for a range of cytokines in flea-allergic and normal dogs, using skin biopsies and peripheral blood mononuclear cells (PBMC). There were no significant differences between the two groups when skin biopsies were challenged with flea allergen *in vitro*. However, when the response of the PBMC to flea antigen was examined, mRNA production

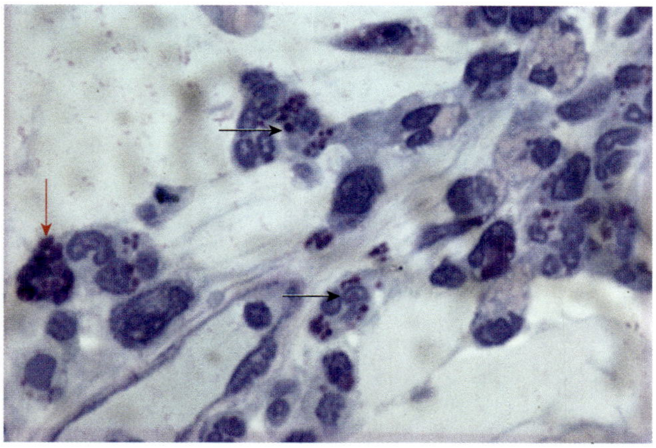

Figure 21.3 Biopsy at 12 hours in Karnovsky's fixative, embedded in methacrylate. Giemsa × 100. Basophils are indicated by arrows with a black border, and a mast cell by an arrow with a red border. Reprinted with permission from the *European Journal of Companion Animal Practice* 19(3).

of IL-4, IL-5, and IL-13 was significantly increased in the allergic group prior to flea exposure when compared to the controls. This could be taken as evidence of Th2 polarization.

Age at which exposure first occurs

Veterinarians practicing in the Southern States of the USA frequently claim anecdotally that many of the worst cases of FAD are seen in dogs born in regions of North America where fleas are sparse to absent and that move to flea-endemic areas later in their life. An epidemiological study conducted in Florida, where fleas are abundant, did indeed conclude that dogs born in the State were less likely to develop severe FAD than were those who were born in the north and who moved south in their later years [4]. This suggests an effect of age on the immune response, and that dogs exposed to fleas early in their life are less likely to develop flea allergy. Interestingly, a directly analogous observation was made in Icelandic horses suffering from *Culicoides* hypersensitivity [17]. Horses born in Iceland (where there are no *Culicoides*) and imported in later years into Sweden are likely to be more frequently affected than are animals born in Sweden, and thus exposed early in their life.

The nature of flea exposure

Halliwell [2] examined the effect of differing flea exposure on 24 stray dogs obtained from a region of the USA that was at that time believed to be flea-free (Cheyenne, Wyoming). Two groups of eight dogs each were exposed to the bites of 25 fleas for 15 minutes once or three times per week and a third group was continually exposed. In order to maintain continual exposure, the area of the kennels on which the dogs slept was kept carpeted, thus enabling completion of the life cycle. All the intermittently exposed dogs showed positive immediate skin test reactivity and detectable flea allergen-specific IgE within 8 weeks. In contrast, such reactivity occurred later and to a lesser extent in the continually exposed dogs. Delayed skin test reactivity followed the same pattern. Nonetheless, some continually exposed dogs did develop hypersensitivity, and thus the distinction was not completely clear-cut. The animals developed immediate and delayed hypersensitivity in random order, with six showing immediate reactivity some time before they evidenced delayed reactions, nine showing delayed reactions before they showed immediate reactions, and in the remaining five immediate and delayed reactivity developed concomitantly. In a similar study, laboratory reared beagles, which were presumed not to have been exposed to fleas, were either given intermittent exposure to 100 fleas applied once weekly and removed after 2 days; or had continual exposure with 16 fleas applied on alternate days [12]. The experimental conditions pertaining to the two studies were thus very different and although the continually exposed dogs had a somewhat delayed onset of clinical signs and a shorter duration and magnitude of lesion scores, the differences were by no means as clear cut as noted in the earlier study.

Two further studies were undertaken to assess the immunological status of dogs naturally continually exposed to fleas and yet showing no clinical evidence of FAD, in the USA. The first study involved stray (pound) dogs in Florida (n = 40), whose history was obviously unknown but who were in all cases observed to be carrying a heavy flea burden [18]. In the second study, client-owned dogs (n = 26) were sampled that had a history of continual and uncontrolled flea exposure for >6 months and no history of skin disease [2]. The levels of flea antigen-specific IgE and IgG were compared to levels in flea-naïve dogs and in dogs presented to the University of Florida in which a diagnosis of FAD was made. In sera from the continually exposed dogs with no signs of FAD, levels of IgE were in most cases undetectable. Levels of IgG in each study were significantly lower than those in the flea-allergic dogs and in some 50% of cases were undetectable.

Taken together, these studies suggest that the immune response and the propensity to develop both immediate and delayed hypersensitivity is dependent upon the nature of flea exposure and that most dogs who fail to develop hypersensitivity when continually exposed to fleas are partially or completely immunologically tolerant.

The atopic state and FAD

In regions where fleas are abundant, FAD is commonly seen as a complicating factor in atopic dermatitis, and it is widely believed that the atopic state predisposes to the development of FAD. In a study attempting to address this issue, the incidence of positive IDT to flea allergen in 120 dogs seen at the University of Florida in which a diagnosis of atopic dermatitis was made was found to be 79% [19]. In contrast, only 9% of 130 atopic dogs in the relatively flea-sparse area of Chicago were positive. One hundred age-matched client-owned normal dogs in the same geographic area of Florida were skin tested and a significantly lower proportion of 39% reacted positively to flea antigen [4], thus confirming the predilection for atopic dogs to develop positive IDTs to flea allergen. However, these data must be interpreted with caution because a positive IDT to flea allergen does not mean that the dog will necessarily suffer from FAD.

Conclusion

The immunopathogenesis of FAD is complex and involves immediate and delayed hypersensitivity as well as cutaneous basophil hypersensitivity. Many animals with FAD also have high levels of flea allergen-specific IgG which could also be pathogenic. The histopathology seen in clinical cases will vary according to the nature of recent flea exposure and the immunologic status. There are a number of factors that are believed to be relevant to the development of FAD and able to affect the outcome either positively or negatively. However, further painstaking work is needed to identify definitively all of these factors and how they interrelate. The fact that a state of partial or complete immunological tolerance is seen in some dogs that are asymptomatic when continually exposed to high flea burdens suggests that attempts to artificially induce tolerance prophylactically might be an avenue worthy of exploration.

References

1. Laffort-Dassot C, Carlotti D-N, Pin D, *et al.* Diagnosis of flea allergy dermatitis: comparison of intradermal testing with flea allergens and a FcεR1α-based IgE assay in response to flea control. *Veterinary Dermatology* 2004; **15**: 321–330.
2. Halliwell REW. Allergic skin diseases in domestic animals. In: Von Tscharner C, Halliwell REW, eds. *Advances in Veterinary Dermatology*, Vol. 1. London: Ballière Tindall, 1990: 91–116.
3. Benjamini E, Feingold BF. Allergy to flea bites. IV. *In vitro* collection and antigenic properties of the oral secretion of the cat flea, *Ctenocephalides felis. Experimental Parasitology* 1963; **13**: 143–154.
4. Halliwell REW, Preston JF, Nesbitt JG. Aspects of the immunopathogenesis of flea allergy dermatitis in dogs. *Veterinary Immunology and Immunopathology* 1987; **17**: 483–494.
5. Greene WK, Carnegie RL, Shaw SE, *et al.* Characterization of the allergens of the cat flea, *Ctenocephalides felis*: detection and frequency of IgE antibodies in canine sera. *Parasite Immunology* 1993; **15**: 69–74.
6. Lee SE, Johnstone IP, Lee RP, *et al.* Putative salivary allergens of the cat flea *Ctenocephalides felis felis. Veterinary Immunology and Immunopathology* 1999; **69**: 229–237.
7. Greene WK, Penhale WJ, Thompson RC. Isolation and *in vitro* translation of messenger RNA encoding allergens of the cat flea. *Veterinary Immunology and Immunopathology* 1993; **37**: 15–23.
8. McDermott MJ, Weber E, Hunter S, *et al.* Identification, cloning and characterization of a major cat flea salivary allergen (Cte f 1). *Molecular Immunology* 2000; **37**: 361–375.
9. Pucheu-Haston CM, Grier TJ, Esch RE, *et al.* Allergenic cross-reactivities in flea-reactive canine sera. *American Journal of Veterinary Research* 1996; **57**: 1000–1005.
10. Gross TL, Halliwell REW. Lesions of experimental flea bite hypersensitivity in the dog. *Veterinary Pathology* 1985; **22**: 78–81.
11. Carlotti DN. Diagnostic de la dermatit par allergie aux piqûres de puces (DAPP) chez le chien. Intérêt des intradermoréactions. *Pratique Médicale et Churgicale de l'Animal de Compagnie* 1985; **20**: 41–47.
12. Wilkerson MJ, Bagladi-Swanson M, Wheeler DW, *et al.* The immunopathogenesis of flea allergy dermatitis in dogs, an experimental study. *Veterinary Immunology and Immunopathology* 2004; **99**: 179–192.
13. von Ruedorffer U, Fisch R, Peel J, *et al.* Flea bite hypersensitivity: new aspects on the involvement of mast cells. *Veterinary Journal* 2003; **165**: 149–156.
14. Halliwell REW, Schemmer KR. The role of basophils in the immunopathogenesis of hypersensitivity to fleas (*Ctenocephalides felis*) in dogs. *Veterinary Immunology and Immunopathology* 1987; **15**: 203–213.
15. Kube P, Audige I, Kuther K, *et al.* Distribution, density and heterogeneity of canine mast cells and influence of staining techniques. *Histochemistry and Cell Biology* 1998; **110**: 129–135.
16. Wuersch K, Brachelente C, Doherr M, *et al.* Immune dysregulation in flea allergy dermatitis—a model for the immunopathogenesis of allergic dermatitis. *Veterinary Immunology and Immunopathology* 2006; **110**: 311–323.
17. Brostrom H, Larsson A, Troedsson M. Allergic dermatitis of Icelandic horses in Sweden: an epidemiological study. *Equine Veterinary Journal* 1987; **19**: 229–236.
18. Halliwell REW, Longino SJ. IgE and IgG antibodies in differing dog populations. *Veterinary Immunology and Immunopathology* 1985; **8**: 215–223.
19. Schick RO, Fadok VA. Responses of atopic dogs to regional allergens: 268 cases 1981–1984. *Journal of the American Veterinary Medical Association* 1986; **189**: 1493–1496.

22

Clinical signs of flea allergy dermatitis in dogs

Emmanuel Bensignor

Dermatology Referral Practice, Rennes-Cesson, France

Conflict of interest: none declared.

Introduction

Despite the wide distribution of modern, effective flea control products around the world, flea allergy dermatitis (FAD) remains one of the most frequent dermatitides in dogs and cats in countries where fleas are endemic [1]. The diagnosis of this condition is mainly based on the recognition of typical clinical signs. A definitive diagnosis can not be established on the basis of the results of intradermal or serological testing (see Chapter 23) [2]. Therefore it is important that veterinary practitioners are familiar with the various clinical presentations of this disease in order to be able to diagnose it early and thereby implement effective treatment and control measures.

Is flea infestation easy to diagnose?

The mere presence of fleas on the dog does not *per se* lead to a diagnosis of FAD. Many dogs can harbour some parasites without substantial clinical signs except mild pruritus. In some instances flea infestation may be overlooked because of parasite ingestion when the dog is pruritic and chewing.

The diagnosis of FAD is supported by demonstrating the presence of adult fleas or their faeces on the dog. This may require a careful search of the whole hair coat for 10 minutes using a flea comb. Flea faeces contain blood and this can be demonstrated using moist white paper; their distinct appearance can also be recognized using microscopy.

Is there a season for flea allergy dermatitis?

In temperate climates FAD is usually, at least initially, diagnosed in the spring, summer, and early autumn periods due to the characteristics of the flea life cycle [1,3] (see Chapter 20). In effect, adult fleas need a temperate climate and are more active with high temperatures and humidity [4]. However, cases may be seen in the colder months of the year, especially if the owner does not use regular antiflea protection on their pet all year round. This is also especially true if the dog lives in contact with cats because they can readily harbour fleas. Consequently, in some cases FAD may be non-seasonal [1].

No epidemiological clues!

Most studies do not indicate a breed or sex predilection. Anecdotal reports have described setters, German shepherds, fox terriers, and chow chows as breeds at risk [1]. Age at diagnosis is highly variable and most cases are seen in young adults (1 to 6 years of age).

'Classical lesions' of flea allergy dermatitis [1–3]

Acute lesions

Pruritus is the rule and it can be severe; the dog may suddenly turn around and bite or scratch; some dogs roll on their back, others rub their rump under trees or bushes.

Veterinary Allergy, First Edition. Edited by Chiara Noli, Aiden Foster, and Wayne Rosenkrantz.

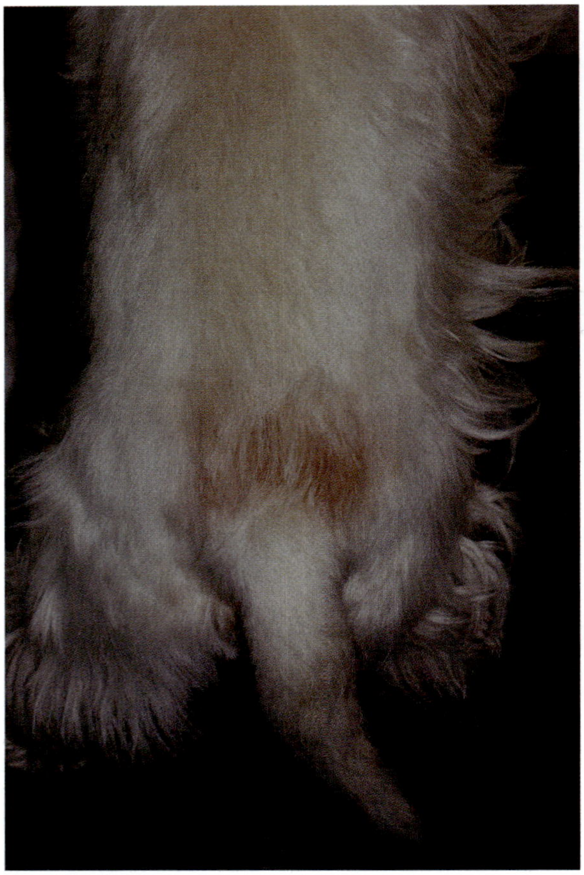

Figure 22.1 Flea allergy dermatitis (initial phase): pruritus is responsible for discolouration of the coat and erythema of the dorsolumbar area.

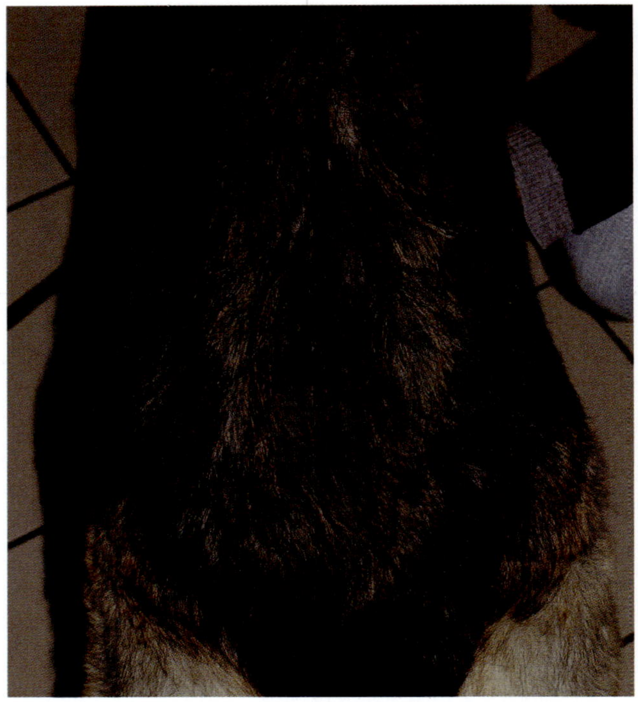

Figure 22.2 Flea allergy dermatitis in a German shepherd: alopecia, erythema, and excoriations on the legs and the dorsal area.

The typical location of the lesions that develop as a result of pruritus is usually on the lower back, at the base of the tail, and on the hindlegs (Figure 22.1). With time they can extend to the abdominal area and the flanks. A recent study has quantified and compared pruritus in FAD, canine atopic dermatitis (CAD) and flea infestation, and suggested that pruritus was more severe in cases of FAD or CAD than in cases of flea infestation without allergy. Moreover, chewing of the dorsolumbar area/back and tail was statistically more frequent in cases of FAD compared to scratching, licking, and rubbing [5].

Flea bites induce papules, erythematous plaques, and wheals. These primary lesions usually persist for 2 to 3 days if left untreated. Therefore initial skin lesions consist of self-inflicted hypotrichosis, erythema, erythematous papules, and plaques (Figure 22.2). Erosions and ulcerations may appear if pruritus is severe and the condition is not rapidly treated. Broken hairs, scales, excoriations, and lichenification are typically present after a few hours or days (Figure 22.3).

Chronic lesions

With time, secondary bacterial pyoderma may develop; signs of lichenification, hyperpigmentation, crusting, and alopecia are also regularly seen (Figures 22.3 and 22.4). Lesions may stay localized to the dorsolumbar area (the typical FAD 'triangle') or may extend to other body areas. In rare cases the lesions may be generalized. It has been demonstrated in a French unpublished study that up to 25% of cases may have lesions localized to the feet or the face or both. It also has been suggested that crusted papules in the umbilical area may be highly suggestive of FAD [1]. For dogs with a white coat there may be reddening of the hairs associated with chronic licking and rubbing (Figure 22.1).

Pyotraumatic dermatitis

The main cause of pyotraumatic dermatitis ('hot spot') in dogs is considered to be FAD [3]. This clinical presentation is mainly seen in dogs with dense coats; golden retrievers and German shepherds may be predisposed. Typically, lesions are localized on the lower rump and in some cases may be seen in other areas such as the cheeks or the flanks (Figure 22.5). The lesions consist of alopecia, erythema, oozing, and finally a large eroded or ulcerated plaque. Pruritus is generally

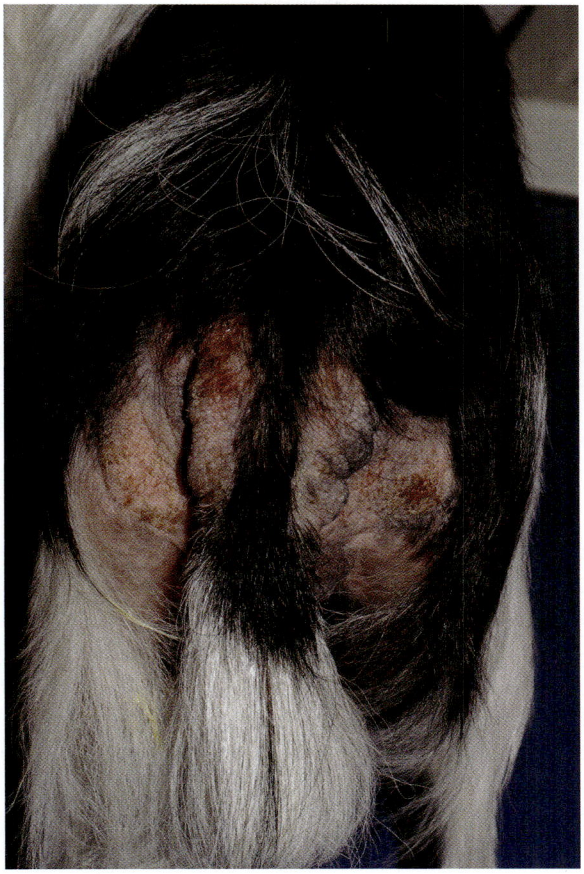

Figure 22.3 Flea allergy dermatitis in a cavalier King Charles: note the chronic lesions with hyperpigmentation and lichenification.

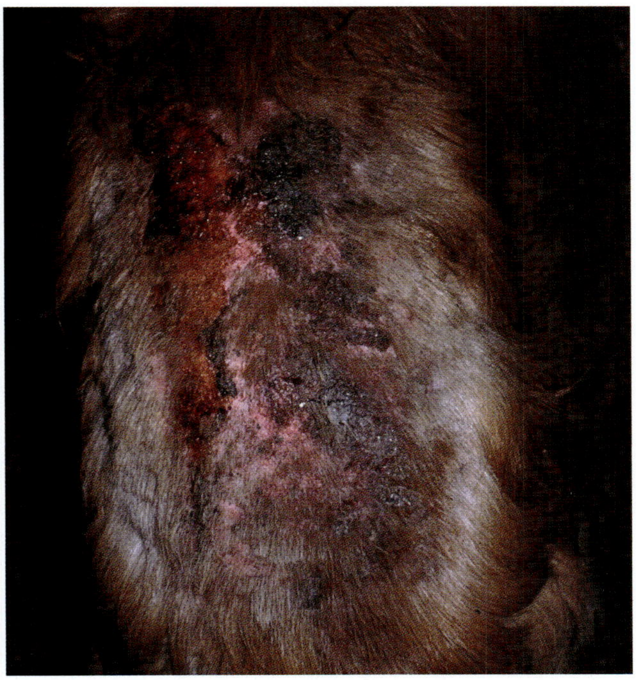

Figure 22.4 Flea allergy dermatitis: chronic phase with alopecia, erythema, excoriations, and crusts.

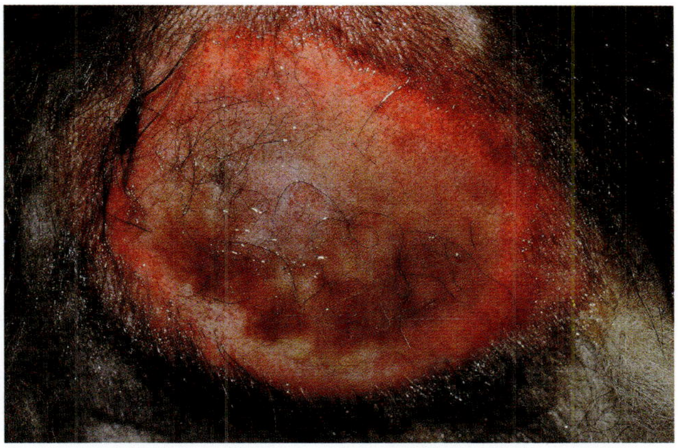

Figure 22.5 Flea allergy dermatitis: hot spot (pyotraumatic dermatitis).

very severe and most lesions are painful. This form is considered to be a pseudopyoderma because the infectious component is usually minimal and the inflammation is responsible for the skin lesions. It should be differentiated from pyotraumatic furunculosis, which is a true deep bacterial infection characterized by a central ulcerated plaque surrounded by deep pustules.

Urticaria

Urticarial reactions characterized by localized or generalized erythematous wheals are rarely seen in FAD [2]. Lesions are typically waxing and waning; pruritus is usually minimal (albeit severe in some cases).

Atopic dermatitis flares

It has been suggested that flea-allergic dogs may be predisposed to atopic dermatitis and also that atopic dogs are predisposed to FAD [6]. This may be due to the direct proinflammatory effects of flea bites and the introduction of antigens contained in flea saliva. Furthermore, dogs may suffer from atopic dermatitis and FAD concurrently (up to 31% in a French study) [7]. Therefore the role of fleas in atopic dermatitis flares should always be considered, and the efficacy of flea treatment carefully monitored as part of the long-term treatment of atopic dogs.

Fibropruritic nodules

This is a rare clinical presentation, most often seen in German shepherd dogs [1,2]. Lesions are characterized by progressive development of small nodules (0.5 to 2 cm) on the dorsolumbar area (Figure 22.6). The

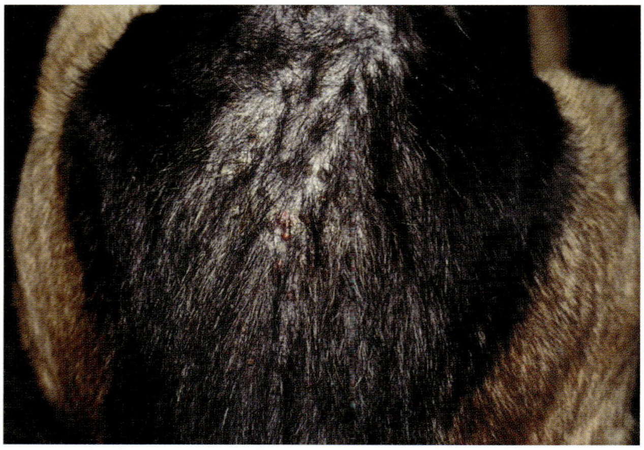

Figure 22.6 Flea allergy dermatitis: fibropruritic nodules on the dorsolumbar area of a German shepherd dog.

Table 22.1 Proposed clinical criteria for the diagnosis of FAD in dogs (reprinted from [2] with permission of Elsevier)

Corticosensitive pruritus
Recurrent pruritus in spring/summer
Increase/decrease of clinical signs depending on the life style (i.e. signs spontaneously improve if the dog is moving to a non-flea-infested environment or vice versa)
Dorsolumbar or tail lesions
Presence of a cat in the environment
Good response to a flea treatment trial

nodules are firm, alopecic, and may be ulcerated. In chronic cases there may be multiple lesions (more than 20). These nodules may need to be distinguished from neoplasms.

Microbial infections

When FAD is not recognized, is not correctly treated, or corticosteroids are administered for long periods, then bacterial or fungal infections may complicate the clinical presentation. Usually, bacterial folliculitis is associated with papules and pustules; however, pruritus is often intense and so epidermal collarettes, crusts, and scales may develop. Deep pyoderma with furuncles, fistulae, and necrosis (bacterial 'cellulitis') may occur in chronic severe cases. FAD should always be suspected in case of recurrent bacterial pyoderma in dogs. *Malassezia* dermatitis may also complicate the clinical presentation. Erythema, hyperpigmentation, lichenification, alopecia, and an unpleasant odour are usually seen with yeast overgrowth (see Chapter 26).

Differential diagnoses

When classical clinical signs are present the clinical diagnosis is easy; however, other causes of skin lesions on the dorsal trunk, such as cheyletiellosis or other allergic skin diseases (atopy, cutaneous adverse food reaction), should be considered [1–3]. It is outside of the scope of this chapter to discuss in detail the clinical diagnostic criteria for CAD. The author has diagnosed CAD in dogs presenting primarily with dorsolumbar lesions, especially in fox terriers and West Highland white terriers. Pediculosis is considered rare in adult dogs, but may be seen in animals residing in welfare shelters, and may be associated with dorsolumbar scaling.

In some terrier breeds, demodicosis due to the long-tailed *Demodex injai* species should also be considered. This form of demodicosis is characterized by greasy erythema on the dorsal part of the back and is usually associated with marked pruritus [3]. In the border terrier breed hyperplasia of the dorsal sebaceous glands has been described, associated with seborrhoea, erythema, and pruritus localized to the dorsal trunk. Histopathological lesions were consistent with a keratinization defect [8]. The author has diagnosed such a condition in other terrier breeds, notably the fox terrier.

Clinical criteria have been proposed to help diagnose FAD (Table 22.1).

References

1. Scott DW, Miller WH, Griffin CE. *Muller and Kirk's Small Animal Dermatology*, 6th edn. Philadelphia: WB Saunders, 2001.
2. Prélaud P. *Allergologie Canine*. Paris: Masson, 2008.
3. Bensignor E, Germain PA. *Dermatologie du Chien et du Chat*. Paris: Med Com edn, 2009.
4. Blagburn BL, Dryden MW. Biology, treatment and control of flea and tick infestations. *Veterinary Clinics of North America: Small Animal Practice* 2009; **39**: 1173–1200.
5. Bruet V, Bourdeau PJ, Roussel A, *et al*. Characterization of pruritus in canine atopic dermatitis, flea bite hypersensitivity and flea infestation and its role in diagnosis. *Veterinary Dermatology* 2012; **23**: 487–e93.
6. Sousa CA, Halliwell REW. The ACVD task force on canine atopic dermatitis (XI): the relationship between arthropod hypersensitivity and atopic dermatitis in the dog. *Veterinary Immunology and Immunopathology* 2001; **81**: 233–237.
7. Carlotti DN, Costargent F. Analysis of positive skin tests in 449 dogs with allergic dermatitis. *European Journal of Companion Animal Practice* 1994; **4**: 42–59.
8. Hill PB, Van den Broek M, Thoday KL. Idiopathic generalized sebaceous gland hyperplasia of the Border terrier: a morphometric study. *Veterinary Dermatology* 2010; **21**: 494–502.

23

Diagnostic investigation of canine flea bite allergy

Dawn Logas

Veterinary Dermatology Center, Maitland, FL, USA

Conflict of interest: none declared.

The diagnosis of canine flea bite allergy begins with the recognition of clinical signs consistent with flea bite allergy together with a history of flea exposure. If fleas or flea faeces are present on examination, or if the client confirms the presence of fleas, then a history of flea exposure is easily established. If no fleas or flea faeces are found on the dog and the client denies the possibility of fleas on their pet, then establishing a history of flea exposure becomes much more difficult. To determine the likelihood of flea exposure for a pet it is important to consider the client's environmental flea control programme and their on-pet flea control for both the affected dog and any other pets in the household. If the client does not have a complete programme then exposure to fleas is much more likely, especially in a flea endemic area. If the client does have what appears to be a complete flea control programme, it is imperative to discover any activities that might lead to the dog's unexpected exposure to fleas or decrease the effectiveness of the flea control programme. Frequent bathing or swimming will dramatically decrease the effectiveness of any of the topically active flea products and will increase the likelihood of flea exposure. The dog's encounters with other pets on a regular basis at the groomer, day care, or the park will increase the chance of flea exposure even with monthly application of a flea preventative. Finally, the dog's exposure to wildlife, including opossums, raccoons, and feral cats or dogs, can increase the chance of flea exposure.

Once a tentative diagnosis of flea bite allergy has been made based on clinical signs and flea exposure, there are several *in vivo* and *in vitro* tests currently available to help diagnose flea bite allergy in the dog. Some of these methods are easily accessible to practicing veterinarians while others are used primarily in research settings. None of these tests should be performed unless there is strong clinical and historical evidence to support the diagnosis of flea bite allergy. Even if these tests are utilized, the diagnosis is ultimately confirmed by the resolution of clinical signs in response to complete flea control and the recrudescence of signs upon re-exposure to fleas.

Live flea challenge test

The live flea challenge test [1,2] is a research tool used as the gold standard for determining the diagnostic value of various assays, including ELISA and intradermal testing. The test consists of placing recently hatched, unfed fleas in a small container with a mesh lid that allows the fleas to feed when placed on the test dog (Figure 23.1). The container is placed mesh side down on a small clipped area of the test dog for 15 to 20 minutes (Figure 23.2). The fleas are then killed and

Veterinary Allergy, First Edition. Edited by Chiara Noli, Aiden Foster, and Wayne Rosenkrantz.

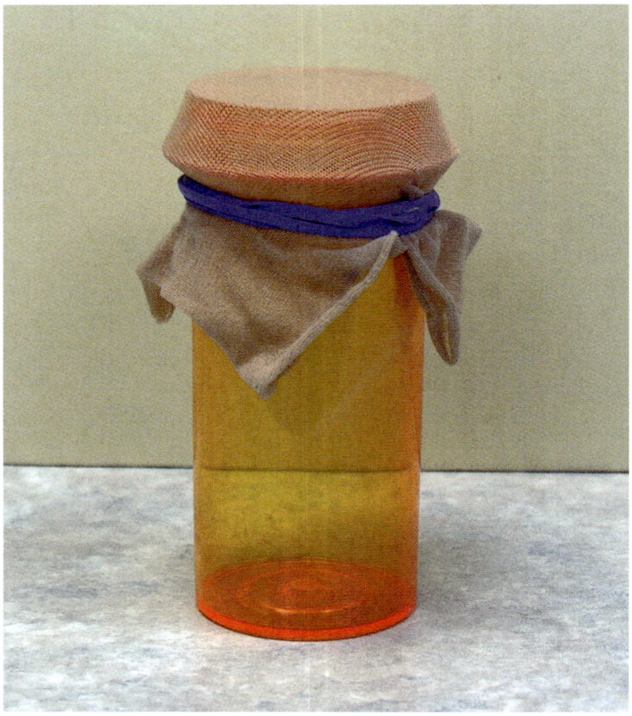

Figure 23.1 Apparatus for live flea challenge test.

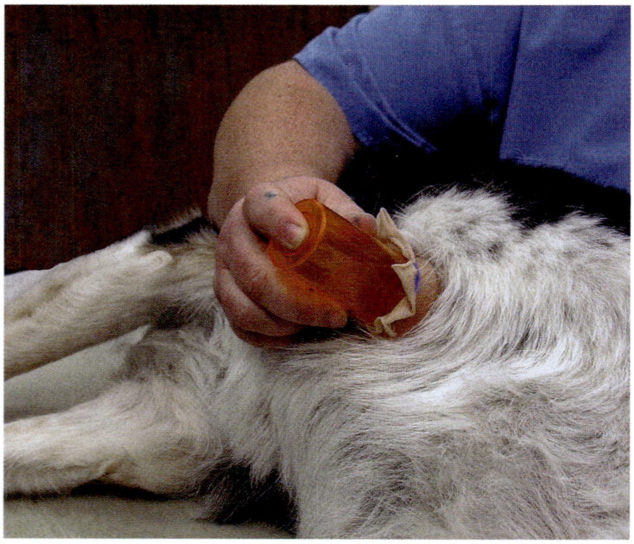

Figure 23.2 Demonstration of how to perform live flea challenge test.

crushed to ensure blood ingestion, thus confirming the test dog's exposure to flea saliva. The test site is inspected at 15 to 20 minutes, and 24 and 48 hours by a trained investigator. Any clinical evidence of immediate, delayed, or both types of hypersensitivity reaction, including erythema, papules, oedema, or crusting, is noted. In some instances the clinical evidence may be extremely mild and may need to be confirmed by histological examination of a skin biopsy from the test site [3].

Intradermal testing

Intradermal testing [4] is fairly easy to perform, but practise is needed to become proficient at interpreting the results. As is the case with aeroallergens, prior glucocorticoid or antihistamine use can cause false-negative reactions to intradermally injected flea antigen. Ideally, the dog should not receive oral glucocorticoids for at least 4 weeks, long-acting injectable glucocorticoids for at least 8 weeks, and antihistamines for at least 7 to 10 days before the test is performed. Whole-body flea extracts are currently available from several companies. These extracts are not standardized and therefore can vary in antigenicity and diagnostic reproducibility [4]. The recommended concentration for testing with whole-body flea extract is 1/1000 w/v. This concentration is non-irritating to the majority of normal dogs but will still produce a strong response in the majority of confirmed flea-allergic dogs [5]. To perform the test, a small area on the lateral thorax or flank is clipped free of hair. Then 0.05 to 0.10 mL of saline (negative control), 1:100 000 histamine phosphate (positive control), and flea antigen are injected intradermally. The flea antigen test site is compared to the control sites 15 to 20 minute after injection. The development of a wheal and flare indicates an immediate (type I) hypersensitivity reaction to the flea antigen. Since 14 to 30% of dogs with flea bite allergy may only have a delayed (type IV) hypersensitivity response to flea antigen, the site must be observed during the following 48 hours for any evidence of oedema, erythema or crusting [4,6].

Intradermal testing should only be performed if there is strong clinical evidence that the dog has flea bite hypersensitivity. This is particularly true in flea-endemic areas. One study from Florida reported up to 24% of clinically normal dogs with no history of dermatologic disease had a positive reaction to intradermally injected whole-body flea extract [7]. A similar study in Norway, a non-flea-endemic area, reported only 2.7% positive reactions in normal dogs [8].

The specificity, sensitivity, and accuracy of intradermal testing also varies depending on the dogs tested (confirmed flea allergic, confirmed atopic, or normal dogs) and the extract used [4,9,10]. In a study, four different types of extracts were compared including two commercially available whole-body extracts and two commercially unavailable products, a purified flea saliva extract and a recombinant flea saliva antigen [10]. The products with the best specificity, sensitivity, and accuracy were the purified flea saliva (93, 90, and 91%)

and one of the whole-body flea extracts (67, 90, and 82%) while the accuracy of the other two products was much lower (64% for the other whole body extract and 73% for the recombinant flea saliva antigen).

Serological testing

There are currently multiple companies providing ELISA IgE testing for flea antigen. The antigens used by these companies vary from whole-body flea extracts to highly purified flea saliva and recombinant flea saliva antigen [4,9,10]. The advantage of serologic testing is its simplicity for the practitioner who only has to collect a blood sample. Since serological testing only identifies IgE-mediated type I hypersensitivity responses, dogs with only a delayed (type IV) reaction will be falsely identified as non-flea allergic. Serological tests are also plagued by varying degrees of accuracy and reproducibility, no matter which antigen or test is utilized. Some studies investigating assays that use whole-body flea extracts found high IgE levels in flea-allergic dogs and low levels in flea-naïve dogs, while other studies found no difference in IgE levels between the flea-allergic and flea-naïve dogs [11,12]. Studies investigating assays that use purified flea saliva or recombinant flea saliva antigens have also produced conflicting results. In one study where the assay compared laboratory sensitized flea-allergic dogs to flea-naïve dogs, the assay's accuracy reached 88% [13]. A second study evaluating the same assay compared naturally occurring flea-allergic dogs to flea-infested dogs with no signs of flea bite allergy. This second study found the assay's accuracy to be only 64% [10].

Histopathology

Collecting skin biopsy samples from suspected flea bite allergy lesions is not recommended as a clinical diagnostic test. The histopathological findings in such lesions consists of a typical type I and/or type IV hypersensitivity reaction [3]. In the research setting when the stimulus for the allergic reaction is known to be a flea bite, histopathology can be useful. In a clinical setting when the exact stimulus for a particular lesion is not known these histological patterns cannot differentiate between flea bite allergy and other canine allergic disease.

Conclusion

The currently available ELISA IgE tests are not recommended to confirm flea bite allergy because of their overall poor accuracy. Intradermal testing with whole-flea antigen is currently the best diagnostic test available for general use. Because currently available whole-body flea extracts are not standardized, the accuracy of intradermal testing varies depending on which extract is used. Accuracy could potentially be improved if purified flea saliva was made commercially available. Therefore, the diagnosis of flea bite allergy must still be confirmed by the resolution of clinical signs in response to flea control and the recurrence of those signs upon re-exposure to fleas.

References

1. Bond Hutchinson MJ. Loeffler A. Serological, intradermal and live flea challenge test in the assessment of hypersensitivity to flea antigen in cats. *Parasitology Research* 2006; **4**: 392–397.
2. Stolper R, Opedebeeck JP. Flea allergy dermatitis in dogs diagnosed by intradermal skin tests. *Research in Veterinary Science* 1994; **57**: 21–27.
3. Gross TL, Halliwell REW. Lesions of experimental flea bite hypersensitivity in the dog. *Veterinary Pathology* 1985; **22**: 78–81.
4. Laffort-Dassot C. Flea allergy in dogs: Clinical signs and diagnosis. *European Journal of Companion Animal Practice* 2009; **19**: 242–248.
5. Willis EL, Kunkle GA, Esch RE, *et al.* Intradermal reactivity to various insect and arachnid allergens among dogs from southeastern United States. *Journal of the American Veterinary Medical Association* 1996; **209**: 1431–1434.
6. Halliwell REW, Gorman NT. Non-atopic allergic skin diseases: hypersensitivity to ectoparasites. In: Halliwell REW, Gorman NT, eds. *Veterinary Clinical Immunology*. Philadelphia: WB Saunders, 1989: 261–267.
7. Kunkle GA, Jones L, Petty P. Immediate intradermal flea antigen reactivity in the clinically normal adult dogs from south Florida, USA. *Veterinary Dermatology* 2000; **11**: 9–12
8. Saevik BK, Ulstein TL. Immediate intradermal flea-antigen reactivity in dogs in a flea-scarce environment. *Veterinary Dermatology* 2002; **13**: 228.
9. Foster AP, Littlewood JD, Webb P, *et al.* Comparison of intradermal and serum testing for allergen specific IgE using a FcεRIα-based assay in atopic dogs in the UK. *Veterinary Immunology and Immunopathology* 2003; **93**: 51–60.
10. Laffort-Dassot C, Carlotti DN, Pin D, *et al.* Diagnosis of flea allergy dermatitis: comparison of intradermal testing with flea antigens and fcεRI α-based assay in response to flea control. *Veterinary Dermatology* 2004; **15**: 321–330.
11. Halliwell REW, Logino SJ. IgE and IgG antibodies to flea antigen in differing dog populations. *Veterinary Immunology and Immunopathology* 1985; **8**: 215–223.
12. McKeon SE, Opdebeeck JP. IgE and IgG antibodies against antigens of the cat flea, *Ctenocephalides felis felis*, in sera of allergic and non-allergic dogs. *International Journal of Parasitology* 1994; **24**: 259–263.
13. McCall CA, Steadman KE, Penner SJ, *et al.* FcεRIα–based measurement of antiflea saliva IgE in dogs. *Compendium on Continuing Education for the Practicing Veterinarian* 1997; **19** (Suppl. *Clinical Advances*): 24–28.

24

Implementing an effective flea control programme

Michael W. Dryden

Department of Diagnostic Medicine and Pathobiology, Kansas State University, Manhattan, KS, USA

Conflict of interest: the author has conducted sponsored research and is sponsored to present lectures at numerous conferences by numerous corporations including Bayer, Ceva, Elanco, IDEXX, Merck, Merial, Novartis, and Pfizer.

Introduction

Since the mid-1990s, great advances have been made in our understanding of the problems encountered in a flea infestation and in the development of effective flea control products. Laboratory and in-home (product performance trials conducted on pets in private residences) investigations have demonstrated that new residual insecticides and insect growth regulators can markedly reduce, if not completely eliminate, fleas from pets and their in-home premises within 2 to 3 months. However, in spite of these advances, flea infestations of dogs and cats and of the premises in which they reside are still a common occurrence and veterinarians often fail to meet client expectations concerning long-term flea control or management of flea allergy dermatitis (FAD).

General control strategies and integrated flea control

Given the high reproductive rate of fleas infesting dogs and cats the most effective modern products and control strategies now involve preventing or markedly reducing flea reproduction [1]. The development of the modern monthly neurotoxic residual flea adulticides such as dinotefuran, fipronil, imidacloprid, indoxacarb, metaflumizone, pyriprole, selamectin, and spinosad has dramatically changed the way flea control is conducted. Prior to the introduction of these highly effective residual adulticides, flea control was attempted through repeated application of organophosphate and pyrethroid based products to dogs and cats [2]. A combination of poor residual activity and selection for resistance often resulted in failed attempts to control flea populations [3]. Failure was due to the fact that some of the fleas within the population could initiate reproduction, laying viable eggs, before being killed by the adulticides [3]. This continued production of eggs would sustain the flea infestation within the premises, often necessitating the repeated application of adulticides and insect growth regulators [2].

Adulticides

The modern monthly residual flea adulticides have enhanced our flea control efforts primarily because of their prolonged residual activity and more rapid residual speed of kill, thus having a much greater impact on continued flea reproduction. Numerous in-home product investigations have demonstrated that when these modern residual flea adulticides, often combined with insect growth regulators, are administered at the appropriate dose and treatment intervals to every dog and cat, they are effective in drastically reducing, if not completely eliminating, flea infestations without the

Veterinary Allergy, First Edition. Edited by Chiara Noli, Aiden Foster, and Wayne Rosenkrantz.

need for direct insecticide treatment of the premises [4–10]. Even though these new adulticides are highly effective, the continued use of these compounds may exert selection pressure on flea populations, resulting in the selection for resistant populations. To delay the development of resistance, ensure suppression of flea reproduction, reduce environmental biomass, and provide for long-term flea control veterinarians may need to consider an integrated strategy [1]. An effective integrated programme should involve: (1) education of veterinary staff and pet owners on the biology of fleas infesting pets, (2) implementation of mechanical control measures, (3) application of insect growth regulators (IGRs), and (4) administration of flea adulticides.

Insect growth regulators

Incorporation of a topical or systemic IGR in a flea control programme provides for potent ovicidal activity. These compounds can generally be grouped into either juvenile hormone analogues, which block development to adults, such as methoprene or pyriproxyfen, or chitin synthesis inhibitors such as lufenuron. A number of studies have documented the prolonged ovicidal effect of these IGRs administered to flea-infested dogs and cats [11–14].

Treatment of dogs with a 1.0% w/v spot-on formulation of pyriproxyfen prevented fleas from producing viable eggs for up to 8 weeks after treatment [13]. Topical methoprene applications also produce prolonged ovicidal activity. A single topical application of a 9% (w/v) methoprene spot-on to flea-infested dogs provided 98.9% inhibition of adult emergence from eggs for 1 month and 92.0% inhibition for 50 days [15]. Systemic IGRs are also effective in preventing fleas from laying viable eggs. When a single oral dose of lufenuron was administered to dogs it almost completely inhibited all eggs and larvae from developing into adult fleas for 1 month following administration [14]. These studies have demonstrated that the ovicidal activity of the IGRs can extend beyond the typical 30-day treatment interval of residual adulticides. Regardless of the variability in susceptibility of fleas to residual adulticides, the incorporation of IGRs into a flea control programme should mean that any surviving fleas will not be capable of producing viable eggs. If the flea population cannot reproduce then eventual elimination of the population is assured.

Non-chemical control

Educating the pet owner on the benefits of mechanical intervention can be very important. Mechanical intervention is designed to reduce biomass in the premises, thus minimizing numbers of emerging fleas biting pets or humans in the home. Pet owners should be asked to list the places that pets spend most of their time resting and sleeping in the home. Examples include pet bedding, couches, chairs, and any bedding materials on furniture including throw rugs and pet carriers. It is in these locations that most flea eggs will be deposited and the potential for flea development is likely greatest. These areas should be cleaned, washed, or vacuumed thoroughly. All pet sleeping and resting areas should be vacuumed thoroughly every day or as often as possible to help remove flea eggs and larvae. Seat cushions and pillows on sofas and chairs should be removed and the areas underneath vacuumed. Vacuuming or steam cleaning should also be directed under sofas, beds, chairs, or other structures where pets may not have direct access but where larvae may have crawled. Cars may also occasionally become infested after transporting flea-infested pets. Removing and washing floor mats and vacuuming out the car interior is recommended.

In one study, a beater-bar type vacuum cleaner removed 15–27% of the larvae and 32–59% of the eggs, with effectiveness decreasing as the density of the carpet pile increased [16]. Vacuuming will also remove a large number of newly emerged adult fleas [17]. Flea traps based on intermittent-light technology can collect a substantial number of newly emergent fleas [18,19]. An intermittent-light trap design collected >86% of the fleas in a 3.1 m × 3.3 m carpeted room during 20-hour trapping periods [18]. In that same study, the intermittent-light trap attracted 57% of the fleas released 8.4 m away from the trap [18]. In a field trial the intermittent-light trap design caught up to 23 times as many fleas when compared to light traps using a continuous light source [19]. This author has observed these traps collecting hundreds of fleas in some homes. While flea traps by themselves will not eliminate an infestation, every flea caught in the trap is one less flea jumping on pets and humans in the home.

Client education

In any flea infestation, client education is essential to the ultimate success of the control programme. This is particularly true in multiple pet households. It must be repeatedly stressed to pet owners that every potential flea host in the household, including ferrets and rabbits, must be treated at prescribed intervals to ensure complete reproductive suppression of the flea population. If a single pet is left untreated, the fleas on that pet will continue producing eggs and the infestation will not be resolved. Many pet owners only worry about flea control during the summer months. However, fleas infestations often escalate during the fall and flea infestations in homes during the winter are not uncommon. In this author's experience modern climate control systems with humidifiers may sustain flea infestations throughout the winter.

It also must be explained to pet owners that elimination of the infestation will not occur immediately due to the presence of the immature flea biomass in the premises. Continued development of immature stages and emergence of fleas is often frustrating for many pet owners [20]. Even if every flea-infested pet in the house is treated correctly it is important to remember that the premises in the home or shaded protected areas in the yard are still going to be infested with immature flea life stages and fleas will continue to emerge for several weeks.

Current flea products do not often repel fleas effectively and they do not kill fleas instantly. It often takes several hours, maybe even a day or two, after these fleas have jumped on treated pets to be killed by the residual insecticide [20]. Therefore pet owners should expect to see some fleas on their pets following treatment. Proper expectations should be set by the well-trained veterinarian or staff and they should never let the pet owner set their own expectations for the elimination of the problem.

Once an infestation has been eliminated most pet owners stop treating their pets. Again client education is important and pet owners should be reminded that there are numerous animals that carry cat fleas that move through the neighbourhood. The reservoir hosts of these fleas will vary depending upon the ecosystem and can include feral cats and dogs, opossums, foxes, mongooses, raccoons, and other urban wildlife depending upon the region [21]. These flea-infested animals are continuously depositing flea eggs in the outdoor environment. If these eggs are deposited into protected microenvironments they may ultimately develop into fleas that jump on our pets. Therefore dogs and cats should be placed on year-round broad-spectrum parasite control that includes activity against fleas [22]. When fleas that have developed from the eggs deposited off these hosts jump on the treated pet, they will either be killed or their eggs destroyed, thus preventing future flea infestations of our pets.

Allergic dogs

In cases of severe flea infestations or in pets with FAD, use of an integrated strategy, particularly those that reduce immature and adult flea biomass, is even more important. In addition, depending upon regulatory requirements and product safety profiles, combining products or increasing frequency of administration may be considered. One compound that is often incorporated into these programmes is nitenpyram. This short-acting compound provides the benefit of rapidly shutting down flea feeding and causing rapid flea death [23]. More recently, oral spinosad has become an effective tool to help manage FAD in dogs. Oral spinosad has been shown to kill 100% of fleas on dogs within 4 hours of administration [24] and has produced marked reduction in pruritus in dogs in a clinical field trial [25].

Perceptions of reduced efficacy

Numerous veterinarians have reported to this author that they think that some of the modern veterinary recommended flea control products may not be controlling some flea infestations as well as in the past, at least in North America. It is apparent that many veterinarians think that resistance to these products has occurred. Historically, insecticide resistance has certainly caused problems in our attempts to control fleas on dogs and cats. Resistance in cat flea populations to carbamates, organophosphates, pyrethroids, pyrethrins, and organochlorines is well established [26]. While selection for resistance must be considered as a possible cause of reported product failures, to date the existence of resistance to the modern residual insecticides dinotefuran, fipronil, imidacloprid, selamectin, and spinosad in cat flea populations has not been conclusively proven.

Most of these 'reported failures' are likely due to lack of client education, lack of understanding of product performance attributes, and compliance issues such as too frequent bathing, not dispensing all of the solution from the package, not depositing the entire contents on the skin, not administering oral products with food to aide in absorption, and not treating all potential flea hosts within the home every month [20]. These are common client compliance issues than need to be addressed through client education. While the above can often be managed by educating clients, there are other problems that may be encountered over which veterinarians have little control, such as a large pre-existing immature flea biomass in the premises, seasonal or yearly fluctuations in flea populations, and naturally occurring differences in flea strain susceptibility to different insecticides [20,27,28].

Likely one of the biggest problems in flea control is the mistaken belief by many pet owners that once treatment is initiated fleas will be rapidly eliminated. Very few pet owners are likely to see the first few fleas that their pets acquire [20]. It seems far more likely that the infestation is not noticed until additional fleas begin to emerge within the premises 1 to 2 months after the initial few fleas were acquired. With female cat fleas beginning egg production within 24 to 48 hours of acquiring a host and producing up to 40 to 50 eggs per day [29], this large-scale reproductive event almost ensures that by the time a pet owner reacts and takes their pet to a veterinarian for treatment, a large 'biomass' of immature fleas already exists within the home. In-home flea product investigations have repeatedly demonstrated that this continued development and emergence of fleas called the 'development window' can continue for 1 to 3 months following administration of topical or systemic flea products [4–10]. Continued presence of fleas following treatment can be quite frustrating to a pet owner who likely had the expectation that the problem would be over quickly. It must be explained to the pet owner that flea eggs laid within the home or outdoor premises (yard or garden) yesterday will continue to develop and fleas will continue to emerge for approximately 1 to 2 more months and maybe even longer in some homes.

The biology of immature flea life stages is actually complex and directly tied to environmental conditions within the microclimate [10]. Temperature dictates the rate of development of the immature stages of the cat flea, with warm temperatures accelerating development and thus shortening the time it takes for eggs to develop to adults. Alternatively, cooler temperatures can markedly delay development of immature flea life stages. It has been noted that in some household investigations, following treatment of all the dogs and cats in a household the level of flea emergence within the premises can actually increase within 1 to 3 weeks following treatment [10,20]. In these so called 'red-line homes' the flea emergence pattern indicates that at the time of initial treatment of the pet or pets the immature life stages in the premises was either in a rapid growth phase, or the development and emergence of fleas was delayed by cool ambient temperatures [10]. Field investigations have demonstrated that fluctuations in temperature and humidity year to year, season to season, or even week to week can dramatically effect flea population development and emergence [9,10,20].

In a 1997 in-home product evaluation study in Tampa, FL, USA where an area finger counting methodology was used, the geometric mean number of fleas on pets prior to treatment was 19.0 and 19.8 in the two treatment groups [5]. Then in a 2010 investigation in the same city the geometric mean number of fleas on pets in the two treatment groups on day 0 was 28.59 and 28.56 [9]. In those same studies the numbers of fleas collected in intermittent-light flea traps was also quite different. In the 1997 Tampa investigation, the geometric mean premise trap counts in the homes in the two treatment groups on day 0 was 14.4 and 10.1 [5], whereas in the 2010 study day 0 premises trap counts in the two treatment groups were 35.3 and 29.7 [9]. Therefore in 2010 in Tampa, pets and their owners were under almost 2.5 to 3 times greater flea pressure than in 1997.

Factors that might affect flea numbers from year to year, season to season, or even household to household include differences in temperature, humidity, and rainfall, treatment history, number of pets in a household, number of indoor or outdoor pets, presence or type of household air conditioning, type of flooring (hardwood floors or carpeting), and numbers of outdoor flea reservoirs. These fluctuations in flea populations can have a major impact on the perception of product performance and client satisfaction.

While resistance to the modern array of flea adulticides has not been proven, natural variability in insecticide susceptibility between flea populations has been demonstrated [3,30–32]. Laboratory investigations have demonstrated that variability in flea strain susceptibility may mean that the expected levels of flea control throughout the month may not always be achieved and that egg production may occur between monthly dosing with some flea strains [3,32]. An example of this variability that has been well documented is the Kansas 1 Colony (KS1) cat flea strain that has been maintained as a closed colony at Kansas State University since 1990. Several insecticides introduced into the US years after this strain was colonized have exhibited poor residual efficacy against the KS1 strain. Laboratory investigations with this flea strain have demonstrated that the efficacy of fipronil against KS1 strain fleas on cats at 1 month post-treatment ranges from 79.3 to 89.9% [30]. The reduced efficacy of fipronil against the KS1 strain is noteworthy when efficacy data from other studies using other flea strains is considered. These studies reported that the efficacy of fipronil against other *C. felis* strains 1 month after application ranged from 95 to 100% [33]. Interestingly, reduced efficacy of imidacloprid against this strain has also been demonstrated. The efficacy of a spot-on formulation of imidacloprid 30 days post-treatment was only 72.6% against the KS1 strain [30]. While other studies evaluating the efficacy of imidacloprid against other *C. felis* strains reported that the efficacy of the spot-on formulation of imidacloprid against *C. felis* 1 month after application ranged from 95.7 to 100% [34].

In addition, reduced susceptibility of the KS1 flea strain to spinosad has also been demonstrated in laboratory investigations. In an investigation of the residual activity of spinosad against the KS1 flea strain, when dogs were infested 28 days following treatment, the efficacy 24 hours later was below 35% [31]. These data are in stark contrast to two other laboratory studies using different flea strains where spinosad was more than 95% effective against experimental flea infestations for a month [35,36]. It is important to note that at this point there are no data to indicate how widespread or how common this variability is within flea populations. However, it must be expected that natural variability might exist and that in some situations one flea product might perform better than another and just the opposite might occur in a different location.

Conclusion

Veterinarians and their staff should have an appreciation for the complexity of flea biology and the problems that can be encountered in flea control. They need to be aware of the effect of temperature and humidity on flea ecology, how the presence of untreated pets and reservoir hosts can impact flea control, how poor compliance and unrealistic expectations can derail a flea control programme from the outset, and how fluctuations in flea populations can dramatically effect perceptions of product performance. Lastly, incorporation of an integrated approach to flea control can be an effective means of reducing flea biomass and provide effective long-term flea control.

References

1. Dryden MW, Broce AB. Integrated flea control for the 21st century. *Compendium of Continuing Education for the Practicing Veterinarian* 2002; **24** (Suppl.): 36–39.
2. Dryden M, Bennett G, Neal J. Concepts of flea control. *Companion Animal Practice* 1989; **19**: 11–22.
3. Dryden MW. Flea and tick control in the 21st century, challenges and opportunities. *Veterinary Dermatology* 2009; **20**; 435–440.
4. Dryden MW, Perez HR, Ulitchny DM. Control of fleas on pets and in homes by use of imidacloprid or lufenuron and a pyrethrin spray. *Journal of the American Veterinary Medical Association* 1999; **215**: 36–39.
5. Dryden MW, Denenberg TM, Bunch S. Control of fleas on naturally infested dogs and cats and in private residences with topical spot applications of fipronil or imidacloprid. *Veterinary Parasitology* 2000; **93**: 69–75.
6. Dryden M, Denenberg TM, Bunch S, *et al.* Control of fleas on dogs and cats and in private residences with the combination of oral lufenuron and nitenpyram. *Veterinary Therapeutics* 2001; **2**: 208–214.
7. Dryden MW, Burkindine T, Lewis L, *et al.* Efficacy of selamectin in controlling natural flea infestations on pets and in private residences in comparison with imidacloprid and fipronil. In: *Proceedings of the American Association of Veterinary Parasitology Annual Meeting*, 2001: 34.
8. Chin A, Lunn P, Dryden M. Persistent flea infestations in dogs and cats controlled with monthly topical applications of fipronil and methoprene. *Australian Veterinary Practitioner* 2005; **35**: 89–96.
9. Robertson-Plouch C, Baker KA, Hozak RR, *et al.* Clinical field study of the safety and efficacy of spinosad chewable tablets for controlling fleas on dogs. *Veterinary Therapeutics* 2008; **9**: 26–36.
10. Beugnet F, Franc M. Results of a European multicentric field efficacy study of fipronil-(S) methoprene combination on flea infestation of dogs and cats during 2009 summer. *Parasite* 2010; **17**: 337–342.
11. Olsen A. Ovicidal effect on the cat flea, *Ctenocephalides felis* (Bouché), of treating fur of cats and dogs with methoprene. *International Pest Control* 1985; **27**: 10–13, 16.
12. Palma KG, Meola SM, Meola RW. Mode of action of pyriproxyfen and methoprene on eggs of *Ctenocephalides felis* (Siphonaptera: Pulicidae). *Journal of Medical Entomology* 1993; **30**: 421–426.
13. Stanneck D, Larsen KS, Mencke N. Pyriproxyfen concentration in the coat of cats and dogs after topical treatment with a 1.0% w/v spot-on formulation. *Journal of Veterinary Pharmacology and Therapeutics* 2003; **26**: 233–235.
14. Hink WF, Zakson M, Barnett S. Evaluation of a single oral dose of lufenuron to control flea infestation in dogs. *American Journal of Veterinary Research* 1994; **55**: 822–824.
15. Young DR, Jeannin PC, Boeckh A. Efficacy of fipronil/(S)-methoprene combination spot-on for dogs against shed eggs, emerging and existing adult cat fleas (Ctenocephalides felis, Bouche). *Veterinary Parasitology* 2004; **125**: 397–407.
16. Byron DW, Robinson WH. Research on household flea control. *Pest Management* 1986; **5**: 29–31.
17. Osbrink WLA, Rust MK, Reierson DA. Distribution and control of cat fleas in homes in southern California (Siphonaptera: Pulicidae). *Journal of Economic Entomology* 1985; **79**: 136–140.
18. Dryden M, Broce A. Development of a flea trap for collecting newly emerged *Ctenocephalides felis* (Siphonaptera: Pulicidae) in homes. *Journal of Medical Entomology* 1993; **30**: 901–906.
19. Müller GC, Dryden MW, Revay EE, *et al.* Understanding attraction stimuli of *Ctenocephalides felis* for non-chemical control methods. *Medical and Veterinary Entomology* 2011; **25**: 413–420.
20. Dryden MW. How you and your clients can win the flea control battle. *Veterinary Medicine* 2009; **March** (Suppl.): 17–26.
21. Blagburn BL, Dryden MW. Biology, treatment and control of flea and tick infestations. *Veterinary Clinics of North America* 2009; **39**: 1173–1200.
22. CAPC. *General Guidelines.* Available at: http://www.capcvet.org/capc-recommendations/capc-general-guidelines. Accessed 01 September 2012.
23. Schenker R, Tinembart O, Humbert-Droz E, *et al.* Comparative speed of kill between nitenpyram, fipronil, imidacloprid, selamectin and cythioate against adult *Ctenocephalides felis* (Bouche) on cats and dogs. *Veterinary Parasitology* 2003; **112**: 249–254.
24. Blagburn BL, Young DR, Moran C, *et al.* Effects of orally administered spinosad (Comfortis) in dogs on adult and immature stages of the cat flea (Ctenocephalides felis). *Veterinary Parasitology* 2010; **168**: 312–317.
25. Dryden MW, Ryan WG, Bell M, *et al.* Assessment of owner-administered monthly treatments with oral spinosad or topical spot-on fipronil/(S)-methoprene in controlling fleas and associated pruritus in dogs. *Veterinary Parasitology* 2013; **191**: 340–346.
26. Rust MK, Dryden MW. The biology, ecology and management of the cat flea. *Annual Review of Entomology* 1997; **42**: 451–473.
27. Dryden MW, Payne PA, Vicki S, *et al.* Efficacy of dinotefuran–pyriproxyfen, dinotefuran–pyriproxyfen–permethrin and fipronil–(S)-methoprene topical spot-on formulations to control flea populations in naturally infested pets and private residences in Tampa Florida. *Veterinary Parasitology* 2011; **82**: 281–286.
28. Dryden M, Carithers D, McBride A, *et al.* A comparison of flea control measurement methods for tracking flea populations in highly infested private residences in Tampa FL, following topical treatment of pets with FRONTLINE® Plus (fipronil/(*S*)-methoprene). *International Journal of Applied Research in Veterinary Medicine* 2011; **9**: 356–367.

29. Dryden MW. Host association, on-host longevity and egg production of *Ctenocephalides felis felis*. *Veterinary Parasitology* 1989; **34**: 117–122.
30. Dryden MW, Smith V, Payne PA, *et al.* Comparative speed of kill of selamectin, imidacloprid, and fipronil–(S)-methoprene spot-on formulations against fleas on cats. *Veterinary Therapeutics* 2005; **6**: 228–236.
31. Dryden MW, Payne PA, Vicki S. *et al*. Efficacy of topically applied dinotefuran formulations and orally administered spinosad tablets against the ks1 flea strain infesting dogs. *International Journal of Applied Research in Veterinary Medicine* 2011; **9**: 123–128.
32. Beugnet F, Doyle V, Murray M, *et al.* Comparative efficacy on dogs of a single topical treatment with the pioneer fipronil/(S)-methoprene and an oral treatment with spinosad against *Ctenocephalides felis*. *Parasite* 2011; **18**: 325–331.
33. Young DR, Jeannin PC, Boeckh A. Efficacy of fipronil/(s)-methoprene combination spot-on for dogs against shed eggs, emerging and existing adult cat fleas (*Ctenocephalides felis*, Bouche). *Veterinary Parasitology* 2004; **125**: 397–407.
34. Hopkins TJ, Kerwick C, Gyr P, *et al.* Efficacy of imidacloprid to remove and prevent *Ctenocephalides felis* infestations on dogs and cats. *Compendium of Continuing Education for the Practicing Veterinarian* 1997; **19**: 11–16.
35. Blagburn BL, Young DR, Moran C, *et al.* Effects of orally administered spinosad (Comfortis) in dogs on adult and immature stages of the cat flea (*Ctenocephalides felis*). *Veterinary Parasitology* 2010; **168**: 312–317.
36. Snyder DE, Meyer J, Zimmermann AG, *et al.* Preliminary studies on the effectiveness of the novel pulicide, spinosad, for the treatment and control of fleas on dogs. *Veterinary Parasitology* 2007; **150**: 345–451.

25

Symptomatic relief for canine flea bite hypersensitivity

Dawn Logas

Veterinary Dermatology Center, Maitland, FL, USA

Conflict of interest: none declared.

Flea bite hypersensitivity is one of the most pruritic skin diseases that can affect the dog. Consistent long-term control of this intense pruritus can only be obtained by minimizing exposure to flea bites through diligent on-pet and environmental flea control. Symptomatic therapy usually allows for a relatively quick and dramatic decrease of the pruritus and inflammation suffered by the flea-allergic dog when exposed to flea bites [1]. It is particularly useful after the diagnosis of flea allergy is made to give the dog that presents with fleas some clinical relief while the environmental infestation is cleared, which in some cases may take weeks to months. It is also helpful as an adjunctive therapy for flea-allergic dogs that have a greater risk of re-exposure to fleas and flea bites.

Antimicrobial agents

Many dogs with active flea bite hypersensitivity have concurrent bacterial or yeast pyodermas. These infections can increase the severity of the pruritus and presenting clinical signs. Treatment with the appropriate antibiotic and antifungal agents allows the clinician to determine what remaining skin lesions and level of pruritus are due strictly to the flea hypersensitivity. Flea-allergic dogs with a light flea burden typically require 3 to 4 weeks of antibiotic or antifungal therapy or both types of therapy for superficial infections. If there is a heavy flea burden or it is difficult to institute a complete flea control quickly, the length of therapy needed may be increased to at least 6 weeks. In either case and particularly for antibiotics, treatment should be continued for 10 to 14 days past resolution of the clinical signs. Once a dog with flea bite allergy is properly managed the need for antimicrobials should be greatly decreased. A recurrence of infection should always be suspected if the dog has a substantial lapse in flea control, active clinical signs, and does not respond favourably to a short course (less than 7 days) of glucocorticoid therapy.

Glucocorticoids

Glucocorticoids [2] are the most effective therapy for controlling the intense pruritus associated with flea bite allergy. Oral preparations are usually recommended over long-acting injectable products, because they are easier to taper and there is no evidence that long-acting injectable preparations provide quicker relief. If the dog is severely pruritic, a relatively high initial dose of prednisone/prednisolone (1–2 mg/kg daily) or methylprednisolone (0.8 to 1.6 mg/kg daily) is recommended for at least the first 3 to 5 days and up to 7 to 10 days. This can be given as a single daily dose but it is usually divided into a twice-daily dose. After this initial loading phase, the dose is then reduced by half to 0.5 to 1 mg/kg given once daily for an additional 7 to 10 days. At this point,

Veterinary Allergy, First Edition. Edited by Chiara Noli, Aiden Foster, and Wayne Rosenkrantz.

if the dog's pruritus has substantially improved the dose is further reduced to every other day. Over the following 2 to 4 weeks, this every day dose may be reduced further or left the same. The length of time the dog needs to remain on the every other day dose depends on overall response to the glucocorticoid therapy and success of the flea control programme.

If the dog has mild to moderate pruritus, the glucocorticoid doses recommended are the same, but the length of therapy is decreased. The initial high dose may only need to be given for 2 to 3 days, then if the dog is still pruritic the glucocorticoids are continued at the half dose daily for another 3 to 7 days. At this point, if the pruritus is substantially decreased, glucocorticoid therapy can be stopped. If not, the dose is reduced to every other day.

Polydipsia, polyuria, polyphagia, and panting are the most common acute adverse effects associated with glucocorticoid use. If these side effects are unacceptable to owners the dose should be decreased faster or an alternative glucocorticoid (triamcinolone, dexamethasone) could be tried. The initial doses used for dexamethasone (0.1 to 0.2 mg/kg once daily) and triamcinolone (0.25 to 1 mg/kg once daily) are lower than prednisone since these are more potent glucocorticoids. The dosage reduction schedules for these steroids remains the same as that of prednisone except they are given at 3-day intervals instead of at 2-day intervals after the first 1 to 2 weeks of therapy.

A small supply of glucocorticoids should be available to most dogs with flea bite allergy, particularly dogs living in flea endemic areas. If there is a known flea exposure or a recurrence of pruritus, the owner can administer the glucocorticoid for 2 to 3 days. Many times this can control the flea allergy flare up and prevent a recurrence of secondary bacterial and yeast infections. It is important that the owner understands the glucocorticoids are only symptomatic therapy and cannot replace diligent flea control. It is also important they understand that if the signs do not abate in a maximum of 5 to 7 days the dog should be re-examined for evidence of infections and other causes of pruritus.

Other systemic antipruritic drugs

None of the other antipruritic drugs commonly used to treat atopy in the dog, including ciclosporin and antihistamines, have been successful in controlling the intense pruritus associated with flea bite allergy. Essential fatty acids alone have also not been successful at controlling the pruritus associated with flea bite allergy although their use may have a mild steroid-sparing effect.

Topical therapy

Non-steroidal topical therapies [3] are most useful for the control of mild to moderate pruritus in flea-allergic dogs. They can reduce the dose of systemic glucocorticoids needed to control severe pruritus, but have little effect when used alone. Topical therapies that are effective for mild flea bite allergy induced pruritus include counter-irritants and anaesthetics. Counter-irritant substances cause a mild inflammatory response in the sensory nerves. The resulting mild numbness, tingling, or cooling sensation helps to override the feeling of pruritus. Phenol and menthol are the most common counter-irritants included in veterinary pharmaceutical products, while mint oils, camphor, eucalyptus, and witch hazel are included in many over the counter preparations. Counter-irritants can be used multiple times daily and normally give a brief respite from the pruritus. Their actual duration of effectiveness is unknown. Pramoxine hydrochloride, derived from morpholine, is a common topical anaesthetic used in veterinary products. The potency of the pramoxine is comparable to benzocaine but it does not have the potential side effect of methemoglobinemia. The onset of action is usually within 3 to 5 minutes while the duration of action varies, but is usually less than 1 hour.

Topical glucocorticoids can be effective for controlling mild to moderate pruritus from flea bite allergy. For mild cases, 1.0% hydrocortisone can provide relief although the duration of action is extremely variable (1 to 48 hours). Topical hydrocortisone is safe even with repeated applications and can therefore be used for extended periods with minimal chance of cutaneous atrophy. Dexamethasone acetate (0.1%), triamcinolone acetonide (0.1%), and betamethasone valerate (0.1%) are all moderately potent topical glucocorticoids that can help control more pruritic cases. Since these glucocorticoids are well absorbed they can have both systemic and cutaneous adverse effects with repeated applications. Therefore they should not be used for extended periods of time. If overused, particularly for long periods of time, they can cause localized cutaneous atrophy and potentially iatrogenic hyperadrenocorticism. Hydrocortisone aceponate (0.584%) [4] and triamcinolone acetonide spray (0.015%) are also moderate potency steroids that are absorbed cutaneously, but are reported to have less systemic effects [5,6]. This may allow them to be used repeatedly over short periods of time with less chance of iatrogenic hyperadrenocorticism. Care should still be taken when using these products long term since cutaneous atrophy can still occur with chronic use [7]. Because of this potential for cutaneous atrophy, it is also recommended that gloves be worn when applying these products.

Immunotherapy

Three different types of immunotherapy [1] have been investigated in the dog in an attempt to either control live fleas on the dog or signs of flea bite allergy. At this time all three types are still in the research stage and are not commercially available.

The first type of immunotherapy investigated was a flea vaccine designed to control flea bite allergy signs. Two double-blinded, placebo-controlled studies compared vaccines made from whole-body flea extract to placebo in dogs with naturally occurring flea allergy [8,9]. No differences were found between the two groups in either study. A third double-blinded, placebo-controlled study compared vaccination with purified *Ctenocephalides felis felis* saliva antigen to placebo in privately owned dogs with naturally occurring flea allergy dermatitis [10]. In this pilot study, clinical signs and pruritus were significantly improved in the test group over the placebo group. Unfortunately, no larger follow-up studies have been conducted to confirm these results and no attempt has been made to make this vaccine commercially available.

The second type of immunotherapy utilized immunomodulators produced by bacteria from the order Actinomycetales to turn off the Th2 response commonly associated with allergic reactions and to promote Th1 reactions. In a small, double-blinded, placebo-controlled clinical trial, 54 flea-allergic dogs were given two intradermal injections of a heat-killed preparation of either *Gordonia bronchialis* or *Rhodococcus coprophilus* or placebo 20 days apart [11]. The dogs were re-evaluated 28 days after the second injection. The dogs who received the injections of heat-killed bacteria had significantly decreased clinical signs and pruritus compared to the dogs who received the placebo injections.

The third type of immunotherapy investigated was immunization directed against the live flea in an attempt to kill the flea and therefore decrease infestation. This type of therapy could decrease the need for chemical flea control in both the flea-allergic and non-flea-allergic dog. One of the largest challenges researchers have faced in the development of this type of vaccine is the apparent absence of natural immunity against fleas in the dog. To overcome this problem, researchers in the field have investigated hidden antigens in the flea gut to incorporate into these vaccines. In one study, fleas exposed to dogs immunized with a flea-midgut extract had a 45% mortality rate and lower fecundity compared to a 29% mortality rate in fleas exposed to control dogs one week postvaccination [12].

Conclusion

Avoidance of flea bites is still the best and only long-term therapy for control of flea-allergy dermatitis. This is accomplished with diligent on-animal and environmental flea control. To help control the severe pruritus that can accompany flea bite dermatitis, glucocorticoids are still the drug of choice for short-term relief. In the future, we may have vaccines that minimize the need for insecticide use, as well as vaccines that may treat the symptoms of flea bite allergy similar to those used for pollen allergies. Long term, such immunotherapies will be better for both the dog and the environment.

References

1. Carlotti DN, Jacobs DE. Therapy, control and prevention of flea allergy dermatitis in dogs and cats. *Veterinary Dermatology* 2000; **11**: 83–98.
2. van den Broek A, Horvath-Ungerboeck C. The use of glucocorticoids in canine dermatology: Part 2. *UK Vet* 2009; **14**: 61–69.
3. Horvath-Ungerboeck C, van den Broek A. The use of glucocorticoids in canine dermatology: Part 3 Topical glucocorticoids. *UK Vet* 2009; **14**: 50–55.
4. Bonneau S, Skowronski V, Sanquer A, *et al.* Therapeutic efficacy of topical hydrocortisone aceponate in experimental flea-allergy dermatitis in dogs. *Australian Veterinary Journal* 2009; **87**: 287–291.
5. DeBoer DJ, Schafer JH, Salsbury CS, *et al.* Multiple-center study of reduced-concentration triamcinolone topical solution for the treatment of dogs with known or suspected allergic pruritus. *American Journal of Veterinary Research* 2002; **63**: 408–413.
6. Reme CA, Dufour P. Effects of repeated topical application of a 0.0584% hydrocortisone aceponate spray on skin thickness in beagle dogs. *International Journal of Applied Research in Veterinary Medicine* 2010; **8**: 1–6.
7. Bizikova P, Linder KE, Paps J, *et al.* Effect of a novel topical diester glucocorticoid spray on immediate- and late-phase cutaneous allergic reactions in Maltese-beagle atopic dogs: a placebo-controlled study. *Veterinary Dermatology* 2010; **21**: 71–80.
8. Halliwell REW. Hyposensitization in the treatment of flea bite hypersensitivity: results of a double-blinded study. *Journal of the American Animal Hospital Association* 1981; **17**: 249–253.
9. Halliwell REW. Clinical and immunological response to alum-precipitated flea antigen in immunotherapy of flea-allergic dogs: results of a double-blind study. In: Ihrke PJ, Mason IS, White SD, eds. *Advances in Veterinary Dermatology*, Vol. 2. Oxford: Butterworth Heinemann, 1993: 41–50.
10. Kwochka KA, McCall CA, Hillier A, *et al.* Flea salivary antigen rush immunotherapy for flea allergy dermatitis in dogs: a double-blinded, placebo–controlled clinical study. *14th Proceedings of the AAVD/ACVD Meeting* (San Antonio, TX USA) 1998, 107–108.
11. Marro A, Pirles M, Schiaffino L, *et al.* Successful immunotherapy of canine flea allergy with injected Actinomycetales preparations. *Immunotherapy* 2011; **3**: 371–378.
12. Heath AW, Arfsten A, Yamanaka M, *et al.* Vaccination against the cat flea *Ctenocephalides felis felis*. *Parasite Immunology* 1994; **16**: 187–191.

Section 4

Complicating Infections in Allergic Dogs

26

Complicating microbial skin infections in allergic dogs

Anette Loeffler

Royal Veterinary College, University of London, London, UK

Conflict of interest: none declared.

Importance and prevalence

Microbial skin infections are amongst the most frequently diagnosed diseases in dogs with dermatological problems [1] and commonly occur with hypersensitivity disorders. Superficial staphylococcal pyoderma was one of the minor Willemse criteria for the diagnosis of canine atopic dermatitis [2], while the 2010 International Task Force guidelines for treatment of canine atopic dermatitis list *Staphylococcus* bacteria and *Malassezia* yeasts as two of the five recognized flare factors [3].

Retrospective surveys investigating allergic skin disease in dogs found concurrent pyoderma in 27 to 36% of atopic dermatitis patients [2,4,5], in around 40% of dogs with adverse food reactions [6,7], and in 10% of 330 dogs with flea allergy dermatitis [8]. *Malassezia* dermatitis was seen in 2 of 91 atopic dogs [5] and in 20% of food-allergic dogs [7], while earlier studies omit yeast-related disease. Frequencies were higher in a recent prospective study where 74% of dogs undergoing allergen-specific immunotherapy over a 9-month period had pyoderma and 67% *Malassezia* dermatitis [9].

Whether microbial infections are truly secondary to allergic disease remains unclear and is discussed in Chapters 7 and 8. In any case, resolution and prevention of recurrent microbial infection are critical for the successful management of an allergic patient because pruritus and erythema are common clinical signs of pyoderma and of *Malassezia* infections in dogs. Furthermore, some cases of so-called 'idiopathic recurrent pyoderma' are likely to be due to underlying hypersensitivity disorders and their successful treatment may be all that is required in the management of an allergic dog. These are cases where clinical signs are absent after resolution of the microbial infection and where recurrence of infection is the only indicator of a hypersensitivity disorder.

Pathogens

Staphylococci colonize the surfaces of most mammals, including dogs, and are therefore ideally suited to cause skin disease when opportunities arise. *Staphylococcus pseudintermedius*, previously *S. intermedius* [10], is the predominant bacterial pathogen in canine skin infections [11,12]. It has been isolated from 90% of superficial pyoderma cases and up to 60% of deep pyoderma cases [12,13]. Laboratory recognition of *S. pseudintermedius* for diagnostic purposes is mainly based on identification of white circular colonies with a characteristic double zone of haemolysis on sheep blood agar, Gram-positive staining, and positive reactions for coagulase, catalase, and mannitol fermentation. The golden pigmented, but otherwise phenotypically very similar, coagulase-positive *S. aureus* is only reported in up to 10% of carriage and clinical isolates from dogs. However, *S. aureus* may have

Veterinary Allergy, First Edition. Edited by Chiara Noli, Aiden Foster, and Wayne Rosenkrantz.

been misdiagnosed in veterinary laboratories based on phenotypic methods alone and attention to accurate species identification is nowadays more important due to the human health implications of meticillin-resistant *S. aureus* (MRSA) [14]. Other staphylococcal species recognized as canine skin pathogens include the coagulase-variable *S. hyicus*, which is probably rare, and *S. schleiferi*, which has recently gained interest due to the high frequency of meticillin resistance, particularly amongst coagulase-positive strains [15–17].

Coagulase-negative staphylococcal species are historically thought to be 'non-pathogenic' but should be considered and treated as pathogens where they are isolated from lesional skin and if cytological evidence supports invasive behaviour, particularly in animals receiving glucocorticoid therapy [18].

The past decade has seen the emergence and spread of multidrug-resistant bacteria, particularly of MRSA and *S. pseudintermedius* (MRSP) [19]. Meticillin-resistant staphylococci (MRS) only differ from their susceptible counterparts in resistance genes and antimicrobial selection pressure will influence their epidemiology and behaviour. MRS were more frequently found in dogs with inflammatory skin disease compared with healthy dogs [20], and chronic concurrent disease, repeated or prolonged exposure to antimicrobial agents, hospitalization, and frequent visits to veterinary clinics have been described as risk factors for MRS acquisition [21–23]. Implications for clinical management of MRSA infections in pets involve most importantly the need for owner and staff awareness about the potential for transmission between humans and pets in both directions. Most MRSA strains isolated from pets are of human origin and thus present a substantial risk to susceptible people in contact with infected pets [24]. In contrast, MRSP are primarily dog-adapted bacteria with a lower zoonotic risk for in-contact humans. MRSP though has the potential to spread easily amongst pets, e.g. susceptible animal patients in veterinary hospitals. It is typically resistant to all clinically relevant antimicrobials and thus calls for rigorous infection control and hygiene measures.

Other bacteria such as streptococci, *Proteus mirabilis*, and *Escherichia coli* are occasionally isolated from skin infections but are thought to occur as opportunists, secondary to *S. pseudintermedius* infection [25]. Skin infection with *Pseudomonas aeruginosa* will typically affect folds and moist areas such as around the face and perineal region. Malodorous green pus is a often a striking feature but infection may be under-recognized as in 4 of 20 dogs, lesions and distribution were described to resemble those of staphylococcal superficial pyoderma [26]. Anaerobic bacteria, such as *Clostridium* spp., *Bacterioides* spp., *Actinomyces* spp., and *Prevotella* spp. are more commonly associated with abscesses, granulomas, or cellulitis but have rarely been isolated from pyoderma and in cases of allergic disease [13].

The yeast *Malassezia pachydermatis* began to be recognized as an important canine skin pathogen in the early 1990s [27]. The species is lipophilic but not lipid dependent, colonizes the stratum corneum of the skin and mucosae in healthy dogs, and preferred niches have been identified such as the anus, external ear canal, lower lip, and interdigital skin [28]. Higher numbers of yeasts have been isolated from lesional and non-lesional skin of atopic dogs compared with those of healthy animals [29]. *Malassezia* yeast can co-exists with staphylococci on healthy skin and in infection [9,30]. While symbiotic or antagonistic effects remain poorly understood, each microbial component needs to be diagnosed and treated individually [31].

Clinical manifestations

Bacterial skin infections are classically differentiated by depth of infection into surface, superficial, and deep pyoderma, although the definition of surface pyodermas remains controversial with evidence of neutrophilic inflammation often lacking [32]. More recently, they were grouped based on a lesion-orientated approach to aid clinical diagnosis [33]. Important characteristics relevant for allergic dogs are summarized in Table 26.1.

Most common in allergic dogs are surface and superficial pyoderma. Neither group extends beyond the basement membrane but pruritus and erythema are common and self-trauma often leads to secondary complications. Surface pyoderma occurs on haired skin (acute moist dermatitis), in folds (intertrigo), in moist areas (mucocutaneous pyoderma), or over larger areas or on paws as in bacterial overgrowth syndrome (Figure 26.1) [34–36]. Superficial pyoderma presents most commonly as folliculitis involving the epidermis and hair follicles, as reflected by the associated lesions (macules, papules, pustules, and epidermal collarettes). Presentations of bacterial folliculitis may vary with coat type, leading to less specific clinical signs of patchy alopecia ('moth-eaten appearance') (Figure 26.2), scaling (Figure 26.3), or stained hairs.

Deep pyoderma is more often thought to be secondary to immune deficiencies rather than hypersensitivity disorders but should be considered in allergic dogs, particularly in patients receiving glucocorticoids [37,38]. Some localized syndromes, such as acral lick dermatitis [13], interdigital nodules [39], and muzzle folliculitis or chin acne (Figure 26.4) [33], are particularly frustrating presentations when they complicate allergic disease. As glucocorticoids are always contraindicated in deep pyoderma, aggressive treatment of the infectious

Table 26.1 Important types of pyoderma and associated characteristics that are seen with hypersensitivity disorders in dogs

Depth	Type	Typical lesions	Important differential diagnoses	Comments and challenges
Surface	Bacterial overgrowth	Erythema, scales, greasy (malodorous) exudate	Uncomplicated allergic skin disease, *Malassezia* dermatitis	Note: no raised lesions on skin and few or no neutrophils on cytology
	Acute moist dermatitis (pyotraumatic dermatitis)	Well-demarcated, moist area of alopecia, erythema, erosion, skin thickening	Pyotraumatic folliculitis and furunculosis Neoplasia	Highly pruritic and often painful
	Intertrigo	Erythema, malodorous exudate in folds		Friction as important contributing factor (face, tail, vulva, skin on ventral neck, obese animals, shar-peis or bloodhounds)
	Mucocutaneous pyoderma	Erythema, swelling, erosions, later crusting, ulceration, fissuring	Immune-mediated or autoimmune disease (e.g. cutaneous lupus), hepatocutaneous syndrome	Most often on lips, other mucocutaneous junctions
Superficial	Bacterial folliculitis (canine superficial pyoderma)	Erythematous macules, papules, pustules (few and transient on canine skin), epidermal collarettes	Demodicosis, dermatophytosis, pemphigus foliaceus, other rare sterile pustular diseases	Classical appearance: papular rash with epidermal collarettes affecting the ventral abdomen and medial thighs Unusual appearances in shorthaired breeds: moth-eaten appearance, scaling, stained hairs
Deep	Furunculosis/ cellulitis	Erythema, haemorrhagic crusts, draining sinuses, ulcers, skin thickening, scarring	Demodicosis, juvenile cellulitis ('puppy strangles'), deep fungal infections	
	Pododermatitis	Interdigital nodules, erythema, with or without draining sinus tracts	Pododemodicosis, foreign bodies, conformational abnormalities, neoplasia, lymphocytic-plasmacytic pododermatitis	
	Acral lick dermatitis	Pruritic nodules on limbs, alopecia, erosion, ulceration, exudation	Neoplasia, fungal granuloma, sterile granuloma	
	Chin acne/ muzzle folliculitis	Erythema, swelling, papules, nodules, alopecia, draining sinus tracts, crusts	Demodicosis, fungal infection, sterile granulomatous disease	
	Pyotraumatic folliculitis and furunculosis	As for acute moist dermatitis but with: satellite lesions in surrounding skin, papules, ulceration	Demodicosis, deep fungal infection, sterile granulomatous disease	Macroscopic signs of deep pyoderma may be subtle or lacking

component is critical before anti-inflammatory treatment can be started. Hallmarks of dermal involvement are haemorrhagic crusts, draining sinus tracts, and more often pain than pruritus (Table 26.1).

Other clinical manifestations of bacterial skin disease that have not been linked explicitly to allergic disease exist and readers are referred to other texts for information [33,40].

Malassezia skin infections are less varied in their clinical presentations. Signs include erythema, yellow or grey greasy exudate, scaling, alopecia, malodour, and hyperpigmentation and lichenification in chronic cases

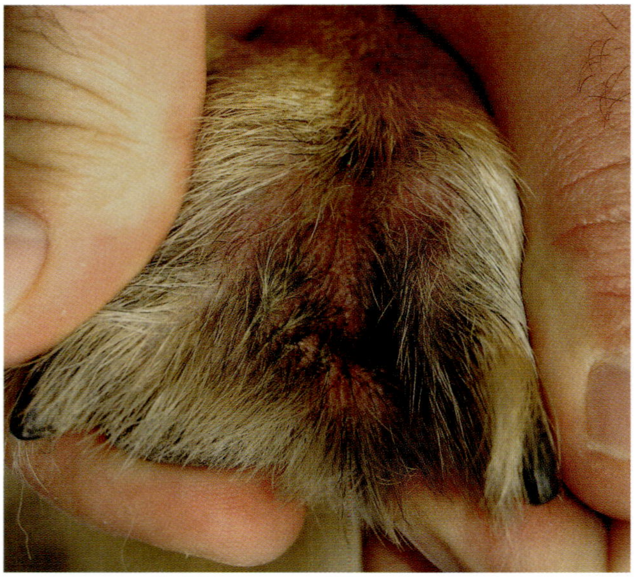

Figure 26.1 Dorsal interdigital aspect of an allergic collie cross with bacterial overgrowth. There is marked interdigital erythema, stained hair, and moisture but no raised lesions that would suggest a bacterial component of disease.

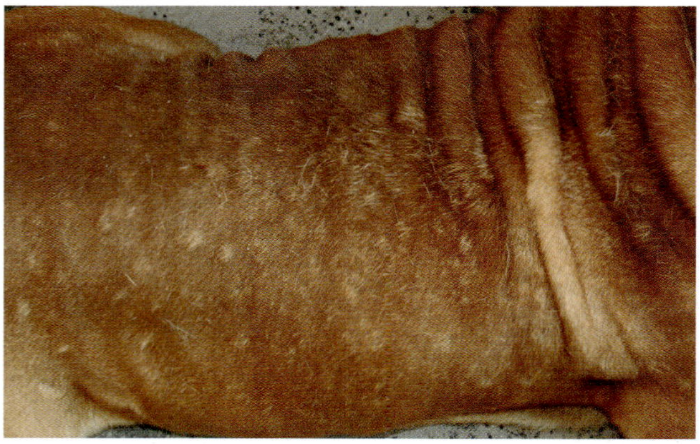

Figure 26.2 Dogue de Bordeaux with widespread lesions suggestive of superficial pyoderma (bacterial folliculitis). Abundant hair loss and small focal areas of alopecia gave the dog a 'moth-eaten' appearance.

(Figure 26.5) [41]. Pruritus is common and may be severe. Areas typically affected are those with a tendency to be moist and warm such as the lip folds, axillae, the groin, interdigital areas, and folds around the perineum and vulva.

Diagnostic approach

Microbial infections should be considered in acute flares of allergic disease and in the long-term management of chronic disease [3]. This involves:

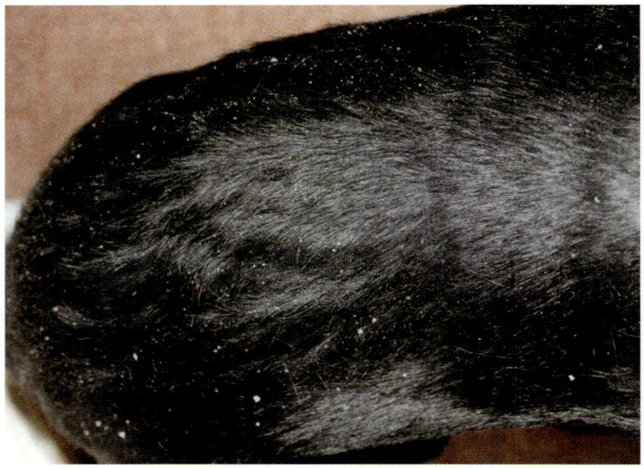

Figure 26.3 Marked scaling on the dorsum of a Labrador with adverse food reaction. Papules and small epidermal collarettes became visible on close inspection, cytology was compatible with bacterial infection, and scaling resolved with 3 weeks of systemic cefalexin therapy.

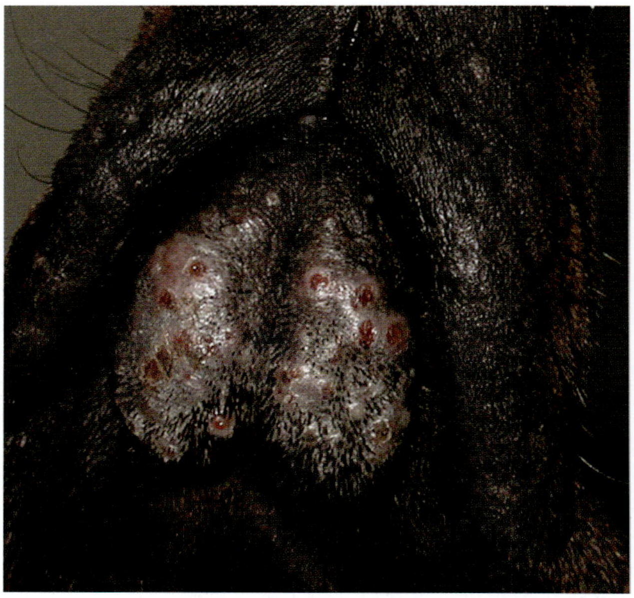

Figure 26.4 Deep pyoderma due to staphylococci affecting the chin of a Doberman with allergic skin disease. Haemorrhagic crusts, swelling, erythema, and pain were the predominant clinical signs.

1 recognition of microbial infection as a flare factor;
2 ruling out differential diagnoses, particularly ectoparasite infestations;
3 correct identification of the type (bacterial, yeast, mixed) and depth (surface, superficial, deep pyoderma) of the infection.

Subsequently, a decision needs to be made on whether empirical treatment will be appropriate. If not, additional sampling and laboratory tests will be required to:

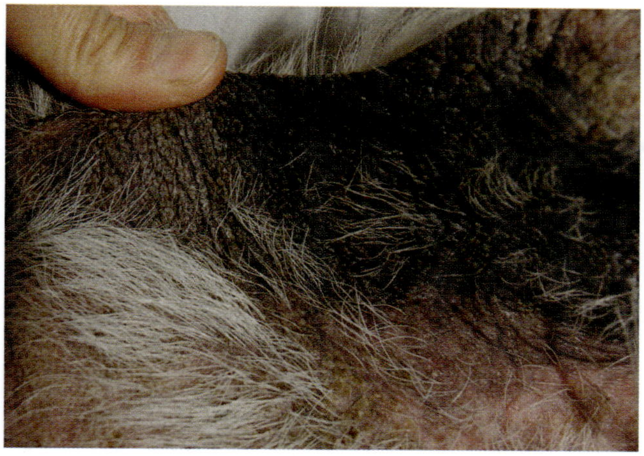

Figure 26.5 Axilla of a West Highland white terrier with *Malassezia* dermatitis. The predominant clinical signs are alopecia, erythema, hyperpigmentation, and lichenification. Note: the clinical signs are indistinguishable from bacterial overgrowth and cytology is required to identify the involved micro-organisms. (Reprinted with permission from Ross Bond.)

4 culture and identify involved pathogens;
5 determine their antimicrobial susceptibilities, including a possible presence of meticillin-resistant bacteria.

Identification of microbial infections

In addition to the baseline information about the patients' allergic disease, assessment of signalment and historical data will inform on frequency and type of flares (e.g. a papular rash observed by owners), and in some cases on response to previous antimicrobial treatment and on ectoparasite control measures.

Clinical signs will be highly suggestive of superficial pyoderma and deep pyoderma (Table 26.1). However, clinical signs are less helpful in the diagnosis of bacterial and yeast overgrowth as erythema and pruritus mimic signs of allergic disease. Cytology will be required to assess the microbial proliferation.

Cytology can confirm an infectious process and will allow identification of the type of infection, i.e. bacterial (cocci, rods), yeast (*Malassezia* spp.), or mixed organisms, combined with inflammatory cells (typically degenerate neutrophils and macrophages) (Figures 26.6 and 26.7) [42]. Cytology would be desirable (but unlikely feasible) for every case prior to prescribing antimicrobial drugs. However, cytology should always be performed where:

1 skin lesions are difficult to interpret, e.g. those associated with microbial overgrowth;
2 sensible empirical antimicrobial therapy was ineffective; if bacteria are still found on cytology, lack of compliance, incorrect prescribing, and multidrug-resistant organisms should be suspected; if inflam-

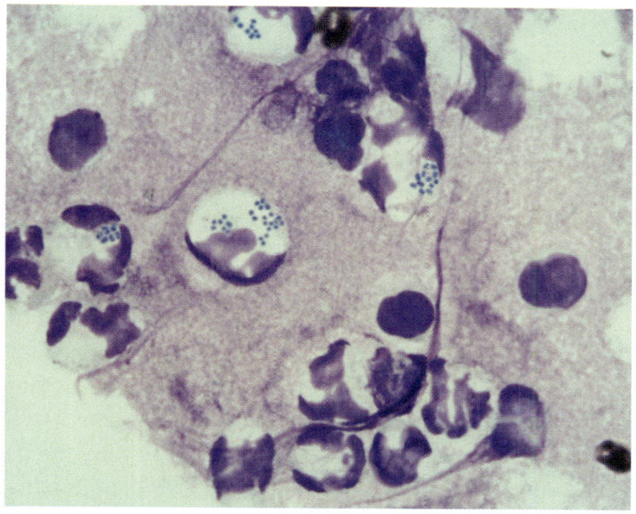

Figure 26.6 Cytological examination of an impression smear from a pustule of a dog with superficial pyoderma. Numerous cocci amongst a background of neutrophils (Romanovsky type stain, ×1000).

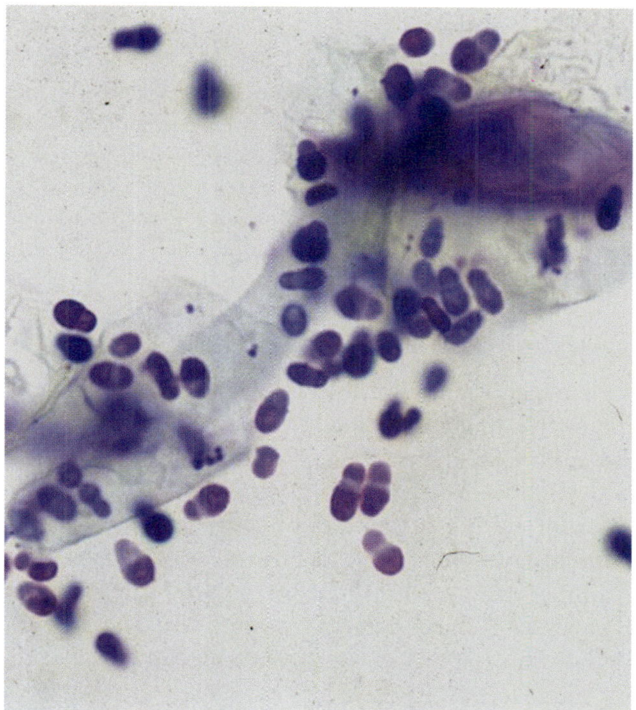

Figure 26.7 Cytological examination of an impression smear from the skin of a dog with *Malassezia* dermatitis. Numerous yeast adhere to the corneocytes (Romanovsky type stain, ×1000).

matory cells persist but no microbes are seen, non-infectious differential diagnoses need to be investigated (e.g. pemphigus);
3 a sample is submitted for bacterial culture so that laboratory results can be interpreted in the light of cytological findings.

Samples can be collected by direct slide impression (most suitable for moist lesions) or adhesive tape impression (dry or greasy areas). These are stained and prepared for examination under oil immersion objective for cellular morphology and numbers of bacteria or yeast organisms [43,44]. While recognition of bacteria and yeast is normally straightforward if they are present in large numbers, diagnosis can be problematic if only a few organisms are seen. Cut-off values for microbes per high-power oil immersion field have been described but this approach is unhelpful because reference ranges for normal microflora counts and invasive behaviour do not exist. If only a few microbes are seen, the diagnosis will rely on a combination of cytology findings (e.g. microbes found within a neutrophilic infiltrate supporting infection) with clinical signs and in some cases response to trial therapy.

As microbial infections may accompany any other skin disease even in allergic patients, ectoparasitoses (e.g. demodicosis, scabies) and dermatophytosis should be considered as additional differential diagnoses in every case. Skin scrapings, hair plucks, coat brushings, Wood's lamp examination and fungal culture will be appropriate. Histopathology from biopsy specimens will rarely be required to diagnose microbial infection but may be necessary to rule out less-common differential diagnoses such as neoplasia, foreign bodies (e.g. for interdigital nodules), or sterile pustular diseases (e.g. pemphigus foliaceus) for pustular, crusting eruptions.

Sampling and in vitro *tests*

Where identification of the bacterial pathogen is essential for treatment decisions, lesions need to be sampled for culture. Although the extra time and cost involved with *in vitro* testing remain practical concerns, indications for culture and susceptibility testing have become particularly important in countries where MRSA and MRSP have emerged. It may be important to ask laboratories to include oxacillin (nowadays used as representative for meticillin) in routine susceptibility testing for staphylococci where this is not done.

Empirical choice of antimicrobial drugs currently remains appropriate for many microbial skin infections, including *Malassezia* dermatitis and for most cases of surface and superficial pyoderma. *In vitro* testing is essential, though, where a substantially increased risk to animal or human health would arise from inappropriate therapy (Table 26.2). Similarly, when empirical treatment fails, culture and susceptibility testing must be initiated without delay (there is currently no evidence that antimicrobial drugs need to be discontinued prior to sampling if resistant organisms are suspected).

Table 26.2 Circumstances for which empirical selection of antimicrobial drugs may be appropriate and for which *in vitro* testing is essential

Empirical choice may be appropriate if	*In vitro* susceptibility test results are essential if
Surface and superficial pyoderma if topical therapy alone will be prescribed	Deep pyoderma (always!)
First occurrence of superficial pyoderma or first use of systemic antimicrobial therapy after topical therapy with cocci confirmed on cytology	History of recurrent pyoderma or repeated systemic antimicrobial therapy
History of only one or two occurrences of pyoderma per year and cocci confirmed on cytology	Rod-shaped bacteria either pure or mixed with other bacteria seen on cytology
	Lack of response to empirically chosen antimicrobial therapy (cytological evidence of persistent bacterial infection)
No increased risk of MRSA or MRSP (no history of MRS in human or animal household contacts)	History of MRSA or MRSP within the household (in humans or animals)
With knowledge of the local resistance pattern of *S. pseudintermedius* and a low local prevalence of MRS	High prevalence of MRSA or MRSP infections within the practice or in the local area
Under consideration of good prescribing principles (e.g. narrow-spectrum, first-tier)	Under consideration of good prescribing principles (e.g. narrow-spectrum, first-tier)

MRSA, meticillin-resistant *S. aureus*; MRSP, meticillin-resistant *S. pseudintermedius.*

Surface and superficial infections and deep infections, if draining sinus tracts yield pus from deeper areas, can be sampled non-invasively using swabs. For deep pyoderma, it is important to culture (and subsequently treat) organisms that are responsible for infection in the dermis rather than surface microbes. In a study of dogs with acral lick granuloma, deep tissue culture was only in agreement with surface culture in 36% of dogs [13]. In these cases, tissue samples obtained by punch or excisional biopsy need to be submitted for macerated tissue culture. It is important to submit samples in a sterile container without formalin (sterile saline can be added to improve transport conditions) and either surgically prepare the area prior to biopsy or remove the epidermis with a sterile scalpel blade in order to eliminate surface bacteria.

Therapy

General approach

Although clearly a day-to-day challenge for veterinary practitioners, most recommendations on the treatment of microbial infections in allergic dogs are based on evidence from expert committee reports or expert opinion rather than from controlled trials [3,45,46]. With antimicrobial use under more and more scrutiny, it has to be considered that staphylococci are transmitted between humans and animals in both directions, that all antimicrobial classes approved for pets are also used in human medicine, and thus that any antimicrobial use in dogs will have implications for human health [47]. Antimicrobials should therefore be dispensed only when infection is highly likely (and ideally confirmed by cytology). Prescribing decisions should be based on the best available evidence.

As a general rule, the deeper the infection, the greater the need for systemic therapy and the longer the required treatment period. In contrast, surface infections such as *Malassezia* dermatitis, bacterial overgrowth, and acute moist dermatitis lend themselves to topical therapy due to the location of pathogens. Antimicrobial treatment may even be avoidable in cases of recurrent intertrigo, if folds can be surgically removed [38].

Topical treatment

Topical antibacterial therapy has long been recommended as an adjunct to systemic drugs in all types of pyoderma [38,48,49]. It has recently gained attention for its potential to reduce the need for systemic antimicrobials, firstly, as the sole antibacterial treatment in surface and superficial pyoderma and secondly, in the treatment of superficial infections due to MRSA or MRSP. In a recent study, 68% of dogs improved or resolved with twice weekly washing with either a 2% chlorhexidine or a 2.5% benzoyl peroxide shampoo alone over a 3-week period, reflected in reduced clinical scores and bacterial counts [50]. For superficial and localized MRSP infections, shampoo therapy produced clinical cure in several studies [51–53], supporting the benefit of achieving high concentrations of active compound through direct local application.

For widespread or generalized infections, shampoos containing antibacterial agents such as 2–4% chlorhexidine formulations or benzoyl peroxide will be most appropriate and good evidence exists to support their use [45]. Ethyl lactate or triclosan are alternatives if the above are not tolerated or available. Shampoos typically need to be applied two to three times a week with a 10-minute contact time before rinsing off. Creams, ointments, gels, or wipes containing antiseptics or antimicrobials, such as fusidic acid, mupirocin, neomycin, or bacitracin, may be effective for localized lesions [54].

As there is currently no concern over clinically relevant antifungal resistance in *Malassezia* species, treatment choices should be based on efficacy, safety, licensing, expected compliance, cost, and availability. There is good evidence to support the use of 2% miconazole nitrate/2% chlorhexidine gluconate shampoos two to three times weekly [55,56]. Other formulations for topical use in *Malassezia* dermatitis include 2–4% chlorhexidine, enilconazole, ketoconazole, 1% selenium sulphide, 2% lyme sulphur, 2.5% acetic acid, and acetic acid/boric acid combinations [57].

Any topical product may have adverse effects, such as most commonly drying and skin irritation, and owners should be encouraged to report these. Due to a known epidermal barrier defect in atopic patients, use of moisturizers may counteract a drying effect of frequent shampooing.

Systemic treatment

Pathogen susceptibility, drug efficacy, safety, availability, and authorization, cost, and practicability are key considerations when choosing antimicrobials for systemic therapy. Recommendations for antimicrobial therapy in animals are repeatedly being updated [38,48,58,59] and, in 2013, international guidelines specifically for canine superficial pyoderma will become available. In allergic patients, *S. pseudintermedius* is the target organism in the vast majority of cases. Surveys from the 1990s reported predictable, 'stable' susceptibility profiles for *S. pseudintermedius* with minor variation between countries which allowed an informed judgement for empirical antibiotic selection [15,60,61]. However, more recent reports from North America, Italy, and Germany have shown that resistance profiles can no longer be reliably predicted as around 20% of *S. pseudintermedius* submissions were MRSP [51,62–64]. As most MRSP isolates are resistant to all β-lactam antibiotics, fluoroquinolones, and lincosamides, and often to tetracyclines and potentiated-sulfonamides, empirical therapy will be unsuccessful in up to one-fifth of patients, prolonging disease and increasing the risk of spread.

Many different antibacterial agents are available and authorized for use in dogs in most countries. In addition, a substantial number of reports and reviews have been published over the past 30 years on use and dosages of antimicrobials [38,48,58]. Surprisingly though, a recent systematic literature review found little good-level evidence to support the use of widely prescribed drugs, which may relate to the many factors that influence bacterial infection and its resolution [46]. In general, narrow-spectrum agents such as lincosamides (e.g. clindamycin 5.5 mg/kg twice daily or 11 mg/kg once daily orally) are preferred against Gram-positive bacteria. However, increased resistance has been seen in isolates from referral practices in the past, indicating that these should only be used for first-time occurrences of pyoderma [12]. Recommended as first-tier drugs are also amoxicillin–clavulanate (12.5 mg/kg twice daily orally) and the first-generation cephalosporins cefalexin (15–30 mg/kg once or twice daily orally) and cefadroxil (22–35 mg/kg twice daily orally); and studies have shown efficacy of trimethoprim (30 mg/kg once or twice daily orally) and ormetoprim (55 mg/kg on day 1, then 27.5 mg/kg once daily orally) potentiated sulfonamides [31,48,58,59]. The third-generation cephalosporins cefovecin (8 mg/kg once every 14 days s.c.) and cefpodoxime (5–10 mg/kg once daily orally) have shown good efficacy in canine pyoderma [46]. However, third-generation cephalosporins have been associated with an increased risk of MRSA acquisition in humans, and should therefore only be used when *in vitro* tests indicate that other drugs are unlikely to be effective or where they are not tolerated. Selection of drugs for MRSA and MRSP infections should always be based on susceptibility testing, which may sometimes require extended testing of 'unconventional' antimicrobials to be requested from laboratories. Most MRSA infections in pets can be treated successfully as strains often remain susceptible to tetracyclines, sulfonamides, or clindamycin, and the prognosis depends on underlying or concurrent diseases. For MRSP, treatment choices are typically more limited and chloramphenicol, amikacin, and rifampicin are the three drugs most commonly reported. These are not authorized in all countries and efficacy and safety data are therefore sparse [65].

For pyoderma, antimicrobials should always be dosed at the higher end of the recommended range in order to achieve sufficient concentrations in the skin. In allergic patients undergoing elimination dietary trials for the diagnosis of adverse food reaction, palatable formulations of antimicrobials should be avoided. It is currently unknown whether shorter courses lead to more frequent recurrences or whether prolonged courses have a greater risk of selecting for resistance amongst the microflora of treated animals. In contrast to the often-prescribed 5-day courses for infections in other organs, it is widely stated that for superficial pyoderma, antimicrobials should be given for 3 weeks, and 5 days beyond clinical resolution. This recommendation dates back to at least 1987, is widely accepted and used in published clinical trials but is supported by little evidence [38]. For deep pyoderma, 4 to 6 weeks or longer and at least 1 to 2 weeks beyond lesion resolution are required. In the absence of firm data, it seems prudent to maintain these recommendations, despite the risk of unnecessarily prolonged exposure of microflora to antibiotics, but in addition to focus on close monitoring of clinical progress and follow-up examination.

In mixed infections where no single antibiotic fits all pathogens, treatment should be aimed initially at the staphylococci. Their elimination may lead to unfavourable conditions for the other opportunists, but additional drugs should be selected if signs of infection persist.

Systemic therapy is only required infrequently for the treatment of *Malassezia* dermatitis, usually in cases where topical treatment is impractical. Azole derivatives, although rarely authorized for systemic use in dogs, can be effective. A recent systematic review of interventions for *Malassezia* dermatitis in dogs found fair evidence for the use of ketoconazole (10 mg/kg/day) and itraconazole (5 mg/kg/day) over 3 weeks [55]. Adverse effects were rare in all studies and included most frequently gastrointestinal disturbances such as vomiting and anorexia. However, they can be more serious and include hepatic toxicosis. Due to inhibition of the P450 enzyme system, drug interactions, particularly with ciclosporin and ivermectin, need to be considered. Monitoring of liver enzymes is recommended and a dose-reduction or temporary (24–48 hour) cessation of therapy has been beneficial in some cases [66].

Combining antimicrobial drugs with glucocorticoids?

Glucocorticoids (and ciclosporin A) are contraindicated in the face of microbial infection due to their immunosuppressive effect and the risk of increasing severity of infection. However, there is little doubt that antimicrobials and glucocorticoids are prescribed concurrently in practice for superficial pyoderma without ill effect in most animals. Although there will be cases where such an approach is justifiable (e.g. in young allergic dogs with concurrent pyoderma that are otherwise healthy but where welfare is compromised by the level of pruritus), there are important arguments against such combination.

The use of glucocorticoids will indeed increase the risk for escalating infection, it may slow resolution of infection and thus prolong duration of antimicrobials required, and it will mask clinical response to antimicrobials because lesions appear less inflamed. In addition though, using glucocorticoids together with antimicrobials will greatly complicate the diagnostic work-up of allergic patients and hinder optimization of long-term medication regimes. Only a step-wise approach, i.e. resolving microbial infections with antimicrobials alone first, then assessing the need for anti-inflammatory medication, will allow assessment of pruritus in the absence of flare factors and thus determination of the lowest necessary doses of anti-inflammatory medication.

Prevention

The aim to prevent recurrences of microbial skin infections in allergic patients should focus in the first instance on an optimization of treatment of the primary hypersensitivity. Thus, in some allergic dogs, once microbial infection has been resolved, relapses of infection may be prevented using anti-inflammatory medications. Where this is not successful, recurrences should be prevented and controlled by topical antimicrobial therapy as a first choice (e.g. regular shampooing).

Owner education

Owners need to be aware that the prognosis for recurrent microbial skin infection is favourable, as effective antimicrobial agents are available for most cases, but that the overall prognosis will depend on concurrent hypersensitivities, and that a long-term commitment for disease management is likely to be required.

Since compliance will be a key factor in the successful management of microbial infections, especially where more labour-intensive topical therapy is chosen, owners need to be closely involved in the decision process about antimicrobial therapy. Owners' enthusiasm for topical therapy may be enhanced if advantages are explained. These include a targeted treatment of the diseased skin without affecting other organs, reduced risk for serious side effects and antimicrobial resistance, scope for tailored dosing by the owner, an overall hygiene effect on the coat, and likely reduced cost. Instructions on how and how often to apply topical treatment need to be clearly explained including the required (often 10-minute) contact time for shampoos.

Immunomodulation

Immunomodulation with staphylococcal vaccines is another alternative for long-term management in poorly controlled allergic dogs and should be considered where topical treatment is inappropriate or ineffective. Reasons for an allergic dog developing microbial infection include skin damage from allergic pruritus, defects in skin barrier function, increased adherence of staphylococci to corneocytes, altered susceptibility to staphylococcal antigens, and the effects of anti-inflammatory medications. The concept of immunomodulation specifically aimed at increasing resistance to recurrent infections is therefore different in allergic patients compared to dogs with presumed immunodeficiencies, such as in German shepherd dog pyoderma [37,67]. There is currently no evidence for the use of drugs with a proposed 'immune-stimulating' effect in the management of allergic dogs. There are, however, promising data from several small studies supporting the use of staphylococcal vaccines. The two most recent studies evaluated a commercial *S. aureus*-based bacterin treatment available in North America (Staphage Lysate, Delmont Laboratories, PA, USA)[68] and an autogenous vaccine, prepared from the patient's infecting *Staphylococcus* [69]. In both studies, systemic antibiotics were given initially to achieve resolution while bacterins were continued, as once or twice-weekly injections, and effect was assessed after 18 and 10 weeks, respectively. Clinical signs were significantly better in the vaccine groups compared with the non-vaccine groups, indicating fewer, slower, or less-severe relapses, treatment was well tolerated and an 18-month follow-up showed that the treatment had been continued in 50% of dogs. Potential adverse effects include cutaneous adverse drug reactions and anaphylaxis.

Long-term use of systemic antimicrobial drugs

Where the above approaches are not sufficient, repeated systemic antibiosis may become unavoidable. However, it was already stated in 1990, that this should be a 'last resort' option due to the risk of promoting drug resistance and the spread of resistant staphylococci [70]. Where cost proved a limiting factor, low-dose and intermittent dosing ('pulse therapy') have been described in the past. Although direct evidence is lacking, it is plausible that both forms will be associated with an even higher risk of selecting for resistance and should therefore not be used [71].

Pulse therapy for yeast infection remains less controversial due to the lack of data supporting resistance in *Malassezia* spp.

Essential follow-up of MRSA/MRSP infections

Dogs with a history of MRSA or MRSP infection require more complex follow-up procedures in order to prevent recurrences of infection with multidrug-resistant bacteria. Around 80% of staphylococcal infections are thought to be caused by endogenous bacteria, i.e. those that are found colonizing the patient as part of the microflora [72,73]. As MRS can persist on skin and mucosal carrier sites of dogs after infection has resolved [22], such carrier animals are at risk of repeated MRS infections during allergic flares. A complete resolution of MRSA or MRSP should only be announced after negative results have been obtained from carrier sites.

Animals can be sampled for carriage by pooling swabs from nostrils, oral mucosa, axillary skin, and perineum. To increase sensitivity, the laboratory can be asked to use selective enrichment culture for MRS. In carrier animals, decolonization, i.e. elimination of MRSA or MRSP from skin and mucosae, may occur spontaneously over a few weeks with subsequent recolonization by less-resistant staphylococci [74,75]. This is more likely in regularly cleaned environments and sensible infection control measures should be implemented concurrently to limit spread and zoonotic transmission, and animals should be monitored weekly. In complicated or more serious cases or where susceptible humans are involved, medical decolonization has been described with antiseptics and topical antibiotics such as fusidic acid and mupirocin [76,77]. However, the use of antimicrobial drugs on healthy animals is controversial, resistance to topical antimicrobials may already exist, and such agents should be used prudently according to local prescribing guidelines. In the UK for example, mupirocin should be reserved for the decolonization of human MRSA carriers prior to elective surgery [78] and its use in animals should therefore be discouraged. Individual cases can be discussed with infection control specialists at referral centres.

References

1. Hill PB, Lo A, Eden CA, *et al.* Survey of the prevalence, diagnosis and treatment of dermatological conditions in small animals in general practice. *Veterinary Record* 2006; **158**: 533–539.
2. Willemse A. Atopic skin disease: a review and reconsideration of diagnostic criteria. *Journal of Small Animal Practice* 1986; **27**: 771–778.
3. Olivry T, DeBoer DJ, Favrot C, *et al.* Treatment of canine atopic dermatitis: 2010 clinical practice guidelines from the International Task Force on Canine Atopic Dermatitis. *Veterinary Dermatology* 2010; **21**: 233–248.
4. Scott DW. Observations on canine atopy. *Journal of the American Animal Hospital Association* 1981; **14**: 766–779.
5. Saridomichelakis MN, Koutinas AF, Gioulekas D, *et al.* Canine atopic dermatitis in Greece: clinical observations and the prevalence of positive intradermal test reactions in 91 spontaneous cases. *Veterinary Immunology and Immunopathology* 1999; **69**: 61–73.
6. Chesney CJ. Food sensitivity in the dog: a quantitative study. *Journal of Small Animal Practice* 2002; **43**: 203–207.
7. Loeffler A, Soares Magalhães R, Bond R, *et al.* A retrospective analysis of case series using home-prepared and chicken hydrolysate diets in the diagnosis of adverse food reactions in 181 pruritic dogs. *Veterinary Dermatology* 2006; **17**: 273–279.
8. Nesbitt GH, Schmitz JA. Fleabite allergic dermatitis: a review and survey of 330 cases. *Journal of the American Veterinary Medical Association* 1978; **173**: 282–288.
9. Colombo S, Hill PB, Shaw DJ, *et al.* Requirement for additional treatment for dogs with atopic dermatitis undergoing allergen-specific immunotherapy. *Veterinary Record* 2007; **160**; 861–864.
10. Devriese LA, Hermans K, Baele M, *et al.* Staphylococcus pseudintermedius versus Staphylococcus intermedius. *Veterinary Microbiology* 2009; **133**: 206–207.
11. White SD, Brown AE, Chapman PL, *et al.* Evaluation of aerobic bacteriologic culture of epidermal collarette specimens in dogs with superficial pyoderma. *Journal of the American Veterinary Medical Association* 2005; **226**: 904–908.
12. Holm BR, Petersson U, Mörner A, *et al.* Antimicrobial resistance in staphylococci from canine pyoderma: a prospective study of first-time and recurrent cases in Sweden. *Veterinary Record* 2002; **151**: 600–604.
13. Shumaker AK, Angus JC, Coyner KS, *et al.* Microbiological and histopathological features of canine acral lick dermatitis. *Veterinary Dermatology* 2008; **19**: 288–298.
14. Bond R, Loeffler A. What's happened to *Staphylococcus intermedius*? Taxonomic revision and emergence of multi-drug resistance. *Journal of Small Animal Practice* 2012; **53**: 147–154.
15. Medleau L, Long RE, Brown J, *et al.* Frequency and antimicrobial susceptibility of *Staphylococcus* species isolated from canine pyoderma. *American Journal of Veterinary Research* 1986; **47**: 229–231.
16. Frank LA, Kania SA, Hnilica KA, *et al.* Isolation of *Staphylococcus schleiferi* from dogs with pyoderma. *Journal of the American Veterinary Medical Association* 2003; **222**: 451–454.
17. May ER, Hnilica KA, Frank LA, *et al.* Isolation of *Staphylococcus schleiferi* from healthy dogs and dogs with otitis, pyoderma, or both. *Journal of the American Veterinary Medical Association* 2005; **227**: 928–931.
18. Rook KA, Brown DC, Rankin SC, *et al.* Case-control study of *Staphylococcus lugdunensis* infection isolates from small companion animals. *Veterinary Dermatology* 2012; **23**: 476–e90.
19. Weese JS, van Duijkeren E. Methicillin-resistant *Staphylococcus aureus* and *Staphylococcus pseudintermedius* in veterinary medicine. *Veterinary Microbiology* 2010; **140**: 418–429.
20. Griffeth GC, Morris DO, Abraham JL, *et al.* Screening for skin carriage of methicillin-resistant coagulase-positive staphylococci and *Staphylococcus schleiferi* in dogs with healthy and inflamed skin. *Veterinary Dermatology* 2008; **19**: 142–149.
21. Soares-Magalhães RJ, Loeffler A, Lindsay JA, *et al.* Risk factors for methicillin-resistant *Staphylococcus aureus* (MRSA) infection in dogs and cats: a case-control study. *Veterinary Research* 2010; **41**: 55.
22. Beck KM, Waisglass SE, Dick HL, *et al.* Prevalence of meticillin-resistant *Staphylococcus pseudintermedius* (MRSP) from skin and carriage sites of dogs after treatment of their meticillin-resistant or meticillin-sensitive staphylococcal pyoderma. *Veterinary Dermatology* 2012; **23**: 369–375.
23. Weese JS, Faires MC, Frank LA, *et al.* Factors associated with methicillin-resistant versus methicillin-susceptible *Staphylococcus pseudintermedius* infection in dogs. *Journal of the American Veterinary Medical Association* 2012; **240**: 1450–1455.
24. Loeffler A, Lloyd DH. Companion animals: a reservoir for methicillin-resistant *Staphylococcus aureus* in the community? *Epidemiology and Infection* 2010; **138**: 595–605.
25. Fortin M, Higgins R. Mixed infection associated with a group B *Streptococcus* in a dog. *Canadian Veterinary Journal* 2001; **42**: 730.
26. Hillier A, Alcorn JR, Cole LK, *et al.* Pyoderma caused by *Pseudomonas aeruginosa* infection in dogs: 20 cases. *Veterinary Dermatology* 2006; **17**: 432–439.
27. Mason KV, Evans AG. Dermatitis associated with *Malassezia pachydermatis* in 11 dogs. *Journal of the American Animal Hospital Association* 1991; **27**: 13–20.
28. Bond R, Saijonmaa-Koulumies LEM, Lloyd DH. Population sizes and frequency of *Malassezia pachydermatis* at skin and mucosal sites of healthy dogs. *Journal of Small Animal Practice* 1995; **36**: 147–150.
29. White SD, Bourdeau P, Blumstein P, *et al.* Comparison via cytology and culture of carriage of *Malassezia pachydermatis* in atopic and

healthy dogs. In: Kwochka KV, Willemse T, von Tscharner C, eds. *Advances in Veterinary Dermatology*, Vol. 3, Boston: Butterworth-Heineman, 1998: 291–298.

30. Mauldin EA, Morris DO, Goldschmidt MH. Retrospective study: the presence of *Malassezia* in feline skin biopsies. A clinicopathological study. *Veterinary Dermatology* 2002; **13**: 7–13.
31. Lloyd DH. Bacterial skin diseases. In: Miller WH, Griffin CE, Campbell KL, eds. *Muller and Kirk's Small Animal Dermatology*, 7th edn. St. Louis, USA: Elsevier Mosby, 2013: 184–222.
32. Lloyd DH. Dealing with cutaneous staphylococcal infection in dogs. *In Practice* 1996; **18**: 223–231.
33. Noli C, Morris DO. Staphylococcal pyoderma. In: Jackson H, Marsella R, eds. *BSAVA Manual of Small Animal Dermatology*, 3rd edn. Quedgeley, UK: British Small Animal Veterinary Association, 2012: 173–187.
34. Holm BR, Rest JR, Seewald W. A prospective study of the clinical findings, treatment and histopathology of 44 cases of pyotraumatic dermatitis. *Veterinary Dermatology* 2004; **15**: 369–376.
35. Pin D, Carlotti DN, Jasmin P, *et al.* Prospective study of bacterial overgrowth syndrome in eight dogs. *Veterinary Record* 2006; **158**: 437–441.
36. Bassett RJ, Burton GG, Robson DC. Antibiotic responsive ulcerative dermatoses in German shepherd dogs with mucocutaneous pyoderma. *Australian Veterinary Journal* 2004; **82**: 485–489.
37. Rosser EJ Jr. German shepherd dog pyoderma: a prospective study of 12 dogs. *Journal of American Animal Hospital Association* 1997; **33**: 355–363.
38. Ihrke PJ. An overview of bacterial skin disease in the dog. *British Veterinary Journal* 1987; **143**: 112–118.
39. Breathnach RM, Fanning S, Mulcahy G, *et al.* Canine pododermatitis and idiopathic disease. *Veterinary Journal* 2008; **176**: 146–157.
40. Gortel K. Recognizing pyoderma, more difficult than it may seem. *Veterinary Clinics of North America, Small Animal Practice* 2013; **43**: 1–18.
41. Bond R, Ferguson EA, Curtis CF, *et al.* Factors associated with elevated cutaneous *Malassezia pachydermatis* populations in dogs with pruritic skin disease. *Journal of Small Animal Practice* 1996; **37**: 103–107.
42. Beco L, Guaguère E, Lorente Méndez C, *et al.* Suggested guidelines for using systemic antimicrobials in bacterial skin infections: part 1- diagnosis based on clinical presentation, cytology and culture. *Veterinary Record* 2013; **172**: 72–78.
43. Forsythe P. Collection and interpretation of clinical samples for dermatological analysis. *In Practice* 2007; **29**: 158–164.
44. Mendelsohn C, Rosenkrantz W, Griffin CE. Practical cytology for inflammatory skin disease. *Clinical Techniques in Small Animal Practice* 2006; **21**: 117–127.
45. Mueller RS, Bergvall K, Bensignor E, *et al.* A review of topical therapy for skin infections with bacteria and yeast. *Veterinary Dermatology* 2012; **23**: 330–341.
46. Summers JF, Brodbelt DC, Forsythe PJ, *et al.* The effectiveness of systemic antimicrobial treatment in canine superficial and deep pyoderma: a systematic review. *Veterinary Dermatology* 2012; **23**: 305–329.
47. World Health Organization. *WHO list of Critically Important Antimicrobials*, 3rd revision, 2011. Available at: http://apps.who.int/iris/bitstream/10665/77376/1/9789241504485_eng.pdf. Accessed 31st January 2013.
48. Lloyd DH. Therapy for canine pyoderma. In: Kirk RW, Bonagura JD, eds. *Kirk's Current Veterinary Therapy XI*. Philadelphia, USA: WB Saunders, 1992: 539–544.
49. Jeffers JG. Topical therapy for drug-resistant pyoderma in small animals. *Veterinary Clinics of North America, Small Animal Practice* 2013; **43**: 41–50.
50. Loeffler A, Cobb MA, Bond R. Comparison of a chlorhexidine and a benzoyl peroxide shampoo as sole treatment in canine superficial pyoderma. *Veterinary Record* 2011; **169**: 249.
51. Loeffler A, Linek M, Moodley A, *et al.* First report of multiresistant, *mecA*-positive *Staphylococcus intermedius* in Europe: 12 cases from a veterinary dermatology referral clinic in Germany. *Veterinary Dermatology* 2007; **18**: 412–421.
52. Murayama N, Nagata M, Terada Y, *et al.* Efficacy of a surgical scrub including 2% chlorhexidine acetate for canine superficial pyoderma. *Veterinary Dermatology* 2010; **21**: 586–592.
53. Bryan J, Frank LA, Rohrback BW, *et al.* Treatment outcome of meticillin-resistant and meticillin-susceptible *Staphylococcus pseudintermedius* pyoderma. *Veterinary Dermatology* 2012; **23**: 361–368.
54. Guaguère E. Topical treatment of canine and feline pyoderma. *Veterinary Dermatology* 1996; **7**: 145–152.
55. Negre A, Bensignor E, Guillot J. Evidence-based veterinary dermatology: a systematic review of interventions for *Malassezia* dermatitis in dogs. *Veterinary Dermatology* 2009; **20**: 1–12.
56. Bond R, Rose JF, Ellis JW, *et al.* Comparison of two shampoos for treatment of *Malassezia pachydermatis*-associated seborrhoeic dermatitis in basset hounds. *Journal of Small Animal Practice* 1995; **36**: 99–104.
57. Miller WH, Griffin CE, Campbell KL. Fungal and algal skin diseases. In: Miller WH, Griffin CE, Campbell KL, eds. *Muller and Kirk's Small Animal Dermatology*, 7th edn. St. Louis, USA: Elsevier Mosby, 2013: 223–282.
58. White SD. Systemic treatment of bacterial infections of dogs and cats. *Veterinary Dermatology* 1996; **7**: 133–143.
59. Beco L, Guaguère E, Méndez CL, *et al.* Suggested guidelines for using systemic antimicrobials in bacterial skin infections: part 2- antimicrobial choice, treatment regimens and compliance. *Veterinary Record* 2013; **172**: 156–160.
60. Lloyd DH, Lamport AI, Feeney C. Sensitivity to antibiotics amongst cutaneous and mucosal isolates of canine pathogenic staphylococci in the UK, 1980–96. *Veterinary Dermatology* 1996; **7**: 171–175.
61. Pellerin JL, Bourdeau P, Sebbag H, *et al.* Epidemiosurveillance of antimicrobial compound resistance of *Staphylococcus intermedius* clinical isolates from canine pyodermas. *Comparative Immunology, Microbiology and Infectious Diseases* 1998; **21**: 115–133.
62. Morris DO, Rook KA, Shofer FS, *et al.* Screening of *Staphylococcus aureus, Staphylococcus intermedius*, and *Staphylococcus schleiferi* isolated obtained from small companion animals for antimicrobial resistance: a retrospective review of 749 isolates (2003–04). *Veterinary Dermatology* 2006; **17**: 332–337.
63. Jones RD, Kania SA, Rohrbach BW, *et al.* Prevalence of oxacillin- and multidrug-resistant staphylococci in clinical samples from dogs: 1,772 samples (2001–2005). *Journal of the American Veterinary Medical Association* 2007; **230**: 221–227.
64. De Lucia M, Moodley A, Latronico F, *et al.* Prevalence of canine methicillin resistant *Staphylococcus pseudintermedius* in a veterinary diagnostic laboratory in Italy. *Research in Veterinary Science* 2011; **91**: 346–348.
65. Frank LA, Loeffler A. Meticillin-resistant *Staphylococcus pseudintermedius*: clinical challenge and treatment options. *Veterinary Dermatology* 2012; **23**: 283–291.
66. Mayer UK, Glos K, Schmid M, *et al.* Adverse effects of ketoconazole in dogs—a retrospective study. *Veterinary Dermatology* 2008; **9**: 199–208.

67. Miller WH. Deep pyoderma in two German shepherd dogs associated with a cell-mediated immunodeficiency. *Journal of the American Animal Hospital Association* 1991; **27**: 513.
68. DeBoer DJ, Moriello KA, Thomas CB, *et al.* Evaluation of a commercial staphylococcal bacterin for management of idiopathic recurrent superficial pyoderma in dogs. *American Journal of Veterinary Research* 1990; **51**: 636–639.
69. Curtis CF, Lamport AI, Lloyd DH. Masked, controlled study to investigate the efficacy of a *Staphylococcus intermedius* autogenous bacterin for the control of canine idiopathic recurrent superficial pyoderma. *Veterinary Dermatology* 2006; **17**: 163–168.
70. DeBoer DJ. Strategies for management of recurrent pyoderma in dogs. *Veterinary Clinics of North America, Small Animal Practice* 1990; **20**: 1509–1524.
71. Nuttall T. Pulse antibiotic therapy: it's time to cut back. *Veterinary Record* 2012; **171**: 472–473.
72. Von Eiff C, Becker K, Machka K, *et al.* Nasal carriage as a source of *Staphylococcus aureus* bacteremia. *New England Journal of Medicine* 2001; **344**: 11–16.
73. Pinchbeck LR, Cole LK, Hillier A, *et al.* Genotypic relatedness of staphylococcal strains isolated from pustules and carriage sites in dogs with superficial bacterial folliculitis. *American Journal of Veterinary Research* 2006; **67**: 1337–1346.
74. Weese JS, Rousseau J. Attempted eradication of methicillin-resistant *Staphylococcus aureus* colonisation in horses on two farms. *Equine Veterinary Journal* 2005; **37**: 510–514.
75. Loeffler A, Pfeiffer DU, Lindsay JA, *et al.* Lack of transmission of methicillin-resistant *Staphylococcus aureus* (MRSA) between apparently healthy dogs in a rescue kennel. *Veterinary Microbiology* 2010; **141**: 178–181.
76. Manian FA. Asymptomatic nasal carriage of mupirocin-resistant, methicillin-resistant *Staphylococcus aureus* (MRSA) in a pet dog associated with MRSA infection in household contacts. *Clinical Infectious Diseases* 2003; **36**: e26–28.
77. Loeffler A, Pfeiffer DU, Lindsay JA, *et al.* Prevalence of and risk factors for MRSA carriage in companion animals: a survey of dogs, cats and horses. *Epidemiology and Infection* 2010; **14**: 1–10.
78. Joint Formulary Committee. Nasal preparations for infection. In: *British National Formulary*, 62nd edn. London, UK: BMJ Group and Pharmaceutical Press, 2011: 692–693.

27

Otitis in the allergic dog

James O. Noxon

Hixson-Lied Small Animal Hospital, Department of Veterinary Clinical Sciences, College of Veterinary Medicine, Iowa State University, Ames, IA, USA

Conflict of interest: none declared.

Introduction

Otitis is defined, for the purposes of this discussion, as inflammation of any component of the ear, including the pinnae, the ear canals, or the middle ear. Inflammation, by definition, includes heat, swelling, redness erythema, pain, and/or loss of function. These classical characteristics, often referred to as the cardinal signs of inflammation, are well represented in the clinical presentation of otitis.

Otitis externa is a common problem in companion animal practice. In two large surveys of general practices in the USA, it represented almost 16% of problems seen in 2.1 million dogs and 13% of 31 484 dogs, and was the second or third most common diagnosis reported in those veterinary practices [1,2]. In addition, Hill *et al.* [3] performed a survey of 20 general veterinary practices in the UK and reported that 24.1% of the 2322 dogs seen in those practices had a dermatological problem. Otitis was the third most common presenting problem (22%) described in those dogs, which reflects an overall prevalence of 5.3% for otitis in those practices. This study most likely underestimates the prevalence of otitis because only 90 out of 795 dogs with dermatological problems in that survey had an otoscopic examination performed.

The cause of otitis externa is often multifactorial. There have been several different classification schemes proposed to explain the pathogenesis of otitis [4,5]. It is well established that there are primary factors or causes of otitis, which initiate the inflammatory process, and perpetuating factors, often called secondary causes or factors, which act to maintain and amplify the inflammatory response. Allergy is considered the pre-eminent primary factor or cause of otitis, with canine atopic dermatitis (CAD), food hypersensitivity, and contact allergic reactions all listed as primary factors in most reviews of otitis [5–11]. The most commonly mentioned perpetuating or secondary factors include bacterial and yeast infections, hyperplastic changes, and otitis media.

The relationship of otitis to allergy

Otitis in atopic dermatitis

Many studies and reviews of allergy and/or otitis in dogs use the term otitis externa to describe any ear abnormalities associated with allergy, while other studies, especially those in recent years, have focused on the changes seen on the pinnae, specifically the erythema. Pinnal erythema is the predominant ear change seen in early and mild cases of allergic otitis [8,9,12]. However, the frequent development of secondary infections in dogs with allergy leads to inflammation and infection of the pinnae and the ear canal, resulting in inflammation extending deep into the canal [9,10,13,14]. With chronicity, most dogs develop secondary bacterial or yeast infections, resulting in more severe erythema, exudation, and proliferative changes characterized by hyperplasia of the epithelium and stenosis [6,8].

Veterinary Allergy, First Edition. Edited by Chiara Noli, Aiden Foster, and Wayne Rosenkrantz.

There have been several proposed diagnostic criteria based on clinical experiences and/or analysis of risk factors to facilitate the clinical diagnosis of atopic dermatitis [12,15,16]. Most of these have recognized the prevalence of otitis in atopic cases and some have specified erythema or dermatitis of the pinnae as a major diagnostic criterion for atopic dermatitis (please refer also to Chapter 10).

Atopic dermatitis (also referred to as non-food-induced atopic dermatitis) has the strongest association of allergy with otitis, with several studies confirming a high incidence of otitis in dogs with atopic dermatitis [8,11,13,15,17–20] (Table 27.1). One unpublished study reported the presence of otitis in up to 83% of dogs with atopic dermatitis, and in that study otitis was the principal or initial complaint in 25% of cases reported [21]. In addition, otitis has been reported to be the sole clinical sign of atopic dermatitis in 3–5% of cases and the initial presenting sign in up to 43% of cases [8,12,20,21]. One study stressed the importance of looking for recurring ear problems as a diagnostic predictor of atopic disease [22]. In that study, significantly more episodes of otitis externa were reported in atopic dogs compared to non-atopic dogs by 12 months of age. Clearly, atopic dermatitis should be considered as a differential diagnosis when otitis externa is the only sign of disease. The high prevalence of otitis externa in CAD is the basis for considering it to be the most common primary factor or underlying disease in chronic otitis externa [5,17,23]. This relationship between atopic dermatitis and otitis is further supported when considering the age of onset reported for cases with otitis, with 50% of dogs developing otitis at 1–5 years of age and an additional 31% had their first episode before 1 year of age [11]. These ages coincide with the ages at which initial signs of atopic dermatitis most often appear in dogs [8,12,13].

Otitis and food hypersensitivity (adverse reactions to food, food allergy)

Food hypersensitivity is reportedly the second most common hypersensitivity to affect the ear [5]. The clinical features of the ear involvement in dogs with food hypersensitivity are very similar to that seen with CAD and may range from erythema of the pinnae to purulent otitis externa with proliferative changes. As seen in dogs with atopic dermatitis, erythema of the pinnae is the most common finding in dogs with food allergy, with 100% of cases with food hypersensitivity showing erythema of the pinnae in one study [24]. Overall, the ears are affected in up to 80% of dogs with food hypersensitivity [23] (Table 27.2). Ear involvement is often the principal problem at the time of presentation and is reported to be the only sign of food allergy in up to 25% of those cases [20,25–30].

Food hypersensitivity should be considered as a possible primary cause in all dogs presenting with otitis, and certainly in those dogs when other history or clinical signs are consistent with an adverse reaction to food. Food hypersensitivity should be strongly considered when otitis or pinnal erythema/pruritus is the only clinical sign. When secondary infections (perpetuating factors) are presented, these must be managed and then controlled with a maintenance programme until a food trial is completed. Ear infections will create clinical signs that can mask any clinical improvement from a dietary trial; therefore, some type of maintenance programme to prevent recurrence of infection is necessary.

Table 27.1 Prevalence of ear involvement in dogs with atopic dermatitis

Author(s)	Location of study	Total dogs	Dogs with otitis (%)	Otitis as initial sign	Otitis as sole sign
Favrot C *et al.* [12]	Switzerland	843*	421 (50)	181 (43)†	NR
Jaeger K *et al.* [35]	Australia Germany USA	552	264 (48)	NR	NR
Muse R *et al.* [21]	USA	54	45 (83)	11 (20)	NR
Scott DW [8]	USA	100	55 (55)	NR	3 (3)
Zur G *et al.* [18]	USA	266	160 (60)	NR	NR
Zur G [13]	Israel	164	81 (49)	NR	NR

*Included all dogs with non-food-induced atopic dermatitis, food-induced-atopic dermatitis, and undetermined atopic dermatitis (dogs not subjected to a food trial).
†Based on percentage reported for all allergic dogs (atopic, food hypersensitivity, and undetermined) with otitis externa.
NR = not reported.

Table 27.2 Prevalence of ear involvement in dogs with food hypersensitivity

Author (s)	Total number of dogs in study	Number with otitis (%)
Carlotti DN *et al.* [26]	33	6 (18)
Chesney CJ [28]	19	5 (26)
Harvey RG [27]	25	14 (56)
Loeffler A *et al.* [29]	181	120 (66)
Muse R *et al.* [21]	17	4 (24)
Rosser EJ [24]	51	41 (80)
White SD [25]	30	1 (3)

Contact hypersensitivities and otitis

Adverse contact reactions in the ears are frequently referred to in veterinary textbooks and written symposia on otitis externa; however, there have been few specific studies to (1) document the initiating cause or substance, and (2) to confirm that the reactions are indeed a hypersensitivity reaction or an irritant reaction. Substances most often cited in such reports include medications, such as neomycin and tetracaine, and vehicles used in commercial formulations, such as propylene glycol [5,6,10,31].

Contact hypersensitivities (i.e. allergic) reactions in the skin of dogs are infrequently documented, but when clinical signs of contact hypersensitivities are reviewed, the medial aspect of the pinna is a common location mentioned for contact hypersensitivity reactions [32–34]. Most veterinarians have recognized an inflammatory reaction in the ears that has resolved by withdrawing topical medication the animal is receiving. Unfortunately, challenges to confirm the specific cause of these reactions are not performed, most often because of concern that a more severe reaction may follow subsequent exposures and/or owner resistance. Propylene glycol, a common ingredient of commercial and compounded otic medications and cleansers, is often mentioned as a cause of contact reactions and otitis [6]. When seen, this reaction is generally accompanied by a creamy, white discharge and varying levels of inflammation; however, the pathogenesis of that reaction is not clear and may have to do with other pharmacologic properties of propylene glycol.

Documentation of topical contact allergic and irritant reactions due to medications is difficult and many cases go unreported. It is likely that these reactions do occur frequently in the ears of dogs; however, more studies are needed identify the incidence and aetiopathogenesis of these reactions. Contact hypersensitivity should be suspected when the pinnae and distal portions of the ear canal are affected along with involvement of other contact areas of the body. Contact hypersensitivity or irritant reactions should be considered when a dog shows clinical improvement while not receiving topic otic medications, followed by recurrence or exacerbation of the otitis while receiving the medication. Cytology will show inflammatory cells, generally neutrophils, with an absence of infectious agents. Resolution of clinical signs should follow discontinuation of the presumed offending substance.

Clinical features of otitis in allergy

Age of onset

One report describes the age of onset of the initial episodes of otitis externa in dogs as follows: 31% <1 year of age, 50% from 1 to 5 years, 19% >5 years of age [11]. In this study, one-half of dogs developed their first episode of otitis during those years in which atopic dermatitis initially develops. These data on age of initial onset of disease provide support for a major role of atopic dermatitis in otitis. One large survey of dogs showed that the age at presentation of dogs with otitis externa was generally evenly distributed among all age groups (0–1 years, 1–3 years, 3–10 years, >10 years) [1]. Statistical analysis of that data was not provided and these were not reported as the *initial* episodes. The age of onset for otitis will depend on the primary or underlying cause.

Breed predispositions

Many purebred dog breeds have been shown to be predisposed to developing otitis, including the basset hound, beagle, bulldog, cocker spaniel, Labrador retriever, Lhasa apso, poodles, pugs, Chinese shar-pei, and springer spaniel [1]. While there are numerous dog breeds reported to be predisposed to otitis externa, it is clear that these same dog breeds are typically those associated with high incidence of allergy [5,8,11,18,23]. Studies looking more closely at allergic dogs have shown predisposition to developing otitis in various breeds, including the Dalmatian, American cocker spaniel, golden retriever, Chinese shar-pei, German shepherd dog, beagle, French bulldog, and Jack Russell terrier [11,18,35] (Table 27.3).

There are also breed variations in the prevalence of otitis externa observed in various studies of atopic dogs based on the country of origin; however, those differences are most thought to be consistent with variations of dogs found in some regions of the world and cultural bias for specific breeds [35,36].

Table 27.3 Dog breeds reported predisposed for otitis externa

Author (s)	Location	Number of dogs	Predisposed breeds
Banfield * [1]	USA	2.1 million	Beagle Bulldog (American and English) Chinese shar-pei German shepherd dog Labrador retriever Lhasa apso Springer spaniel Poodle (all sizes) Pug
Saridomichelakis MN *et al.* [19]	Greece	100	Cocker spaniel Jura des Alpes Brittany spaniel
Jaeger K *et al.* [35]	Germany Australia USA	552	Beagle French bulldog German shepherd dog Jack Russell terrier
Wilhem S *et al.*† [36]	Switzerland (15 countries)	843	Boxer
Zur G *et al.* [18]	USA	266	Dalmatian
Zur G [13]	Israel	117	Chinese shar-pei German shepherd dog Cocker spaniel

*Corporate report. Author(s) not listed. Study done on the general dog population.
†Included dogs with non-food-induced atopic dermatitis, food-induced-atopic dermatitis and undetermined atopic dermatitis (dogs not subjected to a food trial).

Geographical influence

In a large survey of 2.1 million dogs in the USA, the greatest prevalence of otitis externa was found in the states of Florida, Massachusetts, Maryland, New Jersey, and Idaho [1]. Geography affects temperature and humidity, which are often discussed as predisposing factors for otitis [6,17]. Geographical factors that affect these parameters may influence the development of otitis.

Seasonality

There have been some data to support monthly variation in the hospital prevalence of otitis in North America [37]. This variation was felt by the investigators to be related to ambient weather in this population of dogs. However, one study of 266 dogs from California failed to identify seasonal predilection and a survey of data from a large number of dogs showed little seasonal variation of otitis in the USA, though a slight decrease was noted in one study in the months of March and April [1,18]. Statistical evaluation of these data was not reported for the survey. Obviously, seasonality would vary from country to country and even within regions within a country, depending on latitude and other geographical features. In addition, the chronic nature of most cases of otitis, and the time lapse between onset of otitis and the time the dog is presented to the veterinarian may also mask any seasonal effect.

Clinical findings

Otitis is a progressive condition in allergic dogs, starting as erythema and pruritus directed at the pinnae and distal ear canal (Figure 27.1), and progressing with the development of secondary infections to exudative and proliferative forms of otitis. Clinical signs of otitis exhibited by dogs include: pruritus, manifested as rubbing or scratching at the ears, shaking the head, exudation, pain upon manipulation of the pinnae or ear canal, erythema of the pinnae and vertical ear canal, swelling of the canal (best observed with otoscopy), malodour, and head tilt and/or drooping of the ear on the affected side(s). Neurologic signs may be present if there is otitis media.

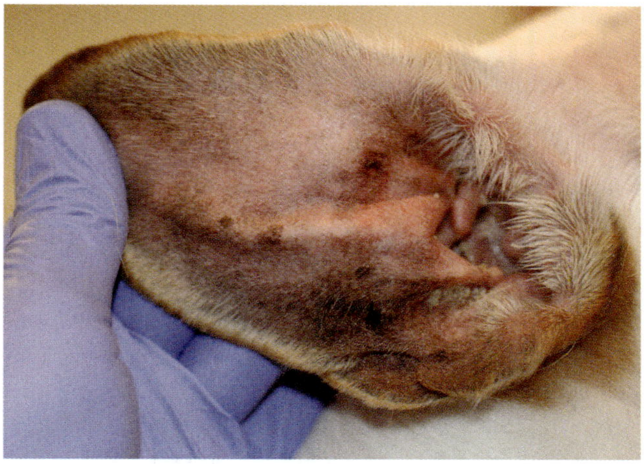

Figure 27.1 Right pinna of an American bulldog with atopic dermatitis. Erythema is visible on the concave aspect of the pinna. No infectious agents were present on cytological evaluation of the pinnae.

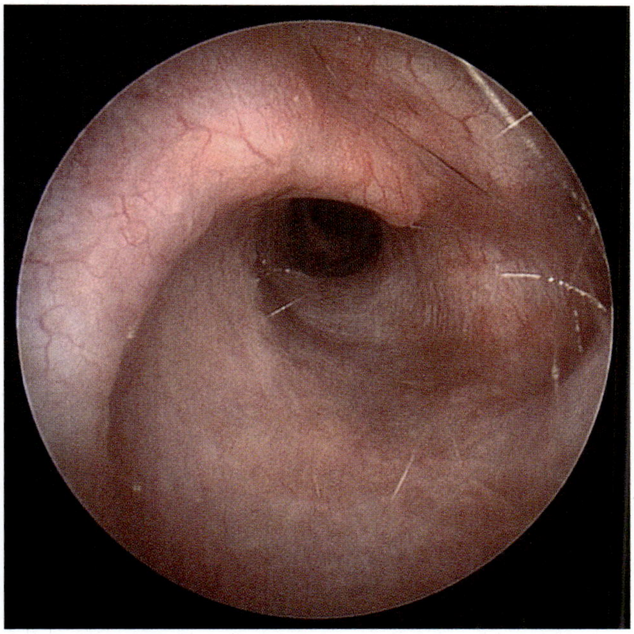

Figure 27.2 Junction of vertical and horizontal components of the left ear canal of the American bulldog seen in Figure 27.1. Erythema of the vertical and horizontal components of the canal is evident.

Otoscopic examination findings will depend on the chronicity of the otitis and the presence or absence of secondary infection. Initially, otoscopic examination of the ear canal may be normal or may show mild erythema of the vertical ear canal (Figure 27.2). As the condition progresses over time, the erythema may progress deeper to more proximal levels of the ear canal and proliferative changes will develop. The nature and amount of exudation will vary with the type and severity of the secondary infections. Cytological findings, in ears uncomplicated by infection, may show numerous keratinocytes and low numbers of inflammatory cells [19]. When infection occurs, micro-organisms may be present and cytology will reflect the severity and types of the organisms involved. Inflammatory cells may or may not be present.

One study of dogs with atopic dermatitis, food hypersensitivity, or both, showed that 58 of 120 dogs (48%) had inflamed ears without exudation and 62 dogs (52%) had otitis with an infectious component [29]. One study of dogs with otitis externa associated with atopic dermatitis showed that 77% had *Malassezia* spp. yeast infections [11]. Another study showed that allergic dogs were more likely to have ear infections associated with *Malassezia* spp. yeast or cocci, while infections with rods were more likely related to more severe underlying conditions [11,18]. These studies may have some bias because they were performed at referral centres; however, it seems clear that secondary infections are common in dogs with otitis and that *Malassezia* spp. yeast play a large role in the pathogenesis of otitis in dogs with atopic dermatitis.

Management of otitis in allergic patients

Managing secondary infections

Infections with bacteria and yeasts are common perpetuating or secondary factors of otitis. The development of infection is accompanied by varying amounts of exudation and involvement of the more proximal (i.e. deeper) areas of the ear canal. It is important to perform proper diagnostic evaluation of the ears, including visual examination, palpation of the pinnae and ear canals, otoscopic examination, and ear cytology. This information should determine the presence of secondary infections. Additional diagnostic information, such as bacterial culture and sensitivity test and diagnostic imaging, may be indicated when atypical organisms are found on cytology, when dogs have failed to respond to appropriate therapy, or other clinical signs suggest middle ear involvement.

Secondary bacterial and yeast infections must be controlled in order to thoroughly evaluate other therapies for allergy. Secondary infections will perpetuate the clinical signs of otitis and make it difficult to evaluate the effectiveness of other interventions for allergy. The pruritus and inflammatory changes associated with the infection will mask possible improvement from the allergy treatment. Therefore, it is important to clear any infection early in the management of allergy cases *and* to prevent recurrence of infection through some maintenance therapeutic programme.

Treatment of existing infection

The goal of treatment should be to clear the infection from the dog. This may be done following standards-of-care for infectious otitis and should include: (1) cleaning of the ear canal to remove debris and infectious material; and (2) specific treatment directed at the infectious agent identified in the dog.

If the tympanic membrane can not be visualized during an otoscopic examination, then cleaning is strongly recommended. Cleaning will remove debris that may obstruct movement of wax out of the canal and of medication into the canal, or that may interfere with the actions of active ingredients utilized for treating infectious agents. Cleaning will also help reduce the population of infectious agents. Ear cleaning may be accomplished using one of several techniques described in the veterinary literature. In general, a deep flushing technique using sterile saline is recommended to achieve a thorough cleaning of the external ear [38]. A ceruminolytic agent may be used if necessary. Systemic corticosteroids are indicated in cases of oedema or hyperplastic changes of the ear canal, prior to ear cleaning, and are usually administered for 1–3 weeks until the ear canal has opened enough to allow a proper flushing and visualization of the tympanic membrane.

Specific therapy for infectious otitis should be based on cytological findings in most cases.

Appropriate therapy for secondary ear infections generally includes topical antimicrobial agents, either an antibiotic or antiseptic agent. These are frequently combined with antifungal and anti-inflammatory agents in commercial otic preparations. Key factors for effective treatment of secondary ear infections with topical medications include proper instillation of the product into the ear canal to ensure deep penetration, the use of an appropriate amount of medication to reach the horizontal ear canal, treatment for a sufficient time to clear the infection, and the use of a medication with active ingredients appropriate for the infectious agents found on cytology or culture. Once-daily application of the appropriate topic agent for 14–30 days is sufficient to eliminate most bacterial and yeast infections.

Systemic therapy for otic infections is indicated when appropriate topical agents are not available, when the owners are unable, or unwilling, to properly instil medications for their animal, when there are hyperplastic changes that restrict the movement of topical agents into the ear canal, when the tympanic membrane is compromised or absent, or when there is co-existing otitis media. The selection of a systemic anti-infective agent should be based on a culture and sensitivity test, which is indicated when: (1) there is a known resistant organism involved (based on past experience with the animal); (2) when the case has failed to respond to appropriate empirical therapy; and (3) when there is a single population of rod-shaped bacteria on cytological examination of exudate collected from the ear. Drugs should be administered according to label guidelines.

A follow-up examination must be performed in 2–4 weeks to confirm that the infection is cleared and not just reduced in severity. Cytology and cultures should be repeated at the follow-up examination to confirm successful treatment. In addition, some dogs with allergic otitis may develop secondary infections even while receiving appropriate treatment for the allergic disease, so diagnostic tests should be performed to monitor for that possibility [39]. Once secondary infections are controlled in allergic dogs with otitis, the pruritus and pain directed at the ears may decrease to acceptable levels. However, many dogs with allergic otitis may continue to exhibit discomfort of the ears after secondary infections are controlled. Those cases require additional therapy for the residual pruritus.

Prevention of recurring infection

Once the infectious agent(s) are cleared from the ears and confirmed with appropriate diagnostic testing, some treatment programme should be initiated to prevent recurrence of the infection and to avoid infection with other agents. Strategies will vary depending on clinician preference and the organisms found on previous tests, but may include: (1) regular or intermittent cleaning of the ears with cleansers documented to possess antimicrobial properties; and (2) intermittent (e.g. once weekly) treatment of the ears with topical antiseptic agents, such as chlorhexidine, chlorhexidine combined with Tris-EDTA, aluminium acetate (Burow's solution), or acetic acid combined with boric acid. Intermittent application of commercial otic medications that contain antibiotics is *not* recommended, to avoid possible amplification of resistance in bacterial populations of the ear.

Managing pruritus

In many dogs, the pruritus caused by allergic otitis will be reduced to acceptable levels with the general treatment prescribed for the allergic disease, including appropriate oral glucocorticoid therapy, ciclosporin therapy, allergen-specific immunotherapy, or adjustments to the diet in dogs with food hypersensitivity. However, some dogs will continue to scratch or rub the ears at a level that is unacceptable to the client, even when the overall level of pruritus is acceptable. Additional treatment is often required to reduce the residual otitis in these cases.

As discussed earlier, the erythema and pruritus of the ears often starts on the concave (i.e. medial) aspect of the pinnae and may involve only the pinnae and the distal-most aspect of the ear canal. If infection is not present, topical glucocorticoids may be helpful to reduce the erythema and pruritus directed at those areas. Medicated wipes or towelettes (such as those containing acetic acid, boric acid, and 1% hydrocortisone) may be sufficient to reduce pruritus and can be used on an as-needed basis. Ointments, creams, or sprays containing pramoxine HCl or hydrocortisone, which is available in various salts including hydrocortisone aceponate, may be applied on an intermittent basis (i.e. one or two times weekly) to reduce the pruritus to acceptable levels.

For dogs with residual pruritus and erythema in the vertical canal, topically administered glucocorticoids may be used to reduce erythema and accompanying pruritus. Topical therapy with a potent glucocorticoid (such as 0.1% dexamethasone, 0.01% fluocinolone or mometasone) is often required for initial treatment to be effective. The frequency of administration should depend on the severity of the signs, although once-daily administration is usually sufficient. These potent glucocorticoids should not be continued long term because the glucocorticoid in the formulation will be absorbed, with subsequent alterations in liver enzyme activities and in the hypothalamic–pituitary–adrenal axis [40–43]. Ideally, the dog should be switched to a less-potent glucocorticoid as quickly as the clinical response permits. Products containing less potent glucocorticoids, such as 1% hydrocortisone, should reduce the likelihood of systemic side effects. Once- or twice-weekly instillation of a less potent topical glucocorticoid is often sufficient to control the residual otitis if infection is not present. This concept was supported in a study by Bensignor *et al.* [44] showing that atopic dogs with recurring otitis were less likely to have relapses of otitis when treated topically with 0.0584% hydrocortisone aceponate drops compared with weekly ear cleaning.

Conclusion

Allergy is a common initiating cause of otitis externa. The strongest relationships are seen with atopic dermatitis and food allergy, where up to 80% of animals with these conditions may have or develop otitis. This relationship is supported by both (1) the prevalence of otitis reported in dogs with confirmed atopic dermatitis and food allergy, and (2) the prevalence of atopic dermatitis in dogs with otitis externa. It is important to consider that otitis may be the only presenting sign of allergy in dogs, especially in cases with food hypersensitivity. In all cases, the management should include: (1) appropriate diagnostic and therapeutic considerations for the otitis, and (2) diagnosis and appropriate treatment of the underlying allergy. Even dogs receiving excellent care for their allergic disease may have relapse of the otitis, and maintenance therapy of the ears to control pruritus and prevent recurrence of infection may be indicated.

References

1. Banfield Pet Hospital®. *State of Pet health: 2011 Report*. Available at: www.banfield.com/banfield/files/bd/bd826667-067d-41e4-994d-5ea0bd7db86d.pdf (accessed Jan 2013).
2. Lund EM, Armstrong PJ, Kirk CA, *et al.* Health status and population characteristics of dogs and cats examined at private veterinary practices in the United States. *Journal of the American Veterinary Medical Association* 1999; **214**: 1336–1341.
3. Hill PB, Lo A, Eden AN, *et al.* Survey of the prevalence, diagnosis and treatment of dermatological conditions in small animals in general practice. *Veterinary Record* 2006; **158**: 533–539.
4. August JR. Otitis externa: a disease of multifactorial etiology. *Veterinary Clinics of North America: Small Animal Practice* 1988; **18**: 731–742.
5. Miller WH, Griffin CE, Campbell KL. *Muller and Kirk's Small Animal Dermatology*, 6th edn. St. Louis: Elsevier, 2013: 741–773.
6. Griffin CE. Otitis externa and otitis media. In: Griffen CE, Kwochka KW, MacDonald JM, eds. *Current Veterinary Therapy: The Science and Art of Therapy*. St. Louis: Mosby Year Book, 1993: 244–262.
7. Rosser EJ. Causes of otitis externa. *Veterinary Clinics of North America: Small Animal Practice* 2004; **34**: 459–468.
8. Scott DW. Observations on canine atopy. *Journal of the American Animal Hospital Association* 1981; **17**: 91–100.
9. Hillier A. Definitively diagnosing atopic dermatitis in dogs. *Veterinary Medicine* 2002; **97**; 198–208.
10. Goth GM. External ear disease in dogs and cats. *Veterinary Focus* 2011; **21**: 2–9.
11. Zur G, Lifshitz B, Bdolah-Abram T. The association between the signalment, common causes of canine otitis externa and pathogens. *Journal of Small Animal Practice* 2011; **52**: 254–258.
12. Favrot C, Steffan J, Seewald W, *et al.* A prospective study on the clinical features of chronic canine atopic dermatitis and its diagnosis. *Veterinary Dermatology* 2010; **21**: 23–31.
13. Zur G, Skorinsky I, Bdolah-Abram T. Canine atopic dermatitis in the Middle East: clinical signs, signalment and common allergens. *Veterinary Medicine* 2012; **57**: 410–419.
14. Logas DB. Disease of the ear canal. *Veterinary Clinics of North America: Small Animal Practice* 1994; **24**: 905–919
15. Willemse T. Atopic skin disease: a review and a reconsideration of diagnostic criteria. *Journal of Small Animal Practice* 1986; **27**: 771–778.
16. Prélaud P, Guaguère E, Alhaidari Z, *et al.* Réévlaution des critères de diagnostic de la dermite atopique. *Revue de Médecine Vétérinaire* 1998; **149**: 1057–1064.
17. Harvey RG, Harari J, Delauche AJ. Etiopathogenesis and classification of otitis externa. In: *Ear Diseases of the Dog and Cat*. Ames: Iowa State University Press, 2001: 81–122.
18. Zur G, Ihrke PJ, White SD, *et al.* Canine atopic dermatitis: a retrospective study of 266 cases examined at the University of

California, Davis, 1992–1998. Part I. Clinical features and allergy testing results. *Veterinary Dermatology* 2002; **13**: 89–102.
19. Saridomichelakis MN, Farmaki R, Leonidas SL, *et al.* Aetiology of canine otitis externa: a retrospective study of 100 cases. *Veterinary Dermatology* 2007; **18**: 341–347.
20. Picco F, Zini E, Nett C, *et al.* A prospective study on canine atopic dermatitis and food-induced allergic dermatitis in Switzerland. *Veterinary Dermatology* 2008; **19**: 150–155.
21. Muse R, Griffin C, Rosenkrantz WS. The prevalence of otic manifestations and otitis externa in allergic dogs. In: *Proceedings of the AAVD/ACVD Annual Meeting*, 1996, Las Vegas, NV, USA: 33–36.
22. Fraser MA, McNeil PE, Girling SJ l. Prediction of future development of canine atopic dermatitis based on examination of clinical history. *Journal of Small Animal Practice* 2008; **49**: 128–132.
23. Griffin CE. Canine atopic disease. In: Griffin CE, Kwochka KW, MacDonald JM, eds. *Current Veterinary Therapy: The Science and Art of Therapy*. St. Louis: Mosby Year Book, 1993: 99–120.
24. Rosser EJ. Diagnosis of food allergy in dogs. *Journal of the American Veterinary Medical Association* 1993; **203**: 259–262.
25. White SD. Food hypersensitivity in 30 dogs. *Journal of the American Animal Hospital Association* 1986; **188**: 695–698.
26. Carlotti DN, Remy I, Prost C. Food allergy in dogs and cats. A review and report of 43 cases. *Veterinary Dermatology* 1990; **1**: 55–62.
27. Harvey RG. Food allergy and dietary intolerance in dogs: A report of 25 cases. *Journal of Small Animal Practice* 1993; **34**: 175–179.
28. Chesney CJ. Food sensitivity in the dog: a quantitative study. *Journal of Small Animal Practice* 2002; **43**: 203–207.
29. Loeffler A, Soares-Magalhaes R, Bond R, *et al.* A retrospective analysis of case series using home-prepared and chicken hydrolysate diets in the diagnosis of adverse food reactions in 181 pruritic dogs. *Veterinary Dermatology* 2006; **17**: 273–279.
30. Jackson HA. Food allergy in dogs-clinical signs and diagnosis. *European Journal of Companion Animal Practice* 2009; **19**: 230–241.
31. Olivry T, Prélaud P, Héripret D, *et al.* Allergic contact dermatitis in the dog: Principles and Diagnosis. *Veterinary Clinics of North America: Small Animal Practice* 1990; **20**: 1443–1456.
32. Nesbitt GH Schmitz JA. Contact dermatitis in the dog: A review of 35 cases. *Journal of the American Animal Hospital Association* 1977; **13**: 155–163.
33. Kunkle GA. Contact dermatitis. *Veterinary Clinics of North America: Small Animal Practice* 1988; **18**: 1061–1068.
34. Grant DI, Thoday KL. Canine allergic contact dermatitis: a clinical review. *Journal of Small Animal Practice* 1980; **21**: 17–27.
35. Jaeger K, Linek M, Power HT, *et al.* Breed and site predispositions of dogs with atopic dermatitis: a comparison of five locations in three continents. *Veterinary Dermatology* 2010; **21**: 119–123.
36. Wilhem S, Kovalik M, Favrot C. Breed-associated phenotypes in canine atopic dermatitis. *Veterinary Dermatology* 2010; **22**: 143–149.
37. Hayes HM, Pickle LW, Wilson GP. Effects of ear type and weather on the hospital prevalence of canine otitis externa. *Research in Veterinary Science* 1987; **42**: 294–298.
38. Nuttall T, Cole LK. Ear cleaning: the UK and US perspective. *Veterinary Dermatology* 2004; **15**: 127–136.
39. Colombo S, Hill PB, Shaw DJ, *et al.* Requirements for additional treatment for dogs with atopic dermatitis undergoing allergen-specific immunotherapy. *Veterinary Record* 2007; **160**: 861–864.
40. Abraham G, Gottschalk J, Ungemach FR. Evidence for ototopical glucocorticoid-induced decrease in hypothalamic-pituitary-adrenal axis response and liver function. *Endocrinology* 2005: **146**; 3163–3171.
41. Aniya JS, Griffin CE. The effect of otic vehicle and concentration of dexamethasone on liver enzyme activities and adrenal function in small breed healthy dogs. *Veterinary Dermatology* 2008; **19**; 226–231.
42. Meyer DJ, Moriello KA, Feder BM, *et al.* Effect of otic medication containing glucocorticoids on liver function test results in healthy dogs. *Journal of the American Veterinary Medical Association* 1990; **196**: 743–743.
43. Reeder CJ, Griffin CE, Polissar NL, *et al.* Comparative adrenocortical suppression in dogs with otitis externa following topical otic administration of four different glucocorticoid-containing medications. *Veterinary Therapeutics* 2008; **9**: 111–121.
44. Besignor E, Pattyn J, Reme C. Reduction of relapses of recurrent otitis externa in atopic dogs with twice-weekly topical application of hydrocortisone aceponate in the ear canal: a randomized, blinded, controlled study. *Veterinary Dermatology* 2012; **23** (Suppl.): 92.

Section 5

Other Allergic Diseases in Dogs

28

Contact allergy

Rosanna Marsella
Department of Small Animal Clinical Sciences, College of Veterinary Medicine, University of Florida, Gainesville, FL, USA

Conflict of interest: none declared.

Is it a rare disease?

Contact allergy is an allergic skin disease whose prevalence greatly varies according to geographical location. Contact allergy was traditionally reported to be a rare disease and some authors still consider it uncommon [1]. In parts of the world (e.g. Florida, USA; Australia) with a tropical climate, contact allergic dermatitis to plants is reported to be very common [2,3]. A frequent reason for the lack of diagnosis sometimes lies in the belief that animals are protected from contact allergy due to the presence of the hair coat. While this may be true for thick and long-coated dogs, this does not apply to short-coated dogs and to glabrous areas of the body where lesions are most commonly found.

Contact allergy can be difficult to diagnose and may be frequently misdiagnosed as atopic dermatitis. In many cases contact allergy actually co-exists with atopic dermatitis and this makes the diagnostic process even more complex and difficult. Although studies to document the exact prevalence and breed predilection are lacking, it is the author's observation that the same breeds that are prone to severe atopic dermatitis (e.g. pit bulls terriers) also appear to be predisposed to contact allergy. One possible explanation for this could be the defective skin barrier that characterizes some subsets of dogs with atopic dermatitis. Skin barrier impairment could lead not only to increased penetration of allergens, including the ones that can cause contact allergy, but also to increased reactivity [4–6]. Another possible explanation, setting aside the issue of a primary skin barrier defect, could be the constant trauma and inflammation present in atopic skin. This in itself may lead to increased ability of the allergens to penetrate and therefore an increased risk for sensitization [7]. It is interesting to note that also in human medicine significant overlap exists between atopic dermatitis and contact allergy [8,9].

In the past, however, atopic dermatitis and contact allergy were considered as being at the opposite ends of the spectrum in terms of hypersensitivities, with atopic dermatitis being presented as a type I hypersensitivity, in which mast cells and histamine play a role, and contact allergy being a type IV hypersensitivity, in which lymphocytes are the main player. The proposed theory was that the atopic state would have a protective effect on contact allergy [10,11]. Currently, as our understanding of these diseases improves, there is the growing realization that these two conditions are not as separate and far from each other as originally thought. Indeed, atopic dermatitis in the chronic phase has some immunologic features not too distant from contact allergy and, interestingly, contact allergy relies, at least in mice, on mast cells as essential promoters of the disease [12].

Causes of contact allergy

Contact allergy is caused by an aberrant response to small molecules called haptens [13,14]. Haptens are too small to be allergenic on their own and need to be conjugated with other proteins in order to elicit an

Veterinary Allergy, First Edition. Edited by Chiara Noli, Aiden Foster, and Wayne Rosenkrantz.

immunologic response. Causes of contact allergy have included topical antibiotics (e.g. neomycin being a common one in both dogs and humans [15]), vehicles used for topical preparations (e.g. propylene glycol [16]), shampoos (e.g. chorhexidine), flea products, carpets, carpet deodorizers [17], metals [18], and plants [19].

In dogs in North America, plants of the Commelinaceae family have been reported to cause contact allergy and represent one of the most common causes of the disease in subtropical climates [20,21]. The Commelinaceae family is composed of about 500 species of monocotyledonous herbs in 38 genera, which grow in tropical and subtropical regions. Several species are commonly grown as houseplants, especially those known as wandering jew (*Tradescantia fluminensis*). The common spiderwort (*Tradescantia virginiana* L.) is extensively grown in gardens. The exact component of the plant responsible for the dermatitis in dogs has not been identified. Contact dermatitis to *Tradescantia* spp. has been occasionally reported in humans [22] but it is not a common cause as it is in dogs exposed to this plant. It is reasonable to speculate that the dermatitis may, at least in part, be caused by calcium oxalate crystals, as they are a common reported cause of dermatitis [23]. In *Tradescantia pallida*, an evergreen perennial plant widely used as an ornamental plant, calcium oxalate crystals occur in the parenchymal tissues of stem, leaf, and root, as well as in flower organs, in the form of either raphides or tetragonal prismatic crystals or both. *Tradescantia* has been reported to also have potassium chloride crystals [24]. It is currently unknown whether these crystals play a role in the canine disease. Interestingly, plants of the Commelineciae family have also been reported to cause immediate reactions in dogs [25].

Pathogenesis

Sensitization

Contact allergy is mediated by activation of $CD8^+$ cytotoxic T cells specific for haptens in contact with the skin. Most studies on the pathogenic mechanisms of contact hypersensitivity have been done in mice [26]. A variable period of exposure to the hapten is needed in order to generate a sensitization. This period of time can range from just a few weeks to months. Extensive studies are done to categorize chemicals based on their ability to induce sensitization [27]. Once the hapten has become allergenic, epidermal Langerhans cells take up the hapten and migrate from the epidermis through the lymph vessels to the paracortical T-cell areas of the skin draining lymph nodes [28]. In this location they differentiate into interdigitating cells, which stimulate naïve T cells to become memory T cells [29].

Elicitation

Once the sensitization has occurred, subsequent exposure to the allergen leads to the recruitment of activated memory T cells to the site of exposure. This is orchestrated by the expression of adhesion molecules. Tumour necrosis factor alpha (TNF-alpha) is rapidly released from Langerhans cells and keratinocytes after hapten exposure and stimulates the expression of E-selectin and VCAM-1 on endothelial cells, facilitating the movement of T cells. Most of the cytokines studies in contact allergy have been done in mice or humans. No study on the kinetics of cytokine release has been done in small animals. In studies dealing with mice, different allergens elicit different patterns of cytokine release, with some inducing both T helper (Th) 1 and Th2 cytokines (IL-4, IL-10) at different stages of the reaction [30,31].

Resolution

This is the last phase of naturally occurring contact hypersensitivity. In this phase, IL-10 may play an important role as it inhibits Th2 cell cytokine production and has a regulatory function. IL-10 is up-regulated in keratinocytes in the late phase of allergic contact reactions. T regulatory lymphocytes (Tregs) play an important function in modulating allergic contact dermatitis [32,33] and humans prone to this condition may have a functional defect of Tregs [34]. $CD4^+$ T cells can function as both regulatory and tolerogenic cells. Several regulatory $CD4^+$ T cell subsets, especially $CD4^+CD25^+$ natural Treg cells, are involved in immunological tolerance and regulation to haptens through the production of the immunosuppressive cytokines IL-10 and TGF-beta. Whether this applies to dogs with contact allergy is unknown at this time.

Clinical presentation

Although contact allergy has been diagnosed in animals as young as 2 months of age, most of the time it is diagnosed in adults (6 months or older). The overlap in age of onset with other allergic diseases such as food-induced dermatitis and atopic dermatitis can increase the diagnostic challenge. The distribution of lesions depends on the eliciting cause. In the event of a shampoo or spray the distribution may be generalized, while in cases caused by plants or carpets the majority of the lesions develop in the contact areas such as the muzzle and periocular area (Figure 28.1), concave surface of the pinnae (Figure 28.2), inguinal area (Figure 28.3), feet, perineal, and genital area (Figure 28.4) [35].

Lesions are particularly evident on glabrous areas. Intense pruritus is common and, in severe cases, this can even lead to a lack of responsiveness to anti-inflammatory

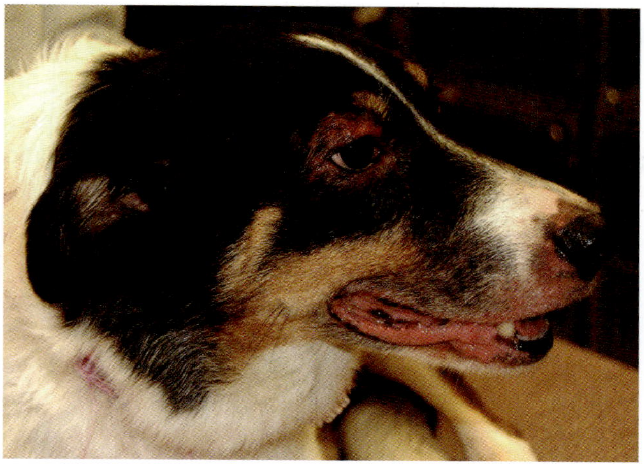

Figure 28.1 Muzzle and periocular lesions in a dog diagnosed with contact allergy to *Commelina diffusa*. Severe erythema, papular eruption, and depigmentation of the lips.

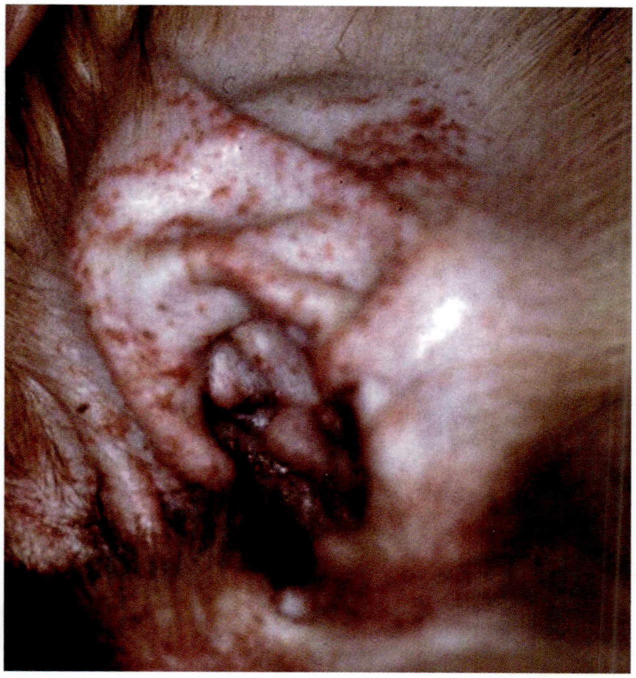

Figure 28.2 Pruritic papular eruption developed after the use of an otic preparation containing neomycin.

doses of glucocorticoids. A primary papular/vesicular eruption is visible in affected areas. With self-trauma secondary microbial infections commonly develop, aggravating even more the level of pruritus. Scrotal dermatitis, in particular, is commonly reported in Europe as a manifestation of contact dermatitis. Commonly reported causes included floor detergents, cement, and bleach [35]. This presentation is most likely a combination of allergic and irritant dermatitis. Pruritus, erythema,

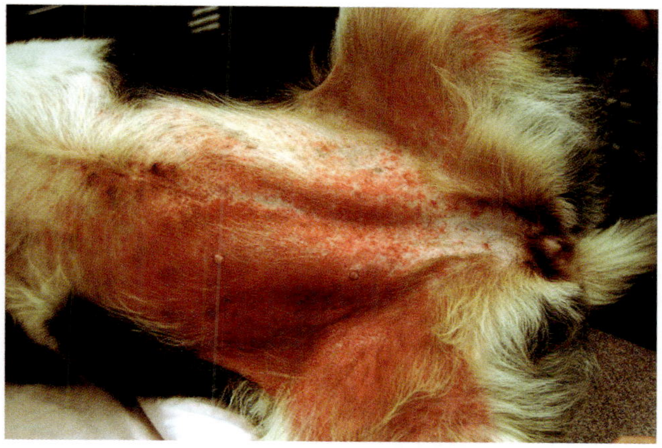

Figure 28.3 Inguinal area. Severe erythematous papular eruption in a dog diagnosed with contact allergy to *Tradescantia fluminensis*.

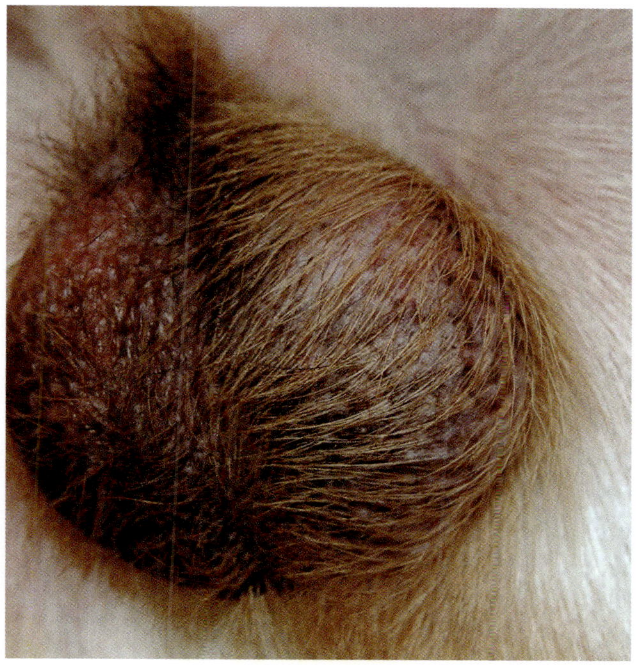

Figure 28.4 Scrotum. Erythema and papular eruption in a dog diagnosed with contact allergy to a floor detergent.

erosions, and ulcerations have been described in these cases. In severe cases pain has also been described.

Diagnosis

Primary differential diagnoses for an intensely pruritic papular dermatitis affecting the pinnae and ventral abdomen include sarcoptes and food-induced dermatitis; also flea allergy, superficial pyoderma, demodicosis, and dermatophytosis. As part of the diagnostic process it is important to first rule out infections and mites. While demodicosis can be ruled out in most cases by a negative skin scraping, sarcoptes cannot be ruled out by a negative skin scraping and trial therapy may be needed. Between contact allergy and food-induced dermatitis, diagnosis of contact can be achieved in a shorter time frame (7–10 days) than food-induced dermatitis (the average duration of food trial being 6–8 weeks).

The diagnosis of contact allergy is usually based on the combination of clinical signs and response to confinement. Confinement is accomplished by thorough bathing and then isolation of the animal in a new environment (this typically requires placement in a kennel in a clinic or animal hospital) to practice allergen avoidance. If complete confinement is not possible, protective gear such as whole body suit and boots can be worn to aid in the diagnosis. In animals without secondary skin infections, allergen avoidance results in complete resolution of clinical signs within 7–10 days. Once complete resolution of clinical signs has occurred, re-challenge is necessary in order to confirm the diagnosis. Atopic dogs may also show some response to confinement, but typically the response is not 100%, because other routes of allergen exposure besides the epicutaneous play a role and some dogs with atopic dermatitis may have a non-allergic (i.e. intrinsic) form [36].

Re-challenge in dogs with contact allergy is done systematically by selectively exposing the dog to either the indoor or the outdoor home environment in order to narrow down the origin of the problem. If contact allergy is the cause and the animal is re-exposed to the offending allergen, signs will reoccur within 24–48 hours. This typically results in pruritus and a papular eruption. An alternative way to diagnose contact allergy, or better, to identify the exact offending allergen once the diagnosis has been made, is the patch test.

In veterinary medicine patch tests are carried out by mincing plant material or carpet fibres (Figure 28.5) and applying those on an area of skin gently clipped 24–48 hours prior to the test. The material is applied to a piece of gauze and placed on the skin. The area is wrapped and the material is left in place for 24–48 hours. Frequently, petroleum jelly is used to mix the material. If so, a separate patch should be prepared for the vehicle to ensure that the reaction is due to the test material and not the vehicle.

A positive reaction is indicated by a papular, pustular/vesicular eruption with intense pruritus (Figure 28.6a,b).

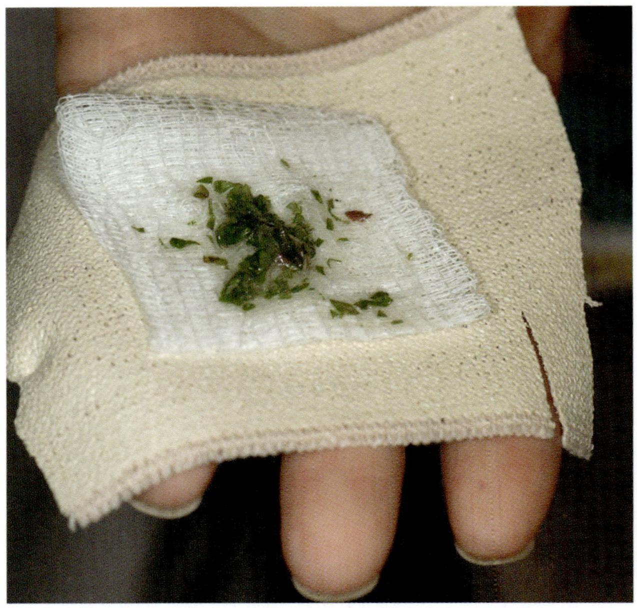

Figure 28.5 Plants are minced, mixed with petroleum jelly, and prepared for a patch test.

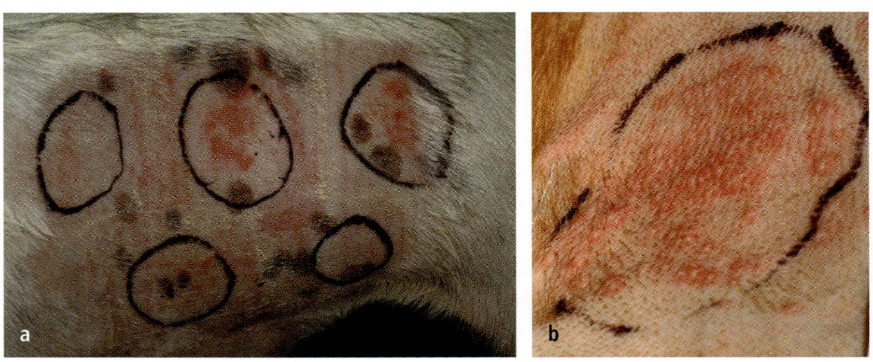

Figure 28.6 (a) Skin of the lateral thorax. Papular eruptions after unveiling the patch test. (b) Close-up of a positive patch test. Note the erythematous papular/vesicular eruption at the site of application of the test material. Intense pruritus was present at the patch test site.

A positive patch test facilitates the identification of the specific offending allergen. A negative patch test does not rule out contact allergy. Indeed, negative patch tests may only mean that the offending allergen was not included in the tested items. This is why typically the confinement is done first and the patch test is considered second, once a diagnosis of contact allergy has been already done and the purpose of the patch test is only the identification of the specific offender. It is important to note that, sometimes, animals can be allergic to multiple items. That is the case with plants, where some cross-reactivity exists between plants belonging to the same family.

Management

In human medicine, numerous attempts have been made with immunotherapy for contact allergy. Previous studies have shown that tolerance to haptens is best induced if it precedes sensitization. Numerous studies have tried to induce tolerance in sensitized individuals and oral immunotherapy has been suggested as a possible strategy [37]. Currently, controversy still exists regarding the efficacy of this approach [38]. Thus, the best approach is still avoidance [39]. When avoidance is not feasible, glucocorticoids can be used either topically or systemically to minimize the severity of clinical signs. It is important to note, however, that the efficacy of this type of approach tends to decrease over time with chronic use, thus great effort should be placed in the identification of the offending allergen and elimination of it.

An alternative to glucocorticoids is offered by pentoxifylline [40,41]. This drug is a methylxanthine derivative and has a multitude of anti-inflammatory effects, also in dogs [42]. The most important mechanism in contact allergy is the suppression of TNF-alpha. Pentoxifylline works best as a preventative rather than treatment and should be started 48 hours prior to exposure [20]. Once contact allergy has flared up, additional therapy with glucocorticoids may be needed. Pentoxifylline can be a gastric irritant and should be given with food. The efficacy seems to be dose dependent. Based on pharmacokinetic studies done in dogs, the dose is best given three times daily at 10–15 mg/kg by mouth [43]. This drug is safe for long-term use and does not decrease in efficacy over time.

Besides systemic therapy, topical therapy is frequently used to treat contact allergy. Crucially important is the removal of the allergen using a soothing and non-irritating product, followed by topical glucocorticoids to decrease the inflammation and pruritus. Ingredients commonly used include oatmeal and pramoxine for the shampoo followed by topical hydrocortisone (as a leave-on conditioner) or hydrocortisone aceponate (as a spray) to decrease inflammation and pruritus. With shampoo therapy it is commonly recommended to leave the medicated shampoo on the skin for 10 minutes before rinsing.

References

1. Olivry T, Prélaud P, Héripret D, *et al.* Allergic contact dermatitis in the dog. Principles and diagnosis. *Veterinary Clinics of North America: Small Animal Practice* 1990; **20**: 1443–1456.
2. Marsella R. Contact allergy. In: Campbell KL, ed. *Small Animal Dermatology Secrets*. Philadelphia, PA: Hanley and Belfus, Elsevier, 2004: 202–207.
3. Queensland Government, Department of Agriculture, Fisheries and Forestry. *Wandering Jew or Trad.* Available at: http://www.daff.qld.gov.au/4790_7385.htm. Accessed October 8, 2012. See also pdf on same website: *Wandering Jew Fact Sheet.*
4. Proksch E, Brasch J. Influence of epidermal permeability barrier disruption and Langerhans' cell density on allergic contact dermatitis. *Acta Dermato Venereologica* 1997; **77**: 102–104.
5. Proksch E, Brasch J, Sterry W. Integrity of the permeability barrier regulates epidermal Langerhans cell density. *British Journal of Dermatology* 1996; **134**: 630–638.
6. Bonnist EY, Gorce JP, Mackay C, *et al.* Measuring the penetration of a skin sensitizer and its delivery vehicles simultaneously with confocal Raman spectroscopy. *Skin Pharmacology and Physiology* 2011; **24**: 274–283.
7. De Benedetto A, Kubo A, Beck LA. Skin barrier disruption: a requirement for allergen sensitization? *Journal of Investigative Dermatology* 2012; **132**: 949–963.
8. Thyssen JP, Linneberg A, Engkilde K, *et al.* Contact sensitization to common haptens is associated with atopic dermatitis: new insight. *British Journal of Dermatology* 2012; **166**: 1255–1261.
9. Spiewak R. Contact dermatitis in atopic individuals. *Current Opinion in Allergy and Clinical Immunology* 2012; **12**: 491–497
10. McFadden JP, White JM, Basketter DA, *et al.* Reduced allergy rates in atopic eczema to contact allergens used in both skin products and foods: atopy and the 'hapten-atopy hypothesis'. *Contact Dermatitis* 2008; **58**: 156–158.
11. McFadden JP, White JM, Basketter DA, *et al.* Does hapten exposure predispose to atopic disease? The hapten-atopy hypothesis. *Trends in Immunology* 2009; **30**: 67–74.
12. Dudeck A, Dudeck J, Scholten J, *et al.* Mast cells are key promoters of contact allergy that mediate the adjuvant effects of haptens. *Immunity* 2011; **34**: 973–984.
13. Martins LE, Reis VM. Immunopathology of allergic contact dermatitis. *Anais Brasileros de Dermatologia* 2011; **86**: 419–433.
14. Zug KA, Warshaw EM, Fowler JF Jr, *et al.* Patch-test results of the North American Contact Dermatitis Group 2005–2006. *Dermatitis* 2009; **20**: 149–160.
15. Lazzarini R, Duarte I, Braga JC, *et al.* Allergic contact dermatitis to topical drugs: a descriptive analysis. *Anais Brasileros de Dermatologia* 2009; **84**: 30–34.
16. Al Jasser M, Mebuke N, de Gannes GC. Propylene glycol: an often unrecognized cause of allergic contact dermatitis in patients using topical corticosteroids. *Skin Therapy Letter* 2011; **16**: 5–7.
17. Comer KM. Carpet deodorizer as a contact allergen in a dog. *Journal of the American Veterinary Medical Association* 1988; **193**: 1553–1554.
18. Kimura T. Contact hypersensitivity to stainless steel cages (chromium metal) in hairless descendants of Mexican hairless dogs. *Environmental Toxicology* 2007; **22**: 176–184.
19. Willemse T, Vroom MA. Allergic dermatitis in a great Dane due to contact with hippeastrum. *Veterinary Record* 1988; **122**: 490–491.

20. Marsella R, Kunkle GA, Lewis DT. Pentoxifylline inhibits contact hypersensitivity reactions to plants of the *Commelinceae* family in dogs. *Veterinary Dermatology* 1997; **8**: 121–126.
21. Kunkle G, Gross TL. Allergic contact dermatitis to *Tradescantia fluminensis* (wandering Jew) in a dog. *Compendium of Continuing Education for the Practising Veterinarian* 1983; **5**: 925–930.
22. Paulsen E, Thormann H. Occupational sensitization from the Tradescantia albiflora cultivar 'Pink Joy'. *Contact Dermatitis* 2010; **62**: 186–188.
23. Julian CG, Bowers PW. The nature and distribution of daffodil pickers' rash. *Contact Dermatitis* 1997; **37**: 259–262.
24. Brizuela M, Montenegro T, Carjuzaa P, *et al.* Insolubilization of potassium chloride crystals in *Tradescantia pallida*. *Protoplasma* 2007; **231**: 145–149.
25. Lee SE, Mason KV. Immediate hypersensitivity to leaf extracts of *Callisia fragrans* (inch plant) in a dog. *Veterinary Dermatology* 2006; **17**: 70–80.
26. Christensen AD, Haase C. Immunological mechanisms of contact hypersensitivity in mice. *Acta Pathologica, Microbiologica, Immunologica Scandinavica* 2012; **120**: 1–27.
27. Kimber I, Basketter DA, Butler M, *et al.* Classification of contact allergens according to potency: proposals. *Food and Chemical Toxicology* 2003; **41**: 1799–1809.
28. Udey MC. Epidermal Langerhans cells tune skin reactivity to contact allergens. *Journal of Clinical Investigation* 2012; **122**: 1602–1605.
29. Kimber I, Maxwell G, Gilmour N, *et al.* Allergic contact dermatitis: a commentary on the relationship between T lymphocytes and skin sensitizing potency. *Toxicology* 2012; **291**: 18–24.
30. Ulrich P, Grenet O, Bluemel J, *et al.* Cytokine expression profiles during murine contact allergy: T helper 2 cytokines are expressed irrespective of the type of contact allergen. *Archives of Toxicology* 2001; **75**: 470–479.
31. Xu H, Banerjee A, Dilulio NA, *et al.* Development of effector $CD8^+$ T cells in contact hypersensitivity occurs independently of $CD4^+$ T cells. *Journal of Immunology* 1997; **158**: 4721–4728.
32. Zielinski CE, Zuberbier T, Maurer M. Immunoregulation in cutaneous allergy: prevention and control. *Current Opinion in Allergy and Clinical Immunology* 2012; **12**: 498–503.
33. Vocanson M, Hennino A, Chavagnac C, *et al.* Allergic contact dermatitis: how to re-induce tolerance? *Medical Science (Paris)* 2006; **22**: 158–163.
34. Reduta T, Stasiak-Barmuta A, Laudańska H. $CD4^+CD25^+$ and $CD4^+CD2^+$ high regulatory T cells in disseminated and localized forms of allergic contact dermatitis: relation to specific cytokines. *Folia Histochemica et Cytobiologica* 2011; **49**: 255–262.
35. Trenti D, Carlotti DN, Pin D, *et al.* Suspected contact scrotal dermatitis in the dog: a retrospective study of 13 cases (1987 to 2003). *Journal of Small Animal Practice* 2011; **52**: 295–300.
36. Fujimura M. The study of canine atopic dermatitis involving the isolation of dogs. *Polish Journal of Veterinary Science* 2011; **14**: 273–277.
37. Bonamonte D, Cristaudo A, Nasorri F, *et al.* Efficacy of oral hyposensitization in allergic contact dermatitis. *Contact Dermatitis* 2011; **65**: 293–301.
38. Spiewak R. Immunotherapy of allergic contact dermatitis. *Immunotherapy* 2011; **3**: 979–996.
39. Alase A, Wittmann M. Therapeutic strategies in allergic contact dermatitis. *Recent Patents on Inflammation and Allergy Drug Discovery* 2012; **6**: 210–221.
40. Schwarz A, Krone C, Trautinger F, *et al.* Pentoxifylline suppresses irritant and contact hypersensitivity reactions. *Journal of Investigative Dermatology* 1993; **101**: 549–552.
41. Saricaoğlu H, Tunali S, Bülbül E, *et al.* Prevention of nickel-induced allergic contact reactions with pentoxifylline. *Contact Dermatitis* 1998; **39**: 244–247.
42. Durgut K, Hosgor K, Gormus N, *et al.* Thecerebroprotective effects of pentoxifylline and aprotinin during cardiopulmonary bypass in dogs. *Perfusion* 2004; **19**: 101–106.
43. Marsella R, Nicklin CF, Munson JW, *et al.* Pharmacokinetics of pentoxifylline in dogs after oral and intravenous administration. *American Journal of Veterinary Research* 2000; **61**: 631–637.

29

Venomous insect hypersensitivity

Mona J. Boord
Animal Dermatology Clinic, San Diego, CA, USA

Conflict of interest: none declared.

Introduction

There are various types of stinging insects that can elicit a hypersensitivity reaction. Hymenoptera are an order of the Insecta class that includes *Apoidea* (bees), *Vespoidea* (wasps, hornets, yellow jackets), and *Formicidae* (fire ants). Due to the direct effects of their venom to humans, Hymenoptera sp. are the most fatal group from the animal kingdom to cause death in humans on a cases per year basis. Hymenoptera account for at least 40 human deaths per year in the United States, with severe anaphylactic reactions in 0.4 to 0.8% in children and 3% in adults reported [1]. These represent the most common life-threatening reactions, but some victims die from lethal toxic doses incurred during massive envenomation obtained in a swarm attack. In dogs and cats, severe systemic reactions, including death, due to venomous insect stings have been reported by veterinarians but the percentage incidence in animal companions is unknown.

Pathogenesis

Once a person or animal is stung there are different immune reactions described. The most common reaction is localized pain and swelling. Depending upon where the sting occurs, the animal may yelp and intensely lick or rub at the affected area. There may be acute lameness if the sting occurred on a paw. This reaction resolves within a few hours.

The next level of reaction is called a large regional or large localized reaction. This involves the swelling extending beyond 10 cm or across multiple joints. This swelling peaks at 48 hours and the reaction lasts a few days. The underlying mechanism of a large reaction is unknown. A large localized reaction involving a vital area, such as the airway, and can result in death, though this occurs only rarely [2].

Anaphylactic reactions are systemic reactions mediated by IgE and sometimes short-term sensitizing IgG antibodies. Complement activation, by IgG–venom complexes, is also reported [2]. There are different classification grades for systemic anaphylactic reactions and most use a I–IV grading scale [2]. Grade I involves generalized skin symptoms of urticaria, pruritus, angioedema, and flushing (Figure 29.1). Grade II additionally includes pulmonary, cardiovascular, and/or gastrointestinal symptoms such as vomiting, diarrhea, dizziness, and/or chest constriction. Grade III additionally includes dyspnea, wheezing, weakness, confusion, or loss of consciousness. Grade IV additionally includes a fall in blood pressure, collapse, cardiac arrest, and/or apnea. Different species have different shock organs and symptoms may vary depending upon the type of animal. Angioedema is the most common presentation in the dog. This presentation seems independent of additional signs such as vomiting, defecation, muscular weakness, and collapse.

A rare reaction pattern reported in humans, and really unknown in animals, is a delayed-type hypersensitivity. This presents within 3 days to 2 weeks following exposure. Patients present with serum sickness-like signs (joint pain, fever, lymphadenopathy, splenomegaly, proteinuria, malaise, and skin rashes). Vasculitis, glomerulonephritis,

Veterinary Allergy, First Edition. Edited by Chiara Noli, Aiden Foster, and Wayne Rosenkrantz.

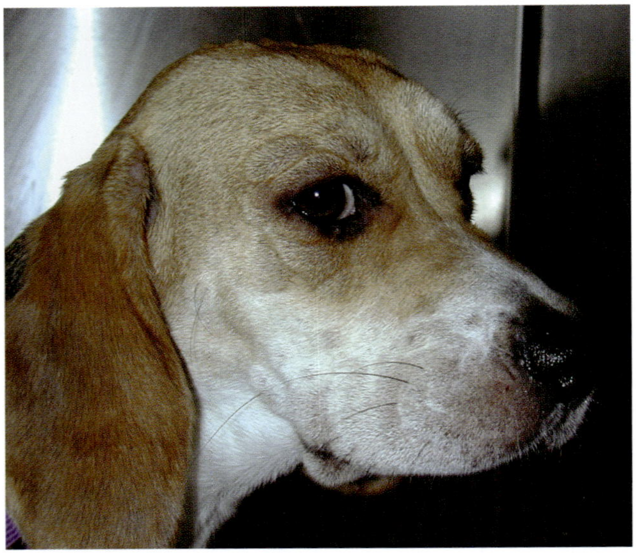

Figure 29.1 Multiple wheals and angioedema in a dog with venomous insect hypersensitivity.

neuropathy, disseminated intravascular coagulation, and arthritis may be associated complications.

Lethal toxic doses may be incurred during massive envenomation obtained in a swarm attack. A honeybee sting injects about 50–147 μg of venom per sting [2] and the lethal dose in humans is about 500 stings [3]. The lethal doses in dogs and cats are unknown, however 20 stings/kg is reported for mammals [4]. A vespid sting typically delivers approximately 3–17 μg venom.

Risk factors

Risk factors for developing a severe sting reaction have been investigated in humans. When patients with a previous history of systemic anaphylactic reaction to a sting were re-stung, 57–75% again developed systemic symptoms [5]. The time interval affected the incidence, with shorter time intervals having a higher risk and the risk lowering to and stabilizing at 20–30% after 10 years [6]. Beekeepers with venom-specific IgE >1.0 kU/L had a 12-fold increased risk of anaphylaxis [7]. In patients previously experiencing a large local reaction, the incidence of a systemic reaction increased to 5–15%. Patients on β-blockers had more severe reactions but no increased incidence of anaphylaxis [8]. The incidence of second reactions in animals is unknown.

Components of venom

The major components of venom from *Apoidea* (honeybee) and *Vespidae* (wasps, hornets, and yellow jackets) are primarily various types of glycoproteins. The more important allergens will be discussed, but a more complete list can be found in a review article by Robert G. Hamilton [9].

Venom from honeybees contains mellitin, phospholipase A_2 (also known as Api m 1), hyaluronidase, biogenic amines, acid phosphatases, apamin, and mast cell degranulating peptide (also known as Peptide 401). Mellitin is a major protein component (50% of dry weight) [2]. It hydrolyzes cell membranes thus altering their permeability. It is thought to be responsible for the pain associated with the sting and for histamine and catecholamine release. Catecholamines act with another major component of the venom, phospholipase A_2, which causes intravascular hemolysis. Hyaluronidase and phospholipase A_2 are the main enzymes of bee venom and are believed to be the major allergens triggering anaphylaxis. Hyaluronidase causes hydrolysis of hyaluronic acid thus disrupting the dermal connective tissue matrix and allowing the venom to disperse in the tissue. Other proteins that are specific to bee venom have been identified including a cysteine-rich trypsin inhibitor (Api m 6). IgE specific antibodies to Api m 6 protein are found in greater than 40% of bee-sensitive human patients and may be helpful in identifying patients more likely to have anaphylactic reactions.

Vespid venom contains phospholipase A_1, hyaluronidase, biogenic amines, acid phosphatases, and antigen 5. Mellitin is not found in their venom. Serotonin, kinins, and acetylcholine are factors contributing to the intense pain from a vespid sting. The major allergens in vespid venom are phospholipase A_1 (Ves v 1), hyaluronidase (Ves v 2), and antigen 5, whose activity is not yet known and is a major allergen in all vespid venom [3,10].

The hyaluronidase of vespid venom shares 50% sequence identity with honeybee venom and is the major cross-reactive protein [2]. Patients can develop true double sensitization to multiple stinging insects or may test positive to more than one stinging insect due to cross-reactivity of hyaluronidase glycopeptides (Api m 2 and Ves v 2) [9]. Thirty to fifty per cent of human patients with skin test sensitivity to honeybee venom also test sensitive to yellow jacket. Serology is used to determine patients with a true sensitivity to both venoms versus those reacting to the cross-reactive hyaluronidase glycopeptide.

Treatment

Treatment recommendations for animals will depend upon the type of reaction the animal is having. As most stings result in localized reactions of short duration, minimal therapy with cool compresses or ice can help alleviate the pain. Diphenhydramine is often helpful and can be given systemically as well as topically. Finding the stinger is helpful in the diagnosis and determining that the sting was from a bee. Most anaphylactic deaths occur quickly, usually within an hour of the sting. Therefore, transportation to an emergency facility and early monitoring and intervention are mandatory. Intubation and oxygen support may be required. An intravenous catheter should be placed, and blood pressure assessed. If venous access is not available, epinephrine 1:1000 (0.1–0.5 mL) subcutaneously or if venous access is available slow administration of epinephrine 1:10 000 (0.5–1.0 mL) intravenously should be given immediately. Crystalloid intravenous fluid therapy should be given to prevent vascular collapse. These animals often respond quickly and completely but need to have additional monitoring to confirm there is good urine production and vascular recovery.

Venom immunotherapy

Venom immunotherapy (VIT) is extremely effective and the treatment of choice in the human medical field to protect patients at risk of anaphylaxis secondary to Hymenoptera hypersensitivity. There is a reduced risk of a subsequent systemic reaction to less than 3% versus up to 75% of untreated patients. This tolerance is well documented; however, the mechanism of action of VIT is unclear. One change documented after VIT therapy is a decreased responsiveness of T cells specifically to phospholipase A allergen. This same decreased responsiveness to phospholipase A occurs with naturally protected hyperimmune individuals such as bee keepers [11]. VIT does appear to shift T-cell cytokine profiles from a Th2 profile to a Th1 profile. VIT administered with a rapid protocol versus a conventional protocol developed the shift to Th1 profile more quickly [11,12]. VIT has not been recommended when the human patient's reaction is a localized reaction or a large localized reaction, although recent research may change this recommendation [11].

Venom immunotherapy in animals

There is little in the veterinary literature to determine the usefulness of VIT in animals. In 2005, the author presented a small pilot study with the following purposes: (1) to determine the usefulness of venom intradermal testing in dogs; (2) to attempt venom immunotherapy; (3) to evaluate response to VIT; and (4) to monitor for side effects from VIT [13]. Five dogs with at least two previous anaphylactic episodes, thought, or known, to be from insect stings and five normal dogs with no known history of an insect sting reaction were administered intradermal tests to honey bee, yellow hornet, yellow jacket, and wasp. The affected dog group included three dogs having had one or more of the following: defecation, urination, vomiting, weakness, collapse, and respiratory changes including respiratory arrest. One of the dogs had developed hives and another facial swelling with other concurrent symptoms listed above. In all affected dogs, the anaphylactic episode occurred more than 4 weeks prior to testing. In human medicine false-negative results are reported when testing is performed within 3 weeks of a systemic reaction.

The protocol recommended by the company providing the testing solutions was modified slightly for use in the dogs. The animals in this study had IV catheters placed, vital parameters were monitored, and they were sedated with atropine and xylazine. They were administered 0.05 mL intradermal injections of saline negative control and histamine positive control, and of the Hymenoptera venom, starting with a concentration of 0.0001 μg/mL. If there was no reaction the venom was then tested at a 10-fold increased concentration up to 10 μg/mL in the affected dogs and up to 100 μg/mL in the normal dogs. A wheal of the same size as the histamine was considered positive. In human medicine the 1.0 μg/mL concentration of honey bee and the 10 μg/mL concentration of vespids may produce an irritant reaction. The irritant reaction concentration in dogs is yet to be determined. In the normal group of our study irritant reactions were observed at antigen concentrations of 10 μg/mL or above depending on the venom tested and 100 μg/mL for honeybee.

All five dogs in the affected group tested positive between 0.001 μg and 10 μg to at least one of the allergens. In the five affected dogs, VIT was started based on a recommended protocol using three different concentrations in gradually increasing amounts over 15 weeks (Table 29.1). This was based on VIT in humans. Three weeks after the 15-week induction schedule these dogs were retested to determine if VIT had affected their

Table 29.1 Venom immunotherapy dosing recommendations

Concentration of allergen					
1 μg/mL		10 μg/mL		100 μg/mL	
Week number	Dosing amount (mL)	Week number	Dosing amount (mL)	Week number	Dosing amount (mL)
1	0.05	5	0.05	9	0.05
2	0.10	6	0.10	10	0.10
3	0.20	7	0.20	11	0.20
4	0.40	8	0.40	12	0.40
				13	0.60
				14	0.80
				15	1.00

sensitivity level. All of the dogs had at least a 10-fold decrease in sensitivity and several tested negative to their treatment allergen.

Interestingly, one dog had an increased sensitivity and with further dilutions tested positive at 0.00001 μg dosing. The dog was then dosed with the buffer saline provided with the testing kit. The test kit saline has human albumin as a stabilizer recommended for the dilutions of the allergens. The dog reacted to the buffered saline solution. It appears the dog was sensitized to human albumin as injections with buffered saline without the human albumin did not elicit a response. The allergens to test this dog were remixed with buffered saline alone without the human albumin. This dog then showed a marked decrease in sensitivity. The author has since had two other dogs develop sensitivity to the buffered saline with human albumin and these dogs are also on remixed VIT.

Two dogs had reactions during the 15-week induction such as pain upon the injections at the injection site, and angioedema on the 0.2 cc of 100 μg concentration. Three of the five dogs had known repeat exposure and developed mild transient swelling. One dog collapsed the day before its monthly VIT was due and the owner found two dead bees in the dog's bedding. That dog's VIT was adjusted to dosing every 15 days.

In 2009, Bryden presented a multicenter retrospective study in which 28 dogs were tested with Hymenoptera allergen [14]. All of these dogs were tested to honey bee and some were tested to wasp and yellow jacket. None of the dogs tested had an adverse reaction following the testing. There is a comment in the paper that a horse tested developed urticaria and a white cheeked gibbon developed anaphylaxis when tested. Of the 28 dogs starting VIT, nine had confirmed challenges with bee and/or wasp stings. Four dogs displayed a reduced intensity of systemic reaction. Two had localized swelling at the site only and two dogs had no reaction. Two of the dogs had an adverse event during therapy and their immunotherapy was modified. One had an episode of anaphylaxis and the other lethargy.

In conclusion, in a small number of veterinary cases it appears Hymenoptera intradermal testing can be performed safely. VIT can decrease the sensitivity to positive intradermal reactions. Patients may sensitize to the human albumin stabilizer used in the diluent provided. It appears that the irritancy testing levels in dogs are similar to humans.

References

1. Golden DBK. Epidemiology of allergy to insect venoms and stings. *Allergy Proceedings* 1989; **16**: 103–107.
2. Bilo BM, Rueff F, Mosbech H, *et al.* Diagnosis of Hymenoptera venom allergy. *Allergy* 2005; **60**: 1339–1349.
3. Vetter RS, Visscher PK. Bites and stings of medically important venomous arthropods. *International Journal of Dermatology* 1998; **37**: 481–496.
4. Manoquerra AS. Hymenoptera stings. In: Ling L, Clark R, Erickson T, *et al.*, eds. *Toxicology Secrets*. Philadelphia: Hanley and Belfus, 2001.
5. Hunt KJ, Valentine MD, Sobotka AD, *et al.* A controlled trial of immunotherapy in insect hypersensitivity. *New England Journal of Medicine* 1978; **299**: 157–161.
6. Golden DBK, Marsh DG, Freidhoff LR, *et al.* Natural history of Hymenoptera venom sensitivity in adults. *Journal of Allergy and Clinical Immunology* 1997; **100**: 760–766.
7. Annila IT, Annila PA, Morsky P. Risk assessment in determining systemic reactivity to honeybee stings in bee-keepers. *Annals of Allergy Asthma and Immunology* 1997; **78**: 473–477.
8. Lantner R, Reisman RE. Clinical and immunologic features and subsequent course of patients with severe insect sting anaphylaxis. *Journal of Allergy and Clinical Immunology* 1989; **84**: 900–906.
9. Hamilton RG. Diagnosis and treatment of allergy to hyenoptera venoms. *Current Opinion in Allergy and Clinical Immunology* 2010; **10**: 323–329.
10. Fitzgerald KT, Flood AA. Hymenoptera stings. *Clinical Techniques in Small Animal Practice* 2006; **21**: 194–204.
11. Bonifazi F, Jutel M, Bilo BM, *et al.* Prevention and treatment of hymenoptera venom allergy: guidelines for clinical practice. *Allergy* 2005: **60**: 1459–1470.
12. Kammerer R, Chvatchko Y, Kettner A, *et al.* Modulationn of T-cell responses to phospholipase A2 and phospholipase A2 derived peptides by conventional bee venom immunotherapy. *Journal of Allergy and Clinical Immunology* 1997; **100**: 96–103.
13. Boord MJ. Sensitivity to hymenoptera venom before and after hymenoptera immunotherapy. *Proceedings American College of Veterinary Dermatology/American Academy of Veterinary Dermatology* 2005
14. Bryden S. Venom allergy in dogs: A multicentre retrospective study. *Proceedings Australia College of Veterinary Science Dermatology Chapter Science Week* 2009.

30

Canine urticaria and angioedema

Peter Hill

Companion Animal Health Centre, School of Animal and Veterinary Sciences, University of Adelaide, Roseworthy, SA, Australia

Conflict of interest: none declared.

Introduction

Urticaria (hives) is a term that refers to the development of multiple cutaneous wheals (Figure 30.1). A wheal is a well-circumscribed, circular, raised lesion caused by oedema within the dermis. Wheals are typically 0.5–3.0 cm in diameter and are either dome-shaped or have a flattened surface. Occasionally, wheals may take on other shapes due to coalescence, or have linear or serpiginous features. Angioedema refers to gross swelling of an extremity such as a distal limb or the face due to more widespread oedema in the deep dermis or subcutis (Figure 30.2). Wheals and angioedema will pit when digital pressure is applied.

Although easily recognized by most practitioners, urticaria and angioedema appear to be relatively uncommon presentations in dogs compared to the high prevalence of other conditions such as flea allergy or canine atopic dermatitis. In a survey of 2322 canine general practice consultations, allergic skin disease was specifically diagnosed in 61 cases but there were no reports of urticaria [1]. Research into these entities in dogs has been almost completely lacking and the veterinary literature is virtually devoid of primary publications relating to their pathogenesis or treatment. The contrast between our knowledge base in canine atopic dermatitis, which is supported by hundreds of studies, investigations, and trials, and that related to urticaria, is stark, and most of the information that does exist is either anecdotal or found in standard textbooks [2–5].

Aetiology

In humans there are numerous pathogenic mechanisms that can lead to urticaria, including allergic reactions to foods, insects, and drugs [6], viral infections [7], autoimmune reactions against the FcεR1 high affinity IgE receptor [8], vasculitis [9], hypocomplementaemia [9], thyroid disease [10], and various environmental stimuli such as cold, heat, pressure, exercise, sunlight, vibration, and water [11–13]. Acute urticaria (defined as episodes that last less than 6 weeks) are usually allergic in origin and a precise aetiology can be elucidated from a detailed history in about 50% of cases. Chronic urticaria refers to episodes that persist for 6 weeks or longer and may occur due to any of the above aetiologies. Thirty to forty per cent of cases are due to autoimmune mechanisms and about 17% are attributable to physical urticarias. However, chronic urticaria in humans is a challenging presentation and many cases remain undiagnosed, despite an extensive investigation by either allergists or dermatologists. Such cases are termed idiopathic [6].

In dogs, urticaria and angioedema are usually caused by acute hypersensitivity reactions, but various non-immunological factors are also reported to be involved in causing an episode. In general practice, allergic reactions to biting or stinging arthropods are considered to be the most common cause of urticaria or angioedema (see also Chapter 29). The offending insects or spiders are rarely seen, but stings from bees, wasps, or hornets, or bites from mosquitoes, black flies, ants, or spiders are considered the most likely causes. In Europe, contact with the hairs from pine or oak processionary moth caterpillars (*Thaumetopoea pityocampa*, *Thaumetopoea*

Veterinary Allergy, First Edition. Edited by Chiara Noli, Aiden Foster, and Wayne Rosenkrantz.

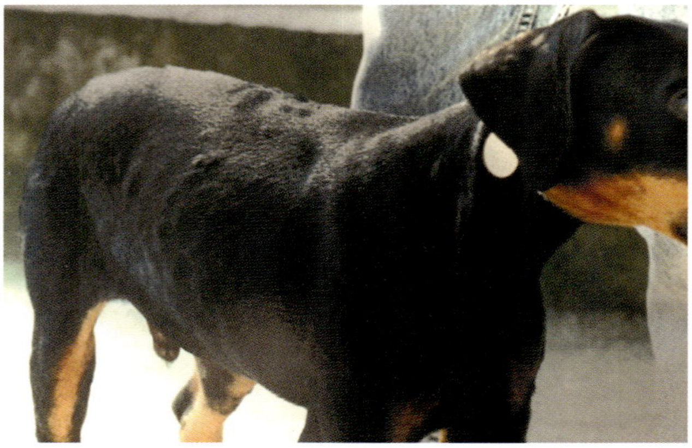

Figure 30.1 Typical appearance of urticaria in a dog. (Reprinted from [5]. © 2011, with the permission of John Wiley & Sons, Ltd.)

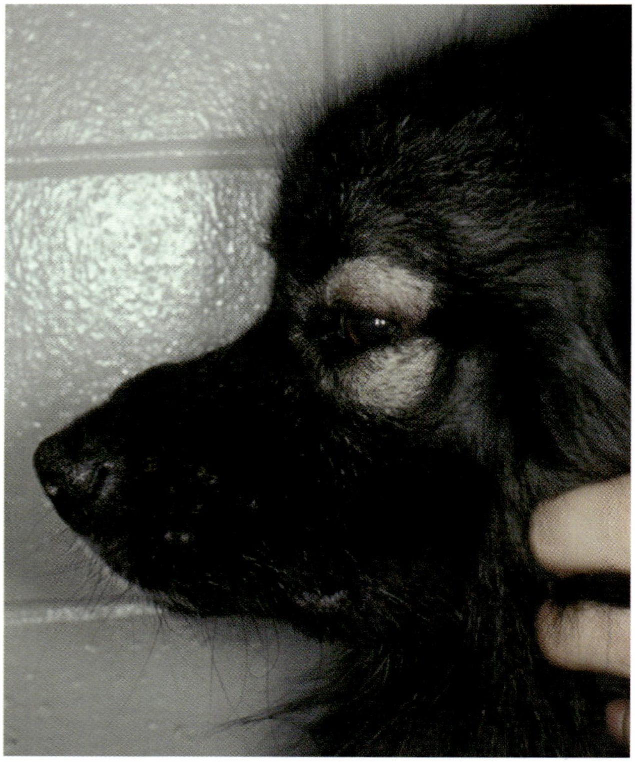

Figure 30.2 Angioedema in a dog that occurred during the performance of an intradermal test.

processionea) or brown-tail moth caterpillars (*Euproctis chrysorrhoea*) can trigger an urticarial or angioedematous reaction in the skin, most commonly around the face (Figure 30.3) [4]. The hairs contain a protein called thaumetopoeine, which can directly trigger mast cell degranulation as well as leading to subsequent allergic sensitization. Bites from fleas can elicit a transient wheal but widespread urticaria is not typically seen in dogs suffering from flea allergic dermatitis [2]. Urticaria has not been reported to occur following infestations with parasitic mites such as *Sarcoptes* or *Cheyletiella*.

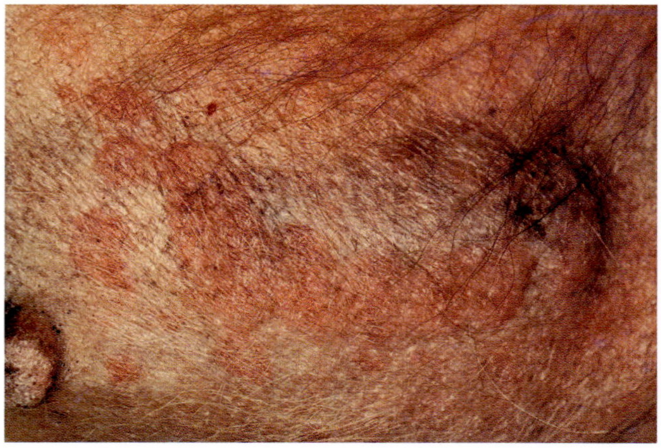

Figure 30.3 Linear urticaria in a dog following contact with a pine processionary caterpillar (*Thaumetopoea pityocampa*). Photo courtesy of Didier N. Carlotti.

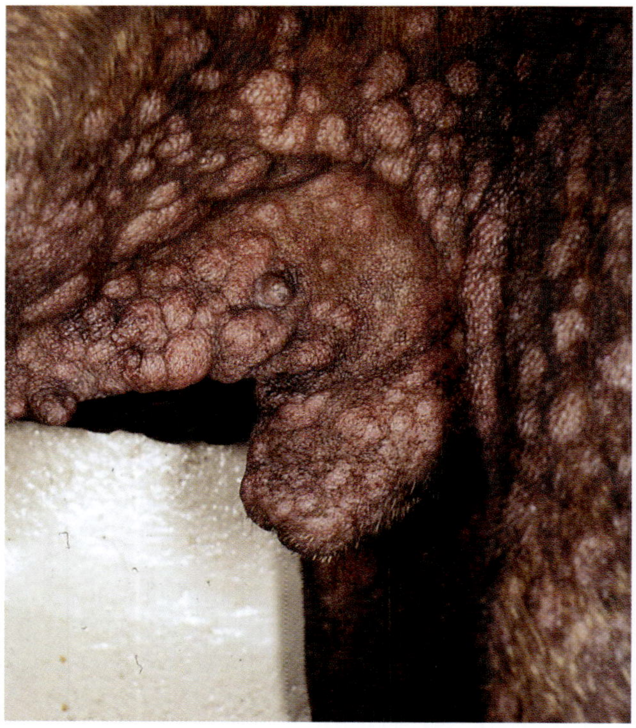

Figure 30.4 Severe urticaria in a dog following administration of a gold injection. (Reprinted from [5]. © 2011, with the permission of John Wiley & Sons, Ltd.)

Various drugs have been anecdotally reported to trigger urticaria, including penicillin, ampicillin, tetracycline, vitamin K, propylthiouracil, amitraz, ivermectin, moxidectin, doxorubicin, and shampoos [2,4]. Generalized urticaria was seen after a dog was given a gold injection (Figure 30.4). One of the few primary case reports in the literature described a case of urticaria and eosinophilic dermatitis in a dog following administration of diethylcarbamazine [14]. Urticaria was also seen in dogs administered a fluorocarbon-based sevoflurane emulsion, which triggered histamine release [15]. Another case of urticaria and bronchospasm occurred in a dog that had received radiographic contrast medium [16].

Allergic reactions to parvovirus, distemper, infectious canine hepatitis, leptospirosis, and rabies vaccines have been reported to trigger urticaria and angioedema in dogs [2,17–20]. In a series of 85 reactions to non-rabies vaccines in Japan, 55 dogs exhibited facial angioedema, with or without urticaria [19]. Analysis of four dogs that developed facial angioedema following vaccination revealed that they had developed IgE antibodies against fetal calf serum, which was used as a stabilizer in the vaccines [21].

In humans, a common cause of urticaria is viral or bacterial infections [7,22]. Some veterinary dermatology texts cite canine distemper or bacterial infections as a cause of canine urticaria [2,4]. However, there are no primary references to support this association and urticaria is not listed as a dermatological sign of canine distemper in these same texts. To date, there appears to be little evidence for a link between urticaria and infectious agents in dogs.

The use of allergen extracts for diagnostic or therapeutic purposes can trigger urticaria or angioedema in dogs. Paradoxically, the injection of allergens during intradermal testing is intended to produce a form of 'iatrogenic urticaria' at the sites of positive reactivity, despite urticaria not being a clinical sign that is seen in naturally occurring atopic dermatitis (Figure 30.5). However, rarely, the injection of such allergens either during testing, or for allergen specific immunotherapy, can elicit more widespread reactions such as urticaria or angioedema (Figure 30.2).

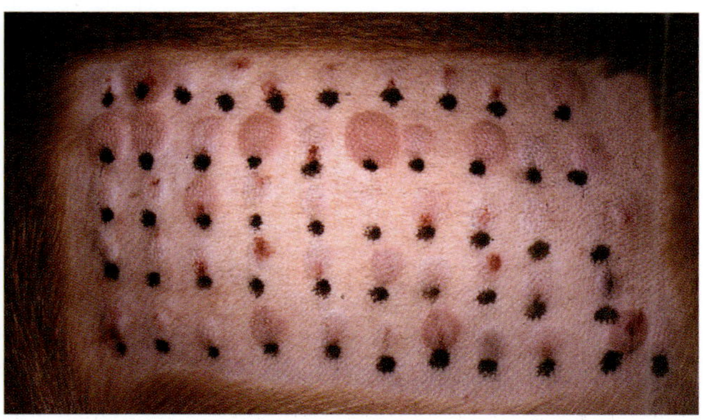

Figure 30.5 Numerous erythematous wheals constitute a positive intradermal test. This is a form of iatrogenic urticaria.

In contrast to atopic dermatitis, urticaria or angioedema can rarely be seen in dogs suffering from cutaneous adverse reactions to food; however, most case series of this dermatosis do not mention either urticaria or angioedema as a clinical sign [23–26]. Allergic contact reactions to plants typically produce an erythematous maculopapular dermatosis, but certain plants can produce irritant substances that elicit urticarial eruptions. In humans, the classic example is the stinging nettle *Urtica dioica* from which the word urticaria is derived. Stinging nettles contain histamine, which can be injected into the skin via hollow hairs present on the leaves and stem. Dogs are less commonly affected by stinging nettles due to the protective effect of the hair coat, but some owners claim their pets are severely affected if contact occurs, especially on the paws and ventrum.

Other factors that have been reported to trigger urticaria in dogs are blood transfusions [27], intestinal parasites, and oestrus [2].

Physical urticarias are rarely seen in dogs compared to their high prevalence in humans. A single case of cold-induced urticaria has been documented in the dog [28]. Other physical urticarias such as those triggered by heat, pressure (dermatographism), exercise, sunlight, vibration, and water are reported anecdotally but primary case reports are lacking [2].

Pathogenesis

Histamine can be injected directly into the skin by stinging nettles. Similarly, various biogenic amines can be present in the venom of bees, wasps, and ants and these can directly affect vascular permeability, resulting in local swellings [29]. Other substances present in arthropods can directly degranulate mast cells causing histamine release. Mellitin, a component of bee venom, can hydrolyse cell membranes and increase membrane permeability resulting in histamine release [29]. Mast cell degranulating peptide (peptide 401) is a protein found in both bee and wasp venom and is the major cause of non-IgE-mediated histamine release following stings from these insects [29]. Thaumetopoeine, which is present in the hairs of processionary caterpillars, is also a mast cell degranulating agent. Certain drugs are also capable of inducing histamine release in dogs. A notable example was the now-withdrawn anaesthetic combination alfaxalone/alfadalone, which contained the solubilizing agent Cremophor EL. This triggered anaphylactoid angioedematous reactions in both dogs and cats, although the severity in dogs was such that the product was never licensed for use in this species [30]. A similar reaction was seen in dogs that received a fluorocarbon-based sevoflurane emulsion, again preventing this product from being developed commercially [15]. Other direct effects of drugs on histamine release are poorly documented in dogs and most drug reactions are probably related to hypersensitivity mechanisms.

It is likely that most cases of urticaria or angioedema that are seen in dogs following insect bites or stings, drugs, vaccines, or food items are due to Type 1 hypersensitivity reactions. This has certainly been proven in the case of vaccine reactions [21]. In such cases the inciting allergens stimulate IgE production, which sensitizes the cutaneous mast cell population. Subsequent exposure to the allergens causes mast cell degranulation and histamine release. Such reactions are one of the few examples of a pure mast-cell-mediated disease, in contrast to the lymphocyte-mediated allergies that typify atopic dermatitis and contact reactions.

To date, no cases of urticaria have been described in dogs due to production of functional autoantibodies against the IgE receptor, despite this being a common cause in humans.

Regardless of the precise trigger, the end result is leakage of fluid from blood vessels that have become more permeable due to the action of histamine or other vasoactive substances. The accumulation of this fluid in the dermis or subcutis results in the pathognomonic swellings that are seen clinically.

History, clinical signs, and differential diagnosis

Most episodes of urticaria or angioedema are acute and are presented as relatively urgent cases. The lesions may or may not be pruritic. In some cases, the likely trigger may be obvious because of the temporal association between an event (e.g. vaccine administration, blood transfusion, dog getting stung in the garden) and the development of lesions. Some potential causes, such as caterpillar-induced angioedema or urticaria, may be particularly common in certain geographical areas. In other cases, there may be no obvious cause in the dog's history. Other than the skin lesions, the dogs are usually otherwise well and general physical examination is normally unremarkable. Some cases of angioedema can affect the upper respiratory tract leading to breathing difficulties.

The lesions of urticaria are pathognomonic as long as they are characterized carefully. The appearance of the wheals should not be confused with any other dermatosis. In short-coated dogs, lesions of staphylococcal folliculitis can lead to raised tufts of hair that could be mistaken for urticaria on a cursory examination. However, closer inspection will readily distinguish between the two conditions. If the lesions are highly inflamed or discoloured, potential differential diagnoses include erythema multiforme minor and vasculitis. Although erythema multiforme can produce urticarial plaques, other lesions will usually be apparent such as erythematous macules, target lesions, crusts, erosions, or ulcers. Vasculitis can have various manifestations, but the type that might be confused with urticaria would typically lead to purpura (dermal haemorrhage) which can be detected using diascopy. The presence of multiple mast cell tumours might be initially confused with urticaria, although these lesions are nodular and will not show marked pitting when pressure is applied.

Potential differential diagnoses for angioedema include juvenile cellulitis, infected cellulitis, snake bite, oedema, lymphoedema, and neoplasia. Juvenile cellulitis is a disease generally seen in puppies (3 weeks to 4 months of age), but it can be seen in adult dogs. It causes acute swelling of the face, eyelids, lips, and pinna. However, in this disease, the dogs are systemically unwell, the submandibular lymph nodes are enlarged, there may be a purulent otitis, and the skin contains papules, pustules, draining tracts, and crusts. Infected cellulitis will be painful and often presents with a bite wound or draining tracts. Snake bites may cause severe local swelling although this is usually accompanied by other systemic signs and is often followed by skin necrosis, something that is not seen with angioedema. Persistent oedematous swelling of an extremity can also be due to hypoalbuminaemia, right-sided heart failure, vasculitis, or lymphoedema, caused by lymphatic obstruction. The latter condition does not have an acute onset and will persist until the underlying cause has been identified and eliminated (primary lymphatic abnormality or obstruction due to neoplasia, surgery, or trauma).

Two further conditions warrant mention, although they should not be confused with classical urticaria. The first is urticarial allergic eruption, a somewhat confusing term that has appeared in the literature [3]. This refers to a histopathological pattern characterized by a combination of dermal oedema and perivascular dermatitis. Clinically, these cases may bear more similarity to dermatoses such as atopic dermatitis, contact dermatitis, staphylococcal skin infection, or vasculopathy. The presence of wheals is reported in some cases, but how these differ from more typical cases of urticaria has not been explained [3]. The second condition is urticaria pigmentosa. In humans, this is a form of cutaneous mastocytosis in which excessive proliferation of mast cells occurs due to mutations in c-kit [31]. Urticaria pigmentosa is recognized in Devon rex and sphynx cats, which have increased numbers of dermal mast cells identified on histopathology, although it is currently not clear if this represents a specific entity or a reaction pattern associated with allergic skin disease [32]. Urticaria pigmentosa has also been described in dogs, although clinically these cases present with a maculopapular eruption that can progress to plaques, nodules, tumours, and bullae, rather than the multiple wheals that occur in classic urticaria [33,34].

Diagnostic evaluation

Although the clinical diagnosis of urticaria or angioedema should be relatively easy in the majority of cases, a search for a specific trigger may be required, especially in recurrent or chronic cases. Many potential causes have been mentioned earlier, but clinicians should be open to the possibility of any exogenous substance or drug acting as a trigger. A detailed history will uncover recent vaccinations, drug administrations, blood transfusions, allergen treatment, or the possibility of environmental contact with arthropods or caterpillars. In cases where these possibilities have been excluded, and the lesions persist or recur, the following tests might be useful in determining the underlying cause.

- Faecal floatation—this can be used to detect intestinal parasites.
- Dietary trials to rule out food allergy/intolerance (see Chapter 18 for details).
- Intradermal testing and/or IgE serology can detect IgE-mediated reactions to biting flies, insects and other aeroallergens (although the latter are rarely implicated as a cause of urticaria).
- Specialized intradermal testing using hymenoptera venoms to detect hypersensitivity to bee and wasp stings (see Chapter 29). This would require referral to a specialist who undertakes such testing.
- Application of an ice cube to the skin for up to 15 minutes to detect cold-induced urticaria.
- Skin biopsy—in classical cases of urticaria this is rarely helpful because dermal oedema is the only change and may be difficult to detect. However, biopsy of atypical cases may reveal alternative causes or patterns such as erythema multiforme, vasculitis, or urticarial allergic eruption.

In humans with chronic urticaria, extensive investigations may be performed to find an underlying cause. These can include various tests to uncover physical urticarias [11], measurement of serum complement components and tryptase, bone marrow biopsies to detect mastocytosis, computed tomography (CT) or magnetic resonance imaging (MRI) scans to detect internal neoplasia, endoscopy to detect inflammatory bowel disease or mastocytosis, and flow cytometry to measure the basophil activation marker CD203c (which correlates with the presence of IgG autoantibodies against the IgE receptor) [35]. In the absence of any primary case reports suggesting the contrary, there is currently no evidence that any of these measures are necessary or beneficial in dogs.

Treatment

Although cases of urticaria or angioedema can be a diagnostic challenge, the treatment of these conditions is relatively easy. Most cases of urticaria are transient and will resolve spontaneously without treatment within 12–48 hours. Many dogs may develop the condition without ever being presented to a veterinarian. For acute cases presented for treatment, the first step is to try and identify and eliminate any causative triggers, which may necessitate termination of drugs.

For symptomatic treatment, a short course of glucocorticoids (2–3 days), given either orally (prednisolone or methylprednisolone at 0.5–1.0 mg/kg/day) or by injection (dexamethasone at 0.05–0.1 mg/kg) is most appropriate. Antihistamines are considered ineffective at treating acute reactions because they cannot control the inflammatory cascade that has already occurred. However, they may help to prevent the further development of lesions if the precipitating allergen is likely to be still present in the dog's system. If this is suspected, antihistamines can be administered concurrently with the initial course of glucocorticoids. They can also be of benefit in chronic or recurrent cases to prevent future episodes. As with atopic dermatitis, a number of different types may have to be tried to find the one that works best for a particular dog. Suitable choices would include chlorpheniramine (0.4 mg/kg q. 8 hours), clemastine (0.05 mg/kg q. 12 hours) or hydroxyzine (2.2 mg/kg q. 8 hours). Cases of urticaria that occur in dogs receiving allergen-specific immunotherapy may benefit from pretreatment with antihistamines prior to each injection, although these dogs should be carefully monitored for signs of a more severe anaphylactic reaction (see Chapter 12).

Mild and uncomplicated cases of angioedema showing no other signs can be treated as for urticaria. If there is severe facial swelling and any respiratory involvement, the dog should be hospitalized, monitored, and treated with epinephrine (0.1–0.5 mL of a 1:1000 solution given subcutaneously) and intravenous glucocorticoids. This should be followed by a short course of oral glucocorticoids.

In humans, chronic urticaria is typically treated with H1 receptor antagonists [6]. If that fails, addition of an H2 receptor antagonist is the next step. If the condition is still refractory, antileukotriene agents (e.g. montelukast) and COX-2 inhibitors (e.g. rofecoxib) can be tried. Glucocorticoids or ciclosporin are generally reserved for refractory cases. Depending on the underlying cause, alternative treatments that have been reported [36] include colchicine, dapsone, sulfasalazine, hydroxychloroquine, methotrexate, cyclophosphamide, interferon alpha, mycophenolate mofetil [37], omalizumab [38], etanercept [39], and rituximab [35]. There appears to be no rationale for the use of any of these latter agents in the treatment of canine urticaria.

References

1. Hill PB, Lo A, Eden CA, *et al.* Survey of the prevalence, diagnosis and treatment of dermatological conditions in small animals in general practice. *Veterinary Record* 2006; **158**: 533–539.
2. Scott DW, WH Miller, Griffin CE. Skin immune system and allergic skin disease. *Muller and Kirk's Small Animal Dermatology, 6th edn.* Philadelphia: W.B. Saunders, 2001: 574–601.
3. Gross TL, Ihrke PJ, Walder E, *et al. Skin Diseases of the Dog and Cat: Clinical and Histopathological Diagnosis*, 2nd edn. Oxford: Blackwell, 2005: 239–241.
4. Préłaud P. Urticaria and angio-edema. In: Guaguère E, Prélaud P, Craig JM, eds. *A Practical Guide to Canine Dermatology*. Paris: Merial, 2008: 265–269.
5. Hill PB. The dog with urticaria or angioedema. In: Hill PB, Warman S, Shawcross G, eds. *100 Top Consultation in Small Animal General Practice*. Oxford: Wiley-Blackwell, 2011: 107–108.
6. Dibbern DA, Dreskin SC. Urticaria and angioedema: an overview. *Immunology and Allergy Clinics of North America* 2004; **24**: 141–162.
7. Clark P. Urticaria. *Australian Family Physician* 2004; **33**: 501–503.
8. Grattan CEH. Autoimmune urticaria. *Immunology and Allergy Clinics of North America* 2004; **24**: 163–181.
9. Davis MD, Brewer JD. Urticarial vasculitis and hypocomplementemic urticarial vasculitis syndrome. *Immunology and Allergy Clinics of North America* 2004; **24**: 183–213.
10. Rumbyrt JS, Schocket AL. Chronic urticaria and thyroid disease. *Immunology and Allergy Clinics of North America* 2004; **24**: 215–223.
11. Dice JP. Physical urticaria. *Immunology and Allergy Clinics of North America* 2004; **24**: 225–246.
12. Lawlor F, Kobza Black A. Delayed pressure urticaria. *Immunology and Allergy Clinics of North America* 2004; **24**: 247–258.
13. Wanderer AA, Hoffman HM. The spectrum of acquired and familial cold-induced urticaria/urticaria-like syndromes. *Immunology and Allergy Clinics of North America* 2004; **24**: 259–286.
14. Vitale CB, Ihrke PJ, Gross TL. Putative diethylcarbamazine-induced urticaria with eosinophilic dermatitis in a dog. *Veterinary Dermatology* 1994; **5**: 197–203.
15. Johnson RA, Simmons KT, Fast JP, *et al.* Histamine release associated with intravenous delivery of a fluorocarbon-based sevoflurane emulsion in canines. *Journal of Pharmaceutical Sciences* 2011; **100**: 2685–2692.
16. Rosenberg M, Patterson R, Kelly JF, *et al.* Acute urticaria and bronchospasm following radiographic contrast media in a dog. *Journal of Allergy and Clinical Immunology* 1977; **59**: 339–340.
17. Brooks R. Adverse reactions to canine and feline vaccines. *Australian Veterinary Journal* 1991; **68**: 342–344.
18. Ohmori K, Masuda K, Sakaguchi M, *et al.* A retrospective study on adverse reactions to canine vaccines in Japan. *Journal of Veterinary Medical Science* 2002; **64**: 851–853.
19. Ohmori K, Sakaguchi M, Kaburagi Y, *et al.* Suspected allergic reactions after vaccination in 85 dogs in Japan. *Veterinary Record* 2005; **156**: 87–88.
20. Miyaji K, Suzuki A, Shimakura H, *et al.* Large-scale survey of adverse reactions to canine non-rabies combined vaccines in Japan. *Veterinary Immunology and Immunopathology* 2012; **145**: 447–452.
21. Ohmori K, Masuda K, Maeda S, *et al.* IgE reactivity to vaccine components in dogs that developed immediate-type allergic reactions after vaccination. *Veterinary Immunology and Immunopathology* 2005; **104**: 249–256.
22. Grattan CEH, Kobza Black A. *Urticaria and mastocytosis.* In: Burns T, Breathnach S, Cox N, *et al.*, eds. *Rook's Textbook of Dermatology*, 8th edn. Oxford: Wiley-Blackwell, 2010: 22.1.
23. Harvey RG. Food allergy and dietary intolerance in dogs: a report of 25 cases. *Journal of Small Animal Practice* 1993; **34**: 175–179.
24. Rosser EJ. Diagnosis of food allergy in dogs. *Journal of the American Veterinary Medical Association* 1993; **203**: 259–262.
25. White SD. Food allergy in dogs. *Compendium on Continuing Education for the Practicing Veterianarian* 1998; **20**: 261–268.
26. Chesney CJ. Food sensitivity in the dog: a quantitative study. *Journal of Small Animal Practice* 2002; **43**: 203–207.
27. Tocci LJ. Transfusion medicine in small animal practice. *Veterinary Clinics of North America: Small Animal Practice* 2010; **40**: 485–494.
28. Willemse A. Acquired cold urticaria in a dog. *Journal of the American Veterinary Medical Association* 1982; **18**: 961–964.
29. Fitzgerald KT, Flood AA. Hymenoptera stings. *Clinical Techniques in Small Animal Practice* 2006; **21**: 194–204.
30. Pawson P. Anaesthetic agents. In: Maddison JE, Page SW, Church D, eds. *Small Animal Clinical Pharmacology*, 2nd edn. Edinburgh: Saunders Elsevier, 2008: 83–112.
31. Brockow K. Urticaria pigmentosa. *Immunology and Allergy Clinics of North America* 2004; **24**: 287–316.
32. Noli C, Colombo S, Abramo F, *et al.* Papular eosinophilic/mastocytic dermatitis (feline urticaria pigmentosa) in Devon rex cats: A distinct disease entity or a histopathological reaction pattern? *Veterinary Dermatology* 2004; **15**: 253–259.
33. Davis BJ, Page R, Sannes PL, *et al.* Cutaneous mastocytosis in a dog. *Veterinary Pathology* 1992; **29**: 363–365.
34. Jeromin AM, Breen PT, Johnson GR. Urticaria pigmentosa-like disease in the dog. *Journal of the American Veterinary Medical Association* 1993; **29**: 508–513.
35. Chakravarty SD, Yee AF, Paget SA. Rituximab successfully treats refractory chronic autoimmune urticaria caused by IgE receptor autoantibodies. *Journal of Allergy and Clinical Immunology* 2011; **128**: 1354–1355.
36. Sheikh J. Advances in the treatment of chronic urticaria. *Immunology and Allergy Clinics of North America* 2004; **24**: 317–334.
37. Zimmerman AB, Berger EM, Elmariah SB, *et al.* The use of mycophenolate mofetil for the treatment of autoimmune and chronic idiopathic urticaria: experience in 19 patients. *Journal of the American Academy of Dermatology* 2012; **66**: 767–770.
38. Metz M, Maurer M. Omalizumab in chronic urticaria *Current Opinion in Allergy and Clinical Immunology* 2012; **12**: 406–411.
39. Gualdi G, Monari P, Rossi MT, *et al.* Successful treatment of systemic cold contact urticaria with etanercept in a patient with psoriasis. *British Journal of Dermatology* 2012; **166**: 1373–1374.

Part 2

Feline Allergy

(Editor: Aiden Foster)

Editor's note

The authors of Part 2 of this book, as elsewhere, have used various terms for cats with allergic skin diseases, including feline allergic dermatitis (FAD), as in Chapter 31, non-flea, non-food hypersensitivity dermatitides (NFNFHD), feline atopic-like dermatitis, feline cutaneous hypersensitivity, and FADS (feline allergic dermatitis syndrome). In general, I have tried to avoid the use of the term feline atopic dermatitis because I do not believe that this accurately reflects the nature of feline allergic skin diseases.

After these chapters were written, the International Committee on Allergic Diseases of Animals (ICADA) considered the terminology for allergic diseases of cats. The consensus of the Committee was to adopt the term 'feline atopic syndrome', which would specifically exclude parasitic causes, but would include environmental allergen causes, and at least some manifestations of asthma, and some manifestations of food reactions, because such manifestations may occur together in one cat. It should be understood that some food-related disease or respiratory disease occurs outside of the feline atopic syndrome 'umbrella'. In the future, the ICADA will be working on refining the terminology for allergic diseases in cats and recommending the terms that should be used as standard in publications. Readers are encouraged to access the ICADA website for more information at: www.icada.info.

Section 1

Cutaneous Allergy in Cats

31

Pathogenesis—immunopathogenesis

Petra J. Roosje

Division of Clinical Dermatology, Department of Clinical Veterinary Medicine, Vetsuisse Faculty, University of Bern, Bern, Switzerland

Conflict of interest: none declared.

The current working hypothesis for feline allergic dermatitis (FAD) is that after exclusion of other skin diseases, a certain subset of cats with defined clinical signs, including chronic or recurrent pruritus that responds to corticosteroids or ciclosporin, has an allergic dermatitis. It is hypothesized that the pathogenesis is comparable to atopic dermatitis (AD) in humans. AD in humans is characterized as a multifactorial disease in which a complex genetic background, immune system, environmental factors, and microbial factors orchestrate the course of AD [1]. Reports on the pathogenesis of FAD in cats have primarily used cats in which fleas and often diet were excluded as causes of the allergic dermatitis. The pathogenesis of flea allergic dermatitis in cats is covered in Chapter 38 of this book. Detailed studies of the pathogenesis of food allergy in cats have not been performed and there are no recognized clinical criteria to distinguish cats with food allergy from those with environmental allergy.

The clinical lesions and distribution pattern are variable in cats with FAD. However, cats with miliary dermatitis, self-induced alopecia, head and neck dermatitis, eosinophilic plaques, or combinations thereof have a comparable histological reaction pattern that may vary in intensity. These histological changes consist of a primarily superficial perivascular to interstitial, mild to moderate inflammatory infiltrate consisting of lymphocytes, mast cells, a variable number of eosinophils, and some histiocytes [2]. Depending on the clinical lesion, the overlying epidermis is usually intact but may be eroded, ulcerated, or have serocellular crusts. The epidermal changes include acanthosis, focal spongiosis, and lymphocytic exocytosis, and vary in severity. These histological changes are comparable to those in humans and dogs with AD [2,3].

Thus, with respect to the working hypothesis, FAD may be the result of several factors influencing the feline immune system that cause a deregulation of the homeostatic balance and lead to the clinical manifestations of FAD.

Genetic background

In humans, studies on twins confirm that a genetic predisposition is important for susceptibility to aeroallergen sensitization and clinical allergic disease including AD [4].

Thus far, primarily null mutations of the filaggrin gene (*FLG*) have been established as major risk factors in humans [5,6]. A recent genome-wide association meta-analysis of healthy humans and human AD replicated identification of the *FLG* locus and two other earlier described loci but also found additional signals of genes associated with epidermal proliferation and differentiation and a signal located in a region that has been linked to inflammatory diseases, including Crohn's disease, asthma, and psoriasis [7].

The rise in occurrence of human allergic diseases cannot be explained by a genetic predisposition alone. Therefore epigenetic mechanisms may help to explain the gene–environment interaction. In particular, the prenatal and early life environment is thought to be a very sensitive period for the influence of environmental factors on shaping of the immune response in children [8].

Veterinary Allergy, First Edition. Edited by Chiara Noli, Aiden Foster, and Wayne Rosenkrantz.

In cats, only one anecdotal report on familial involvement with pruritic allergic dermatitis exists [9]. Interestingly, the involved kittens where born to a cat with miliary dermatitis but were hand-raised, which does not exclude the possibility that environmental factors may have influenced disease development.

Feline skin barrier and exposure to allergens

In human AD, skin barrier disturbance is thought to play a strong role and facilitate antigen transfer and induction of the inflammatory response [10]. Increased transepidermal water loss (TEWL) is regarded as a marker for skin barrier dysfunction and correlates with disease severity in human AD [11].

Little is known about the early events and it is the subject of discussion whether the aberrant skin barrier function precedes skin inflammation and initiates development of AD or that the inflammatory reaction induces the epidermal barrier defect in humans with AD [12]. In any case, it was shown in mice that skin barrier disruption by tape stripping could initiate a T helper cell 2 (Th2) reaction by induction of eosinophil- and Th2-attracting epidermal chemokines and cytokine expression [13]. The cytokine TSLP (thymic stromal lymphopoietin) seems to be particularly important [14].

In cats, trauma to the skin, by licking and scratching, is one of the hallmark signs of allergic dermatitis and may facilitate allergen penetration. Prevention of self-trauma to the skin induces regression of skin lesions and underlines the importance of trauma in the pathogenesis of FAD.

Currently, it is unknown whether aeroallergens can reach and penetrate the skin surface of cats under natural circumstances. Although house dust mites (HDM) or HDM allergens were demonstrated in dust samples from sleeping/resting areas in cat households, their presence on the feline skin was not described [15].

Although little is known about the epidermal barrier function in healthy cats and cats with allergic skin diseases, one study described TEWL, skin hydration, and pH at different body regions of healthy cats [16]. Additionally, allergens applied to tape-stripped skin can induce an inflammatory infiltrate comparable to that found in spontaneous AD cats, as was shown in a study using an adapted atopy patch test (APT) [17]. In this study, three out of six AD cats had macroscopically positive reactions at 24 and/or 48 hours with relevant allergens in the highest concentrations, whereas healthy control cats did not display any positive reactions and none of the AD cats had a reaction to the negative control [17]. A macroscopically positive reaction against *Dermatophagoides farinae* and *D. pteronyssinus* contained a cellular infiltrate comparable to the infiltrate found in lesional skin of AD cats [17]. This infiltrate was characterized by immunohistochemical staining for IL-4, CD4, CD3, MHC class II, and CD1a.

Interestingly, it was demonstrated that cats with ulcerated skin lesions of eosinophilic dermatitis can react to Fel d 1. In this report it was hypothesized that Fel d 1 allergen may function as an autoallergen through aberrant exposure of the immune system to this allergen [18]. Of note is that Fel d 1 is not an enzymatic allergen and it was reported that autoallergens in humans can evoke a Th2, but also a Th1, response [19,20].

Antigen-specific immunoglobulin E

Sensitization to environmental allergens has been the focus of many studies trying to elucidate the immunopathogenesis of AD in human patients. Although it is clear that antigen-specific immunoglobulin E (IgE) can amplify the local inflammatory response, there is also evidence from human patients ('intrinsic AD') and mouse models that AD symptoms can occur without the presence of increased antigen-specific IgE, total IgE, and also IgG [21].

Initial studies in cats therefore focused on detection of antigen-specific IgE. These early studies in cats used *in vivo* tests for the demonstration of antigen-specific IgE, such as the intradermal (skin) test (IDT), Prausnitz–Küstner (PK) test, and passive cutaneous anaphylaxis (PCA) test [22,23]. In the latter two tests, serum and heat-inactivated serum of a hypersensitive/allergic cat are injected into the skin of a healthy cat and after 24 hours a relevant allergen is injected intradermally (PK test) or intravenously (PCA test). The skin is evaluated for a local wheal and flare reaction. Heating the serum at 56°C inactivates IgE, but not IgG, enabling these tests to determine the presence of these two antibody classes. Interestingly, in FAD cats, positive PK reactions are mostly IgE-mediated but can also be mediated by IgG [23,24]. Moreover, in hypersensitized laboratory cats, positive PK tests are only obtained from cats with positive IDT results and reactivity is abolished by heating of the serum [25]. Positive IDT reactions correlate well with positive PK tests but animals with negative IDT and positive serum allergen-specific IgE assessed by ELISA do not have PK reactivity [25]. The authors hypothesized that this poor correlation between serum IgE and mast cell degranulation could be explained by heterogeneity of feline IgE [26]. Another explanation may be the presence of allergen-specific immunoglobulin light chains but this has not been investigated in cats [27].

It proved difficult to develop reliable, well-validated monoclonal or polyclonal antibodies against feline IgE and to the best of the author's knowledge no studies have been published demonstrating IgE in FAD skin or healthy cat skin by immunohistochemistry.

Later, the feline epsilon chain was cloned and sequenced, and showed a high homology with the canine analogue [28,29]. The role of antigen-specific IgE in the immunopathogenesis of FAD remains obscure because the presence of allergen-specific IgE in serum does not correlate with the presence of clinical signs of AD in cats [30,31]. Moreover, there are no significant differences between house dust mite-specific IgE levels in serum of FAD cats and clinically healthy cats [25,30]. Parasitism was found to enhance the IgE response to orally administered antigens in laboratory animals [32]. These findings were confirmed in a study of pet cats with pruritus of different causes [31].

Further, as IgG antibodies are formed during sensitization, feline house dust-specific IgG levels were significantly higher in FAD cats compared to cats with non-dermatological illness or cats with undefined pruritus but levels where not different from normal cats [33]. Additionally, a correlation between IDT-positive results and serum allergen-specific IgG level was not observed.

Thus, the role of antigen-specific IgE in the immunopathogenesis of FAD remains unclear.

Dendritic cells

Dendritic cells (DCs) link the innate and adaptive immune system. They interact with many other cells of the skin immune system and facilitate recognition, phagocytosis, and transmission of information of antigens from the environment to the innate and adaptive immune system [34]. In order to fulfil all these tasks a number of DC subtypes, including Langerhans cells (LCs), exist which are characterized by expression of different markers. DCs contribute to both tolerance and the generation of allergic skin inflammation.

Increased numbers of activated intraepidermal dendritic-shaped cells, characterized by CD1a and MHC class II staining, are present in FAD skin [35]. Some of these intraepidermal cells could be definitely identified as LCs as they contained Birbeck granules visualized by electron microscopy [35]. In the dermis of FAD skin, increased numbers of dendritic cells are recognized by their morphology and positive staining for CD1a and MHC class II [35]. Based on morphology, the main cell population expressing MHC class II in the dermis consisted of dendrocytes, indicating participation of DCs in the pathogenesis [35,36]. This population was much larger than the dermal CD1a$^+$ cell population, which can be explained by activation and influx of other DCs. As not only LCs but also other DC subtypes express CD1a in human patients with AD, it is also not possible to say that all CD1a$^+$ cells were LCs [34]. Of note is that the MAC387 staining, which is often used for identification of macrophages, labelled only few monocytes and macrophages and stained primarily eosinophils in the allergic feline skin [36].

T cells

T-cell responses mediate AD and the initial hypothesis that AD was mediated by Th2 cells has been adapted. Depending on the chronicity, different T-cell subsets play a role and include primarily Th2, T22, and Th1 cells [37].

Lymphocytes are part of the cellular infiltrate in allergic cats and subsets were visualized by immunohistochemistry. An increased number of T cells is observed in lesional and non-lesional FAD skin compared to healthy cats and consists of more CD4$^+$ cells compared to CD8$^+$ cells [38]. Healthy control skin is nearly devoid of CD4$^+$ cells and CD8$^+$ cells are not found [38]. Moreover, an increased number of IL-4$^+$ T cells, indicative of Th2 cells, could be demonstrated in lesional and non-lesional skin of FAD cats [39]. Whereas an increased CD4$^+$/CD8$^+$ cell ratio is present in the skin of FAD cats, this ratio is unchanged in the peripheral blood when comparing healthy and FAD cats [38].

Unfortunately, real-time RT-PCR assays for measurement of various feline interleukins (IL-2, IL-4, IL-5, IL-6, IL-10, IL-12 (p35 and p40)), IL-18, tumour necrosis factor-alpha (TNF-α), transforming growth factor-beta (TGF-β), and interferon-gamma (IFN-γ) could not detect a significantly increased gene expression or skewing of the cytokine gene transcription profile in normal, lesional, and non-lesional FAD skin [40]. Based on this information, it is not possible to elucidate which type of T-cell populations are involved in the cellular infiltrate in FAD. Additionally, when biopsies are used from cats with spontaneous FAD, cytokine and chemokine expression is influenced by chronicity of the lesion and clinical type of lesion, including skin barrier impairment induced by licking or scratching.

Only limited information exists on the role of chemokines in a subgroup of FAD cats. In cats with eosinophilic plaques increased RANTES (regulated upon activation, normal T-cell expressed, and secreted) and TARC (thymus and activation-regulated chemokine) expression was described [41,42]. RANTES is a chemokine produced by many cell types and induces chemotaxis and activation of eosinophils, also memory T cells and monocytes [43,44]. TARC induces its own production in keratinocytes and stimulates a Th2-dominated inflammatory reaction [45].

Eosinophils

Eosinophils are important effector cells in parasitic defence and are also associated with allergic disease. They contribute to tissue inflammation through their released granule proteins and cytokine expression [46].

Eosinophils are prominent cells in the inflammatory infiltrate in FAD, and in FAD cats with miliary dermatitis they are a more specific indicator for a hypersensitivity reaction than mast cells [47].

Feline eosinophil granules contain major basic protein, and granule proteins have peroxidase, ribonuclease, and bactericidal activities [48]. Piecemeal degranulation was described in stimulated circulating eosinophils [49], but was also noticed in electron microscopic evaluation of FAD tissue (Roosje, unpublished data). Tissue damage has been studied in cats selected for eosinophilic dermatitis lesions, but not per se in cats selected for signs of FAD [50].

Eosinophils are recruited by several chemokines (e.g. eotaxin and RANTES) and Th2 cytokines (e.g. IL-4 and IL-5)[46]. In feline eosinophilic plaques, increased expression of RANTES mRNA was reported [41]. Under the influence of Th2 cytokines, eosinophils produce IL-12, IL-13, IL-16, and TGF-β1, and influence the local T-cell response [46]. IL-12 promotes a switch from a Th2 to a Th1-like immune response in chronic lesions in human AD patients [51].

Mast cells

Skin mast cells can be sensitized via the high-affinity IgE receptor on the cell surface. Upon binding of antigens recognized by surface bound IgE, mast cells release their preformed granule content, synthesize prostaglandins and leukotrienes, and produce cytokines, chemokines, and growth factors. However, they can also serve as effector cells by IgE-independent mechanisms. Through their released products they can influence keratinocytes, LCs, DCs, T cells, and can even present antigens directly to T cells [46,52], although this has not been demonstrated in cats.

Although mast cells are often prominently present in FAD skin, they are not specific for hypersensitivity reactions and can be seen in conjunction with other histological patterns such as pemphigus foliaceus [53]. Nevertheless, there is evidence for an active participation of mast cells in FAD. Subepidermal oedema and changed granularity of mast cells can be observed in haematoxylin and eosin sections of FAD skin and the mast cell count in skin of AD cats is significantly higher compared to healthy cats, although with a wide range in their number [47]. Additionally, a correlation between the number of mast cells and eosinophils within the same biopsy could not be found [47].

Changes in protease content of mast cell granules in lesional and non-lesional skin are found, indicating a generalized effect of mast cells in FAD. In FAD cats, a significantly lower number of mast cells was observed with tryptase staining compared to staining for chymase and Astra blue staining [47]. Additionally, a substantial number of chymase-positive mast cells contained coarse granules but only in lesional skin. In healthy cat skin, all mast cells stained positive for tryptase and around 90% stained positive for chymase [54]. Moreover, in a study using a double labelling technique for chymase and tryptase in cats with different types of eosinophilic dermatitis, three different types of mast cells (only chymase, chymase–tryptase, and only tryptase) were identified [55].

In humans with AD, mast cell protease content changes as well [56]. Tryptase activates keratinocytes, primary nerve cells, and endothelial cells through binding to the surface proteinase-activated receptor-2 (PAR-2) [57]. Intracutaneous injection of endogenous PAR-2 agonists provoked enhanced and prolonged itch when applied intralesionally and thus PAR-2 signalling is seen as one of the links between inflammation and pruritus in human AD patients [58]. Moreover, an oral chymase inhibitor ameliorated pruritus and skin inflammation in a mouse model for AD [59].

Role of microbial factors

Whereas there is clinical evidence for bacterial or yeast infections in some cats with FAD, their influence on the immunopathogenesis of FAD is unknown. Moreover, at present the role of the feline skin microbiome in health and allergic disease has not been investigated.

The complexity and redundancy in the pathogenesis of canine or human atopic dermatitis are in contrast to the scant number of reports on cats with allergic dermatitis. Currently, there is only little evidence to support the hypothesis that the immunopathogenesis of FAD is analogous to AD in humans. Moreover, the interaction between the immune system and the nervous system resulting in pruritus, the hallmark of FAD, is a terra incognita.

References

1. Werfel T. The role of leukocytes, keratinocytes, and allergen-specific IgE in the development of atopic dermatitis. *Journal of Investigative Dermatology* 2009; **129**: 1878–1891.
2. Gross TL, Ihrke PJ, Walder EJ, *et al. Skin diseases of the dog and cat*, 2nd edn. Oxford: Blackwell Publishing, 2005: 118–122.

3. Sowden JM, Powell RJ, Allen BR. Selective activation of circulating CD4+ lymphocytes in severe adult atopic dermatitis. *British Journal of Dermatology* 1992; **127**: 228–232.
4. Strachan DP, Wong HJ, Spector TD. Concordance and interrelationship of atopic diseases and markers of allergic sensitization among adult female twins. *Journal of Allergy and Clinical Immunology* 2001; **108**: 901–907.
5. Palmer CN, Irvine AD, Terron-Kwiatkowski A, *et al.* Common loss-of-function variants of the epidermal barrier protein filaggrin are a major predisposing factor for atopic dermatitis. *Nature Genetics* 2006; **38**: 441–446.
6. Rodriguez E, Baurecht H, Herberich E, *et al.* Meta-analysis of filaggrin polymorphisms in eczema and asthma: robust risk factors in atopic disease. *Journal of Allergy and Clinical Immunology* 2009; **123**: 1361–1370, e7.
7. Paternoster L, Standl M, Chen CM, *et al.* Meta-analysis of genome-wide association studies identifies three new risk loci for atopic dermatitis. *Nature Genetics* 2012; **44**: 187–192.
8. North ML, Ellis AK. The role of epigenetics in the developmental origins of allergic disease. *Annals of Allergy, Asthma and Immunology* 2011; **106**: 355–361; 62.
9. Moriello KA. Feline atopy in three littermates. *Veterinary Dermatology* 2001; **12**: 177–181.
10. De Benedetto A, Kubo A, Beck LA. Skin barrier disruption: a requirement for allergen sensitization? *Journal of Investigative Dermatology* 2012; **132**: 949–963.
11. Gupta J, Grube E, Ericksen MB, *et al.* Intrinsically defective skin barrier function in children with atopic dermatitis correlates with disease severity. *Journal of Allergy and Clinical Immunology* 2008; **121**: 725–730.
12. Boguniewicz M, Leung DY. Atopic dermatitis: a disease of altered skin barrier and immune dysregulation. *Immunological Reviews* 2011; **242**: 233–246.
13. Onoue A, Kabashima K, Kobayashi M, *et al.* Induction of eosinophil- and Th2-attracting epidermal chemokines and cutaneous late-phase reaction in tape-stripped skin. *Experimental Dermatology* 2009; **18**: 1036–1043.
14. Oyoshi MK, Larson RP, Ziegler SF, *et al.* Mechanical injury polarizes skin dendritic cells to elicit a T(H)2 response by inducing cutaneous thymic stromal lymphopoietin expression. *Journal of Allergy and Clinical Immunology* 2010; **126**: 976–984.
15. Loft KE, Rosser EJ, Jr. Group 1 and 2 Dermatophagoides house dust mite allergens in the microenvironment of cats. *Veterinary Dermatology* 2010; **21**: 152–158.
16. Szczepanik MP, Wilkołek PM, Adamek ŁR, *et al.* The examination of biophysical parameters of skin (transepidermal water loss, skin hydration and pH value) in different body regions of normal cats of both sexes. *Journal of Feline Medicine and Surgery* 2011; **13**: 224–230.
17. Roosje PJ, Thepen T, Rutten VP, *et al.* Immunophenotyping of the cutaneous cellular infiltrate after atopy patch testing in cats with atopic dermatitis. *Veterinary Immunology and Immunopathology* 2004; **101**: 143–151.
18. Wisselink MA, van Ree R, Willemse T. Evaluation of *Felis domesticus* allergen I as a possible autoallergen in cats with eosinophilic granuloma complex. *American Journal of Veterinary Research* 2002; **63**: 338–341.
19. Chapman MD, Wunschmann S, Pomes A. Proteases as Th2 adjuvants. *Current Allergy and Asthma Reports* 2007; **7**: 363–367.
20. Heratizadeh A, Mittermann I, Balaji H, *et al.* The role of T-cell reactivity towards the autoantigen alpha-NAC in atopic dermatitis. *British Journal of Dermatology* 2011; **164**: 316–324.
21. Roguedas-Contios AM, Misery L. What is intrinsic atopic dermatitis? *Clinical Reviews in Allergy and Immunology* 2011; **41**: 233–236.
22. Reedy LM. Results of allergy testing and hyposensitization in selected feline skin diseases. *Journal of the American Animal Hospital Association* 1982; **18**: 618–623.
23. Roosje PJ, Willemse T. Cytophilic antibodies in cats with miliary dermatitis and eosinophilic plaques: passive transfer of immediate-type hypersensitivity. *Veterinary Quarterly* 1995; **17**: 66–69.
24. Schleifer SG, Willemse T. Evaluation of skin test reactivity to environmental allergens in healthy cats and cats with atopic dermatitis. *American Journal of Veterinary Research* 2003; **64**: 773–778.
25. Gilbert S, Halliwell RE. Feline immunoglobulin E: induction of antigen-specific antibody in normal cats and levels in spontaneously allergic cats. *Veterinary Immunology and Immunopathology* 1998; **63**: 235–252.
26. Halliwell RE, Gilbert S, Mei L. Induced and spontaneous IgE antibodies to *Dermatophagoides farinae* in dogs and cats: evidence of functional heterogeneity of IgE. *Veterinary Dermatology* 1998; **9**: 179–184.
27. Groot Kormelink T, Thio M, Blokhuis BR, *et al.* Atopic and non-atopic allergic disorders: current insights into the possible involvement of free immunoglobulin light chains. *Clinical and Experimental Allergy* 2009; **39**: 33–42.
28. Griot-Wenk ME, Obexer-Ruff G, Fluri A, *et al.* Partial sequences of feline and caprine immunoglobulin epsilon heavy chain cDNA and comparative binding studies of recombinant IgE fragment-specific antibodies across different species. *Veterinary Immunology and Immunopathology* 2000; **75**: 59–69.
29. Weber ER, Helps CR, Foster AP, *et al.* Molecular cloning and phylogenetic analysis of a cDNA encoding the cat (*Felis domesticus*) Ig epsilon constant region. *Veterinary Immunology and Immunopathology* 2000; **76**: 299–308.
30. Taglinger K, Helps CR, Day MJ, *et al.* Measurement of serum immunoglobulin E (IgE) specific for house dust mite antigens in normal cats and cats with allergic skin disease. *Veterinary Immunology and Immunopathology* 2005; **105**: 85–93.
31. Belova S, Wilhelm S, Linek M, *et al.* Factors affecting allergen-specific IgE serum levels in cats. *Canadian Journal of Veterinary Research* 2012; **76**: 45–51.
32. Gilbert S, Halliwell RE. The effects of endoparasitism on the immune response to orally administered antigen in cats. *Veterinary Immunology and Immunopathology* 2005; **106**: 113–120.
33. Foster AP, O'Dair HA, DeBoer DJ. Allergen-specific IgG antibodies in cats with allergic skin disease. *Research in Veterinary Science* 1997; **63**: 239–243.
34. Novak N. An update on the role of human dendritic cells in patients with atopic dermatitis. *Journal of Allergy and Clinical Immunology* 2012; **129**: 879–886.
35. Roosje PJ, Whitaker-Menezes D, Goldschmidt MH, *et al.* Feline atopic dermatitis. A model for Langerhans cell participation in disease pathogenesis. *American Journal of Pathology* 1997; **151**: 927–932.
36. Taglinger K, Day MJ, Foster AP. Characterization of inflammatory cell infiltration in feline allergic skin disease. *Journal of Comparative Pathology* 2007; **137**: 211–223.
37. Guttman-Yassky E, Nograles KE, Krueger JG. Contrasting pathogenesis of atopic dermatitis and psoriasis—part II: immune cell subsets and therapeutic concepts. *Journal of Allergy and Clinical Immunology* 2011; **127**: 1420–1432.

38. Roosje PJ, van Kooten PJ, Thepen T, *et al.* Increased numbers of $CD4^+$ and $CD8^+$ T cells in lesional skin of cats with allergic dermatitis. *Veterinary Pathology* 1998; **35**: 268–273.
39. Roosje PJ, Dean GA, Willemse T, *et al.* Interleukin 4-producing $CD4^+$ T cells in the skin of cats with allergic dermatitis. *Veterinary Pathology* 2002; **39**: 228–233.
40. Taglinger K, Van Nguyen N, Helps CR, *et al.* Quantitative real-time RT-PCR measurement of cytokine mRNA expression in the skin of normal cats and cats with allergic skin disease. *Veterinary Immunology and Immunopathology* 2008; **122**: 216–230.
41. Kimura T, Kano R, Maeda S, *et al.* Expression of RANTES mRNA in skin lesions of feline eosinophilic plaque. *Veterinary Dermatology* 2003; **14**: 269–273.
42. Maeda S, Okayama T, Ohmori K, *et al.* Molecular cloning of the feline thymus and activation-regulated chemokine cDNA and its expression in lesional skin of cats with eosinophilic plaque. *Journal of Veterinary Medical Science* 2003; **65**: 275–278.
43. Rot A, Krieger M, Brunner T, *et al.* RANTES and macrophage inflammatory protein 1 alpha induce the migration and activation of normal human eosinophil granulocytes. *Journal of Experimental Medicine* 1992; **176**: 1489–1495.
44. Schall TJ, Bacon K, Toy KJ, *et al.* Selective attraction of monocytes and T lymphocytes of the memory phenotype by cytokine RANTES. *Nature* 1990; **347**: 669–671.
45. Vestergaard C, Deleuran M, Gesser B, *et al.* Thymus- and activation-regulated chemokine (TARC/CCL17) induces a Th2-dominated inflammatory reaction on intradermal injection in mice. *Experimental Dermatology* 2004; **13**: 265–271.
46. Liu FT, Goodarzi H, Chen HY. IgE, mast cells, and eosinophils in atopic dermatitis. *Clinical Reviews in Allergy and Immunology* 2011; **41**: 298–310.
47. Roosje PJ, Koeman JP, Thepen T, *et al.* Mast cells and eosinophils in feline allergic dermatitis: a qualitative and quantitative analysis. *Journal of Comparative Pathology* 2004; **131**: 61–69.
48. Fondati A, Carreras E, Fondevila MD, *et al.* Characterization of biological activities of feline eosinophil granule proteins. *American Journal of Veterinary Research* 2004; **65**: 957–963.
49. Fondati A, Fondevila D, Ferrer L. Piecemeal degranulation (PMD) morphology in feline circulating eosinophils. *Research in Veterinary Science* 2003; **75**: 127–132.
50. Fondati A, Fondevila D, Ferrer L. Histopathological study of feline eosinophilic dermatoses. *Veterinary Dermatology* 2001; **12**: 333–338.
51. Grewe M, Czech W, Morita A, *et al.* Human eosinophils produce biologically active IL-12: implications for control of T cell responses. *Journal of Immunology* 1998; **161**: 415–420.
52. Mazzoni A, Siraganian RP, Leifer CA, *et al.* Dendritic cell modulation by mast cells controls the Th1/Th2 balance in responding T cells. *Journal of Immunology* 2006; **177**: 3577–3581.
53. Preziosi DE, Goldschmidt MH, Greek JS, *et al.* Feline pemphigus foliaceus: a retrospective analysis of 57 cases. *Veterinary Dermatology* 2003; **14**: 313–321.
54. Beadleston DL, Roosje PJ, Goldschmidt MH. Chymase and tryptase staining of normal feline skin and of feline cutaneous mast cell tumors. *Veterinary Allergy and Clinical Immunology* 1997; **5**: 54–58.
55. Noli C, Welle M, Scarampella F, *et al.* Quantitative analysis of tryptase- and chymase-containing mast cells in eosinophilic conditions of cats. *Veterinary Pathology* 2003; **40**: 219–221.
56. Jarvikallio A, Naukkarinen A, Harvima IT, *et al.* Quantitative analysis of tryptase- and chymase-containing mast cells in atopic dermatitis and nummular eczema. *British Journal of Dermatology* 1997; **136**: 871–877.
57. Steinhoff M, Corvera CU, Thoma MS, *et al.* Proteinase-activated receptor-2 in human skin: tissue distribution and activation of keratinocytes by mast cell tryptase. *Experimental Dermatology* 1999; **8**: 282–294.
58. Steinhoff M, Neisius U, Ikoma A, *et al.* Proteinase-activated receptor-2 mediates itch: a novel pathway for pruritus in human skin. *Journal of Neuroscience* 2003; **23**: 6176–6180.
59. Terakawa M, Fujieda Y, Tomimori Y, *et al.* Oral chymase inhibitor SUN13834 ameliorates skin inflammation as well as pruritus in mouse model for atopic dermatitis. *European Journal of Pharmacology* 2008; **601**: 186–191.

32

Clinical presentations and specificity of feline manifestations of cutaneous allergies

Claude Favrot

Vetsuisse Faculty, University of Zurich, Zurich, Switzerland

Conflict of interest: none declared.

Classical presentations of feline atopic-like disease and cutaneous adverse reactions to food: eosinophilic dermatitis, miliary dermatitis, self-induced alopecia, and head and neck pruritus

Most of the cats with cutaneous hypersensitivity disorders (HD) present with one of the following reaction patterns: miliary dermatitis, various forms of eosinophilic dermatitis (see section 'Classical presentations of atopic-like disease and cutaneous adverse reactions to food'), self-induced symmetrical alopecia, and head and neck pruritus [1–4]. In fact, in previous studies only 6% presented with none of these patterns and exhibited signs such as pododermatitis (including plasma cell pododermatitis), seborrhoeic reactions, exfoliative dermatitis (mural folliculitis), facial erythema, pruritus without any obvious skin changes, and ceruminous otitis [2,3,5–10]. This chapter will focus on the classical presentations of feline atopic-like disease (ALD) and cutaneous adverse reactions to food (CARF); other hypersensitivity disorders and less classical presentations will only be discussed for comparison purposes. It is worth noting that ALD and CAFR are indistinguishable clinically and consequently will be discussed together. When differences between these two conditions were reported in studies, they will be mentioned in this chapter or in Chapter 33.

Signalment and history of cats with atopic-like disease and/or cutaneous adverse reactions to food

A familial predisposition has been observed by some authors and a breed predisposition (Abyssinian) has been suggested for ALD [1,3,11]. These data collectively support an association of HD with a hereditary background, although proper genetic studies have not been carried out in allergic cats. A gender predisposition has not been demonstrated, although females represented 59% of a panel of 161 ALD and/or CAFR cats [3]. The majority of HD cats seem to exhibit the first clinical signs before 3 years of age, although some studies suggest a wider range of age at onset of signs of disease [1,2,12]. In one study the age at onset was 3.4 years, with cats demonstrating CAFR being slightly older (mean 4 years old with 52% less than 3 years of age at onset) than those with ALD (mean 3 years old with 72% less than 3 years of age at onset) [3]. In the same study seasonality was a feature of the disease in less than 10% of cats (only 3% in CAFR cats).

Classical presentations of atopic-like disease and cutaneous adverse reactions to food

In one study, including more than 500 cats, 59% of the cats with CAFR or ALD or both conditions presented with head and neck pruritus, 52% with self-induced symmetrical alopecia, 25% with eosinophilic dermatitis,

Veterinary Allergy, First Edition. Edited by Chiara Noli, Aiden Foster, and Wayne Rosenkrantz.

19% with military dermatitis, and 46% with at least two of these four patterns [3]. It should, however, be kept in mind that cats included in this study were mostly presented in referral centres; consequently, the proportion of the clinical presentations in general practice may be quite different. In the same study, miliary dermatitis was more often seen in flea bite hypersensitive cats (35%); miliary dermatitis was less frequently associated with multiple patterns (28%).

Cats with CAFR or ALD or both conditions usually present with pruritus. In one study, owners evaluated the itching as 5 or above 5 in a scale ranging from 0 to 10 in 88% of the cats [3]. Pruritus is, however, not always recognized by owners, especially in cats with self-induced alopecia; trichoscopy (to demonstrate broken hair tips) is useful in such cases to demonstrate over grooming.

- **Miliary dermatitis** refers to a papulocrustous dermatitis that usually develops on the face and dorsal aspects of the body (Figure 32.1). Primary lesions consist of small papules topped by yellow to brown-crust. Given their small size the lesions may be difficult to see but are easily palpated. Miliary dermatitis is often associated with other facial lesions or alopecia or both.

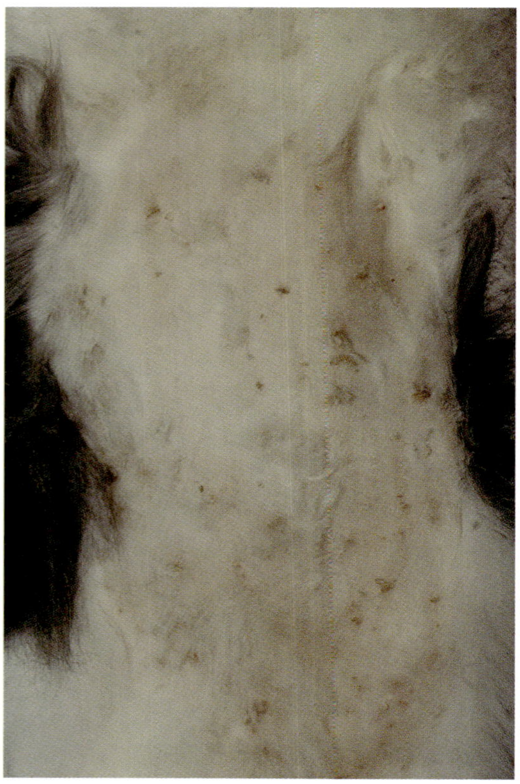

Figure 32.1 Miliary dermatitis. Reprinted from [3]. © 2011, with the permission of John Wiley & Sons, Inc.

- **Head and neck pruritus** refers to papular and erythematous changes occurring on the face and neck of non-flea hypersensitivity dermatitis (NFHD; namely, ALD and CAFR) cats often in association with self-induced excoriations (Figure 32.2), alopecia (Figure 32.3), crusts (Figure 32.4), miliary dermatitis, and/or seborrhoeic changes.
- **Self-induced alopecia** is characterized by usually symmetrical changes occurring mostly on the flanks, abdomen, and dorsum and caused by excessive licking; the hair tips in and around the lesions are broken (Figure 32.5).
- **Eosinophilic dermatitides** consist of eosinophilic plaques or granulomas and/or indolent ulceration.
  - **Indolent ulcer** (also called eosinophilic or rodent ulcer, some authors favour the term lip ulcer) is a

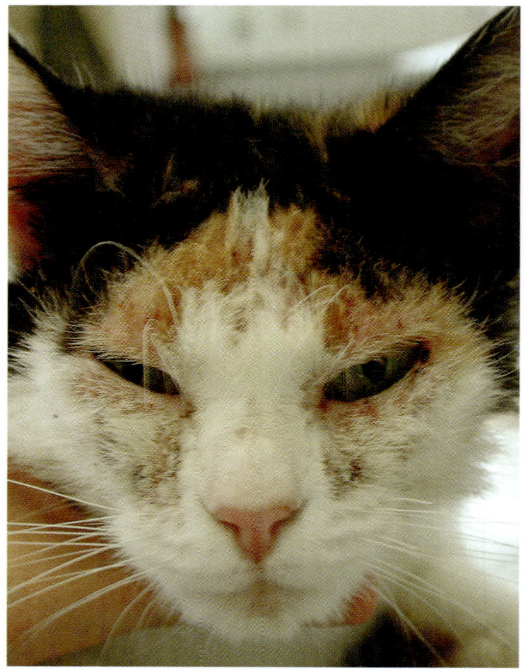

Figure 32.2 Head and neck pruritus: erosions.

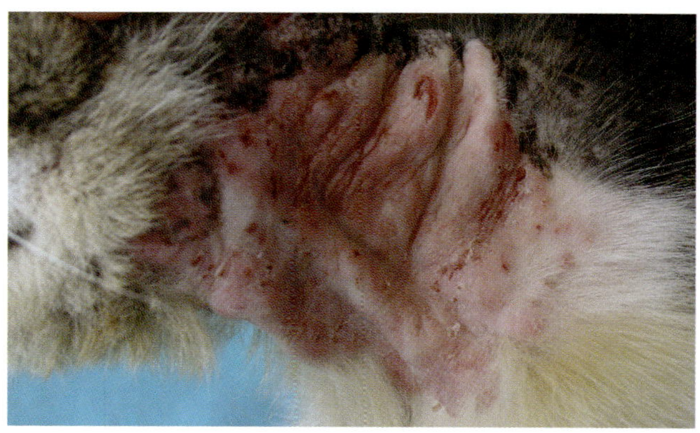

Figure 32.3 Head and neck pruritus: alopecia.

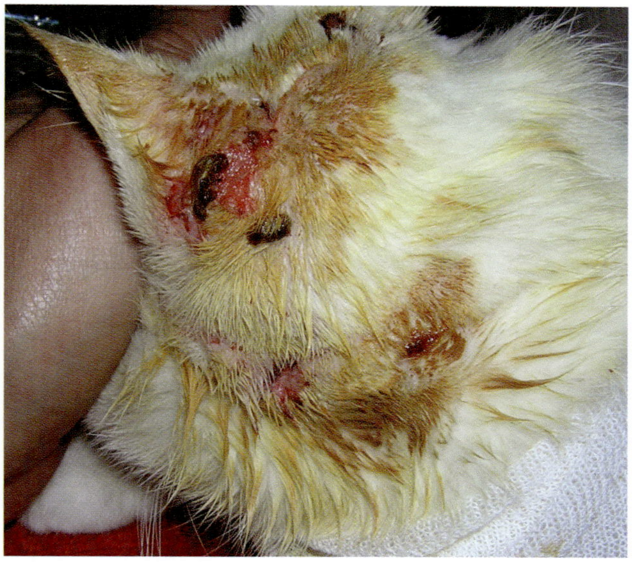

Figure 32.4 Head and neck pruritus: ulcerations and crusts.

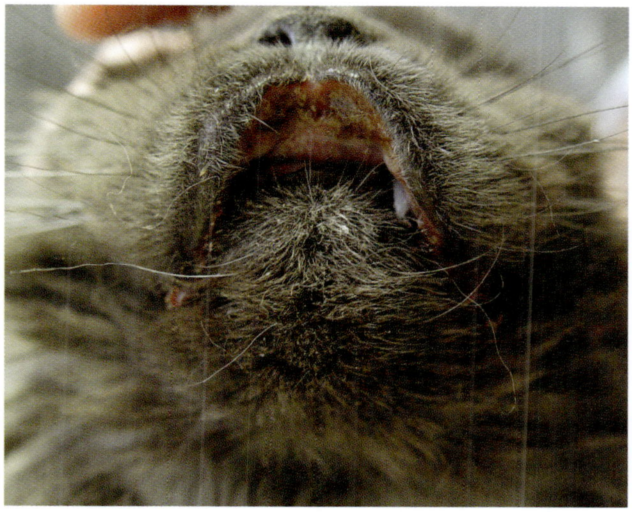

Figure 32.6 Indolent ulcer.

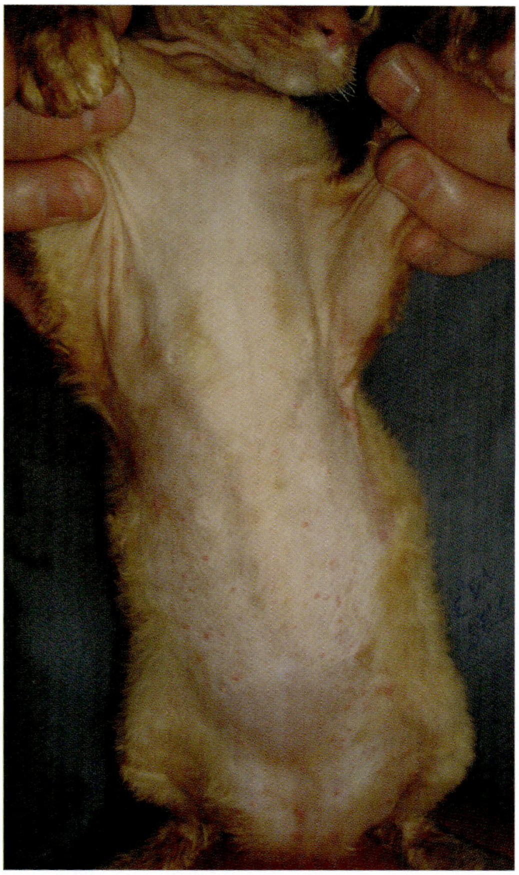

Figure 32.5 Self-induced alopecia.

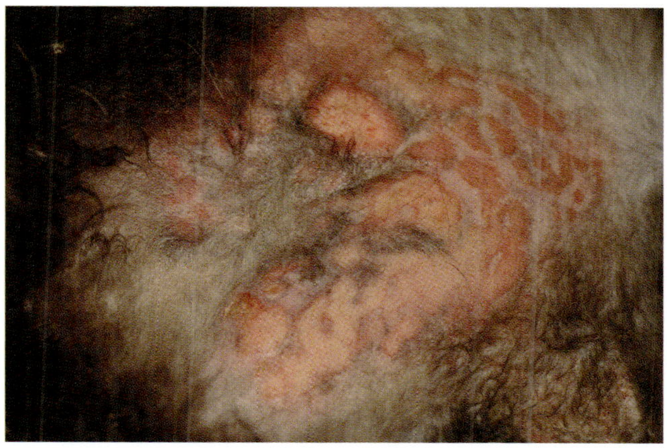

Figure 32.7 Eosinophilic plaques.

unilateral or bilateral erosive to ulcerative lesion of the upper lips (Figure 32.6).

- **Eosinophilic plaques** are raised, erythematous, exudative, and intensely pruritic lesions developing on the abdomen, inguinal, medial, and caudal aspects of the thigh area, and less frequently on the neck and face (Figure 32.7) [13].
- **Eosinophilic granulomas** may present as linear, diffuse to nodular swollen, and usually firm lesions occurring mostly in the oral cavity, interdigital areas, chin (fat chin; Figure 32.8a), and limbs (linear granulomas; Figure 32.8b).

Distribution patterns

In the study mentioned previously, two body areas were affected in more than 50% of cats with CAFR and/or ALD: face/head and abdomen [3]. Additionally, ears, neck, and hind limbs were affected in about one-third of the patients. In comparison, flea hypersensitivity dermatitis cats present less frequently with facial,

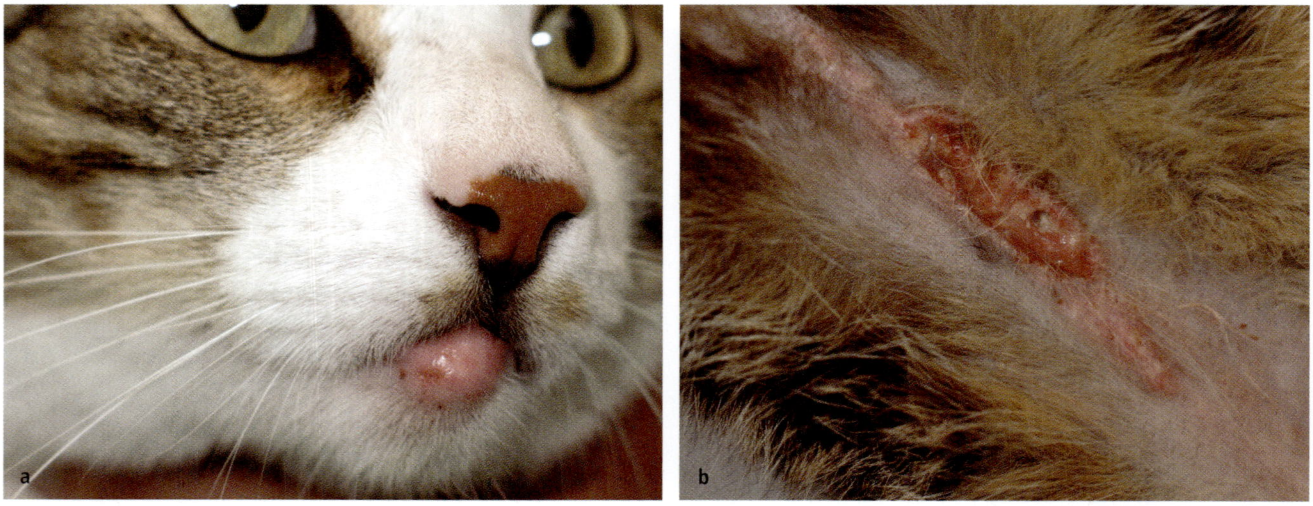

Figure 32.8 Eosinophilic granuloma: fat chin (a) and linear granuloma (b).

lips, and ear lesions but more often with changes on the dorsum, rump, and flanks. When CAFR and ALD are compared, limbs and abdomen are more frequently affected in ALD cats. Interestingly, the face and head appear to be more represented in cats with CAFR, although not significantly (Table 32.1 and Figure 32.9).

Other signs

Cats with HD may also present with some non-dermatological signs. In one study, 6% presented with sneezing or coughing or both, 14% with digestive signs (soft tools, diarrhoea, vomiting), 7% with conjunctivitis, and 16% with otitis externa or media or both [3]. These results should be compared to those provided by Carlotti and Prost, who suggested that up to 50% of allergic cats may show some degree of sneezing [14]. Blood eosinophilia has also been suggested to be a non-specific but helpful diagnostic criterion [4]. In the study mentioned above, eosinophilia was present in the majority of tested cats but was also detected in flea allergic cats and numerous pruritic cats with non-hypersensitivity skin diseases [3].

Specificity of reaction patterns

Even though each of these patterns can be seen in association with numerous causes, some of them are typical of specific aetiologies (Table 32.2). For example, miliary dermatitis is more often associated with flea HD than CAFR or ALD. It is worth mentioning that the proportions of each pattern are not significantly different when CAFR and ALD cats are compared.

Table 32.1 Affected areas in cats with hypersensitivity dermatitis (reprinted from [3] © 2011, with permission of John Wiley & Sons, Inc.)

	CAFR and ALD (%)	ALD (%)	CAFR (%)	Flea HD (%)	OD (%)
Head/face	58	56	61	42	47
Ears	34	32	36	21	48
Chin	17	17	18	14	12
Lips	14	15	13	5	6
Oral/mouth	7	2	15	4	2
Neck	40	36	50	36	20
Rump/tail	15	18	10	53	8
Front limbs	26	34	13	21	15
Hind limbs	32	40	18	21	12
Front paws	7	6	8	4	12
Hind paws	6	1	13	4)	7
Lateral thorax	15	17	11	10	10
Sternum/axilla	11	10	11	8	7
Flanks	10	14	5	20	7
Abdomen	53	59	43	50	22
Perineum	12	14	10	12	4
Dorsum	19	23	11	42	15

CAFR, cutaneous adverse food reaction; ALD, atopic-like dermatitis; HD, hypersensitivity dermatitides; OD, other dermatoses.

The specificity of feline manifestations of cutaneous allergy

Differential diagnoses

Cats with HD usually present with one of the reaction patterns described above; however, none of these patterns

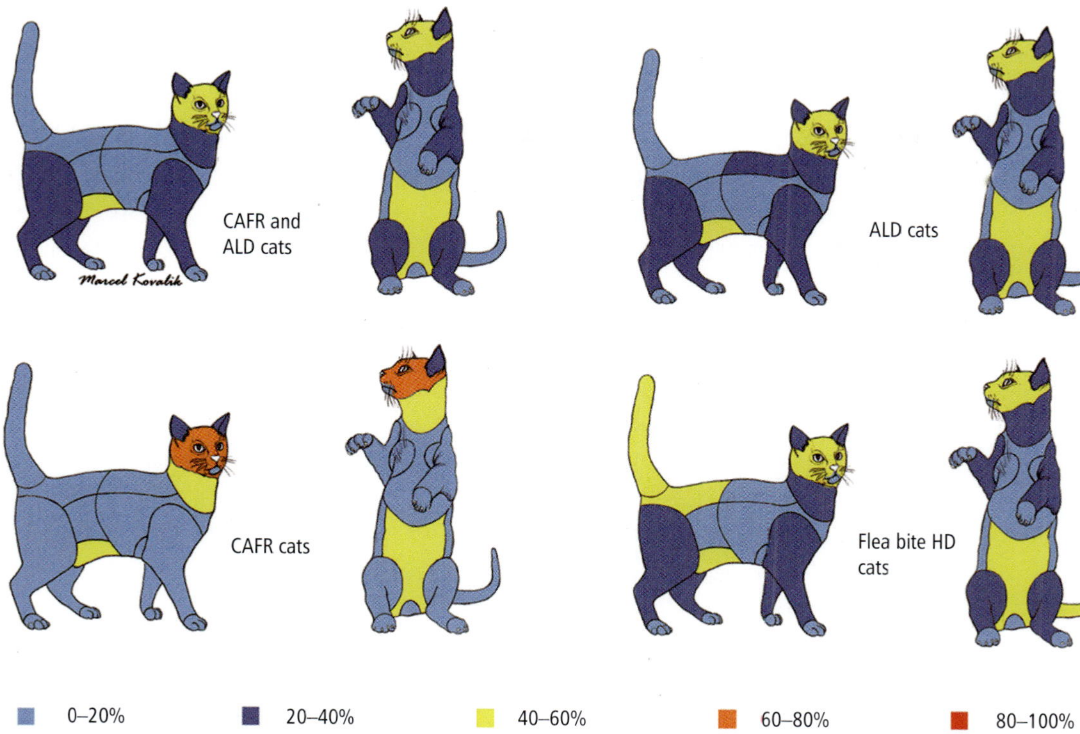

Figure 32.9 Cats with hypersensitivity dermatitis: percentage of cats affected for each body area. CAFR, cutaneous adverse food reaction; ALD, atopic-like dermatitis; HD, hypersensitivity dermatitides; OD, other dermatoses. (Reprinted from [3] © 2011, with permission of John Wiley & Sons, Inc.)

Table 32.2 Frequency of each reaction pattern for each type of hypersensitivity dermatitis (reprinted from [3] © 2011, with permission of John Wiley & Sons, Inc.)

	ALD and CAFR (%)	ALD (%)	CAFR (%)	Flea HD (%)	Other pruritic cats (%)
Miliary dermatitis	19	18	20	35	9
Eosinophilic granuloma complex	25	26	25	14	2
Erosions/ulcerations face & neck	59	56	64	38	55
Symmetrical alopecia	52	57	43	39	18
At least 1 of previous 4	94	95	47	91	74
Multiple patterns	46	46	46	28	7

CAFR, cutaneous adverse food reaction; ALD, atopic-like dermatitis; HD, hypersensitivity dermatitides.

is pathognomonic and the exact same clinical changes may be associated with a rather wide range of possible causes, allergic and non-allergic. Some of these causes may also be associated with all of these patterns, especially ectoparasites, while some others are specific for one clinical presentation. The main consequence is that each of these patterns is associated with a specific list of differential diagnoses that should be ruled out before making a diagnosis of feline cutaneous allergy.

It is usually assumed that ectoparasites such as fleas, mites such as *Otodectes*, *Notoedres* and *Demodex*, lice, *Neotrombicula*, together with bacterial and fungal diseases, should be ruled out in all cats where hypersensitivity dermatitides are suspected [1–4,12,13]. Additionally, depending on the clinical presentation, some other differential diagnoses should be considered and appropriate diagnostic investigations should be carried out (Table 32.3).

Table 32.3 Reaction patterns in pruritic cats: main differential diagnoses and corresponding tests

Reaction pattern	Main differential diagnoses	Test
Miliary dermatitis	Fleas	Comb, therapeutic trial
	Ectoparasites: cheyletiella, lice, notoedres, sarcoptes	Scrapings, therapeutic trial
	Dermatophytes	Cultures, trichoscopy, Wood's lamp
	Bacterial folliculitis (rare)	Cytological examination
Self-induced alopecia	Internal diseases including hyperadrenocorticism and liver or pancreatic carcinoma	Trichoscopy (hair tips are usually not broken)
	Bacterial folliculitis	Cytological examination
	Psychogenic alopecia	Diagnosis of exclusion, therapeutic trial
	Ectoparasites (*Demodex*)	Skin scrapings
Eosinophilic dermatitis	Gingivitis	Histopathology
	Fleas	Flea comb and therapeutic trial
	Skin tumours (mast cell tumour, cutaneous lymphoma, metastases)	Histopathology
	Bacterial diseases (staphylococci, mycobacteriosis, nocardiosis)	Cytological examination, histological examination, culture, PCR
	Xanthomatosis	Histopathology
Head and neck pruritus	Ectoparasites including *Notoedres*, *Demodex*, *Otodectes*, *Sarcoptes*, lice, cheyletiella, fleas	Flea comb, scrapings, therapeutic trial
	Fungal diseases (dermatophytes, *Malassezia*)	Cytological examination, Wood's lamp, trichoscopy, culture
	Bacterial diseases	Cytological examination, culture
	Viral diseases (herpesvirus, papillomavirus, calicivirus, poxvirus, feline leukaemia virus)	Histological examination, PCR
	Mosquito bite dermatitis	
	Skin tumours (cutaneous lymphoma, squamous cell carcinomas, mast cell tumours)	Histopathological examination

References

1. Foster AP. Diagnosing and treating feline atopy. *Veterinary Medicine* 2002; **97**: 226–240.
2. Foster AP, Roosje PJ. Update on feline immunoglobulin E (IgE) and diagnostic recommendations for atopy. In: August JR, ed. *Consultations in Feline Internal Medicine*, Vol. 5. Philadelphia: Saunders WB, 2005: 229–238.
3. Hobi S, Linek M, Marignac G, *et al*. Clinical characteristics and causes of pruritus in cats: a multicentre study on feline hypersensitivity-associated dermatoses. *Veterinary Dermatology* 2011; **22**: 406–413.
4. O'Dair H, Markwell P, Maskell I. An open prospective investigation into aetiology in a group of cats with suspected allergic skin disease. *Veterinary Dermatology* 1996; **7**: 193–202.
5. Prélaud P, Guaguère E, Freiche V, *et al*. The allergic cat. *Pratique Médicale et Chirurgicale de l'Animal de Compagnie* 1999; **34**: 437–447.
6. Prost C. Les dermatoses allergiques du chat. *Pratique Médicale et Chirurgicale de l'Animal de Compagnie* 1993; **28**: 151–164.
7. Scott DW, Miller WH, Griffin CE. Skin immune system and allergic skin diseases. *Muller and Kirk's Small Animal Dermatology*, 6th edn. Philadelphia: WB Saunders Co, 2001: 543–666.
8. Bryan J, Frank L. Food allergy in the cat: a diagnosis of elimination. *Journal of Feline Medicine and Surgery* 2010; **12**: 861–866.
9. Declercq J. A case of diet-related lymphocytic mural folliculitis in a cat. *Veterinary Dermatology* 2000; **11**: 75–80.
10. Saridomichelakis MN, Koutinas AF. A retrospective study of 10 spontaneous cases of feline atopic dermatitis. *European Journal of Companion Animal Practice* 2001; **11**: 177–183.
11. Moriello KA. Feline atopy in three littermates. *Veterinary Dermatology* 2001; **12**: 177–181.
12. Roosje PJ, Thepen T, Rutten VPMG, *et al*. Feline atopic dermatitis. In: Thoday KL, Foil CS, Bond R, eds. *Advances in Veterinary Dermatology*, Vol. 4. Oxford: Blackwell Sciences, 2002: 178–187.
13. Young KM, Moriello KA. Eosinophils and eosinophilic diseases. In: August JR, ed. *Consultations in Feline Internal Medicine*, Vol. 5. Philadelphia: WB Saunders, 2005: 236–246.
14. Carlotti D, Prost C. L'atopie feline. *Point Vétérinaire* 1989; **20**: 777–784.

33

Complications of cutaneous skin allergies (skin infections)

Laura Ordeix

Department of Animal Medicine and Surgery, Veterinary School, Autonomous University of Barcelona; Dermatology Service, Hospital Ars Veterinaria, Barcelona, Spain

Conflict of interest: none declared.

Introduction

The cat has received relatively little attention in veterinary medicine compared to the dog. Although published information on feline medicine, and in particular on dermatology, is continually growing, research into feline dermatology is, in some respects, well behind research into canine dermatology. As a consequence, veterinarians may practise feline dermatology as they do canine dermatology. However, this may not always be helpful. Cats can be presented with distinct dermatological diseases, making them dissimilar to dogs. There are two features of canine dermatology, particularly with regard to cutaneous allergy, that are not commonly present in the feline counterpart.

Firstly, in dogs, cutaneous allergic diseases have characteristic clinical presentations, which can be suggestive of the underlying aetiology. Conversely, in cats the presentation of allergic diseases is not, usually, typical of the underlying aetiology. Secondly, dogs with allergic skin diseases, including atopic dermatitis and cutaneous adverse food reaction, are predisposed to secondary microbial infection of the skin [1].

In the author's experience the dermatological problems most frequently observed in cats are head and/or neck pruritus, symmetrical autoinduced alopecia, papulonodular mucocutaneous dermatitis (lesions of the eosinophilic granuloma complex), and papulocrusted dermatitis (miliary dermatitis). All of these reaction patterns have been associated with cutaneous allergic diseases. In addition, the same allergic disease may cause different dermatological problems (i.e. clinical polymorphism). Moreover, the prevalence of superficial skin infections, in particular feline pyoderma and *Malassezia* dermatitis, is relatively lower in the cat compared with the dog and, in particular, in the allergic cat. The reasons for this decreased susceptibility have not been fully elucidated. Anecdotally, biological differences between species in epidermal barrier function, local microenvironment, and in innate and adaptive immunity have been suggested as causes for this relative resistance to skin infection. Furthermore, it has been reported that there is poor adherence of a range of staphylococcal species to feline corneocytes compared to corneocytes in dogs or humans [2]. It is not clear if these observations are clinically significant, although it is assumed that there is a correlation between bacterial adherence and the susceptibility of the host to infection.

In both dogs and humans beings the relationship between superficial infections and cutaneous allergic diseases is considered to be reciprocal. Allergic patients have an increased susceptibility to recurrent infections and clinical and experimental evidence suggest that secondary infections can influence the severity of allergic dermatitis [1,3]. Unfortunately, little information is available on microbial diseases of allergic cats and about

Veterinary Allergy, First Edition. Edited by Chiara Noli, Aiden Foster, and Wayne Rosenkrantz.

the role of secondary cutaneous infections contributing to the severity of the pruritus and to the development of skin lesions in allergic cats.

This chapter discusses the pathogenesis, clinical presentation, diagnosis, and treatment of superficial skin infections in allergic cats.

Superficial bacterial infections

Aetiopathogenesis

Superficial bacterial infections mainly involve micro-organisms that are either part of the cutaneous or mucosal microbiota, or are introduced into a cutaneous lesion from the environment or from carrier sites.

In cats, as in dogs or human beings, the most common cause of superficial bacterial skin infections is staphylococci infections. Coagulase-positive and coagulase-negative species of *Staphylococcus* have been isolated from healthy and diseased feline skin and mucosae. It is considered that the group *S. felis/S. simulans*, both coagulase-negative species with similar biochemical properties, has a resident status, being isolated from skin and mucosal sites in both healthy and diseased cats [4]. *Staphylococcus pseudintermedius* and *S. aureus* are the coagulase-positive species most often isolated from healthy cats and from cats with skin lesions [5]. However, the residency status of *S. pseudintermedius* in cats remains unclear.

Adherence of bacteria to host tissues is an essential step in the colonization process and therefore in causing infection. *Staphylococcal* adherence to epidermal cells from atopic dogs is significantly greater than those from normal dogs. Although staphylococcal adherence to corneocytes from healthy cats has been investigated, adherence studies involving cats with inflammatory allergic skin conditions have not been reported. Other factors that may influence the pathogenesis of feline skin infections, such as host immune competence, are not known. However, clinical evidence suggest that, as in dogs, reduced immune response due to the chronic use of glucocorticoids may result in secondary bacterial skin infection in allergic cats.

Less commonly, *Pasteurella multocida*, a common inhabitant of the oral cavity and respiratory tract of cats, can transiently infect the skin of allergic cats. This micro-organism may infect skin lesions caused by excessive self-grooming.

Aggravating factor of allergy

In atopic dogs, staphylococcal superficial skin infections occur more frequently than in cats and bacterial products are known to augment cutaneous inflammation and pruritus. Therefore, treatment of such infections has been shown to improve the severity of atopic dermatitis [1]. In feline dermatology similar observations are lacking, although one study reported a beneficial response for cats with eosinophilic plaques with amoxicillin trihydrate–clavulanate potassium as the sole therapy [6]. This study demonstrated not only that eosinophilic plaques were frequently associated with secondary bacterial infections but also may suggest a role of bacterial infections in the pathogenesis of cutaneous allergic diseases in some cats.

The potential role of bacterial infections, in particular of staphylococci, in perpetuating skin lesions resulting from excessive grooming as a result of allergic disease should be considered in all feline cases.

Clinical signs

Contrary to what happens in dogs, superficial staphylococcal infections in cats rarely present with the typical clinical picture characterized by pustules and epidermal collarettes. When present these lesions tend to be associated with cats that have received glucocorticoids (Figure 33.1). Cutaneous lesions suggestive of superficial bacterial infection in cats include crusted papules, excoriations, ulcerations, and eroded or ulcerated plaques or nodules.

Allergic cats with secondary bacterial folliculitis may present with crusted papules on the trunk, mainly on the dorsum, encompassed in a reaction pattern known as miliary dermatitis (Figure 33.2). In allergic cats, bacterial skin infections are more likely to be diagnosed with cutaneous lesions secondary to scratching, such as head and neck excoriations or ulcerations, or from licking, such as abdominal excoriations or from the surface of

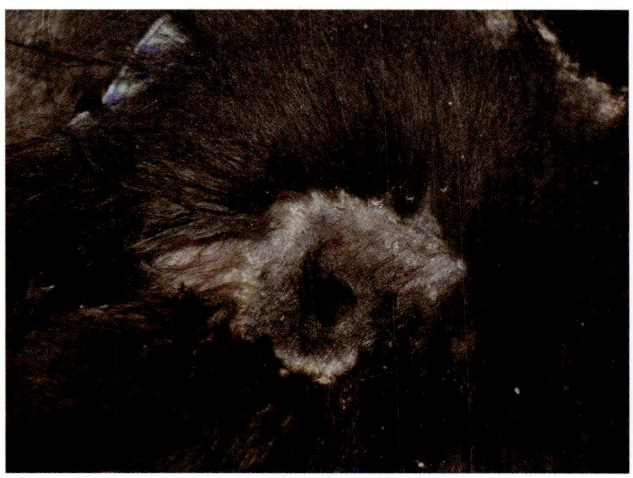

Figure 33.1 Epidermal collarette on the top of the head in an allergic Persian cat receiving methylprednisolone acetate therapy.

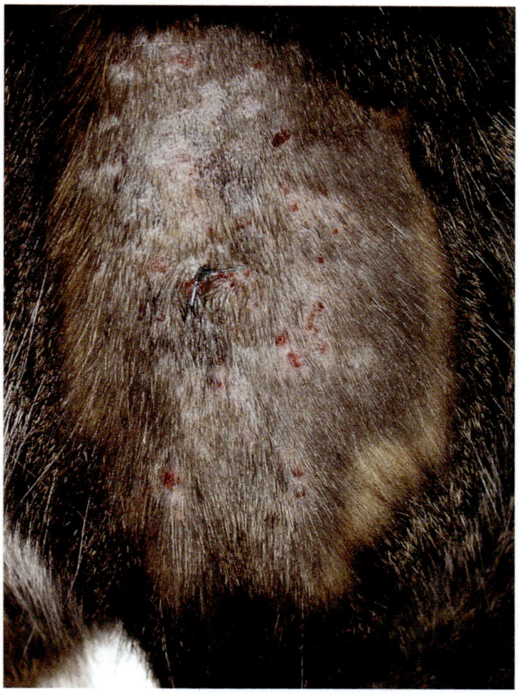

Figure 33.2 Papulocrusting dermatitis (miliary dermatitis) in a non-flea, non-food allergic cat. The cat was shaved to photograph the lesions.

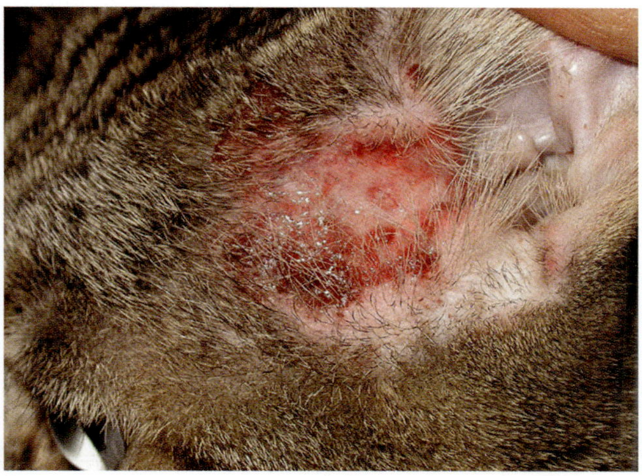

Figure 33.3 Superficial staphylococcal infection in an allergic cat with facial pruritus and consequent excoriations.

skin lesions associated with pruritic lesions of the eosinophilic granuloma complex (Figure 33.3).

Rarely, some allergic cats may be presented with bacterial paronychia secondary to excessive claw licking characterized by alopecia, erythema, erosion or ulceration, and purulent discharge around the claw and claw fold (Figure 33.4). Bacterial infections associated with otitis externa in allergic cats are also rare.

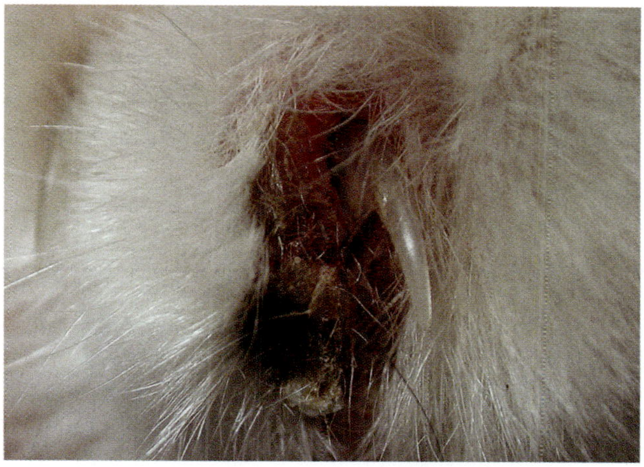

Figure 33.4 Bacterial paronychia due to *Pasteurella multocida* in a non-flea, non-food allergic cat, with constant pedal licking.

Diagnosis

The diagnosis of superficial bacterial infections in cats is based on the cytological examination of material collected from the skin surface. Direct impression smears are usually preferred to collect material from exudative lesions such as excoriations, erosions, and ulcers. Collection of material using an adhesive tape is preferred for those skin areas that would be hard to reach using a direct impression smear technique, including interdigital spaces, eyelids, lips, and the perianal area, or in the presence of less exudative or encrusted lesions.

Smears are air-dried, except for samples collected using adhesive tape, and stained with a Romanovsky-type panoptic stain such as Diff Quick® (Medion Diagnostics AG, Düdingen, Switzerland). Preparations are initially examined microscopically at a low magnification (40×) to determine the sample area for more detailed study. By moving up to a higher magnification (100×) the cell population can be determined, evaluating the numbers and type of inflammatory cells such as neutrophils and eosinophils. With higher magnification (400×) some bacteria can be identified; however, for more accurate identification of some infectious agents, such as small bacilli, the sample should be examined under an oil immersion lens (1000×).

Published data regarding cytological criteria useful to diagnose bacterial overgrowth or infection in cats are scarce. It is conventionally accepted that the presence of degenerate neutrophils, with or without eosinophils, and intracellular cocci or bacilli or both are diagnostic of bacterial infection (Figure 33.5). The presence of extracellular bacteria mixed with granulocytic cells is considered to be suggestive of bacterial infection. Numerous bacteria in the absence of an inflammatory response would be compatible with bacterial overgrowth.

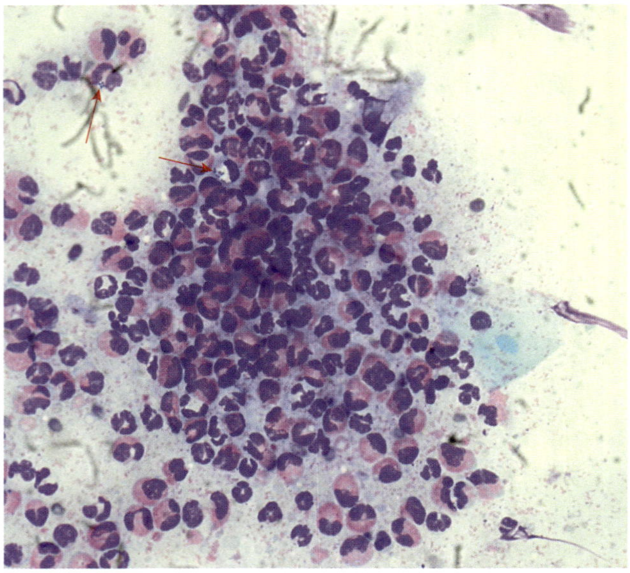

Figure 33.5 Cytological examination of a plaque on the abdomen of an allergic cat showing eosinophilic inflammation; arrows indicate intracellular cocci.

Bacterial culture to confirm the identity of bacteria, particularly when rods are seen on cytology and to provide sensitivity data, may be necessary in some severe or unresponsive cases.

Treatment

Superficial bacterial infections in cats are commonly treated with systemic antibiotics, given the relatively difficulty of treating cats with topical medications due to self-grooming and the difficulty in bathing them. In some circumstances, such as localized lesions with compliant cats, topical treatment such as 2–3% chorhexidine solution or gel, could be tried.

Oral treatment in cats may be difficult to administer, and given that many pharmacological products are devised for use in dogs the formulation and palatability may be inappropriate for cats. These features may cause the cat to salivate after which administration of the medication is impossible. Therefore, in some cases, parenteral administration may be the required.

Few reports exist regarding the antibacterial susceptibilities of the staphylococci isolated from cats [4]. As in dogs, antibiotics used empirically for the treatment of superficial infections due to cocci may include amoxicillin–clavulanic acid (12.5–25 mg/kg twice daily per os (p.o.), cephalexin (15–20 mg/kg twice daily p.o.), cefadroxil (20 mg/kg twice daily p.o.), and clindamycin (5.5 mg/kg twice daily p.o.). Other antibiotics should be chosen on the basis of the results of sensitivity testing, which should be carried out whenever the identity and sensitivity of infecting organisms cannot be predicted, such as bacilli infections, or when previous empiric treatment does not yield the expected response.

Unfortunately, the majority of allergic cats with superficial bacterial infections secondary to self-induced lesions, contrary to what happens in dogs, do not show a marked improvement in their pruritus after antibacterial treatment alone, suggesting that secondary bacterial infections do not play a significant role in the cat's discomfort. In the author's experience, most allergic cats need concurrent anti-inflammatory treatment to reduce pruritus and resolve skin lesions.

Superficial fungal infections

Superficial fungal infections described in cats include *Malassezia* spp. overgrowth and dermatophytosis.

Dermatophytosis

Dermatophytosis is the most pleomorphic disease in feline dermatology and is usually considered a differential diagnosis for any dermatological problem including those associated with allergic cutaneous diseases. Interestingly, with miliary dermatitis and with papular eosinophilic or mastocytic dermatitis of the Devon rex, both reaction patterns are clinically suggestive of an allergic disease and dermatophytosis [7]. Although dermatophytosis may be diagnosed in cats with concurrent allergic dermatitis, it is usually associated with glucocorticoid or ciclosporin therapy rather than being a consequence of the allergic disease.

Malassezia overgrowth

Malassezia spp. overgrowth, with or without dermatitis, may be observed in allergic cats. In contrast to allergic dogs, in which *Malassezia* spp. overgrowth is frequently diagnosed, this condition is apparently less common in allergic cats. This discrepancy may be due to different or fewer changes in the cutaneous microenvironment secondary to the allergic disease in cats compared to dogs. *Malassezia pachydermatis* is the most frequently isolated species from the skin, mucosae, or ear canals of healthy cats; other yeasts of the genus *Malassezia*, including *M. sympodialis*, *M. globosa*, *M. furfur*, and *M. nana*, have been isolated [8].

Aggravating factor of allergy

In dogs, the most common predisposing factor for *Malassezia* overgrowth is hypersensitivity disorders, especially atopic dermatitis [9]. Moreover, analogous to what happens for superficial bacterial infections in allergic dogs, treatment of such infections may result in an improvement in the severity of atopic dermatitis [1]. A favourable response to antifungal treatment as the sole therapy in allergic cats has been also reported [8]. This observation may suggest that infection with *Malassezia* spp. may be partly responsible for both pruritus and cutaneous lesions in some allergic cats.

Malassezia overgrowth has also been associated with severe systemic diseases (e.g. paraneoplastic syndromes and retroviral infections). Consequently, a diagnosis of *Malassezia* overgrowth may indicate, where the clinical signs and history are compatible, the need to investigate for underlying systemic disease.

Clinical signs

Malassezia spp. dermatitis may affect allergic cats of any age and of both sexes, although it is more often diagnosed in mature adult cats. Skin lesions related to *Malassezia* spp. dermatitis commonly occur on the face, ventral neck, abdomen, and ear canals, a distribution that seems to parallel that of feline allergic pruritus [8]. These lesions are characterized by some degree of alopecia, erythema, greasy adherent brownish scales, increased cerumen, hyperpigmentation, easily plucked hair, and follicular casts (Figures 33.6 and 33.7). Hyperpigmentation and lichenification, contrary to what happens in dogs, are rarely observed. These clinical features may suggest that feline skin responds to a chronic inflammatory stimulus in a different manner from canine skin.

Diagnosis

Cytological examination is the most useful technique for the assessment of *Malassezia* density on the skin surface. Collection using adhesive tape is preferred by the author; some clinicians use direct impression smears and heat fixation may aid uptake of stain and examination for yeast organisms.

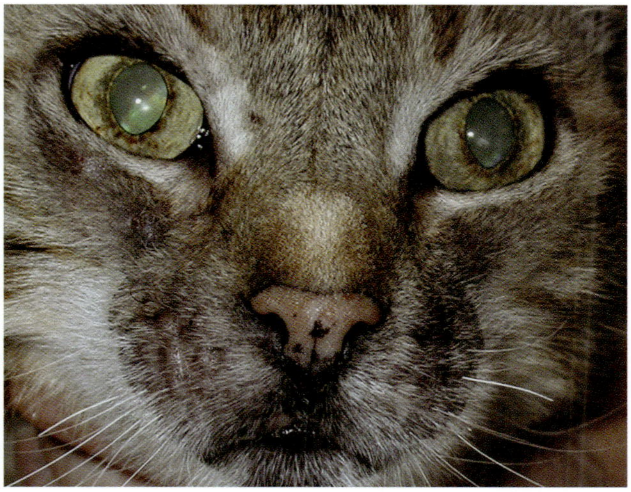

Figure 33.6 Alopecia, hyperpigmentation and greasy adherent brownish scales in an allergic cat with *Malassezia* dermatitis.

Although *Malassezia* spp. are part of the microflora of the skin of clinically normal cats, when using the adhesive tape method in healthy cats *Malassezia* organisms are not always observed or are found in low numbers (i.e. one yeast per 10 oil-immersion fields) and predominantly in only one anatomical site [8]. Therefore, finding more that one micro-organism per, at least, 10 oil-immersion fields (1000×) is compatible with yeast overgrowth (Figure 33.8).

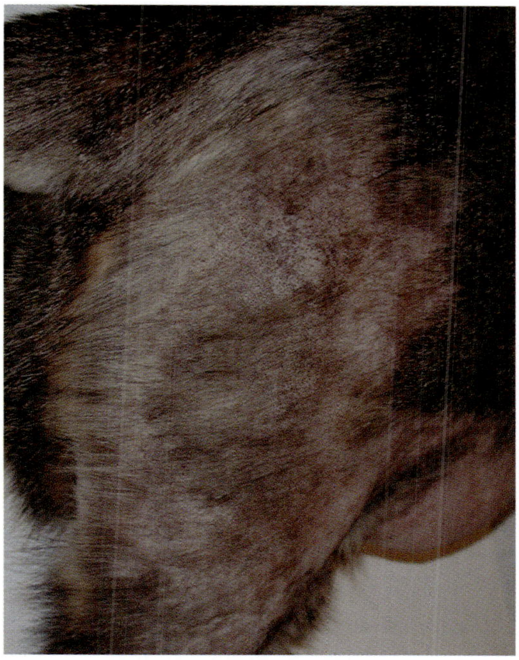

Figure 33.7 Alopecia with easily plucked hair and follicular casts in an allergic cat with *Malassezia* dermatitis.

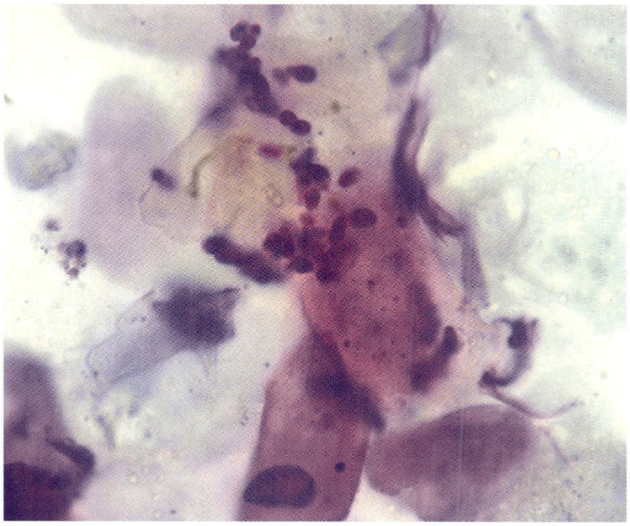

Figure 33.8 Cytological examination of lesional skin surface of cat from Figure 33.6 using acetate tape technique. Presence of abundant yeast organisms compatible with a *Malassezia* overgrowth.

Treatment

There are few studies assessing the efficacy of antifungal treatment of *Malassezia* overgrowth in cats. Reduction in the yeast counts and an associated marked clinical improvement of seborrhoeic dermatitis associated with *M. pachydermatis* in Devon rex cats has been reported with oral itraconazole therapy (5 mg/kg once daily, 7 days on, 7 days off, 7 days on) [10]. In a case series of 18 allergic cats with *Malassezia* dermatitis, seven cats were treated with azoles as the sole oral therapy (itraconazole 5 mg/kg once daily or ketoconazole 6–10 mg/kg once daily) and 11 with a combination of azoles and antibiotic with or without glucocorticoid therapy. Adjunctive topical therapy with chlorhexidine was used in some cats. After 3–4 weeks of treatment, substantial reduction in pruritus and skin lesions was observed in five of seven cats treated solely with azoles. No adverse effects were described [8].

Viral infections

The clinical course in human beings with atopic dermatitis can also be complicated by both localized and disseminated cutaneous viral infections, most often caused by herpesvirus (eczema herpeticum), human papilloma virus, or molluscum virus. It has been suggested that a defective skin barrier can contribute to this infectious complication [3]. In veterinary medicine a relationship between cutaneous viral infections and allergic dermatitis has not been described to date.

Cats can be subclinical carriers of several viruses (feline herpesvirus 1, feline calicivirus, feline leukaemia virus, and feline immunodeficiency virus) [11]. Therefore, the veterinary clinician should be aware of the potential for activation of viral-associated clinical diseases in allergic cats treated long-term with glucocorticoids or ciclosporin.

References

1. DeBoer DJ, Marsella R. The ACVD task force on canine atopic dermatitis (XII): the relationship of cutaneous infections to the pathogenesis and clinical course of canine atopic dermatitis. *Veterinary Immunology and Immunopathology* 2001; **81**: 239–249.
2. Woolley KL, Kelly RF, Fazakerley J, *et al.* Reduced *in vitro* adherence of *Staphylococcus* species to feline corneocytes compared to canine and human corneocytes. *Veterinary Dermatology* 2008; **19**: 1–6.
3. Boguniewicz M, Leung D. Recent insights into atopic dermatitis and implications for management of infectious complications. *Journal of Allergy and Clinical Immunology* 2010; **125**: 4–13.
4. Patel A. Bacterial pyoderma. In: August JR, ed. *Consultations in Feline Internal Medicine*, Vol. 5. Missouri, USA: Elsevier Saunders, 2006: 251–259.
5. Abraham JL, Morris DO, Griffeth GC, *et al.* Surveillance of healthy cats and cats with inflammatory skin disease for colonization of the skin by meticillin-resistant coagulase-positive staphylococci and *Staphylococcus schleiferi* ssp. *schleiferi*. *Veterinary Dermatology* 2007; **18**: 252–259.
6. Wildermuth BE, Griffin CE, Rosenkrantz WS. Response of feline eosinophilic plaques and lip ulcers to amoxicillin trihydrate-clavulanate potassium therapy: a randomized, double-blind placebo-controlled prospective study. *Veterinary Dermatology* 2012; **23**: 110–118.
7. Colombo S, Scarampella F, Ordeix L, *et al.* Dermatophytosis and papular eosinophilic/mastocytic dermatitis (urticaria pigmentosa-like dermatitis) in three Devon rex cats. *Journal of Feline Medicine and Surgery* 2012; **14**: 498–502.
8. Ordeix L, Galeotti F, Scarampella F, *et al.* *Malassezia* spp. overgrowth in allergic cats. *Veterinary Dermatology* 2007; **18**: 316–323.
9. Chen T, Hill P. The biology of *Malassezia* organisms and their ability to induce immune response and skin disease. *Veterinary Dermatology* 2005; **16**: 4–26.
10. Ahman S, Perrins N, Bond R. Treatment of *Malassezia pachydermatis*-associated seborrhoeic dermatitis in Devon rex cats with itraconazole-a pilot study. *Veterinary Dermatology* 2007; **18**: 171–174.
11. Lappin MR. Infectious disease consequences in cats treated with cyclosporine. *Proceedings of the Continuing Education Programme, 7th World Congress of Veterinary Dermatology*, 2012: 408–413.

34

Diagnostic investigation of the allergic feline

William E. Oldenhoff and Karen A. Moriello

Department of Medical Sciences, School of Veterinary Medicine, University of Wisconsin–Madison, Madison, WI, USA

Conflict of Interest: Bill Oldenhoff received a research salary stipend from Delmont Laboratories and has received unrestricted gift monies from HESKA. Karen Moriello has received research funding from the Winn Foundation for Feline Research, American College of Veterinary Dermatology, Companion Animal Fund-University of Wisconsin, Industry Research Grants from Pfizer Animal Health, Alpharma, Novartis, and DVM/TEVA. Karen Moriello has been a consultant for HESKA Corporation and Bayer Corporation. In addition, she is co-editor of the journal of Veterinary Dermatology.

Introduction

Pruritic cats are a diagnostic challenge. Although the hallmark of allergic dermatitis is pruritus many other conditions can present in similar ways. A recent multicentre study investigating the aetiology of 'hypersensitivity' in more than 500 cats revealed that there was no one pattern or presentation classic to cats for allergic disease and the underlying cause could only be identified via the use of core diagnostic investigations and response to treatment trials [1]. The goal of this chapter is to outline a diagnostic protocol for pruritic cats. Unlike dogs, where most allergic dogs follow common patterns of dermatitis and pruritus [2,3], this is not the situation in the cat.

Key aspects of the history

Cat owners vary widely in their observational and historical contributions to the evaluation of pruritus in cats. This is in part because behaviours in cats, such as grooming, are considered normal and owners may not differentiate excessive grooming from 'meticulous care of his hair coat'. Unlike the situation in dogs, it is unlikely owners will have much information about littermates, although atopic dermatitis has been documented in a litter of kittens [4]. Key questions that an owner should answer include the life style of the cats (indoors or outdoors), number of cats in the home (affected and unaffected), whether or not the pruritus is acute or chronic (>2 months or repeated episodes), and whether all animals are currently receiving routine flea control.

Client education

One of the most challenging aspects of investigating the pruritic cat is managing the owner's preconceived expectations or prejudices for or against a particular disease. It cannot be emphasized enough that delay in diagnosis is due to haphazard diagnostics, lack of a plan, and lack of client cooperation. Visual aids that show the relative commonalities of causes are often helpful. (Figure 34.1 shows a pie graph of the causes of feline pruritus to make the point of starting with the most likely cause.)

Eliminate parasites. Skin scrapings, acetate tape preparations, trichogram, flea combing, or brushing to identify parasites, ear swabs for mites, and response to a treatment trial should be assessed.

In Hobi's study [1], flea allergy dermatitis (FAD) was the most common hypersensitivity dermatosis of cats; however, when all of the data were carefully examined,

Veterinary Allergy, First Edition. Edited by Chiara Noli, Aiden Foster, and Wayne Rosenkrantz.

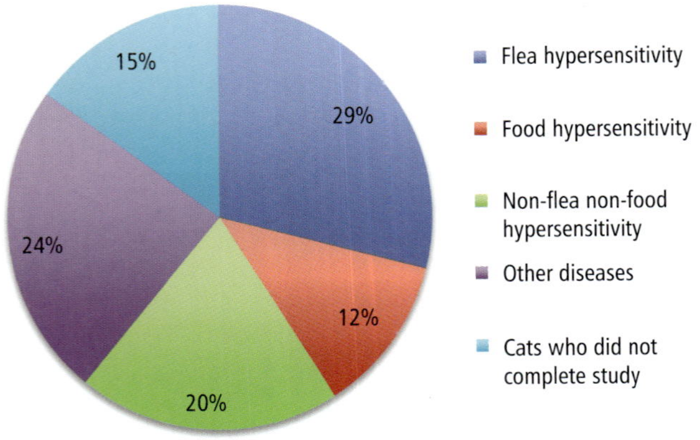

Figure 34.1 Causes of pruritus in 502 cats (Hobi *et al.* 2011 [1]).

parasitic causes of pruritus accounted for almost 39% of pruritus in 502 cats (Figure 34.1). The largest subgroup (29%) consisted of cats with FAD and the remaining was caused by other parasites. This emphasizes two major points of discussion with owners. First, the diagnosis of FAD is often made via a response to a treatment trial and, given the high percentage of cats with FAD, this is a cost-effective step in the investigation of the pruritic cat. Second, routine diagnostic tests such as skin scrapings, ear swab cytology, coat brushings, and faecal examinations are important for any cat with acute or, especially, chronic pruritus.

Although FAD commonly presents as miliary dermatitis of the dorsal midline and tail base, it can also manifest as head and neck excoriations, eosinophilic diseases, or symmetrical alopecia [1]. The variable appearance of FAD underscores the importance of flea prevention in all pruritic cats. Fleas can be particularly difficult to identify because cats will remove and ingest fleas through grooming. Identification of *Dipylidium caninum* segments in the perineal area suggests flea exposure because fleas are an intermediate host for this tapeworm. A positive reaction to flea saliva on intradermal testing is useful to demonstrate flea exposure but does not prove current clinical disease [5]. FcE-RI based ELISA testing is available and demonstrated an 82% predictive value when compared to intradermal testing [6].

Because flea allergy dermatitis is a true hypersensitivity disorder, a small population of fleas can cause a pruritus flare in cats with FAD. A variety of effective topical products are available and monthly usage should be recommended for all animals in the household of a pruritic cat. Many owners are reluctant to pursue a flea control for two reasons. First is the 'it is not fleas, I do not see fleas' attitude and second is concern over the repeated use of pesticides. Both issues require client education and selection of products with a high margin of therapeutic safety. Clients must be assured of the safety of these products and clinicians must ensure that clients understand that a cat may present with FAD without direct evidence of fleas in the household. Please refer to Chapter 41 for more information on flea control.

Table 34.1 Guidelines for intradermal testing with fluorescein

1. Sedate the cat using a sedative that does not interfere with intradermal test results†
2. Shave lateral thorax, mark the injection sites in a grid pattern with a permanent marker pen
3. Inject 5 mg/kg i.v. fluorescein
4. Administer saline, histamine, and allergens via intradermal injections
5. Measure the diameter of injection sites between 5 and 20 minutes after injection*

† Drug availability varies by country. Drugs that have antihistaminic activity or profound vasodilatory activity, such as acepromazine, should be avoided. The authors use the following drug combination in their practice:
Butorphanol: 0.2–0.4 mg/kg
Dexmedetomidine: 2.0–5.0 μg/kg
Ketamine: 2 mg/kg
These drugs are then administered intravenously.
* In the authors' experience, positive IDT reactions in cats often do not persist as long as those in dogs. It is standard practice to stop after half of the allergens have been injected and score the test and then again at the end of the procedure. Positive IDT reactions can be scored objectively or subjectively depending upon the clinician.

Otodectes will often respond to common flea control products; however, if head and neck pruritus are prominent, additional otic parasiticidal therapy is warranted. In general, mites such as *Notoedres*, *Sarcoptes* (rare but with regional variation), and *Cheyletiella* spp. are very responsive to flea-related products or the use of other protocols (Table 34.1), as are lice such as *Felicola subrostratus*. *Demodex gatoi* can cause severe pruritus and it can be easy or difficult to find mites depending upon the case. Diagnosis via response to treatment trial is not uncommon.

Wide superficial skin scrapings, faecal flotations, hair trichograms, and evidence of contagion may be helpful in making a definitive diagnosis of a parasitic infestation. Much like the situation in dogs with *Sarcoptes*, parasitic causes of pruritus are important to rule out before pursing expensive and time consuming 'allergy' diagnostics. While some of these mites can be difficult to identify, there are several treatment regimens that have been described to rule out contagious ectoparasites. The reader is directed to other sources that discuss treatment regimens for the different contagious parasites [7,8]. Treatment regimens may vary by geographic locale due to regulations and product labelling in different countries. Typically, this may rely on topical application of products containing fipronil, imidacloprid, moxidectin, and selamectin, amongst others.

Rule out 'other' causes of pruritus. This includes a physical examination focusing on both dermatologic and non-dermatologic causes, skin cytology, Wood's lamp examination, direct examination of hairs, fungal culture, and collection of skin biopsies.

In Hobi's study [1], diseases other than parasites were common causes of pruritus. Although parasites are the most common cause of pruritus, the initial history and physical examination may reveal that the cause is a non-parasitic, non-hypersensitivity aetiology such as dermatophytosis, autoimmune, or neoplastic conditions. The clinician's acumen, not a diagnostic flow chart, is more important.

Of note is the recent recognition that bacterial and yeast overgrowth may be causes of pruritus in cats, in association with an underlying trigger. A study has highlighted the importance of bacteria in the pathogenesis of eosinophilic plaques [9]. In the study, cats with eosinophilic plaques and/or lip ulcers were treated solely with amoxicillin trihydrate/clavulonate potassium. Cats with eosinophilic plaques had significant reduction in lesion size compared with the placebo group.

The recognition of *Malassezia* overgrowth as a contributing cause of pruritus has been increasing [10,11]. Clinical signs consistent with yeast overgrowth include erythema, greasy scales, and excessive cerumen. The classic clinical signs of yeast overgrowth in the dog, hyperpigmentation and lichenification, are not frequently observed in the cat [10]. Yeast organisms may be difficult to identify via cytological skin impression smears from a normal cat. The contribution of microbial overgrowth to pruritus may not be determined except by response to treatment trial (see Chapter 33).

After eliminating parasites and infections as causes of pruritus, the diagnosis is likely a food or environmental hypersensitivity. Attempts have been made to produce criteria for the diagnosis of non-flea hypersensitivity in cats. Favrot and others [12] identified the following criteria that can be used as an aid in the diagnosis of the pruritic cat:

- At least two body parts involved
- At least two of the following clinical presentations:
  - symmetrical alopecia
  - eosinophilic dermatitis
  - erosions on head and neck
  - miliary dermatitis
- Symmetrical alopecia
- Any lesion on the lips
- Erosions or ulcerations on chin or neck
- No lesions on the dorsal trunk
- Absence of non-symmetrical alopecia on back and tail
- Absence of nodules or tumours.

The presence of five of these eight diagnostic criteria gives 75% sensitivity and 76% specificity for the diagnosis of non-flea hypersensitivity. It is important to note that these criteria are unable to distinguish between food hypersensitivity and environmental hypersensitivity. The clinician's acumen and skill is the most important tool for diagnosing hypersensitivity in cats.

Rule out food allergy. An elimination diet trial should be carried out to investigate food allergy.

The prevalence of food allergy in the cat is unknown. In Hobi's study [1] it was 12%; however, it is important to note that the participants were from referral practices. The true prevalence in cats based on combined primary and referral care populations is unknown. However, the authors strongly recommended performing a food trial prior to pursuing testing for allergic disease in any cat with non-seasonal pruritus.

Cats with food allergy can be clinically indistinguishable from cats with environmental allergies [1,12]. Attempts to develop criteria to distinguish food-allergic cats from environmentally allergic cats have not been successful thus far [12].

Food allergies can develop at any age. Hobi *et al.* [1] found that the mean age of initial signs was the same with food-allergic and environmentally allergic cats, with most cats exhibiting initial signs prior to 3 years of age. However, 26% of food-allergic cats experienced their first clinical signs after 6 years of age, in contrast to only 12% of environmentally allergic cats. The study also found that food-allergic cats were presented more frequently with gastrointestinal signs, although this still only accounted for 21% of food-allergic cats. Although food-allergic cats may be clinically indistinguishable from environmentally allergic cats, it is reported that cats with food allergy exhibit lesions of the head, face, and neck more frequently, although this is clearly not diagnostic for food allergies [1].

The only way to diagnose food allergies is through an appropriate elimination diet trial. To date, there is no *in vitro* diagnostic test to identify food allergies. The gold standard considered by many clinicians is a home-cooked novel protein diet. In reality, there is no such thing as a truly 'hypoallergenic' protein source [13]. One must pick a protein source that the cat has never been exposed to; so, a thorough dietary history is needed. The current trend among commercial over-the-counter diets is to include a variety of exotic protein sources such as salmon, duck, venison, bison, etc. As a result, it has become increasingly difficult to find a true 'novel' protein that is appropriate for an elimination trial. Furthermore, one needs an owner who is willing to cook for their cat and a cat that is willing to eat the home-cooked diet. Owing to these difficulties, many owners pursue commercially available diets for diagnosing food allergies. Alternatives to the home-cooked novel protein diet are the commercial novel protein diets and the commercial hydrolysed diets.

There are caveats that should be kept in mind when choosing a commercial elimination diet trial. Commercial novel protein diets should be prescription diets obtained from the veterinarian. Many over-the-counter, apparently novel protein dry dog foods contain detectable levels of contaminant proteins that are not listed among the ingredients [14]. One should assume this is the case for cat food as well, highlighting the fact that over-the-counter 'novel protein' foods are not appropriate to diagnose food allergies. Again, a thorough dietary history is indicated.

Hydrolysed protein diets have proteins that are broken down to smaller peptides in order to reduce allergenicity [13]. In theory, these peptides are too small to elicit an immune response. In practice, there is variability to the size of protein molecules in hydrolysed diets [15]. Additionally, if the animal is sensitive to the native protein, it may also be sensitive to the hydrolysed diet made from the native protein [16]. Thus, a thorough dietary history is also important for choosing the correct hydrolysed diet. Historically, many authors consider hydrolysed diets to be unpalatable [15,17,18]. In the authors' experience, most cats will accept hydrolysed diets.

The diet trial should initially be conducted for a minimum of 6 to 8 weeks. Considerable debate exists in the veterinary literature about the duration of a diet trial [13,18]. In animals with gastrointestinal manifestations of food allergy, improvement in gastrointestinal signs may be seen within a few days of starting a diet trial [19]. If improvement is seen with the diet trial, an adverse reaction is diagnosed by relapse upon challenging with the old diet.

Clearly there is no such thing as the perfect elimination diet trial. If there is strong suspicion of food allergy and the cat does not respond to one diet trial, a second diet trial to definitively rule out food allergy is indicated.

Environmental allergy

If infections, parasites, and food allergies have been ruled out and pruritus remains, then the likely diagnosis is environmental allergies. As stated previously, pruritic cats can be presented with several different clinical manifestations (miliary dermatitis, eosinophilic disease, self-induced symmetrical alopecia, head/neck pruritus). None of these patterns is considered to be diagnostic for environmental allergies [1,12]. The diagnostic criteria for environmental allergies in the cat is elimination of other causes of pruritus (especially adverse reactions to food), compatible clinical signs, and response to glucocorticoids, ciclosporin, or antihistamines [1].

Allergic skin disease due to environmental allergens is a clinical diagnosis; 'allergy' testing is potentially useful for identifying causative sensitivities in a cat that has a clinically sound diagnosis of allergic skin disease. This is illustrated by several studies that demonstrate that even normal healthy cats can have 'positive allergy test' results using commercially available *in vitro* tests [20–23]. Thus, the main indication for such 'allergy' testing is to identify relevant allergens for immunotherapy. Two main testing types are available: intradermal tests and serum tests.

Intradermal testing is useful in many species but the thin skin of the cat, as well as the transient, often poor, wheal formation may limit its use. The use of fluorescein can significantly improve the ability to identify positive reactions [24,25]. The protocol we recommend for fluorescein use is modified from Kadoya-Minegishi *et al.* 2002 [24] and can be found in Table 34.1.

Fluorescein use and measurement of wheal diameters have been associated with high intertest and intraobserver agreement [25]. Intravenous fluorescein use in the cat is considered to be safe because there is only one report in the literature of an adverse event [26].

There are many commercial companies offering *in vitro* tests and variable methodologies to measure IgE; however, discussion of each test is beyond the scope of this chapter. These tests are attractive because they are easier to perform than intradermal tests. The most widely used and studied *in vitro* test is an ELISA that utilizes the cloned alpha chain of the human high affinity IgE receptor (FcE-RI). Immunotherapy can be formulated based on the results of intradermal or serum testing. The reader is directed to Chapter 36 for more details on immunotherapy in the cat.

Owing to the many potential causes of pruritus, a stepwise approach to the pruritic cat is indicated. This can take time and requires a degree of patience from the client, but ultimately this provides the best patient care and is most cost effective. Excellent client communication is imperative in order to set proper expectations for their pet's care.

References

1. Hobi S, Linek M, Marignac G, *et al.* Clinical characteristics and causes of pruritus in cats: a multicentre study on feline

hypersensitivity-associated dermatoses. *Veterinary Dermatology* 2011; **22**: 406–413.
2. Favrot C, Steffan J, Seewald W, *et al.* A prospective study on the clinical features of chronic canine atopic dermatitis and its diagnosis. *Veterinary Dermatology* 2010; **21**: 23–31.
3. Wilhem S, Kovalik M, Favrot C. Breed-associated phenotypes in canine atopic dermatitis. *Veterinary Dermatology* 2011; **22**: 143–149.
4. Moriello KA. Feline atopy in three littermates. *Veterinary Dermatology* 2001; **12**: 177–181.
5. Moriello KA, McMurdy MA. The prevalence of positive intradermal skin test reactions to flea extract in clinically normal cats. *Companion Animal Practice* 1989; **19**: 298–302.
6. McCall C, Stedman K, Bevier D, *et al.* Correlation of Feline IgE, determined by FceR1α-Based ELISA technology, and IDST to *Ctenocephalides felis* salivary antigens in a feline model of flea bite allergic dermatitis. *Compendium on Continuing Education for the Practicing Veterinarian* 1997; **19**: 29–32.
7. Fisher MA, Shanks DJ. A review of the off-label use of selamectin (Stronghold/Revolution) in dogs and cats. *Acta Veterinaria Scandinavia* 2008; **50**: 46.
8. Merola VM, Eubig PA. Toxicology of avermectins and milbemycins (macrocylic lactones) and the role of P-glycoprotein in dogs and cats. *Veterinary Clinics of North America: Small Animal Practice* 2012; **42**: 313–333.
9. Wildermuth BE, Griffin CE, Rosenkrantz WS. Response of feline eosinophilic plaques and lip ulcers to amoxicillin trihydrate–clavulanate potassium therapy: a randomized, double-blind placebo-controlled prospective study. *Veterinary Dermatology* 2012; **23**: 110–e25.
10. Ordeix L, Galeotti F, Scarampella F, *et al.* Malassezia spp. overgrowth in allergic cats. *Veterinary Dermatology* 2007; **18**: 316–323.
11. Bond R. Superficial veterinary mycoses. *Clinics in Dermatology* 2010; **28**: 226–236.
12. Favrot C, Steffan J, Seewald W, *et al.* Establishment of diagnostic criteria for feline nonflea-induced hypersensitivity dermatitis. *Veterinary Dermatology* 2012; **23**: 45–50, e11.
13. Verlinden A, Hesta M, Millet S, *et al.* Food allergy in dogs and cats: a review. *Critical Reviews in Food Science and Nutrition* 2006; **46**: 259–273.
14. Raditic DM, Remillard RL, Tater KC. ELISA testing for common food antigens in four dry dog foods used in dietary elimination trials. *Journal of Animal Physiology and Animal Nutrition* 2011; **95**: 90–97.
15. Cave NJ. Hydrolyzed protein diets for dogs and cats. *Veterinary Clinics of North America: Small Animal Practice* 2006; **36**: 1251–1268.
16. Ricci R, Hammerberg B, Paps J, *et al.* A comparison of the clinical manifestations of feeding whole and hydrolysed chicken to dogs with hypersensitivity to the native protein. *Veterinary Dermatology* 2010; **21**: 358–366.
17. Bryan J, Frank LA. Food allergy in the cat: a diagnosis by elimination. *Journal of Feline Medicine and Surgery* 2010; **12**: 861–866.
18. Miller WH, Griffin CE, Campbell KL. In: *Muller and Kirk's Small Animal Dermatology*, 7th edn. Elsevier Mosby: St. Louis, 2013, p. 402.
19. Guilford WG, Jones BR, Markwell PJ, *et al.* Food sensitivity in cats with chronic idiopathic gastrointestinal problems. *Journal of Veterinary Internal Medicine* 2001; **15**: 7–13.
20. Diesel A, DeBoer DJ. Serum allergen-specific immunoglobulin E in atopic and healthy cats: comparison of a rapid screening immunoassay and complete-panel analysis. *Veterinary Dermatology* 2011; **22**: 39–45.
21. Bexley J, Hogg JE, Hammerberg B, *et al.* Levels of house dust mite-specific serum immunoglobulin E (IgE) in different cat populations using a monoclonal based anti-IgE enzyme-linked immunosorbent assay. *Veterinary Dermatology* 2009; **20**: 562–568.
22. Gilbert S, Halliwell REW. Feline immunoglobulin E: induction of antigen-specific antibody in normal cats and levels in spontaneously allergic cats. *Veterinary Immunology and Immunopathology* 1998; **63**: 235–252.
23. Taglinger K, Helps CR, Day MJ, *et al.* Measurement of serum immunoglobulin E (IgE) specific for house dust mite antigens in normal cats and cats with allergic skin disease. *Veterinary Immunology Immunopathology* 2005; **105**: 85–93.
24. Kadoya-Minegishi M, Park SJ, Sekiguchi M, *et al.* The use of fluorescein as a contrast medium to enhance intradermal skin tests in cats. *Australian Veterinary Journal* 2002; **80**: 702–703.
25. Schleifer SG, Willemse T. Evaluation of skin test reactivity to environmental allergens in healthy cats and cats with atopic dermatitis. *American Journal of Veterinary Research* 2003; **64**: 773–778.
26. Davidson M, Baty K. Anaphylaxis associated with intravenous fluorescein administration in a cat. *Progress in Veterinary and Comparative Ophthalmology* 1991; **1**: 127–128.

35

Symptomatic treatments

Alison B. Diesel

Department of Small Animal Clinical Sciences, College of Veterinary Medicine and Biomedical Sciences, Texas A&M University, College Station, TX, USA

Conflict of interest: none declared.

Although controversy exists in regard to the comparative pathogenesis of canine atopic dermatitis and feline cutaneous allergies (also referred to as non-flea, non-food hypersensitivity dermatitis), the principles and practices of managing allergic skin disease in cats and dogs remains somewhat similar. Therapy is typically tailored to the individual based on severity and duration of clinical signs, owner preference, and taking into account patient disposition. Compared to dogs, few controlled studies have been performed in cats with cutaneous allergies; much of the information presented throughout the literature with regard to disease management has been based on anecdotal findings, clinical preferences, the results of open-enrolment field trials, and case reports.

As in the dog, the goal of managing cutaneous allergies in cats is to minimize the presence and persistence of pruritus and other clinical manifestations of allergic skin disease (e.g. eosinophilic skin lesions). Attention should be paid to providing improved comfort and quality of life for the allergic cat. Identification of flare factors and secondary complications is just as important in the management of the allergic cat as it is in the management of the allergic dog. Each individual animal has a specific hypersensitivity threshold; this threshold is defined by the level of stimuli that results in clinical signs associated with pruritus or other manifestations of cutaneous allergy [1,2]. Pruritus and manifestation of allergic skin disease is an additive process with contributions not only from the underlying allergy but also secondary pruritic conditions such as bacterial infection, yeast overgrowth, and parasitic infestation. Some factors are more important for certain cats than for others; determining which factors are present and may be aggravating underlying cutaneous allergy is central to developing a therapeutic plan for the individual patient.

Managing secondary pruritic conditions

Flea infestation

One of the more common reasons for a flare in cutaneous allergy in the cat is the secondary occurrence of flea infestation. This may be confirmed on physical examination by the presence of live fleas or flea faeces. Due to the fastidious grooming behaviour of most cats, however, evidence of fleas may not be readily found. It is not uncommon for a cat with cutaneous allergy to have concurrent flea allergy dermatitis. In geographic areas where fleas are considered to be endemic, it is recommended to initiate and maintain treatment with adulticidal flea prevention; this should be continued year-round to minimize infestation and flare (see Chapter 41).

Microbial overgrowth/infection

Historically, secondary bacterial overgrowth and pyoderma have been considered to be an uncommon to rare finding in cats with cutaneous allergy [3,4]. Other sources, however, suggest that feline pyoderma may be more prevalent than previously reported, particularly in cats with underlying allergic skin disease [5–7]. As with

Veterinary Allergy, First Edition. Edited by Chiara Noli, Aiden Foster, and Wayne Rosenkrantz.

bacterial skin infection, secondary *Malassezia* overgrowth has historically been considered uncommon to rare in cats with cutaneous allergy; the presence of *Malassezia* was more frequently attributed to severe underlying systemic illness [8,9]. More recent sources, however, suggest that yeast overgrowth may be more common than previously recognized in allergic cats [10].

For more information about the diagnosis and treatment of microbial infections see Chapter 33.

Allergen avoidance

From a practical standpoint, avoidance of environmental allergens is essentially impossible for most cats with cutaneous allergy. Cats are almost never allergic to allergens that can readily be avoided or eliminated from the environment, unless concurrent cutaneous adverse reaction to food exists or food has previously been determined to be a contributing flare factor. As with dogs and people, house dust mite is considered to be an important and common environmental allergen in cats with cutaneous allergy. Although frequently recommended as an adjunct therapy, practices designed to reduce the number of house dust mites in the environment (e.g. regular and improved ventilation with allergen-reducing filters, utilizing insecticides and insect growth regulators in resting areas, steam cleaning and frequent washing of bedding in hot water, etc.) are generally not effective on their own for managing the allergic feline patient. For more information on allergen avoidance see Chapter 11.

Medical management of cutaneous allergy

In the absence of secondary complications, options for management of cutaneous allergy in cats include the use of medication and/or allergen-specific immunotherapy. The latter will be discussed further in the next chapter. Medical options for cutaneous allergy include administration of essential fatty acids (EFA), antihistamines, glucocorticoids, and ciclosporin.

Essential fatty acids

The benefits of essential fatty acid supplementation have been assessed in several older studies on cats with allergic skin disease; various preparations have been evaluated with regards to their effects on lesion improvement and reduction in pruritus [11–17]. Most of the studies, however, were not controlled nor randomized with unclear inclusion and exclusion criteria. Although the responses were variable among all of the studies, clinical improvement was reported for most cats with regard to lesion resolution and pruritus reduction; statistical significance, however, was questionable. In dogs with atopic dermatitis, the benefits of EFA appear to contribute to skin barrier function restoration [18,19]; barrier function has become increasingly important with regard to managing the atopic canine patient. Although this has not been investigated thoroughly, defects in cutaneous barrier function may also contribute to feline cutaneous allergy; preliminary data on transepidermal water loss from the skin of normal cats may well help future assessment of cats with allergic skin disease [20]. Whether clinical improvement from EFA supplementation in cats with cutaneous allergy is related to improved barrier function, the anti-inflammatory effects of fatty acids [21], or simply an improved quality of overall hair coat is uncertain. The relative safety of EFA supplementation (occasional vomiting is the only reported side effect), however, makes this option appealing as part of the management strategy for the allergic cat. Their proposed synergistic effects with antihistamines [12] may also provide an option for conservative medical therapy, particularly in the mildly affected allergic cat. Various dosing formulations exist, which may be added to the food (capsule, oil, spray) or potentially applied topically; efficacy should be assessed after at least 4 to 6 weeks of administration.

Antihistamines

As in dogs, antihistamines show variable efficacy overall for the management of pruritus and cutaneous lesions in cats with allergic skin disease; success has been reported anywhere from 20 to 73%. Table 35.1 lists several antihistamines that have been used in cats for the management of cutaneous allergy. Most of the information is anecdotal or based on open trials. A single randomized, double-blinded, placebo-controlled, crossover study evaluated cetirizine administration in cats with mild to moderate cutaneous allergy; no improvement was noted, however, in the population at the dose evaluated [22]. Anecdotally, antihistamines may be more efficacious in cats with both cutaneous allergy and allergic asthma. It is important to remember, however, that every animal is different; an antihistamine that is beneficial for one animal may not be beneficial for another and vice versa. Typically, it is recommended to trial antihistamine administration for at least 2 to 3 weeks to determine efficacy. Sequential administration of different antihistamines is often necessary to find the best option in a particular patient [23–25]. The relatively mild and infrequent side effects make antihistamine administration a reasonable option to consider, especially in patients with mild allergic disease. As with EFA, antihistamines may work synergistically with other therapeutic options (EFA, glucocorticoids) to allow for

Table 35.1 Antihistamines used in the management of feline cutaneous allergy

Antihistamine	Dosage	Side effects
Clemastine	0.25–0.68 mg/cat per o.s., twice daily	Diarrhoea, lethargy, fixed drug eruption
Hydroxyzine	5–10 mg/cat p.o., twice or three times a day	Behavioural changes (hyperexcitability, depression), teratogenic
Chlorpheniramine	2–4 mg/cat p.o., once, twice, or three times a day	Transient drowsiness, unpalatable (bitter)
Cyproheptadine	2 mg/cat p.o., twice daily	Polyphagia, behavioural changes, vocalization, vomiting, sedation, increased affection
Fexofenadine	30–60 mg/cat p.o., once daily 2 mg/kg p.o., once or twice daily	
Diphenhydramine	2–4 mg/cat p.o., twice daily 1–2 mg/kg p.o., twice or three times a day	Unpalatable (liquid form = alcohol based)
Cetirizine	1 mg/kg p.o., once daily 5 mg/cat p.o., once daily	
Amitriptyline	5–10 mg/cat p.o., once or twice daily	

Adapted in part from Vidémont and Pin 2009, Jackson and Foster 2006, and Scott and Miller 1999 [8,23–25].

improved efficacy and potential dose reduction of additional medication.

Glucocorticoids

One of the most commonly utilized treatments for cats with cutaneous allergy is the administration of glucocorticoids. Indeed, until recently, steroids were considered to be a 'mainstay' of therapy for most allergic cats [23]. Their highly effective nature in most cats still keeps glucocorticoids high on the list of options for rapid resolution of an allergic flare. For cats with seasonal manifestation of allergy, lasting only a few months, steroids are considered to be a very reasonable choice for maintenance therapy. Although glucocorticoids are typically tolerated better by cats than dogs, with fewer adverse effects reported even with long-term administration [26], they are not without risk and may become less effective with regards to disease management over time (tachyphylaxis). Side effects of glucocorticoid administration in cats include polydipsia, polyuria, diabetes mellitus, weight gain, cutaneous atrophy, hyperadrenocorticism with skin fragility syndrome, congestive heart failure, and urinary tract infections [26]. The obese feline patient is particularly at risk for development of irreversible diabetes mellitus secondary to glucocorticoid administration; caution should be exercised with steroid administration (particularly injections or high doses) in these cases.

Formulation options for glucocorticoids include injections, oral medication, and topical preparations. Although topical therapy is used less frequently in allergic cats than in dogs due to their fastidious grooming behaviour, the availability of rapidly absorbed products makes this option more appealing. Efficacy has been shown with the administration of 0.0584% hydrocortisone aceponate spray in the management of feline allergic skin disease [27]; this compound acts specifically in the epidermis with minimal to no systemic absorption (metabolized in the skin). Care must be taken though with frequent application at the same spot as cutaneous atrophy has been reported with repeated use [28]. Although the product is currently not licensed for use in cats, it appeared to be well tolerated, safe, and effective in the population treated. Oral preparations are generally preferred by many dermatologists over injectable formulations due to the ability to taper the dose of medication over time. Most of the dosing recommendations are based on clinical experience and extrapolated from canine studies. Cats respond more favourably to prednisolone than to the prodrug prednisone; the latter is not nearly as bioavailable and is ineffectively metabolized by most cats due to their relatively poor glucuronidation ability [26]. Prednisolone or methylprednisolone is typically dosed orally 1–2 mg/kg per day to initiate therapy, then tapered to 0.5–1.0 mg/kg every 48 hours for maintenance; dosing for glucocorticoids is generally higher in cats compared to dogs to achieve the same clinical effect. Alternatively, dexamethasone administered 0.1–0.2 mg/kg every 3 days (or less) may be effective for many patients.

Triamcinolone is also used fairly commonly; dosing is generally initiated at 0.1–0.2 mg/kg per day, and then tapered to every 48–72 hours for maintenance. In earlier literature, there was a great deal of variability with regards to the relative potency of triamcinolone compared to other glucocorticoids. A more recent study, however, determined triamcinolone to be approximately seven times as potent as methylprednisolone in allergic cats [29].

In general, it is recommended to taper the dose of steroid over time to the minimal effective dose that maintains relative comfort in the patient. This will decrease the risks of adverse effects, especially for long-term administration. Although there is no rhyme or reason, many practitioners start the dose taper approximately 7 to 10 days after initiating therapy. The goal is to achieve the lowest possible alternate day (or less) dose in the patient that maintains comfort. When longer-duration steroids are used, the interval between medication administrations can be extended further.

Intolerance of oral medication is a frequent treatment consideration for allergic cats; many cats are rather resentful of being administered pills on a frequent basis. Injectable therapy is typically used in such cases; however, care must be exercised in these cases as repeated injections (especially repository formulations) can increase the chance for development of diabetes mellitus and skin fragility syndrome. When frequent, repeated injections are necessary to control allergic skin disease, alternative therapies with fewer side effects (e.g. oral ciclosporin) should be considered. Methylprednisolone acetate is one of the most commonly used injectable glucocorticoid preparations in allergic cats; treatment has been successful at 20 mg/cat (4 mg/kg) administered every 2 to 3 weeks for a total of three injections. Although either subcutaneous or intramuscular injection is acceptable and effective, some clinicians prefer the intramuscular route to avoid the potential for injection site reactions [30]. Often, an initial positive response is reported, which is followed by a decrease in therapeutic benefit; this typically results in administration of higher doses at more frequent intervals, thereby increasing the risk of adverse effects. In cases where this phenomenon (called tachyphylaxis) occurs, it is recommended to reassess therapeutic options as this is not considered to be adequate long-term management in cats with cutaneous allergies.

Ciclosporin

More recently, ciclosporin has gained favour for the medical management of cutaneous allergy in cats. A liquid formulation is labelled and approved for the treatment of feline cutaneous allergy; it is available in the United States, Europe, and Japan (Atopica® for Cats, Novartis Animal Health). This microemulsion formulation of ciclosporin (often referred to as ciclosporin (modified)) has more predictable pharmacokinetics and is more bioavailable in dogs and cats. Ciclosporin, especially compared to glucocorticoids, has more specific anti-inflammatory effects with regards to the treatment of cutaneous allergy. This calcineurin inhibitor is a potent effector of cell-mediated immunity, having more targeted effects on T lymphocytes; the drug stabilizes mast cells and eosinophils and decreases cytokine production and adhesion by keratinocytes and endothelial cells [31].

Ciclosporin has been shown to be effective when, initially, dosed at 5–10 mg/kg once daily for cats [32,33]. The manufacturer recommends dosing at 7 mg/kg once daily. As compared to glucocorticoids, ciclosporin takes several days to achieve therapeutic concentrations in the serum; clinical improvement is typically reported between 2 and 3 weeks. After about 4 to 6 weeks, the medication appears to reach a steady state, at which time the dose may be tapered in most patients. Most practitioners have found that the majority of cats with cutaneous allergy can be maintained at the same dose (5–10 mg/kg) on alternate days without a relapse of clinical signs. In some cases, the dose may be tapered even further; anecdotally, some cats can be maintained on twice-weekly administration for long-term management. This additional dose reduction is typically attempted after at least 2 months on alternate-day dosing. Although somewhat unpalatable, the liquid formulation of ciclosporin can be mixed with and administered in food; this does not appear to affect the clinical response in cats [34]. Up to one-third of cats will ingest the ciclosporin when mixed into food; the other two-thirds may require direct oral administration. If hypersalivation occurs following administration, a syringe of fresh water can be dispensed into the mouth.

Compared to glucocorticoids, ciclosporin appears to be tolerated relatively well for the long-term management of feline cutaneous allergy [35]. Gastrointestinal upset (vomiting, diarrhoea, decreased appetite) are reported most frequently and are more common during initiation of therapy [36]. Although no clinical studies exist, there is concern for an increased risk of contracting viral diseases (FeLV, FIV) in cats being administered ciclosporin. Fatal toxoplasmosis has been reported in a few cats treated with ciclosporin [37,38]; seroconversion of toxoplasma antibody titres has been reported in the absence and presence of clinical illness. In general, it is recommended that cats being managed with ciclosporin for cutaneous allergy have serology evaluated for toxoplasma and FeLV/FIV prior to initiating therapy and periodically during treatment. If IgM titres are greater than 1 : 64, this is potentially indicative of active toxoplasma infection. Increasing IgG titres (persistently high titres, or increase by fourfold or greater) is indicative of seroconversion; this would be seen in cases where cats have previously been exposed to toxoplasma but they were not actively infected. When seroconversion or significant increases in toxoplasma antibody titres are noted (either IgG or IgM) along with clinical signs of infection, therapy for toxoplasmosis should be initiated immediately. Scavenging, hunting, and consuming raw or undercooked meat should also be discouraged. For cats that are allowed to go outside and cannot be kept indoors, the application of one or two bells around the neck should make it impossible for them to successfully hunt.

Other therapeutic options

Older therapeutics, which have fallen out of favour for the management of feline cutaneous allergy, include progestagens (e.g. megestrol acetate), gold salts, and chlorambucil. No trials evaluated any of these options; response was generally variable and required careful monitoring. With the availability of safer treatments, these options should no longer be considered for the allergic cat.

Other therapeutics, however, may have potential, especially when more standard therapy has not shown beneficial results. An analogue of palmitoylethanolimide, named palmidrol, which binds cannabinoid receptors on mast cells, has been evaluated for the treatment of eosinophilic lesions; beneficial results were noted in several cats; however, this option requires further evaluation [39]. Tyrosine kinase inhibitors have been beneficial for the treatment of canine atopic dermatitis; these options may likewise prove effective in cats although studies have yet to be published. In cats with more recalcitrant eosinophilic lesions (eosinophilic granuloma, indolent ulcer), low-dose radiation therapy has also been anecdotally successful; however, again, studies are necessary to evaluate long-term and comparative efficacy. Laser ablation has also been reported successful for recalcitrant eosinophilic lesions in cats, particularly in difficult to manage locations (e.g. oral cavity) [40]; this modality may be considered where standard therapy has not been effective although studies are necessary to document efficacy for long-term control.

As in dogs with atopic dermatitis, the management of clinical signs of cutaneous allergy in cats requires careful consideration of the various therapeutic options. More conservative, safer options should be considered first, particularly if clinical signs are relatively mild. Care must be taken to monitor adverse reactions and side effects of long-term administration of glucocorticoids or ciclosporin. A combination of therapeutics is often necessary in the allergic cat to achieve the most beneficial results; there is no single best option for allergy management in any species.

References

1. Halliwell REW. Pathogenesis and treatment of pruritus. *Journal of the American Veterinary Medical Association* 1974; **164**: 793–796.
2. Scott DW, Miller WH. Medical management of allergic pruritus in the cat, with emphasis on feline atopy. *Journal of the South African Veterinary Association* 1993; **62**: 103–108.
3. Scott DW, Miller WH, Griffin CE. Skin immune system and allergic skin diseases. In: *Small Animal Dermatology*, 6th edn. Philadelphia PA: WB Saunders, 2001: 601–608.
4. Marsella R, Olivry T. Animal models of atopic dermatitis. *Clinical Dermatology* 2003; **21**: 122–133.
5. Yu HW, Vogelnest LJ. Feline superficial pyoderma: a retrospective study of 52 cases (2001–2011). *Veterinary Dermatology* 2012; **23**: 448–e86.
6. Wildermuth BE, Griffin CE, Rosenkrantz WS. Response of feline eosinophilic plaques and lip ulcers to amoxicillin trihydrate-clavulanate potassium therapy: a randomized, double-blind placebo-controlled prospective study. *Veterinary Dermatology* 2011; **23**: 110–e25.
7. Wildermuth BE, Griffin CE, Rosenkrantz WS. Feline pyoderma therapy. *Clinical Techniques in Small Animal Practice* 2006; **21**: 150–156.
8. Mauldin EA, Morris DO, Goldschmidt MH. Retrospective study: the presence of *Malassezia* in feline skin biopsies. A clinicopathological study. *Veterinary Dermatology* 2002; **13**: 7–13.
9. Sierra P, Guillot J, Jacob H, *et al.* Fungal flora on cutaneous and mucosal surfaces of cats infected with feline immunodeficiency virus or feline leukemia virus. *American Journal of Veterinary Research* 2000; **61**: 158–161.
10. Ordeix L, Galeotti F, Scarampella F, *et al. Malassezia* spp. overgrowth in allergic cats. *Veterinary Dermatology* 2007; **18**: 316–323.
11. Lechowski R, Sawosz E, Klucinski W. The effect of the addition of oil preparation with increased content of n-3 fatty acids on serum lipid profile and clinical condition of cats with miliary dermatitis. *Journal of Veterinary Medicine Series A-Physiology Pathology Clinical Medicine* 1998; **45**: 417–424.
12. Scott DW, Miller WH. The combination of an antihistamine (chlorpheniramine) and an omega-3/omega-6 fatty acid containing product for the management of pruritic cats—results of an open clinical-trial. *New Zealand Veterinary Journal* 1995; **43**: 29–31.
13. Miller WH, Scott DW, Wellington JR. Efficacy of DVM Derm Caps Liquid™ in the management of allergic and inflammatory dermatoses in the cat. *Journal of the American Animal Hospital Association* 1993; **29**: 37–40.
14. Logas DB, Kunkle GA. Double-blinded study examining the effects of evening primrose oil on feline pruritic dermatitis. *Veterinary Dermatology* 1993; **4**: 181–184.
15. Harvey RG. A comparison of evening primrose oil and sunflower oil for the management of papulocrustous dermatitis in cats. *Veterinary Record* 1993; **133**: 571–573.
16. Harvey RG. Effect of varying proportions of evening primrose oil and fish oil on cats with crusting dermatosis ('miliary dermatitis'). *Veterinary Record* 1993; **133**: 208–211.

17. Harvey RG. Management of feline miliary dermatitis by supplementing the diet with essential fatty acids. *Veterinary Record* 1991; **128**: 326–329.
18. Marsella R, Genovese D, Gilmer L, *et al.* Investigations on the effects of a topical ceramide and free fatty acid solution (Allerderm Spot-On) on clinical signs and skin barrier function in dogs with atopic dermatitis: a double-blinded, randomized, controlled study. *Veterinary Dermatology* 2012; **23** (Suppl. 1): 66–67.
19. Piekutowska A, Pin D, Rème CA, *et al.* Effects of a topically applied preparation of epidermal lipids on stratum corneum barrier of atopic dogs. *Journal of Comparative Pathology* 2008; **138**: 197–203.
20. Szczepanik MP, Wilkolek PM, Adamek LR, *et al.* The examination of biophysical parameters of skin (transepidermal water loss, skin hydration and pH value) in different body regions of normal cats of both sexes. *Journal of Feline Medicine and Surgery* 2011; **13**: 224–230.
21. Park HJ, Park JS, Hayek MG, *et al.* Dietary fish oil and flaxseed oil suppress inflammation and immunity in cats. *Veterinary Immunology and Immunopathology* 2011; **141**: 301–306.
22. Wildermuth K, Zabel S, Rosychuk RA. The efficacy of cetirizine hydrochloride on the pruritus and dermatitis of cats with mild to moderate atopic dermatitis; a randomized, double-blinded, placebo-controlled, cross-over study. *Veterinary Dermatology* 2012; **23** (Suppl. 1): 66.
23. Vidémont E, Pin D. How to treat atopy in cats? *European Journal of Companion Animal Practice* 2009; **19**: 276–282.
24. Jackson A, Foster A. Management of feline miliary dermatitis: a clinical update. *In Practice* 2006; **28**: 147–151.
25. Scott DW, Miller WH. Antihistamines in the management of allergic pruritus in dogs and cats. *Journal of Small Animal Practice* 1999; **40**: 359–364.
26. Lowe AD, Campbell KL, Graves T. Glucocorticoids in the cat. *Veterinary Dermatology* 2008; **19**: 340–347.
27. Schmidt V, Buckley LM, McEwan NA, *et al.* Efficacy of a 0.0584% hydrocortisone aceponate spray in presumed feline allergic dermatitis: an open label pilot study. *Veterinary Dermatology* 2011; **23**: 11–e4.
28. Bizikova P, Linder KE, Paps J, *et al.* Effect of a novel topical diester glucocorticoid spray on immediate- and late-phase cutaneous allergic reactions in Maltese–beagle atopic dogs: a placebo-controlled study. *Veterinary Dermatology* 2010; **21**: 71–80.
29. Ganz EC, Griffin CE, Keys DA, *et al.* Evaluation of methylprednisolone and triamcinolone for the induction and maintenance treatment of pruritus in allergic cats: a double-blinded, randomized, prospective study. *Veterinary Dermatology* 2012; **23**: 387–e72.
30. Foster A. Diagnosing and treating feline atopy. *Veterinary Medicine* 2002; **97**: 226–240.
31. Robson D. Review of the properties and mechanisms of action of cyclosporine with an emphasis on dermatological therapy in dogs, cats and people. *Veterinary Record* 2003; **152**: 758–772.
32. King S, Favrot C, Messinger L, *et al.* A randomized double-blinded placebo-controlled study to evaluate an effective ciclosporin dose for the treatment of feline hypersensitivity dermatitis. *Veterinary Dermatology* 2012; **23**: 440–e84.
33. Wisselink MA, Willemse T. The efficacy of cyclosporine A in cats with presumed atopic dermatitis: a double blind, randomized prednisolone-controlled study. *Veterinary Journal* 2009; **180**: 55–59.
34. Steffan J, King S, Seewald W. Ciclosporin efficacy in the treatment of feline hypersensitivity dermatitis is not influenced by the feeding status. *Veterinary Dermatology* 2012; **23** (Suppl. 1): 64–65.
35. King S, Van Lare KA, Heward JK. A six-month repeated-dose toxicity study of ciclosporin A oral solution in cats. *Veterinary Dermatology* 2012; **23** (Suppl. 1): 64.
36. Heinrich NA, McKeever PJ, Eisenschenk MC. Adverse events in 50 cats with allergic dermatitis receiving ciclosporin. *Veterinary Dermatology* 2011; **22**: 511–520.
37. Barrs VR, Martin P, Beatty JA. Antemortem diagnosis and treatment of toxoplasmosis in two cats on cyclosporine therapy. *Australian Veterinary Journal* 2006; **84**: 30–35.
38. Last RD, Suzuki Y, Manning T, *et al.* A case of fatal toxoplasmosis in a cat being treated with cyclosporine A for feline atopy. *Veterinary Dermatology* 2004; **15**: 194–198.
39. Scarampella F, Abramo F, Noli C. Clinical and histological evaluation of an analogue of palmitoylethanolamide, PLR 120 (comicronized Palmidrol INN) in cats with eosinophilic granuloma and eosinophilic plaque: a pilot study. *Veterinary Dermatology* 2001; **12**: 29–39.
40. Kovács K, Jakab C, Szász AM. Laser-assisted removal of a feline eosinophilic granuloma from the back of the tongue. *Acta Veterinaria Hungarica* 2009; **57**: 417–426.

36

Allergen-specific immunotherapy

Alison B. Diesel

Department of Small Animal Clinical Sciences, College of Veterinary Medicine and Biomedical Sciences, Texas A&M University, College Station, TX, USA

Conflict of interest: none declared.

As discussed in Chapter 35, the principles and practices of managing allergic skin disease in cats and dogs are similar despite differing opinions with regard to the pathogenesis of canine atopic dermatitis and feline cutaneous allergy. As there is no cure for allergy in any species; the goal of therapy is to minimize clinical signs associated with allergy, and provide improved comfort and enhanced quality of life. Therapeutic options are generally divided into medical options (as discussed in Chapter 35) and allergen-specific immunotherapy (ASIT); treatments may be used solely or in combination to provide the maximum clinical benefit. As with medical options, the decision to pursue immunotherapy for feline cutaneous allergy is partially dependent on the severity and duration of clinical signs, owner preference, and taking into account the cat's disposition. Much of what is known in regard to ASIT for cutaneous allergies in the cat is extrapolated from canine studies and based on anecdotal findings and clinical preferences. There are reports of controlled trials with immunotherapy for feline asthma and these will be discussed in Chapter 37.

Principles and considerations for allergen-specific immunotherapy

ASIT is defined as the incremental administration of increasing quantities of an allergen extract(s) to an allergic patient. The goal of successful therapy is to reduce or eliminate the clinical signs associated with repeated exposure to the causative allergen(s) (WHO definition) [1]. Compared to humans, there are few studies investigating the mechanism of action of ASIT in veterinary medicine; a few studies have evaluated the mechanism of action of ASIT in atopic dogs [2,3] and feline asthma [4]; however, no such studies have been performed with regard to immunotherapy in cats with cutaneous allergy.

Although much of what has been reported in cats is based on open trials and anecdotal information [5–7], ASIT is considered to be a safe and effective treatment option for cutaneous allergy in cats. Efficacy is considered to be similar to that reported in atopic dermatitis in dogs; success rates range from 50 to 100% in the literature [8,9]. Clinical improvement is often noted between 3 and 6 months following initiation of immunotherapy; however, maximal benefits can take 12–18 months to become apparent. Side effects are considered to be relatively rare for cats administered conventional ASIT. Anecdotal reports of localized pruritus and anaphylaxis have been noted, although are considered to be less frequent than in dogs [9].

As in dogs, no single or standardized immunotherapy administration protocol exists for cats with cutaneous allergy. Interval between injections, injection volume, and even allergen concentration are all highly variable between dermatologists; the schedule of administration is typically extrapolated from the preferred canine protocol. Most clinicians specializing in dermatology recommend a trial of administration for at least 1 year to evaluate efficacy in the particular feline patient. Once efficacy is documented at the end of the year trial, many practitioners will attempt to reduce the frequency of

Veterinary Allergy, First Edition. Edited by Chiara Noli, Aiden Foster, and Wayne Rosenkrantz.

injections while still maintaining remission/control of clinical signs; this may allow for improved client and patient compliance. Although typically recommended to continue life-long in cats where immunotherapy has proven to be beneficial for controlling cutaneous allergies, a small percentage of cats may remain in remission without recurrence of allergic skin disease if immunotherapy is discontinued after some years [8].

Allergens should be selected for ASIT based on the results of 'allergy testing' and most dermatologists limit the number of allergens to 10 or 12. Testing is used as an aid for the formulation of ASIT, rather than as a diagnostic tool. Options for testing include intradermal and serum testing, as were discussed in Chapter 34. The selection of allergens should take into account the clinical history and the feasibility of environmental exposure to allergens implicated by positive test reactions.

Options for allergen-specific immunotherapy

Historically, the only option available for ASIT in the allergic cat was via injection using either aqueous or alum precipitated allergens (conventional ASIT). Newer, alternative options, however, are also available. These include rush immunotherapy and sublingual immunotherapy.

Conventional injection allergen-specific immunotherapy

Conventional injection ASIT has historically been the only option available for immunotherapy in veterinary medicine. Different geographical regions use either alum precipitated or aqueous allergen extracts for inclusion in a patient-specific immunotherapy 'cocktail', which is administered subcutaneously. The injection schedule is generally borrowed from the preferred canine injection protocol. This will typically depend on the company formulating treatment or the preferences of the practitioner. The injection schedule is broken into two phases. During the induction phase, gradually increasing amounts of allergen are administered over a period of several weeks; this is accomplished by administering larger injection volumes of gradually more concentrated allergen mixtures. During the maintenance phase, the interval between injections is lengthened (injections typically administered every 1 to 3 weeks, depending on preferred protocol) while continuing to administer the same volume of the 'maintenance' concentration of allergen (most commonly 20 000 PNU/mL). Therapy is continued for at least a year to evaluate efficacy.

Owners should monitor improvement based on a decrease in pruritus and clinical signs, decreased necessity for other medications (dose, frequency), and ability to replace more 'risky' treatment options (e.g. glucocorticoids) with 'safer' alternatives (e.g. antihistamines). In patients with only minimal to moderate improvement after 1 year therapy should be reassessed based on the client's perceived benefits. The efficacy of ASIT is reported to be up to 78% for conventional injectable immunotherapy in cats with cutaneous allergy. Side effects are rare and may include localized pruritus or anaphylaxis. Injection site fibrosarcoma development has not been evaluated in cats administered either aqueous or alum precipitated ASIT.

Rush immunotherapy

An alternative option to conventional injection immunotherapy is rush immunotherapy. While still administering immunotherapy via subcutaneous injection, this method essentially eliminates the induction phase of the immunotherapy protocol. Gradually increasing amounts of allergen are administered over several hours as opposed to several weeks until the maintenance dose is reached. Rush immunotherapy should be administered in a hospital or clinic setting; careful monitoring of adverse reactions and vital parameters is recommended during administration. This option for immunotherapy administration has been evaluated in dogs and people, with few adverse reactions reported. A pilot study evaluated rush immunotherapy in cats [10]; although only a small number of cats were included, it appeared to be safe and effective for reaching maintenance therapy. Anecdotally, adverse reactions reported are similar to those seen with conventional immunotherapy; increased localized (and more generalized) pruritus as well as anaphylaxis has been noted in cats with cutaneous allergy administered rush immunotherapy. It is uncertain whether improved efficacy is noted with this method as compared to conventional administration protocols. The benefit of rush immunotherapy, however, is it condenses the induction phase into only a few hours; this eliminates the need for frequent injections to be administered at home. Rather, the frequent injections are administered under clinical supervision and owners can start immediately on a maintenance injection schedule (every 1 to 3 weeks); this sort of protocol may promote improved client compliance.

Sublingual immunotherapy

A very different option for ASIT administration is sublingual immunotherapy. As opposed to either conventional or rush injectable immunotherapy, sublingual offers a 'needle-free' option. Small drops of allergen extract are administered under the tongue or onto the oral mucosa. This may be a preferred option for clients with a fear of needles or who may have physical or emotional difficulty injecting their pets. The frequency of administration, however, is vastly different; administration is recommended twice daily for sublingual immunotherapy. This option is relatively new in veterinary medicine; it was developed from studies performed in humans documenting efficacy for allergic diseases. Little information exists with regard to sublingual immunotherapy in veterinary medicine; one study documented efficacy for controlling canine atopic dermatitis [11]. Although the exact mechanism of action is uncertain, there appear to be immunologic changes that are different to those observed with injectable immunotherapy; dogs that had failed conventional ASIT previously still potentially showed a beneficial response to sublingual immunotherapy in the study population. In dogs, therapeutic efficacy is similar to that reported for conventional immunotherapy as well as the time to see clinical improvements.

There are no studies evaluating sublingual immunotherapy in cats with cutaneous allergy. Anecdotally, benefits have been observed for some cats where sublingual immunotherapy was used as part of the therapeutic protocol. It appears to be well tolerated by most cats, although the twice-daily oral administration may not be appreciated by all cats. The formulation is palatable and even 'picky' felines may tolerate the small volume necessary for administration. Studies are needed to evaluate the relative efficacy and safety profile in a large number of allergic cats to compare sublingual versus conventional immunotherapy.

Concurrent medication administration

There are no studies evaluating a difference in efficacy with any form of ASIT, whether concurrent antipruritic medications were or were not administered. For most allergic cats, concurrent medication is necessary especially during the induction and early maintenance phase of immunotherapy administration. Whether this leads to a different immunologic response and outcome is uncertain. Many dermatologists, however, have no problem administering concurrent medications, including antihistamines or glucocorticoids or ciclosporin, as needed to provide humane relief of pruritic skin disease. This will generally prevent self-trauma and relapse, which may otherwise contribute to client frustration and non-compliance. Efficacy can still be assessed based on the ability to lower concurrent medication doses and potentially discontinue certain medications in favour of safer options.

As in dogs with atopic dermatitis, the management of clinical signs of cutaneous allergy in cats requires careful consideration of the various therapeutic options. Allergen-specific immunotherapy should especially be considered in cats whose season lasts more than 4 months and in cats less than 3 years of age. In older cats with concurrent medical conditions (e.g. diabetes mellitus), ASIT may be the safest option as opposed to other medical interventions. The various options for conventional or rush injectable immunotherapy versus sublingual immunotherapy should be discussed with the client and evaluated based on owner preference and the disposition of the cat.

References

1. Bousquet J, Lockey R, Malling HJ, *et al.* Allergen immunotherapy: therapeutic vaccines for allergic diseases. World Health Organization. American Academy of Allergy, Asthma, and Immunology. *Annals of Allergy, Asthma and Immunology* 1998; **81**: 401–405.
2. Shida M, Kadoya M, Park SJ, *et al.* Allergen-specific immunotherapy induces Th1 shift in dogs with atopic dermatitis. *Veterinary Immunology and Immunopathology* 2004; **102**: 19–31.
3. Keppel KE, Campbell KL, Zuckermann FA, *et al.* Quantitation of canine regulatory T cell populations, serum interleukin-10 and allergen-specific IgE concentrations in healthy control dogs and canine atopic dermatitis patients receiving allergen-specific immunotherapy. *Veterinary Immunology and Immunopathology* 2008; **123**: 337–344.
4. Reinero CR, Byerly JR, Berghaus RD, *et al.* Rush immunotherapy in an experimental model of feline allergic asthma. *Veterinary Immunology and Immunopathology* 2006; **110**: 141–153.
5. Löewenstein C, Mueller RS. A review of allergen-specific immunotherapy in human and veterinary medicine. *Veterinary Dermatology* 2009; **20**: 84–98.
6. Bettenay SV. Response to hyposensitization in 29 atopic cats. In: Kwochka KW, Willemse T, von Tscharner C, eds. *Advances in Veterinary Dermatology*, Vol. 3. Oxford, UK: Butterworth Heinemann, 1998: 517–518.
7. Carlotti D, Prost C. L'atopie féline. *Le Point Vétérinaire* 1988; **20**: 777–784.
8. Vidémont E, Pin D. How to treat atopy in cats? *European Journal of Companion Animal Practice* 2009; **19**: 276–282.
9. Trimmer AM, Griffin CE, Rosenkrantz WS. Feline immunotherapy. *Clinical Techniques in Small Animal Practice* 2006; **21**: 157–161.
10. Trimmer AM, Griffin CE, Boord MJ, *et al.* Rush allergen specific immunotherapy protocol in feline atopic dermatitis: a pilot study of four cats. *Veterinary Dermatology* 2005; **16**: 324–329.
11. DeBoer DJ, Morris M. Multicentre open trial demonstrates efficacy of sublingual immunotherapy in canine atopic dermatitis (abstract). *Veterinary Dermatology* 2012; **23** (Suppl. 1): 65–66.

Section 2

Feline Asthma

37

Feline asthma

Carol R. Reinero

Department of Veterinary Medicine and Surgery, University of Missouri, Columbia, MO, USA

Conflict of interest: funding or provision of drug for the various research studies cited from the author's laboratory came from the Morris Animal Foundation, Winn Feline Foundation, AB Science, Kansas City Area Life Sciences Institute, Imulan Biotherapeutics, and the College of Veterinary Medicine at the University of Missouri, all except AB Science (France) based in the USA.

Introduction

Feline asthma is a chronic lower airway disorder associated with clinical signs of cough, wheeze, and expiratory respiratory distress. Its hallmark features include eosinophilic airway inflammation, airflow limitation at least in part reversible with bronchodilators, and structural changes in the lung termed remodeling. It is believed, as in humans, that the single most common cause of asthma in cats is a type I hypersensitivity response to aeroallergens. Evidence for an allergy as the predominant cause of asthma is based on data from epidemiologic studies [1–3] and experimental asthma models [4,5], along with some empiric evidence that allergen avoidance or allergen-specific immunotherapy (ASIT) have resulted in beneficial clinical responses in pet cats [6–8]. Other causes in humans, including pharmacologic stimuli, environmental substances/air pollutants (e.g. ozone, environmental tobacco smoke), occupational factors, exercise (especially but not exclusively in cold air), emotional stress, and infections (in particular certain viruses), are not well substantiated to cause feline asthma (reviewed in [9]).

Immunopathology

In susceptible individuals with appropriate genetic and environmental influences, inhalation of what should be benign antigens leads to a local hypersensitivity response. Aeroallergens are taken up by antigen presenting cells (dendritic cells) that sample antigens from the airway lumen. Allergens are processed and presented in conjunction with MHCII to naïve T helper 0 (Th0) cells in mucosal inductive sites below the epithelial surface. A polarized Th2-mediated immune response results in production of cytokines, which orchestrate the allergic inflammatory response. Key cytokines include interleukin-5 (IL-5), critical for eosinophil maturation, differentiation, and survival, and IL-4, 6, and 13, which allow B cells to undergo a class switch and terminally differentiate into IgE-secreting plasma cells. Allergen-specific IgE is avidly bound to high-affinity FcεRI receptors on mast cells and basophils, which upon re-exposure to allergen leads to degranulation and further exacerbation of the inflammatory cascade. Chronically, the cat develops hallmark features of asthma: eosinophilic airway inflammation, airway hyper-responsiveness/airflow obstruction and airway remodeling. Experimentally, an asthmatic phenotype could be reproduced in cats by sensitizing and challenging with the clinically relevant allergens house dust mite and Bermuda grass, leading to eosinophilic airway inflammation, allergen-specific bronchoconstriction, a Th2 cell cytokine profile in blood and bronchial alveolar lavage fluid (BALF), induction of allergen-specific IgE, and airway remodeling [5].

Veterinary Allergy, First Edition. Edited by Chiara Noli, Aiden Foster, and Wayne Rosenkrantz.

Clinical presentation

Cats with asthma can present with a cough, wheeze, or episodic respiratory distress (with increased effort on exhalation). Additionally, they may have a history of what owners perceive as gastrointestinal signs, namely 'hacking up hairballs', which may actually represent a cough. Finally, exercise intolerance, especially in younger or more active cats, may be noted.

Diagnosis

In practice, diagnosis of asthma is made using a combination of signalment, history, clinical signs, thoracic radiography, exclusion of respiratory parasites, BALF cytology demonstrating airway eosinophilia, and response to empiric therapy with bronchodilators and glucocorticoids. Diseases that may mimic many of the clinicopathologic features of asthma include chronic bronchitis, heartworm-associated respiratory disease (HARD), *Aelurostrongylus abstrusus*, and ascariasis. Rigorous discrimination of these disorders from asthma may be challenging and the limitations of currently available diagnostics are beyond the scope of this chapter. In practice, ancillary tests may include a complete blood count, fecal flotation, fecal Baermann, and heartworm antibody and antigen tests. Empiric therapy with an appropriate antihelmintic may also be used diagnostically to help rule out parasitic diseases. Thoracic radiography classically demonstrates a bronchial or bronchointerstitial pattern (Figure 37.1a,b), sometimes with evidence of hyperinflated lungs or collapse of a lung lobe (most commonly the right middle and caudal portion of the left cranial lobes). However, radiographs are neither sensitive nor specific for asthma and may in fact be normal [10]. In the author's experience, if radiographic evidence of hyperinflation is documented to be transient (that is at least in part reversible with bronchodilators or after resolution of the acute and late phase IgE-mediated responses), that would support a diagnosis of asthma. Bronchoalveolar lavage fluid cytology, with identification of increased percentage/numbers of airway eosinophils in asthma (Figure 37.2), remains a crucial diagnostic test to discriminate from chronic bronchitis but not respiratory parasites. While bacterial culture of the lavage fluid can help determine if there is secondary infection complicating management of the clinical signs, it must be remembered that overall infection is uncommon in feline asthma.

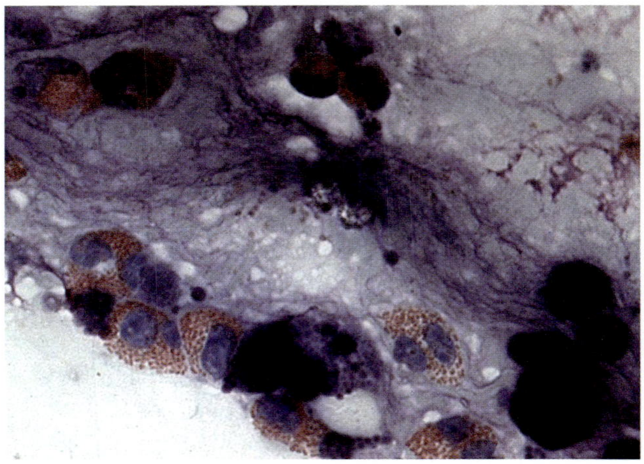

Figure 37.2 Cytologic examination of bronchoalveolar lavage fluid from a cat with asthma shows increased numbers of eosinophils scattered on a dark blue mucinous background.

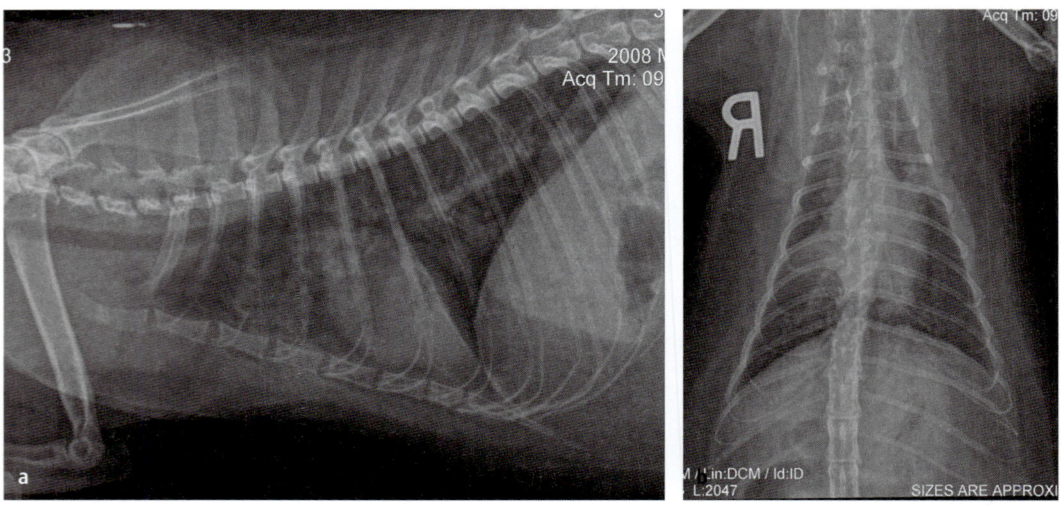

Figure 37.1 Lateral (a) and dorsoventral (b) thoracic radiographs taken from a cat with feline asthma demonstrate a bronchointerstitial pattern and collapse of the right middle lung lobe.

Because feline asthma is postulated to be allergic in nature, allergen-specific IgE testing can be performed to help identify clinically relevant allergens. This can be done either by intradermal testing, which evaluates IgE bound to mast cells in the dermis, or by serum testing, which evaluates circulating IgE. Care must be taken in selecting the laboratory for serum testing because there are no regulatory agencies ensuring accurate results and widely discrepant results between laboratories have been found [11]. False-positive and false-negative test results are not uncommon. Concurrent use of oral glucocorticoids has been shown to diminish skin test positivity to allergens in experimentally asthmatic cats; a 2-week withdrawal is adequate to restore skin reactivity [12]. In contrast in this same study, glucocorticoids did not appear to impact serum allergen-specific IgE testing. It is not known what effect oral steroids administered for longer than 2 weeks, or injectable steroids, might have on the results of tests in experimental cats with asthma. The impact of steroids on test values in cats with allergic skin diseases may be different. The value of running skin and serum allergen-specific IgE tests is to try to determine which allergens are implicated in disease. This is important in trying to make recommendations for allergen avoidance. Additionally, in the future, allergen-specific immunotherapy [11,13,14] may become a viable option for pet cats with this disease and knowing which allergens to use in the 'allergy shots' is important.

In humans, measuring lung mechanical function is a common, simple, and non-invasive test that aids in the diagnosis of asthma. Direct (e.g. ventilator acquired pulmonary mechanics; Figure 37.3) or indirect (barometric whole body plethysmography) techniques to estimate pulmonary function in pet cats are not widely available at this time and the reader is referred to other manuscripts on this topic [15–17].

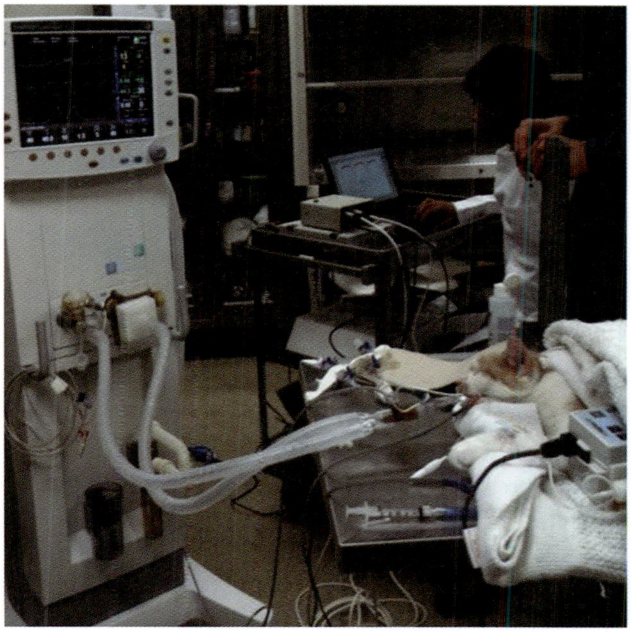

Figure 37.3 Information on the function of the lung in feline asthmatics can be determined by use of ventilator-acquired pulmonary mechanics. While this technique is currently used in research settings, it is feasible to perform these types of measurements in pet cats with spontaneous asthma.

Treatment

Palliative therapies

There is no cure for feline asthma at this time. The standard of therapy in practice includes three major recommendations for cats: environmental modulation, bronchodilators, and glucocorticoids. These treatments focus on decreasing environmental triggers of allergic signs, reducing bronchoconstriction, and blunting airway inflammation. Bronchodilators and glucocorticoids unfortunately work only after the allergic cascade has already been well established and thus are only palliative.

Since asthma is triggered by inhalation of and an inappropriate response to aeroallergens, it would be ideal to remove the clinically relevant allergen(s) from the cats' environment. In practice, that can rarely be done either because the allergen(s) are ubiquitous, or because they are not accurately identified with available testing. It is more realistic to modify the environment so the cat has minimal contact with non-allergenic stimuli that could trigger airflow limitation in a non-specific manner, such as powders, dusts (toilet/kitty litter), aerosols, and smoke. Hepa-type air filters may also prove beneficial.

Bronchodilators are critically important in the management of asthmatics in respiratory distress ('status asthmaticus') to reverse the bronchospasm mediated by specific allergen or non-specific irritants; they may also be beneficial in chronic management of this disorder. However, given their lack of potent anti-inflammatory effects they should not be used as monotherapy in asthmatics. This is because airway inflammation is a key event, which further exacerbates airway hyper-reactivity and airway remodeling and must be addressed directly. The major classes of bronchodilators used in pet cats or experimental models include methylxanthines, short-acting and long-acting beta-2 agonists (SABA and LABA, respectively), and anticholinergics [18–21]. Depending on the drug, oral and/or inhaled formulations are available. Inhaled formulations can be administered

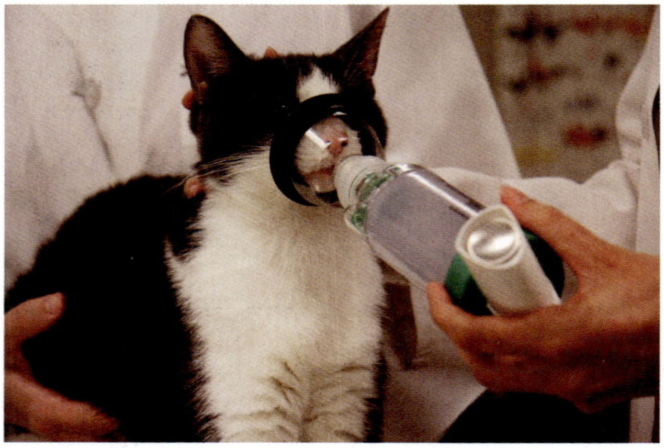

Figure 37.4 Inhaled bronchodilators or glucocorticoids can be delivered to cats by using a holding chamber (spacer) fitted to a metered dose inhalant canister on one side and a face mask on the other. Cats should take seven to ten deep breaths after actuation of the metered dose inhalant drug.

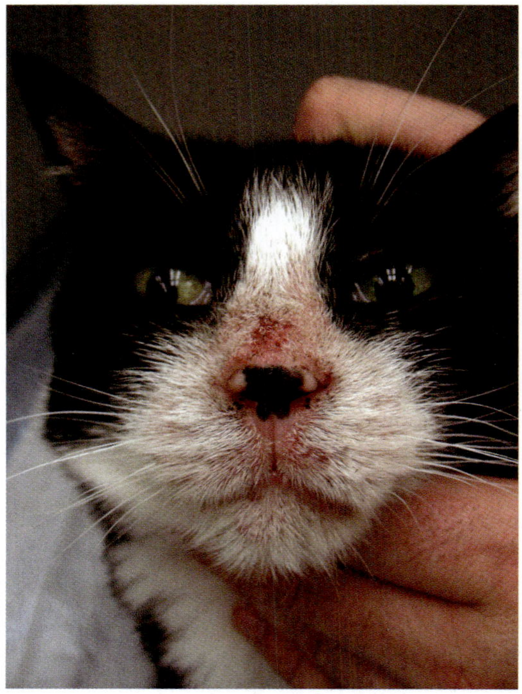

Figure 37.5 A pet cat receiving chronic inhalant glucocorticoids developed skin lesions of the muzzle under the area enclosed by the tight fitting face mask. Skin scraping documented the presence of *Demodex*. Reprinted with permission from Richard Meadows, Veterinary Medical Teaching Hospital, University of Missouri, USA.

using a spacer with a tightly fitting face mask (Figure 37.4). Regular use (likely >2–3 times/week) of inhaled racemic albuterol, consisting of two isomer forms (R-albuterol and S-albuterol) is not recommended because it has been shown to exacerbate eosinophilic airway inflammation in experimentally asthmatic cats [20]; this formulation is best suited for acute 'rescue' for cats in acute respiratory distress. Proinflammatory and airway constrictive properties of the S-albuterol isomer, which is cleared more slowly from the respiratory tract, accumulate over time. A commercially available single isomer preparation of inhaled R-albuterol (levalbuterol) can be used safely in a chronic fashion in place of racemic albuterol.

Glucocorticoids are considered the mainstay of therapy for feline asthma because they suppress airway eosinophilia. Inhaled steroids are preferred over oral steroids in humans because topical deposition is associated with fewer systemic side effects. In healthy cats, inhaled fluticasone is associated with fewer systemic immunologic and, to a lesser extent, endocrine effects [22]. A prospective, randomized, placebo-controlled, cross-over study in experimentally asthmatic cats confirmed that oral prednisone (10 mg/day) and inhaled flunisolide delivered though a pediatric holding chamber (500 μg/day) significantly decreased eosinophilic airway inflammation compared with placebo [23]. A subsequent study using this model compared different doses of inhaled fluticasone (44, 110, or 220 μg twice daily) and showed all were equipotent in controlling airway inflammation [24]. Thus, as is true in humans receiving inhaled steroids, efficacy may plateau and giving more is not always better. Clinical side effects of inhaled steroids are not common. Oral thrush, which has been described in humans who actuate the metered dose inhalant directly into their oral cavity, has not been described in cats, probably because a face mask is employed. However, *Demodex* infection of the muzzle of a cat in contact with the area of deposition of the inhalant steroid has been seen at the author's institution (Figure 37.5).

Other drugs evaluated in experimental feline asthma include the antiserotonerigic drug cyproheptadine (4 mg/day orally) and the cysteinyl leukotriene (cysLT) antagonist zafirlukast (20 mg/day orally), neither of which significantly reduced airway eosinophilia compared with placebo [23]. A later study examined a higher dose of cyproheptadine (16 mg/day) and the second generation histamine 1 receptor antagonist cetirizine (10 mg/day) compared with placebo, and also found a lack of significant reduction in eosinophilic airway inflammation with either drug [25]. Immunomodulatory therapy with feG-COOH (a salivary tripeptide involved in neuroendocrine immunology) (1 mg/kg/day for 2 weeks) also lacked significant effects on eosinophilic airway inflammation or clinical signs compared with placebo [26]. Ciclosporin has also been used in experimental feline asthma and was shown to not inhibit the early phase asthmatic response (i.e. as occurs during an acute asthma attack), but may be beneficial to ameliorate chronic pathologic changes associated with asthma. While not routinely advocated to treat asthma, ciclosporin may be tried in cases not responding to standard therapies.

Dietary consumption of omega-3 polyunsaturated fatty acids (ω3 PUFAs) in combination with the antioxidant luteolin was investigated in experimentally asthmatic cats and found to blunt production of bioactive eicosanoids contributing to airway inflammation after 4 weeks [27]. While it was disappointing that there was no significant difference in airway inflammation in treated versus untreated asthmatic cats, there was a reduction in airflow limitation measured by barometric whole body plethysmography. While dietary supplementation with ω3 PUFAs and luteolin is clearly inadequate to treat asthma by itself, future studies in pet cats could be performed to determine if it may be a useful adjunct, perhaps allowing for reduction in glucocorticoid dose. Another recent study showed that the tyrosine kinase inhibitor masitinib blunted airway eosinophilia and improved lung function in experimental feline asthma; however, toxicity was a major limitation in the study [17]. Other small molecule inhibitors may be of interest if they target relevant signaling pathways. Stem cell therapy is also undergoing pilot investigation.

'Curative' therapy

All of the aforementioned treatments act relatively late in the allergic inflammatory cascade and thus are only palliative, doing nothing to restore immunologic tolerance to allergen. To date, the only curative therapy for any type of allergy is allergen-specific immunotherapy (ASIT). This treatment normalizes a dysregulated immune response to allergen, restoring immunologic tolerance. An abbreviated protocol for ASIT called rush immunotherapy (RIT) allows for rapid loading of increasing doses of allergen to which a patient has been sensitized before initiation of maintenance therapy. The first protocol used in experimentally asthmatic cats involved alternating intranodal and subcutaneous allergen injections; this protocol, while leading to significant reductions in airway eosinophilia, was associated with (some severe) side effects [14]. Safety was improved by eliminating the intranodal injections, as did use of the adjuvant, CpG-ODN [13]. Because asthma is triggered by allergens delivered to the mucosa, a comparison of the safety and efficacy of mucosal versus subcutaneous RIT protocols was performed [28]. While both protocols decreased eosinophilic airway inflammation, the subcutaneous protocol subjectively demonstrated more consistent resolution of clinical signs of bronchospasm after aerosol challenge with allergen.

A major challenge for translational application of ASIT from research to pet cats is the accurate identification of allergens to which a pet cat has become sensitized. While it is straightforward to assess ASIT in experimental asthma because the sensitizing allergens are known, in pet cats allergenic triggers may be intermittent (e.g. seasonal) or their identification hampered by concurrent therapy. Additionally, identification of allergen-specific IgE does not necessarily imply that allergen is the cause of the lower airway inflammation meaning that 'allergy testing' must be interpreted in light of all the clinical and pathologic features consistent with asthma. Using an experimental model of allergic asthma in the cat where sensitizing allergens were known, intradermal testing (IDT) and serum allergen-specific IgE determination using a commercial FcϵR1α-based ELISA were compared [11]. While the sensitivity of the IDT was greater than serum allergen-specific IgE determination, both were specific. This suggests that IDT might serve as a better screening test but either can be used to guide selection of allergens for ASIT. Importantly, this study also evaluated a different commercial laboratory using an enzymoimmunometric assay for feline allergen-specific IgE determination and found that this laboratory had unreliable results, including failure to detect Bermuda grass allergen-specific IgE as well as inappropriate identification of allergens to which the cats had not been sensitized even in samples in which IgE had selectively been destroyed by heat inactivation [11]. If ASIT is to become a viable treatment option for pet cats with allergic asthma future studies should be performed to more rigorously evaluate the accuracy of diagnostic laboratories offering allergen-specific IgE testing.

Another question that arises pertaining to allergen-specific IgE testing is the effect of concurrent glucocorticoid therapy on skin reactivity and serum IgE concentrations. Many pet cats with asthma are being administered glucocorticoids to control their clinical signs at the time allergen identification is considered. In an experimental asthma model, 1 month of oral or inhaled glucocorticoids failed to diminish serum allergen-specific IgE [12]. In comparison, IDT reactivity was dampened in asthmatic cats receiving these treatments, although reactivity was restored after a 2-week withdrawal from glucocorticoid therapy.

Because there is likely to be some difficulty in appropriately identifying sensitizing allergens in pet cats with allergic asthma, the question arises as to whether inadvertent 'inappropriate' selection of allergens would confer cross-protection against the clinically relevant allergens. This was addressed in an additional study in which experimentally asthmatic cats were sensitized with one allergen and administered a different allergen for RIT [29]. Results showed that airway eosinophilia was dampened when either sensitizing or unrelated allergens were used for RIT. The scenario in which a pet cat could be polysensitized and receiving only a partial repertoire of sensitizing allergens in RIT was also mimicked in this study. Cats sensitized to both house dust mite and Bermuda grass receiving only one of those allergens in RIT demonstrated reduction in eosinophilic airway inflammation compared with cats administered placebo RIT. Thus, allergens used in RIT do not have to be identical to sensitizing allergens in order to dampen airway eosinophilia, the cardinal hallmark feature of allergenic asthma. Interestingly, this study showed that closely matching the sensitizing and treating allergens appears to induce immunologic tolerance (indicated by allergen-specific lymphocyte hypoproliferation and increases in IL-10 producing cells and regulatory T cells), which could ultimately allow discontinuation of RIT. However, use of a non-sensitizing allergen in RIT while still conferring benefit, does not dampen allergen-specific lymphocyte proliferation or increase IL-10 producing cells. This could suggest that an active immune response requiring indefinite immunotherapy may be required.

Prior to its use in pet cats, it is also critical to determine if glucocorticoids diminish efficacy of RIT since pet cats will need concurrent glucocorticoid treatment during the months it will take immunotherapy to work. This makes sense because ASIT modulates the immune system to induce immunologic tolerance and glucocorticoids suppress immune responses. Results in experimental feline asthma show that oral, but not inhaled, glucocorticoids negatively impact RIT efficacy [30]. Inhaled glucocorticoids should thus be considered as the mainstay of anti-inflammatory therapy during immunotherapy in asthmatic cats.

Although there is substantial evidence in *experimental* feline asthma that RIT holds promise, it must be recognized that this is a model of asthma and a variety of factors are more carefully controlled than in the pet cat counterpart. Because pet cats are likely to have more complex genetics, environmental influences, concurrent therapies and other illness, and allergen exposures, carefully controlled clinical trials must be performed in pet cats with spontaneous asthma to prove safety and efficacy before immunotherapy can be routinely advocated.

References

1. Ranivand L, Otto C. Feline asthma trends in Philadelphia, Pennsylvania 1896–2007. In: *26th Annual Symposium of the Veterinary Comparative Respiratory Society*, 2008; Oklahoma City, OK, 2008.
2. Reinero C, DeClue A, Rabinowitz P. Asthma in humans and cats: is there a common sensitivity to aeroallergens in shared environments? *Environmental Research* 2009; **109**: 634–640.
3. Schafer T, Merkl J, Klemm E, *et al.* We and our pets: allergic together? *Acta Veterinaria Hungarica* 2008; **56**: 153–161.
4. Kirschvink N, Leemans J, Delvaux F, *et al.* Functional, inflammatory and morphological characterisation of a cat model of allergic airway inflammation. *Veterinary Journal* 2007; **174**: 541–553.
5. Norris Reinero C, Decile K, Berghaus R, *et al.* An experimental model of allergic asthma in cats sensitized to house dust mite or bermuda grass allergen. *International Archives of Allergy and Immunology* 2004; **135**: 117–131.
6. Corcoran B, Foster D, Fuentes V. Feline asthma syndrome: a retrospective study of the clinical presentation in 29 cats. *Journal of Small Animal Practice* 1995; **36**: 481–488.
7. Halliwell R. Efficacy of hyposensitization in feline allergic diseases based on upon results of in vitro testing for allergen-specific immunoglobulin E. *Journal of the American Animal Hospital Association* 1997; **33**: 282–288.
8. Prost C. Treatment of feline asthma with allergen avoidance and specific immunotherapy: experience with 20 cats. *Revue Francaise d'Allergologie et d'Immunologie Clinique* 2008; **48**: 409–413.
9. Reinero C. Advances in the understanding of pathogenesis, and diagnostics and therapeutics for feline allergic asthma. *Veterinary Journal* 2011; **190**: 28–33.
10. Adamama-Moraitou K, Patsikas M, Koutinas A. Feline lower airway disease: a retrospective study of 22 naturally occurring cases from Greece. *Journal of Feline Medicine and Surgery* 2004; **6**: 227–233.
11. Lee-Fowler T, Cohn L, DeClue A, *et al.* Comparison of intradermal skin testing (IDST) and serum allergen-specific IgE determination in an experimental model of feline allergic asthma. *Veterinary Immunology and Immunopathology* 2009; **132**: 46–52.
12. Chang C, Lee-Fowler T, DeClue A, *et al.* The impact of oral versus inhaled glucocorticoids on allergen specific IgE testing in experimentally asthmatic cats. *Veterinary Immunology and Immunopathology* 2011; **144**: 437–441.
13. Reinero C, Cohn L, Delgado C, *et al.* Adjuvanted rush immunotherapy using CpG oligodeoxynucleotides in experimental feline allergic asthma. *Veterinary Immunology and Immunopathology* 2008; **121**: 241–250.
14. Reinero CR, Byerly JR, Berghaus RD, *et al.* Rush immunotherapy in an experimental model of feline allergic asthma. *Veterinary Immunology and Immunopathology* 2006; **110**: 141–153.
15. Kirschvink K. Barometric whole body plethysmography and enhanced pause (PENH): how relevant are they? *Veterinary Journal* 2008; **176**: 125–126.
16. Kirschvink N, Leemans J, Delvaux F, *et al.* Non-invasive assessment of airway responsiveness in healthy and allergen-sensitized cats by use of barometric whole body plethysmography. *Veterinary Journal* 2007; **173**: 343–352.
17. Lee-Fowler T, Guntur V, Dodam J, *et al.* The tyrosine kinase inhibitor masitinib blunts airway inflammation and improves associated lung mechanics in a feline model of chronic allergic asthma. *International Archives of Allergy and Immunology* 2012; **158**: 369–374.
18. Kirschvink N, Leemans J, Delvaux F, *et al.* Bronchodilators in bronchoscopy-induced airflow limitation in allergen-sensitized cats. *Journal of Veterinary Internal Medicine* 2005; **19**: 161–167.

19. Leemans J, Kirschvink K, Clercx C, *et al.* Functional response to inhaled salbutamol and/or ipratropium bromide in *Ascaris suum*-sensitised cats with allergen-induced bronchospasms. *Veterinary Journal* 2010; **186**: 76–83.
20. Reinero C, Delgado C, Spinka C, *et al.* Enantiomer specific effects of albuterol on airway inflammation in healthy and asthmatic cats. *International Archives of Allergy and Immunology* 2009; **150**: 43–50.
21. Leemans J, Kirschvink N, Bernaerts F, *et al.* A pilot study comparing the antispasmodic effects of inhaled salmeterol, salbutamol and ipratropium bromide using different aerosol devices on muscarinic bronchoconstriction in healthy cats. *Veterinary Journal* 2009; **180**: 236–245.
22. Reinero CR, Brownlee L, Decile KC, *et al.* Inhaled flunisolide suppresses the hypothalamic-pituitary-adrenocortical axis, but has minimal systemic immune effects in healthy cats. *Journal of Veterinary Internal Medicine* 2006; **20**: 57–64.
23. Reinero C, Decile K, Byerly J, *et al.* Effects of drug treatment on inflammation and hyperreactivity of airways and on immune variables in cats with experimentally induced asthma. *American Journal of Veterinary Research* 2005; **66**: 1121–1127.
24. Cohn L, DeClue A, Cohen R, *et al.* Effects of fluticasone propionate dosage in an experimental model of feline asthma. *Journal of Feline Medicine and Surgery* 2010; **12**: 91–96.
25. Schooley E, McGee Turner J, Jiji R, *et al.* Effects of cyproheptadine and cetirizine on eosinophilic airway inflammation in cats with experimentally induced asthma. *American Journal of Veterinary Research* 2007; **68**: 1265–1271.
26. Eberhardt J, DeClue A, Reinero C. Chronic use of the immunomodulating tripeptide feG-COOH in experimental feline asthma. *Veterinary Immunology and Immunopathology* 2009; **132**: 175–180.
27. Leemans J, Cambier C, Chandler T, *et al.* Prophylactic effects of omega-3 polyunsaturated fatty acids and luteolin on airway hyperresponsiveness and inflammation in cats with experimentally-induced asthma. *Veterinary Journal* 2010; **184**: 111–114.
28. Lee-Fowler T, Cohn L, DeClue A, *et al.* Evaluation of subcutaneous versus mucosal (intranasal) allergen-specific rush immunotherapy in experimental feline asthma. *Veterinary Immunology and Immunopathology* 2009; **129**: 49–56.
29. Reinero C, Lee-Fowler T, Chang C, *et al.* Beneficial cross-protection of allergen-specific immunotherapy on airway eosinophilia using unrelated or a partial repertoire of allergen(s) implicated in experimental feline asthma. *Veterinary Journal* 2012; **192**: 412–416.
30. Chang CH, Cohn LA, DeClue AE, Liu H, Reinero CR. Oral glucocorticoids diminish the efficacy of allergen-specific immunotherapy in experimental feline asthma. *Veterinary Journal* 2013; **197**: 268–272.

Section 3

Flea Bite Allergy

38

Pathogenesis

Ross Bond

Department of Clinical Sciences and Services, Royal Veterinary College, Hatfield, UK

It is commonly stated that flea allergy dermatitis (FAD) is the commonest allergic disorder recognized in cats in geographical areas where fleas are present. This view is supported by a recent European multicentre study of more than 500 pruritic cats examined by veterinary dermatologists where FAD accounted for 29% of cases [1]. It is currently thought that dogs and cats do not show significant signs of skin disease associated with fleas unless they are allergic to components of flea saliva, although extreme flea burdens are likely to induce discomfort due to mechanical irritation. This section aims to review the immunological mechanisms involved in the development of FAD in cats and other relevant species (for comparative purposes), as essential background for the following sections on clinical signs and diagnostic testing.

Flea saliva

In common with other blood-sucking insects, flea saliva comprises a complex cocktail of substances that improve feeding success by interference with blood clotting and inflammatory pathways. During the process of feeding, the adult flea inserts its mouthparts through the epidermis, wherein a tube termed the epipharynx penetrates capillaries and blood is siphoned by the flea. The process of penetration is aided by salivary components that soften and spread dermal tissue; anticoagulants aid withdrawal of blood. Amongst the proteins and histamine-like compounds in flea saliva, up to 15 fractions can be identified by chromatography [2,3]. Salivary apyrase enzymes are ubiquitous in haematophagous insects, including cat [4] and rat fleas [5]; these enzymes hydrolyse ATP and ADP in the presence of Ca^{2+} and Mg^{2+} and may prevent ADP-induced platelet aggregation at the site of feeding [5,6]. Napthyl esterase and platelet-activating factor (PAF)-acetylhydrolase activity has also been demonstrated in salivary gland homogenates from cat fleas; PAF-acetylhydrolase activity may confer an advantage to fleas by down-regulating PAF-mediated inflammatory processes [7].

More recently, a molecular analysis of the salivary transcriptome of the oriental rat flea, *Xenopsylla cheopis*, has provided great detail on the complexity of flea saliva with the identification of phosphatase, esterase, apyrase, and adenosine deaminase enzymes, along with mucins (likely lubricants of the insect feeding canal) and novel polypeptides of the FS family [6].

Allergenicity of flea saliva

Components of flea saliva induce pathological effects by acting as allergens in sensitized hosts, in addition to their direct chemical assault on the skin. Whilst early reports suggested that the flea allergen was a hapten that bound to dermal collagen, this could not account for the immediate (wheal) responses observed on flea exposure and intradermal testing observed in cats and dogs [8]. There are no reports of detailed studies of the allergenic components of flea saliva in relation to the feline host; studies in other species illustrate general concepts but cannot be assumed to apply specifically to cats without further investigation. Studies of this nature are required for the development of optimal diagnostic and flea-specific immunotherapeutic reagents for cats [9].

Veterinary Allergy, First Edition. Edited by Chiara Noli, Aiden Foster, and Wayne Rosenkrantz.

Given the complex mix of substances within flea saliva, it is likely that a variety of allergens will be important in hypersensitivity responses amongst the population of sensitized cats. Lee *et al.* identified fractions of 40 and 12–8 kDa molecular weight as potential allergens in fractions of flea salivary glands in dogs [3]. In a study of nine dogs deemed to be hypersensitive to fleas based on the results of live flea challenge, three reacted to the 40 kDa protein, five reacted to the 12–8 kDa fraction, and one reacted to both fractions when intradermally tested. Dogs non-reactive to live flea challenge did not react to intradermal tests with these fractions [3]. Frank *et al.* reported that fractions of 12, 18, and 42 kDa frequently induced positive intradermal test responses in dogs experimentally sensitized to fleas [2]. The proteins of 12 and 18 kDa were cloned and expressed in *E. coli* and the recombinant proteins were found to retain their allergenic properties in the sensitized dogs. Subsequent studies have indicated that the recombinant 18 kDa protein (then termed rCte f 1) is expressed and secreted in a fully processed, correctly refolded, and fully active form from yeast (*Pichia pastoris*), and insect cells (*Trichoplusia ni*) using a baculovirus vector [10]. The function of Cte f 1 is unknown because it lacks homology with protein and DNA sequences in the major databases. More recently Jin *et al.* [9] cloned and expressed this protein (now referred to as FSA 1) from the original DNA sequence in an *E. coli* system and utilized it in a co-immunization DNA vaccine protocol that ameliorated clinical signs and allergic responses in experimentally sensitized laboratory cats [9]. These studies suggest that FSA1 is a major allergen in both dogs and cats, but the significance of this and other allergenic components of flea saliva in hypersensitivity responses in a wider population of naturally sensitized cats remains to be determined. It has been suggested that naturally sensitized animals may react to a wider array of allergenic fractions than laboratory animals, possibly due to longer flea exposure and more genetic variability in the pet population [3,10].

Immune responses to flea saliva in cats and other species

Classically, the response of a host to an ectoparasitic visitor may be classified as: (1) histaminic, due to the direct effects of histamine-like substances in venom or saliva; (2) enzymatic, due to proteolytic or cytolytic action of insect secretions; (3) hypersensitive or allergic; or (4) immune and non-responsive [11]. Close inspection of the skin at the site of a flea bite will normally reveal a tiny red mark in the non-sensitized individual, presumably reflecting mechanical trauma and histaminic or enzymatic effects. Hypersensitivity and tolerant immunological responses are of greater significance to veterinary dermatologists. The immunopathogenesis of FAD is multifaceted and varies between species. For more information about the immunopathogenesis of FAD in dogs see Chapter 21.

Guinea pigs

The original investigations on the immunopathogenesis of FAD were performed in guinea pigs by Benjamini *et al.* [12]. These authors found that guinea pigs exposed to fleas developed different immune responses in an ordered and sequential manner. Following an induction phase of 1–4 days, delayed, cell-mediated immune reactivity associated with lymphocyte recruitment was noted from days 5–9. After a further 2–5 days, immediate responses characterized by erythema and wheals within 1 hour of flea exposure were observed; these co-existed with delayed responses for a period of about 50 days. This was followed by a period (days 60–90) when only immediate reactions were observed. Intriguingly, no reactivity was observed after 90 days, indicating that a state of tolerance had developed. However, hypersensitivity persisted in guinea pigs for more than 12 months in the absence of repeated flea exposure.

Cats

Less data are available on the immunopathogenesis of flea allergy in cats. In a study involving small numbers of cats, Colombini *et al.* concluded that intermittent flea exposure neither favoured nor reduced the tendency to develop flea sensitization when assessed by intradermal testing and serological testing for IgE antibodies to flea saliva [13]. In another small study, early exposure of kittens to fleas did not appear to influence the likelihood of subsequent development of sensitization following continuous flea exposure [14]. Continuous flea exposure from weeks 16 to 43 of age led to the development of immediate reactivity following live flea challenge in 16 cats, and delayed reactivity in eight cats, although a smaller number of cats with immediate/IgE-mediated sensitization were detected by intradermal or serological testing. More recently, Jin *et al.* induced hypersensitivity in 18 cats by four cycles of flea exposure for a 3-day period, every other week; fleas were removed 23 days after application by oral treatment with nitenpyram [9]. Immediate intradermal test reactivity in sensitized cats was reported to persist for more than 90 days after the fourth cycle of flea exposure.

The lack of clear correlation between the clinical outcome following flea exposure and the results of intradermal and serological testing in two of these studies

[13], and in a subsequent investigation [15], indicates that live flea challenge should be considered the 'gold-standard' method for assessing flea sensitization in cats. These studies also clearly demonstrate that hypersensitivity to flea saliva in cats may reflect immediate or delayed hypersensitivity responses or both.

Both clinical and experimental studies have demonstrated that cats may develop immediate and delayed hypersensitivity responses to components of flea saliva. More detailed investigations are required to elucidate the factors that promote allergic sensitization in cats, and to identify the major allergens at the molecular level so that reagents for diagnosis and immunoprophylaxis can be developed and optimized for clinical use.

References

1. Hobi S, Linek M, Marignac G, *et al.* Clinical characteristics and causes of pruritus in cats: a multicentre study on feline hypersensitivity-associated dermatoses. *Veterinary Dermatology* 2011; **22**: 406–413.
2. Frank GR, Hunter SW, Stiegler GL, *et al.* Salivary allergens of *Ctenocephalides felis*: collection, purification and evaluation by intradermal skin testing in dogs. In: Kwochka KW, Willemse T, von Tscharner C, eds. *Advances in Veterinary Dermatology*, Vol. 3. Oxford: Butterworth Heinemann, 1998: 201–212.
3. Lee SE, Johnstone IP, Lee RP, *et al.* Putative salivary allergens of the cat flea, *Ctenocephalides felis felis*. *Veterinary Immunology and Immunopathology* 1999; **69**: 229–237.
4. Cheeseman MT. Characterization of apyrase activity from the salivary glands of the cat flea *Ctenocephalides felis*. *Insect Biochemistry and Molecular Biology* 1998; **28**: 1025–1030.
5. Ribeiro JM, Vaughan JA, Azad AF. Characterization of the salivary apyrase activity of three rodent flea species. *Comparative Biochemistry and Physiology B* 1990; **95**: 215–219.
6. Andersen JF, Hinnebusch BJ, Lucas DA, *et al.* An insight into the sialome of the oriental rat flea, *Xenopsylla cheopis* (Rots). *BMC Genomics* 2007; **8**: 102.
7. Cheeseman MT, Bates PA, Crampton JM. Preliminary characterisation of esterase and platelet-activating factor (PAF)-acetylhydrolase activities from cat flea (*Ctenocephalides felis*) salivary glands. *Insect Biochemistry and Molecular Biology* 2001; **31**: 157–164.
8. Halliwell REW. Managing flea allergy dermatitis 3. *Veterinary Medicine/Small Animal Clinician* 1984; **79**: 1273–1278.
9. Jin J, Ding Z, Meng F, *et al.* An immunotherapeutic treatment against flea allergy dermatitis in cats by co-immunization of DNA and protein vaccines. *Vaccine* 2010; **28**: 1997–2004.
10. McDermott MJ, Weber E, Hunter S, *et al.* Identification, cloning, and characterization of a major cat flea salivary allergen (Cte f 1). *Molecular Immunology* 2000; **37**: 361–375.
11. Gaafar SM. *Pathogenesis of ectoparasites*. In: Soulsby EJL, ed. *Biology of Parasites*. New York: Academic Press, 1966: 229–236.
12. Benjamini E, Feingold BF, Kartman L. Skin reactivity in guinea pigs sensitised to flea bites: the sequence of reactions. *Proceedings of the Society for Experimental Biology and Medicine* 1961; **108**: 700–702.
13. Colombini S, Hodgin EC, Foil CS, *et al.* Induction of feline flea allergy dermatitis and the incidence and histopathological characteristics of concurrent indolent lip ulcers. *Veterinary Dermatology* 2001; **12**: 155–161.
14. Kunkle GA, McCall CA, Stedman KE, *et al.* Pilot study to assess the effects of early flea exposure on the development of flea hypersensitivity in cats. *Journal of Feline Medicine and Surgery* 2003; **5**: 287–294.
15. Bond R, Hutchinson MJ, Loeffler A. Serological, intradermal and live flea challenge tests in the assessment of hypersensitivity to flea antigens in cats (*Felis domesticus*). *Parasitology Research* 2006; **99**: 392–397.

39

Clinical presentations

Dawn Logas
Veterinary Dermatology Center, Maitland, FL, USA

Conflict of interest: none declared.

Flea allergy dermatitis (FAD) is one of the most common allergic skin diseases of cats, especially in areas where fleas are endemic [1,2]. In a multicentre European study of 502 cats with pruritic dermatitis, 29% were diagnosed with flea allergy while 12% were diagnosed with food allergy and 20% with non-flea, non-food hypersensitivity dermatitides (NFNFHD) [3]. As in the dog, pruritus is the primary clinical sign of flea bite allergy in cats. However, pruritus can be more difficult to recognize in the cat because of their normal grooming behaviour and the fact that cats perform much of their grooming in private. If an owner notices their cat grooming excessively, scratching excessively, or pulling out hair, the cat should be considered very pruritic.

Unlike dogs that have a fairly typical clinical presentation associated with FAD, cats can present with a variety of clinical signs. In the previously mentioned study of 502 cats, four common reaction patterns were identified: miliary dermatitis, symmetric alopecia, head and neck excoriations, and eosinophilic granuloma complex [3]. These patterns were mainly seen alone, but 25% of the flea-allergic cats presented with a combination of patterns.

Miliary dermatitis

Miliary dermatitis [4,5] is a unique clinical pattern seen in cats and is a common clinical presentation for FAD. In the study of 502 cats, 35% of cats with flea bite allergy presented with miliary dermatitis as part or all of their clinical signs [3]. The lesions consist of multiple, small, crusted papules that may be easier to feel than to see in their early stages. As the dermatitis progresses, the small papules can coalesce to form larger crusted papules and plaques that are easy to visualize. As the cat licks, bites, and scratches at these lesions they become excoriated and more crusted. Miliary dermatitis lesions in flea-allergic cats are most often found on the caudal dorsum, caudal thighs, or in a generalized distribution. Less frequently, the distribution of papules is confined to a very distinct area of the body such as the pinnae, the forelimbs, or preauricular area. Alopecia may or may not accompany miliary dermatitis. Although FAD is one of the common inciting causes of miliary dermatitis, many other differential diagnoses should be considered if the cat does not improve with adequate flea control.

Symmetrical alopecia

Symmetrical alopecia [6] is a common sign of FAD. In the study of 502 cats, 39% of flea-allergic cats presented with symmetrical alopecia [3]. The distribution of the alopecia can vary. Bilaterally symmetrical alopecia of the caudal dorsum and flank area is the most common distribution (Figure 39.1). The ventrum, forelimbs, head, and neck are also commonly affected. Signs of inflammation, such as erythema, erosions, or crusting, are not usually observed or alopecia may be associated with miliary dermatitis. In cases with just alopecia many owners are convinced that the fur is falling out rather than being traumatically removed by the cat because cats can be extremely secretive about their excessive grooming. However, individual hairs from these cats do not epilate easily and when examined microscopically the hairs have

Veterinary Allergy, First Edition. Edited by Chiara Noli, Aiden Foster, and Wayne Rosenkrantz.

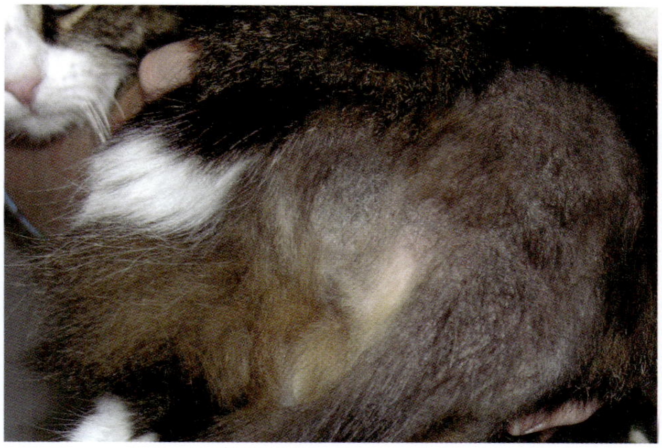

Figure 39.1 Hind quarters of a cat with flea allergic dermatitis; alopecia and broken hairs secondary to excessive grooming.

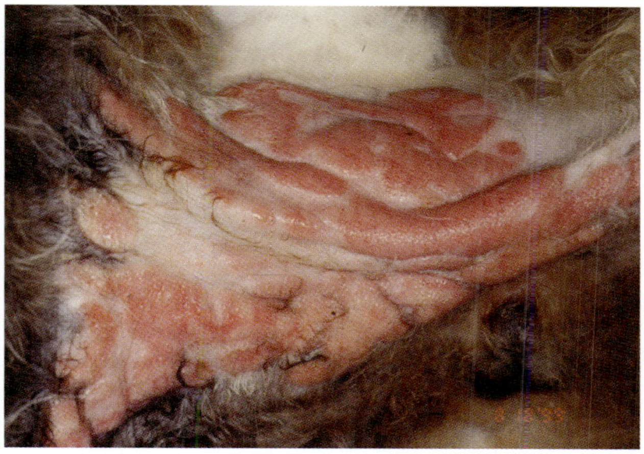

Figure 39.2 Ventral abdomen of a cat with multiple eosinophilic granulomas secondary to flea allergy dermatitis.

blunted or fractured ends instead of tapered ends. This indicates the hairs were traumatically removed. If these cats are prevented from grooming by wearing an Elizabethan collar their fur regrows.

Head and neck excoriations

Excoriations, erosions, ulcers, and crusting of the face, head, and neck are included in this reaction pattern. In the study of 502 cats, these lesions were most commonly associated with food hypersensitivity (64%), but flea-allergic cats also presented with this pattern (38%) [3].

Eosinophilic granuloma complex

The eosinophilic granuloma complex [7] is another unique reaction pattern seen in the cat. Three clinical entities comprise the eosinophilic granuloma complex (ECG) including lip ulcers (also called rodent, eosinophilic, or indolent ulcer) (Figure 39.2), eosinophilic plaques, and eosinophilic granulomas (Figure 39.3). These entities can occur alone or in combination with each other. In some cases of feline flea bite allergy, rodent ulcers, or eosinophilic granulomas of the hard palate are the only clinical signs present. In the study of 502 cats, only 14% of FAD cats presented with ECG compared to 26% of the so-called NFNFHD cats and 25% of food-allergic cats [3]. Therefore, as with miliary dermatitis, it is recommended to investigate flea allergy in cases of ECG. An exception to this was observed in one study in which five of eight research cats with laboratory-induced FAD developed rodent ulcers along with other dermatologic signs [8]. In this case, genetics along with hypersensitivity may have played a role in the development of these ulcers because all the cats affected were related and had been obtained from a cat colony with an increased incidence of rodent ulcers.

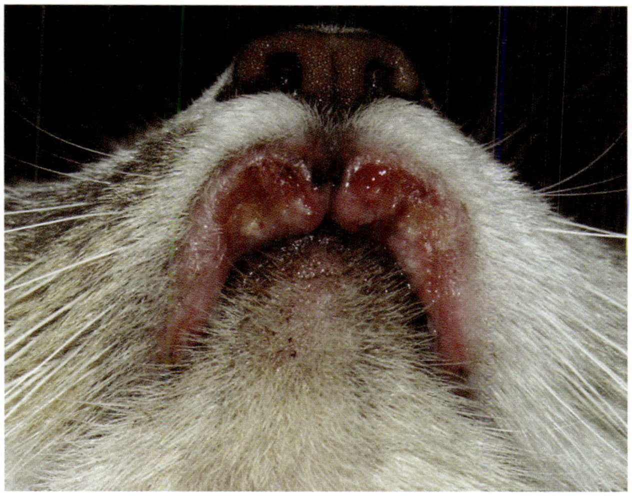

Figure 39.3 Upper lip of cat. Large rodent ulcer secondary to flea allergy dermatitis.

Other signs

Cats may also have otitis externa (3%) and non-dermatologic signs (30%) associated with flea bite allergy [3]. The non-dermatologic signs include respiratory signs, conjunctivitis, and gastrointestinal signs such as vomiting, diarrhoea, and soft stools.

The clinical presentation of flea bite allergy in the cat is extremely variable. Therefore, flea bite allergy should be considered as a differential diagnosis for almost any pruritic cat. One's suspicion of flea bite allergy should increase if the cat lives in an endemic flea area and the cat has lesions on the rump, tail head, dorsum, or flanks.

References

1. Horvath C, van den Broek A. Feline flea allergy dermatitis. *UK Vet* 2006; **11(6)**: 55–62.
2. Craig M. Flea allergic dermatitis in cats. *UK Vet* 2008; **13(5)**: 43–48.
3. Hobi S, Linek M, Marignac G, *et al.* Clinical characteristics and causes of pruritus in cats: a multicentre study on feline hypersensitivity associated dermatoses. *Veterinary Dermatology* 2011; **22**: 406–413.
4. Noli C. Flea allergy in cats—clinical signs and diagnosis. *European Journal of Companion Animal Practice* 2009; **19**: 249–253.
5. Coatesworth J. Feline miliary dermatitis. *UK Vet* 2007; **12(7)**: 73–76.
6. Coward P. A clinician's approach to feline alopecia. *UK Vet* 2010; **15(6)**: 31–36.
7. Oliveira A, van den Broek A. The feline eosinophilic granuloma complex. *UK Vet* 2006; **11(1)**: 48–55.
8. Colombini S, Hodgin EC, Foil CS, *et al.* Induction of feline flea allergy dermatitis and the incidence and histopathological characteristics of concurrent indolent lip ulcers. *Veterinary Dermatology* 2001; **12**: 155–161.

40

Diagnostic workup

Dawn Logas

Veterinary Dermatology Center, Maitland, FL, USA

Conflict of interest: none declared.

The diagnosis of feline flea bite allergy is based on the potential for flea exposure, compatible clinical signs, and consistent history. In flea-endemic areas, flea bite allergy is one of the most common hypersensitivities diagnosed in cats [1]. Because the clinical signs are extremely variable, flea bite allergy should be placed on the differential diagnosis list for any pruritic cat with potential flea exposure. If the dorsum, rump, and tail base areas are affected, flea bite allergy should move higher in the differential diagnoses list; however, this pattern of distribution is not exclusive to flea allergy so it does not rule out other types of hypersensitivity. If there is a history of flea exposure, or if fleas or flea faeces are observed on physical examination, the diagnosis of flea bite allergy is also more likely. Unfortunately, the reverse is not true. Many flea bite allergic cats have no known history of flea exposure and no evidence of fleas on examination. There are several reasons why this may occur. Owners may not notice fleas on their cats because of their thick hair coat and the fact that many cats do not like to be closely examined, groomed, or bathed. In addition, in one study, flea bite allergic cats were found to be significantly better at mechanically removing fleas from their coat compared to non-flea-allergic cats (65.4% of fleas removed after 4 days versus 57% of fleas removed after 4 days) [2]. In the same study, fleas that fed on flea-allergic cats had significantly lower egg production then those that fed on non-flea-allergic cats [2]. This leads to fewer fleas on the cat and in the environment to be noticed by the owner, particularly on a flea-allergic cat.

Once a tentative diagnosis of flea bite allergy is made there are several *in vivo* and *in vitro* tests that can be used to help confirm the diagnosis. Some of these methods are readily available to practising veterinarians while others are mainly used in research settings. None of these tests should be performed unless there is strong evidence to support the diagnosis of flea bite allergy. The diagnosis of flea allergy is ultimately confirmed by the resolution of clinical signs in response to complete flea control and the recrudescence of signs if re-exposure to fleas occurs.

Live flea challenge test

The live flea challenge test [2–5] is a research tool used as the gold standard when evaluating the diagnostic value of various assays, including ELISA and intradermal testing (see Figure 23.2). The test consists of placing recently hatched, unfed fleas in a small container with a mesh lid that allows the fleas to feed when placed on the test cat. The container is placed mesh side down on a small clipped area of the test cat for 15 to 20 minutes. The fleas are then killed and crushed to ensure blood ingestion, thus confirming the test cat's exposure to flea saliva. The test site is inspected at 15 to 20 minutes, 6, 24, and 48 hours by a trained investigator. Any clinical evidence of immediate or delayed hypersensitivity reactions, including erythema, papules, oedema, or crusting, is noted. In some instances the clinical evidence may be extremely mild and may need to be confirmed by histological examination of skin tissue obtained from the test site.

The accuracy of the live flea challenge in the cat depends on whether or not the flea allergy is laboratory-induced

Veterinary Allergy, First Edition. Edited by Chiara Noli, Aiden Foster, and Wayne Rosenkrantz.

or naturally occurring, and how long the signs have been present. In one study in which cats with clinically confirmed flea bite allergy were evaluated, the live flea challenge was found to be a very specific and sensitive test [3]. Another study in which flea bite allergy was induced in kittens, six of eight asymptomatic cats had positive live flea challenge results [4]. It is possible that the live flea challenge was identifying very early flea allergy in these kittens. Unfortunately, it is impossible to know if these kittens later developed clinical signs because the study ended at this point. In another study it was more difficult to interpret the results of the flea bite challenge because the diagnosis of flea bite allergy was assumed simply because of previous flea exposure [5]. In this study, 14/17 cats with previous flea exposure had an immediate or delayed positive live flea challenge even though none of the cats had documented flea bite allergy. At the time of examination only seven cats had any evidence of skin disease, all of which was considered very mild and five cats were infested with fleas without notable dermatologic lesions.

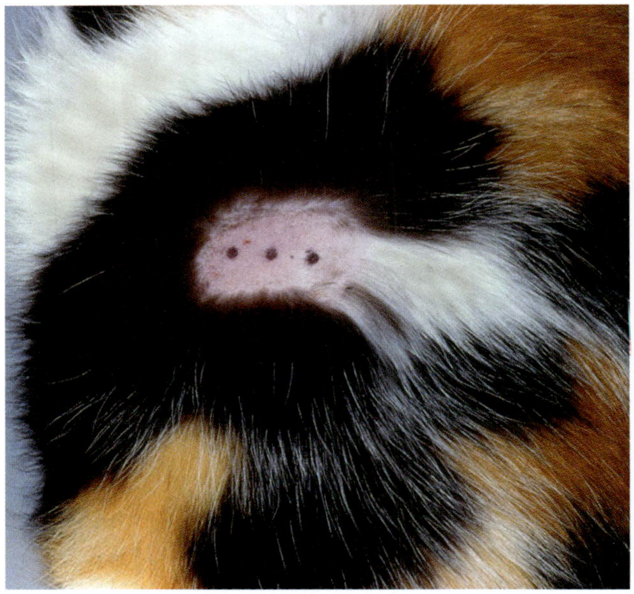

Figure 40.1 Lateral chest wall of cat. Positive skin test reactions to flea, mosquito, and *Culicoides* allergens.

Intradermal testing

Intradermal testing is fairly easy to perform but practice is needed to become proficient at interpreting the results. As in the case of aeroallergens, prior glucocorticoid or antihistamine use can cause false-negative reactions to intradermally injected flea antigen. If possible, a cat should not receive oral glucocorticoids for at least 4 weeks, long acting injectable glucocorticoids for at least 8 weeks, and antihistamines for at least 7 to 10 days before the test is performed. Whole-body flea extracts are currently available from several companies. These extracts are not standardized and therefore can vary in antigenicity and diagnostic reproducibility. A more standardized flea saliva antigen preparation is only available for research purposes. The currently recommended concentration for whole-body flea antigen is 1/1000 w/v. To perform the test, a small area on the lateral thorax or flank is clipped free of hair. Then 0.05–0.1 mL of saline (negative control), histamine (positive control), and flea antigen are injected intradermally. The flea antigen test site is compared to the control sites 10 to 15 minutes after injection. The development of a wheal and flare indicates an immediate (type I) hypersensitivity response to the flea antigen (Figure 40.1). Since some cats may only have a delayed (type IV) hypersensitivity response to flea antigen, the site must be observed during the following 48 hours for any evidence of oedema, erythema, or crusting [5]. Sedation is usually not required to conduct this test on the majority of cats. If the cat is fractious, ketamine or dexmedetomidine may be administered because neither drug will interfere with the test results. With fractious cats it is preferable to rely directly on the response to flea control to diagnosis flea bite allergy.

The documented accuracy of intradermal testing in the cat with flea antigen varies greatly depending on the study and which antigen is used. In two studies evaluating cats with naturally occurring flea allergy or cats with long standing laboratory-induced flea allergy, all cats (total of 15) reacted within 15 minutes to intradermal injection of 1/1000 w/v of whole flea antigen with a +2 or greater reaction. None of the flea-naïve cats (total of 13) in these studies reacted to the intradermal injection of 1/1000 w/v of whole-flea antigen [2,3]. In another study, flea bite allergy was induced in 10 flea-naïve cats [6]. At the beginning of the study, all 10 cats had negative skin test results. At the end of the 240-day study, there was no correlation between the presence of clinical signs consistent with flea bite allergy and a +2 or greater, 15-minute skin test reaction. In this study the sites were not examined at 24 or 48 hours for delayed reactions. In a second study in which flea allergy was induced in kittens, a positive immediate intradermal test also did not correlate with the clinical signs of flea allergy [4]. However, seven out of ten cats with clinical signs had delayed reactions, while only one out of eight asymptomatic cats had a delayed reaction. In a final study, the intradermal and live flea challenge reactions of eight flea-naïve cats and 27 cats with previous flea exposure were compared [5]. In this study, the specificity of intradermal testing compared to live flea challenge ranged from 90 to 100% while the sensitivity was only 33% at best. If the number of immediate and delayed positives were taken together, 17/27 cats had a positive response to one or more of the three commercial whole-body flea extracts tested. A major flaw in this study, as mentioned in Section Live flea challenge test, was that the cats in the test group were not documented by clinical signs as being flea allergic. This puts the assumption that these cats were actually flea allergic in question and therefore makes interpretation of the results of the study difficult.

In several of the studies described above, a proprietary purified flea saliva antigen was used along with the whole-body flea antigens for intradermal testing [2,5,6]. It was hoped that this more purified antigen would give more consistent and accurate results than the whole-body flea antigens. There were no differences observed between the results obtained using either antigen.

Another confounding factor with intradermal flea testing in cats is that the concentration of allergen being used may not be optimal. The current standard 1/1000 w/v concentration for flea antigen has been extrapolated from the dog and some early studies in the cat. A more recent study found the irritant threshold concentration for flea antigen in cats to be higher than 1/750 w/v [7]. This would suggest that cats may need to be tested with a higher concentration of flea antigen to more accurately identify flea bite allergic cats. More research is needed in this area to define the optimal concentration of flea antigens for intradermal testing in the cat.

Serological testing

There are currently multiple companies providing ELISA IgE testing for flea antigen. The antigens used by these companies vary from whole-body flea extracts to highly purified flea saliva to recombinant flea saliva antigen. The advantage of serological testing is that it is a relatively easy test to perform, only involving the collection of a blood sample. Serological testing reputedly only identifies IgE-mediated hypersensitivity, therefore cats with only delayed (cell-mediated) reactions will be incorrectly labelled as non-flea allergic by serological testing. Serological tests are also plagued with varying accuracy and reproducibility no matter which antigen or test is utilized. Two studies demonstrated no correlation between positive ELISA test results (using either whole body flea extract or flea saliva antigen) and clinical evidence of flea allergy in cats [4,6]. In another study, ELISA testing using flea saliva antigen was more sensitive than intradermal testing when compared to live flea challenge [5].

Functional *in vitro* test

The functional *in vitro* test (FIT) for sensitized type I allergic effector cells monitors the blood for allergic effector cells (mainly basophils) with bound allergen-specific antibodies on their surface [8,9]. As with the ELISA IgE testing, all that is required from the cat is a blood sample. The blood cells are washed and incubated with the selected antigen. If membrane-bound antibodies on the basophils are cross-linked by the antigen there is immediate release of histamine. This histamine is quantified and compared to the relevant maximal histamine release. A histamine release of ≥20% is considered to be a positive response. In a study designed to investigate the usefulness of FIT in the diagnosis of feline flea allergy, 14 cats were sensitized to *Ctenocephalides felis* over a 28-weeks period [9]. FITs were performed weekly and compared to both intradermal and serology testing. The results of FITs were comparable to intradermal testing but discordant with the ELISA IgE testing. At this point more research is needed to see if FIT is a viable alternative to intradermal testing and is more accurate than ELISA IgE testing.

Histopathology

Taking skin biopsy samples from suspected flea bite allergy lesions is not recommended as a clinical diagnostic test. Histopathology of these lesions shows changes consistent with immediate or delayed or both types of hypersensitivity reaction [3]; it cannot differentiate between flea allergy and other allergic diseases. In the research setting when the stimulus for the allergic reaction is known to be a flea bite, histopathology can be useful.

In vivo and *in vitro* flea 'allergy' testing in cats should only be used if a tentative diagnosis of flea bite allergy is made based on consistent history and clinical signs. A positive result for any of these tests helps to confirm the diagnosis of flea bite allergy, but a negative result does not rule out flea bite allergy. Ultimately, the diagnosis is confirmed by response to flea control and recurrence of signs with re-exposure to fleas.

References

1. Hobi S, Linek M, Marignac G, *et al.* Clinical characteristics and causes of pruritus in cats: a multicentre study on feline hypersensitivity-associated dermatoses. *Veterinary Dermatology* 2011; **22**: 406–413.
2. McDonald BJ, Foil CS, Foil LD. An investigation on the influence of feline flea allergy on the fecundity of the cat flea. *Veterinary Dermatology* 1998; **9**: 75–79.
3. Lewis DT, Ginn PE, Kunkle GA. Clinical and histological evaluation of immediate and delayed flea antigen intradermal skin test and

flea bite sites in normal and flea allergic cats. *Veterinary Dermatology* 1999; **10**: 29–37.

4. Kunkle GA, McCall CA, Stedman KE, *et al.* Pilot study to assess the effects of early flea exposure on the development of flea hypersensitivity in cats. *Journal of Feline Medicine and Surgery* 2003; **5**: 287–294.
5. Bond R, Hutchinson MJ, Loeffler A. Serological, intradermal and live flea challenge tests in the assessment of hypersensitivity to flea antigen in cats. *Parasitology Research* 2006; **99**: 392–397.
6. Colombini S, Hodgin EC, Foil CS, *et al.* Induction of feline flea allergy dermatitis and the incidence and histopathological characteristics of concurrent indolent lip ulcers. *Veterinary Dermatology* 2001; **12**: 155–161.
7. Austel M, Hensel P, Jackson D, *et al.* Evaluation of three different histamine concentrations in intradermal testing of normal cats and attempted determination of the irritant threshold concentrations of 48 allergens. *Veterinary Dermatology* 2006; **17**: 189–194.
8. Stuke K, von Samson-Himmelstjerna G, Mencke N, *et al.* Flea allergy dermatitis in cats: establishment of a functional *in vitro* test. *Parasitology Research* 2003; **90**: S129–131.
9. Stuke K, von Samson-Himmelstjerna G, Dreesman J, *et al.* Monitoring of basophil sensitization to antigens of the cat flea: a new tool for the diagnosis of feline flea bite hypersensitivity? *Parasitology Research* 2008; **103**: 807–820.

41

Therapy

Marie-Christine Cadiergues

Toulouse Veterinary School, Toulouse, France

Conflict of interest: Marie-Christine Cadiergues has served as a study investigator with Merial, Novartis, and Intervet; she has received honoraria for consulting and lectures from Bayer, Elanco, Merial, Novartis, Pfizer, Vétoquinol, and Virbac.

Introduction

Flea allergy dermatitis (FAD) remains the most common allergic skin disease of dogs and cats, although its frequency varies according to geographical location. The past 20 years have brought important advances in flea biology as well as better insecticides [1]. Nevertheless, flea control in general, and more specifically in cats with FAD, remains a real challenge for vets and owners. The goal is to minimize flea bites, i.e. to minimize the amount of saliva injected by fleas in order to be under the allergic threshold.

Main difficulties and pitfalls

Convincing the owner and customizing flea control measures

Surprisingly, one major difficulty in FAD control is convincing the owner (and sometimes the referring practitioner) that FAD is the correct diagnosis. It is rather common to be faced with owner disbelief or scepticism. Because fleas are not seen by the owner, and their presence is difficult to prove on animals with FAD, the owner is sometimes absolutely convinced that fleas cannot be the cause of his/her cat's dermatitis. Some people associate fleas with a lack of hygiene and cannot accept that their pet(s) might have fleas. Other people, who recognize fleas in cats to be common, doubt that their pet would present with a flea-related skin disease when other pets with fleas do not have a skin problem. Furthermore, why should pruritus be so severe if only a few fleas are present? Owners may be sceptical because they think, or have been told, that they are doing everything they can to kill fleas and/or that they have used the 'wonder' product.

Once convinced, the owner needs guidance and motivation. A clear explanation of the flea life cycle combined with information on the way products work is usually helpful. Demonstrating how to apply the product(s) correctly is recommended; a small area on the skin of the back of the neck could be shaved to ensure that a spot-on formulation is applied onto the skin and not in the fur.

The therapeutic regimen should always be customized, necessitating a thorough cat history and details of the owner's circumstances.

Skin lesions and excessive grooming

Excessive grooming, cutaneous inflammation, and secondary cornification disorders (scaling) should be considered when applying a topical flea product. Not only may the product irritate the skin but its diffusion may also be impaired by the skin changes. Excessive grooming, which is very common in cats with FAD, might reduce the amount of insecticide present on the skin thereby reducing or delaying its efficacy. Consequently, systemic products would be the type of product of choice because they would be at a sufficient concentration despite over-grooming and/or skin lesions.

Veterinary Allergy, First Edition. Edited by Chiara Noli, Aiden Foster, and Wayne Rosenkrantz.

In-contact animals and premises

All the in-contact animals should be treated, albeit less strictly perhaps than the cat with FAD. Other cats, in particular, are easily forgotten either because they live outdoors or because they may not be around when it is time to treat the patient. Cats can also be difficult to medicate and are sometimes not considered by owners to be part of the problem. All areas regularly visited by the pet with FAD (including cars and sheds) should be treated with a suitable product at an appropriate frequency. Visiting pets inadequately treated for fleas represent a risk as they can re-introduce fleas (mainly immature stages which can develop and lead to delayed re-infestations but possibly also adults) in a well-controlled household. Similarly, visiting infested places can trigger a flare. When such possibilities cannot be avoided, strict preventive treatment, similar to a trial therapy regimen, should be recommended.

Maintaining consistency of flea control

After a while, particularly when there is clinical improvement, attention given to flea control tends to flag. However, this must not be allowed to happen. The practitioner and/or well-trained nurses from the practice must regularly emphasize the importance of consistent flea control. Reminders can be sent using modern communication forms (text messages, Multimedia Messaging Services on mobile phones, emails). These are sometimes offered free of charge by pharmaceutical companies.

Over-the-counter products

Extensive and long-term flea control measures require considerable effort and expense. This can produce a progressive reduction in compliance, and may also explain why over-the-counter (OTC) products are sometimes preferred by owners. Some OTC products, with natural active ingredients (herbal, essential oils) do not have the efficacy, residual activity, or safety profile of the veterinary products. With time, substitution of OTC products could lead to poor control of FAD, owner frustration, or even suspicion of resistance.

Active ingredients and formulations

Neonicotinoids

This class of insecticides was developed for crop protection and subsequently found to be highly effective for flea control in dogs and cats, with an excellent tolerance. Imidacloprid, nitenpyram, and dinotefuran are the active ingredients available for pets.

Imidacloprid has a high affinity for the nicotinergic acetylcholine receptors in the postsynaptic region of the central nervous system (CNS) in insects. The ensuing inhibition of cholinergic transmission in insects results in paralysis and death of the parasite. It is only available as a spot-on with surface action. It is effective against adult fleas, requiring 8 hours of contact [2–4]. It also has, in common with most insecticidal products, a larvicidal effect [5,6].

Nitenpyram is a fast-acting, orally administered flea treatment. Like imidacloprid, it acts on the nicotinic acetylcholine receptor channel. It is readily absorbed with peak plasma levels reached within 30 minutes and a half-life of about 8 hours [7,8]. The first signs of efficacy are seen 15 minutes or more after ingestion. Fleas are dislodged after 30 minutes, and within 6 hours, over 95% are killed. The effect is prolonged for 24–48 hours [8].

Dinotefuran is a third-generation neonicotinoid; dinotefuran was synthesized with acetylcholine as the lead compound whereas imidacloprid was based on nicotine. It is also a fast-killing insecticide, effective for 30 days following application [9]. It is available for cats in the USA as a spot-on, combined with pyriproxyfen. In dogs it is also combined with permethrin. The owner should be reminded that permethrin-containing products marketed for dogs are toxic in cats. The owners should be discouraged from using such products in a household where cats and dogs cohabit to avoid accidental intoxication.

Phenylpyrazoles

Introduced in Europe in 1994, fipronil has been a market leader ever since. First available as a spray, fipronil later became available in a spot-on formulation, eventually being combined with methoprene, still as a spot-on. Now that fipronil's patent has expired, generic products have appeared on the market and are now available OTC in the USA. Phenylpyrazoles block the gamma-aminobutyric acid (GABA)-gated chloride channels of neurons in the central nervous system, sharing a common binding site with cyclodienes. Fipronil also binds to two different glutamate-gated chloride channels [10,11]. The efficacy of fipronil was evaluated in cats with FAD. The 10% fipronil solution applied monthly to cats with FAD reduced flea counts by 94% on day 90 with pruritus reduced or absent in 78% of cats [12]. In a study comparing the fipronil-based original product and a generic, despite comprising different vehicles, the two formulations were equally able to eradicate flea infestation, to prevent new infestations, and they were equally well-tolerated [13].

Avermectins

Selamectin is believed to bind to glutamate-gated chloride channels in the parasite's nervous system, increasing permeability and allowing the rapid and continued influx of chloride ions into the nerve cell. This inhibits nerve activity thereby causing paralysis [14]. Selamectin is applied topically, is rapidly absorbed through the skin, and is distributed via the blood. It has activity against both internal and external parasites. Several studies have been published supporting its efficacy against fleas [5,15–19]. Topical application was over 98% effective after 24 hours in cats [18,19]. A study performed in dogs and cats with FAD housed in flea-infested, simulated home environments showed a significant reduction in clinical signs after two applications, 1 month apart [20].

Metaflumizone

Metaflumizone is derived from pyrazoline and acts by binding the voltage-dependent sodium channels in insects. Studies in controlled environment (experimental infestations, comb-counts 48 hours after treatment and re-infestations) showed over 90% efficacy for 7 weeks in cats [21]. Speed of kill was evaluated in adult cats and compared with a product containing a combination of fipronil-(S) and methoprene, it was found to be slower [22].

Spinosad

Spinosad is an aerobic fermentation product of the soil bacterium, *Saccharopolyspora spinosa*. Spinosad kills insects through activation of the acetylcholine nervous system through nicotinic receptors. A chewable tablet is indicated for the treatment and prevention of flea infestations caused by *C. felis*, was first introduced for dogs to the US market in 2007 and in Europe in 2011, followed by the approval for cats in USA, Canada, and Japan in 2012. Its excellent efficacy against fleas and its rapid killing effect that is observed in dogs are also reported in cats [23,24]. Spinoram, a spinosin, is available for cats in the USA as a spot-on.

Oxadiazines

Indoxacarb is a novel oxadiazine insecticide which has good field activity against a number of pests including Lepidoptera, as well as certain Homoptera and Coleoptera. Its main mode of action is via blocking of sodium nerve channels. Following application, indoxacarb is taken up by fleas where it is converted into a highly active metabolite. This metabolite causes fleas to stop feeding and they die within hours. Unlike insects, mammals mainly convert indoxacarb into non-toxic metabolites so they are not exposed to the active insecticide. It has been licensed for cats as a spot-on formulation.

One study was carried out in the EU (Spain, France, and Germany) with the final formulation. A total of 110 dogs and 97 cats were included in the indoxacarb group; 101 dogs and 85 cats were kept as per protocol efficacy analysis. A total of 97 dogs and 100 cats were included in the control group, treated with an authorized reference product containing fipronil; 89 dogs and 85 cats were kept as per protocol efficacy analysis. Animals were treated every 4 weeks with a total of three treatments. Counting of fleas, flea allergy dermatitis assessment, observations on local reaction at the application site, and general attitude were carried out on Day 0 and every two weeks on Days (+2) 14, 28, 42, 56, 70, and 84. In both groups the percentage of dogs and cats with flea allergy dermatitis decreased markedly over time. In the indoxacarb-treated group, dogs and cats were considered cured from signs of FBA from the sixth visit in dogs and the fourth visit in cats. At the end of the observation period (visit seven), one dog and one cat still had signs of FAD in the fipronil group. The number of dogs and cats with signs of flea allergy dermatitis was not different between the two treatment groups at each of the seven visits [25].

Juvenile hormone analogues

The pharmacological properties of juvenile hormone analogues (JHAs) are characterized by mimicking the juvenile hormones of insects resulting in interference with metamorphosis and reproduction. Prevention of larval development breaks the flea life cycle. Due to the specificity of juvenile hormone for insects, pyriproxyfen has virtually no effects on mammals. Two products, methoprene and pyriproxyfen, are used for flea control, either administered to the animal or applied in the environment.

Insect developmental inhibitors

Lufenuron is a systemic insect developmental inhibitor (IDI) which interferes with chitin synthesis, polymerization, and deposition [26]. Lufenuron has no effect on adult fleas. Excreted in flea faeces, it prevents normal pupation of larvae feeding on those flea faeces. Numerous studies have shown its efficacy either administered orally or injected to cats [14,27–29].

Recommendations

As yet, the ideal product does not exist

Flea avoidance is certainly the goal for a cat with FAD. This is difficult and takes time. Symptomatic, antipruritic therapy is often necessary. Furthermore, there are so many opportunities for a cat to pick up fleas (e.g. environment, neighbourhood, occasional visiting pets, and wildlife) that even if flea control is considered optimal, it may still fail. Allergen-specific immunotherapy has, to date, not been helpful.

The ideal product to protect an animal with FAD against fleas would be one with repellent action, i.e. a product that ideally would prevent fleas (mainly newly emerged adults but also fleas coming from infested animals) from jumping on, or at least disturbing any fleas that did arrive in the coat so that they would leave immediately without biting (flushing effect). Unfortunately, although such products are effective against some insects (e.g. mosquitoes), they are not very helpful in flea control. The best repellent against fleas is permethrin, which is toxic for cats.

One should remember that a newly emerged flea will start feeding within a few minutes of its arrival on the host. The first blood meal lasts from 10 minutes (males) to 25 minutes (females) [30]. It is, therefore, not surprising that none of the aforementioned products is able to kill fleas before the fleas start to bite. However, some of them (nitenpyram and spinosad) can certainly shorten the blood meal duration thereby reducing the amount of saliva injected and consequently minimizing the allergenic stimulus. The once perceived dogma of the single flea bite concept is behind us. The goal when managing FAD should be to rapidly reduce flea numbers and flea feeding rather than preventing flea bites, which is virtually impossible. It is the author's opinion that fast-acting products will potentially be more helpful at reducing antigen exposure because the total duration of feeding is decreased.

A female flea starts laying eggs within 24–36 hours and then continues to do so for the rest of its life. Consequently, to prevent additional environmental contamination, a product that becomes effective in less than 24 hours should be recommended.

Adulticidal products on the animal with flea allergy dermatitis

Given what has already been said about the testing and evaluation of antiparasitic substances, and also the effects of over-grooming and skin inflammation on reducing product efficacy, it might be wise to recommend systemic products. Some practitioners use products more frequently but when doing so this may be against manufacturer and country recommendations. The author prefers alternating, every 2 weeks, between two different products each with a different mode of action. The efficacy of insecticidal products is dose-dependent. The dose itself is time-dependent, varying according to whether the product is applied all over the body surface or to a more restricted area. Systemic products have the advantage of not being altered by any skin change/action.

Treatment of in-contact animals

All must be treated, including other cats. Their treatment regimen does not have to be as strict as that of the pet with FAD. A single adulticidal product (instead of possibly two on the animal with FAD), applied according to the manufacturer's recommendations (instead of every 14 days) might be suggested. Should the animal with FAD be treated with a systemic (or possibly topical) insect growth regulator (IGR) such as lufenuron (or methoprene/pyriproxyfen), all in-contact animals should also be treated.

Targeting the different steps of the life cycle: integrated control

An insect growth regulator—JHA or an IDI—should be combined with an adulticide(s), either on the animal or in the environment. Prior to application of flea control products in the environment, hygienic measures should be recommended, bearing in mind the relative lack of efficacy of vacuuming against larvae. Prior steam cleaning should be suggested.

When premises are too large, or when young children are at high risk of coming in contact with the products (particularly pyrethroids) whilst playing on carpets, the IGR should be administered directly to the animal, preferably systemically.

Customizing flea control

Factors that may influence failure in a flea control programme may be product-related or animal and/or owner-related. Client compliance, short-term and long-term, is essential in FBA cases. Therefore, any control plan has to be practical for the owner and must be adapted to individual circumstances. Compliance, ability, health, financial resources, presence of young children, and degree of pet and owner contact must all be taken into consideration.

Antipruritic therapy

Symptomatic therapy may be needed to relieve pruritus, particularly in the induction phase, as the antiparasitic treatment may take time to be fully effective, and when the condition flares up (visiting pets, antiflea treatment less drastic). Glucocorticosteroids (GCS) are most commonly used. Although cats tend to tolerate GCS better than dogs and humans, adverse effects do occur including: obesity, diabetes mellitus, alopecia, skin fragility, aggravation of heart failure, behavioural changes, and predisposition to infection. Usual active ingredients are:

- prednisolone: 1–2 mg/kg once daily per os then wean;
- methylprednisolone: 0.8–1.5 mg/kg once daily per os then wean;
- dexamethasone: 0.1–0.2 mg/kg once daily per os then wean.

Should the cat tolerate topical therapy, a hydrocortisone aceponate spray can be used [31].

Despite the availability of safe, effective products, treating FAD remains a challenge. This challenge should be more readily overcome once both practitioner and owner(s) are entirely convinced of the diagnosis. Appropriate knowledge of the flea life cycle and flea-related biology, an understanding of the mode of action of flea control products, and motivation are all required. An integrated approach to treatment should be adopted, involving all the players in the flea life cycle—the FAD patient, all in-contact pets, and the environment. Each case must be customized, with effective flea control products used in combination with cleaning measures such as steaming, vacuuming, and regular grooming.

References

1. Rust MK. Advances in the control of *Ctenocephalides felis* (cat flea) on cats and dogs. *Trends in Parasitology* 2005; **21**: 232–236.
2. Dryden MW, Denenberg TM, Bunch S. Control of fleas on naturally infested dogs and cats and in private residences with topical spot applications of fipronil or imidacloprid. *Veterinary Parasitology* 2000; **93**: 69–75.
3. Ritzhaupt LK, Rowan TG, Jones RL. Evaluation of efficacy of selamectin, fipronil, and imidacloprid against *Ctenocephalides felis* in dogs. *Journal of the American Veterinary Medical Association* 2000; **217**: 1669–1671.
4. Schenker R, Tinembart O, Humbert-Droz E, *et al.* Comparative speed of kill between nitenpyram, fipronil, imidacloprid, selamectin and cythioate against adult *Ctenocephalides felis* (Bouche) on cats and dogs. *Veterinary Parasitology* 2003; **112**: 249–254.
5. Mehlhorn H, Hansen O, Mencke N. Comparative study on the effects of three insecticides (fipronil, imidacloprid, selamectin) on developmental stages of the cat flea (*Ctenocephalides felis* Bouche 1835): a light and electron microscopic analysis of in vivo and in vitro experiments. *Parasitology Research* 2001; **87**: 198–207.
6. Fourie LJ, Kok DJ, Peter RJ. Control of immature stages of the flea *Ctenocephalides felis* (Bouche) in carpets exposed to cats treated with imidacloprid. *Journal of the South African Veterinary Association* 2000; **7**: 219–221.
7. Dobson P, Tinembart O, Fisch RD, *et al.* Efficacy of nitenpyram as a systemic flea adulticide in dogs and cats. *Veterinary Record* 2000; **147**: 709–713.
8. Rust MK, Waggoner MM, Hinkle NC, *et al.* Efficacy and longevity of nitenpyram against adult cat fleas (Siphonaptera: Pulicidae). *Journal of Medical Entomology* 2003; **40**: 678–681.
9. Correia TR, Cruz VP, Ribeiro Fde A, *et al.* Residual activity in vitro of treated dog's hair coat with dinotefuran on larvae and adults of *Ctenocephalides felis felis* (Bouche, 1835) (Siphonaptera: Pulicidae). *Revista Brasileirade Parasitologia Veterinaria* 2008; **17**: 195–199.
10. Zhao X, Yeh JZ, Salgado VL, *et al.* Fipronil is a potent open channel blocker of glutamate-activated chloride channels in cockroach neurons. *Journal of Pharmacology and Experimental Therapeutics* 2004; **310**: 192–201.
11. Zhao X, Salgado VL, Yeh JZ, *et al.* Differential actions of fipronil and dieldrin insecticides on GABA-gated chloride channels in cockroach neurons. *Journal of Pharmacology and Experimental Therapeutics* 2003; **306**: 914–924.
12. Medleau L, Hnilica KA, Lower K, *et al.* Effect of topical application of fipronil in cats with flea allergic dermatitis. *Journal of the American Veterinary Medical Association* 2002; **221**: 254–257.
13. Cadiergues MC, Bonneau SG, Fourier JJ. Assay of two 10% (w/v) fipronil spot-on formulations against feline infestations with *Ctenocephalides felis*. *Journal of Feline Medicine and Surgery* 2011; **13**: 304–308.
14. Zakson-Aiken M, Gregory LM, Meinke PT, *et al.* Systemic activity of the avermectins against the cat flea (Siphonaptera: Pulicidae). *Journal of Medical Entomology* 2001; **38**: 576–580.
15. Ritzhaupt LK, Rowan TG, Jones RL, *et al.* Evaluation of the comparative efficacy of selamectin against flea (*Ctenocephalides felis felis*) infestations on dogs and cats in simulated home environments. *Veterinary Parasitology* 2002; **106**: 165–175.
16. Shanks DJ, Rowan TG, Jones RL, *et al.* Efficacy of selamectin in the treatment and prevention of flea (*Ctenocephalides felis felis*) infestations on dogs and cats housed in simulated home environments. *Veterinary Parasitology* 2000; **91**: 213–222.
17. Benchaoui HA, Clemence RG, Clements PJ, *et al.* Efficacy and safety of selamectin against fleas on dogs and cats presented as veterinary patients in Europe. *Veterinary Parasitology* 2000; **91**: 223–232.
18. McTier TL, Jones RL, Holbert MS, *et al.* Efficacy of selamectin against adult flea infestations (*Ctenocephalides felis felis* and *Ctenocephalidescanis*) on dogs and cats. *Veterinary Parasitology* 2000; **91**: 187–199.
19. McTier TL, Shanks DJ, Jernigan AD, *et al.* Evaluation of the effects of selamectin against adult and immature stages of fleas (*Ctenocephalides felis felis*) on dogs and cats. *Veterinary Parasitology* 2000; **91**: 201–212.
20. Dickin SK, McTier TL, Murphy MG, *et al.* Efficacy of selamectin in the treatment and control of clinical signs of flea allergy dermatitis in dogs and cats experimentally infested with fleas. *Journal of the American Veterinary Medical Association* 2003; **223**: 639–644.
21. Holzmer S, Hair JA, Dryden MW, *et al.* Efficacy of a novel formulation of metaflumizone for the control of fleas (*Ctenocephalides felis*) on cats. *Veterinary Parasitology* 2007; **150**: 219–224.
22. Franc M, Beugnet F. A comparative evaluation of the speed of kill and duration of efficacy against weekly infestations with fleas on cats treated with fipronil-(S)-methoprene or metaflumizone. *Veterinary Therapeutics* 2008; **9**: 102–110.
23. Robertson-Plouch C, Baker KA, Hozak RR, *et al.* Clinical field study of the safety and efficacy of spinosad chewable tablets for controlling fleas on dogs. *Veterinary Therapeutics* 2008; **9**: 26–36.
24. Franc M, Bouhsira E. Evaluation of speed and duration of efficacy of spinosad tablets for treatment and control of *Ctenocephalides canis* (Siphonaptera: Pulicidae) infestations in dogs. *Parasite* 2009; **16**: 125–128.
25. European Medicines Agency. *Activyl: EPAR-Scientific Discussion*. Available at: http://www.ema.europa.eu/ema/index.jsp?curl=pages/medicines/veterinary/medicines/000163/vet_med_000229.jsp&mid=WC0b01ac058001fa1c#authorisation (accessed 24 November 2012).

26. Dean SR, Meola RW, Meola SM, *et al.* Mode of action of lufenuron in adult *Ctenocephalides felis* (Siphonaptera: Pulicidae). *Journal of Medical Entomology* 1999; **36**: 486–492.
27. Dryden MW, Perez HR, Ulitchny DM. Control of fleas on pets and in homes by use of imidacloprid or lufenuron and a pyrethrin spray. *Journal of the American Veterinary Medical Association* 1999; **215**: 36–39.
28. Jacobs DE, Hutchinson MJ, Fox MT, *et al.* Comparison of flea control strategies using imidacloprid or lufenuron on cats in a controlled simulated home environment. *American Journal of Veterinary Research* 1997; **58**: 1260–1262.
29. Franc M, Cadiergues MC. Use of injectable lufenuron for treatment of infestations of *Ctenocephalides felis* in cats. *American Journal of Veterinary Research* 1997; **58**: 140–142.
30. Cadiergues MC, Hourcq P, Cantaloube B, *et al.* First bloodmeal of *Ctenocephalides felis felis* (Siphonaptera: Pulicidae) on cats: time to initiation and duration of feeding. *Journal of Medical Entomology* 2000; **37**: 634–636.
31. Schmidt V, Buckley LM, McEwan NA, *et al.* Efficacy of a 0.0584% hydrocortisone aceponate spray in presumed feline allergic dermatitis: an open label pilot study. *Veterinary Dermatology* 2012; **23**: 11–6, e3–4.

Section 4

Mosquito Bite Allergy

42

Mosquito bite

Masahiko Nagata

ASC Dermatology Service, Tokyo; Synergy Animal General Hospital Dermatology Service, Saitama, Japan

Conflict of interest: none declared.

Pathogenesis

Mosquitoes are common insects that affect both humans and animals. While generally harmless, mosquito bites have been associated with eosinophilic dermatitis in some cats [1–7]. This condition can probably be seen in any location where mosquitoes are found; cases have been reported in Australia, Japan, New Zealand, and North America. Cutaneous allergic reactions to mosquito bites and their antigens in cats have been investigated using mosquito bite exposure, intradermal tests, and Prausnitz–Küstner tests (P-K tests) [2,5].

Mosquito bite exposure with *Aedes albopictus* on lesional and unaffected skin in allergic cats showed wheals within 20 minutes. Papules developed over a 12 to 48-hour period, which consisted of a dense eosinophilic infiltrate. Control cats showed only slight and transient erythema after being bitten. Intradermal tests in allergic cats with an extract of *A. albopictus* and P-K tests, both following *A. albopictus* bites, showed wheals in some cases although papules were not observed. Intradermal tests in control cats and P-K tests with saline and healthy cat serum failed to produce positive reactions. These findings indicate that dermatitis due to mosquito bites in cats is triggered by a type I hypersensitivity reaction to mosquito antigens. However, the delayed papule reactions are more difficult to categorize, indicating that saliva toxins and/or cutaneous late-phase reactions do not represent papule reactions.

In humans, cutaneous responses to mosquito bites are determined by previous exposure. Normal cutaneous reactions to mosquito bites have been divided into five stages based on experimental studies [8]. After the initial non-reactive stage (stage 1), subsequent bites cause a delayed cutaneous reaction (stage 2). Several months after the exposure an immediate wheal develops (stage 3). Thereafter, the delayed bite disappears (stage 4) and, finally, the immediate reaction disappears (stage 5). These reactions are generally considered to be immunological in nature and it is suspected that the sequence of change is due to a process of sensitization and desensitization. Studies of the bite reaction in relation to age have shown an increase in immediate reactions from early childhood to adolescence, which decrease thereafter. In cats this reaction is not thoroughly understood; it is predicted that a relationship between the clinical reactions and frequency of exposure are similar to normal mosquito bite reactions in humans.

Clinical features

The most striking clinical features include miliary dermatitis and/or eosinophilic granuloma on the outer pinnae, nasal bridge, and outer margins of footpads in cats sensitized to mosquito bites (Figures 42.1, 42.2, and 42.3). The skin lesions consist of papules, erosions, crusts, and nodules, which lead to mild or severe pruritus. Regional lymphadenopathy is also noted in some cases. Most cases involve short-haired, free-roaming cats. It is clear that affected cats have a high risk of mosquito bites during their lives. Mosquitoes are attracted to hosts by a number of factors [9], with dark colour acting as an important visual attractant [10]. The development and severity of the lesions appears to be directly associated

Veterinary Allergy, First Edition. Edited by Chiara Noli, Aiden Foster, and Wayne Rosenkrantz.

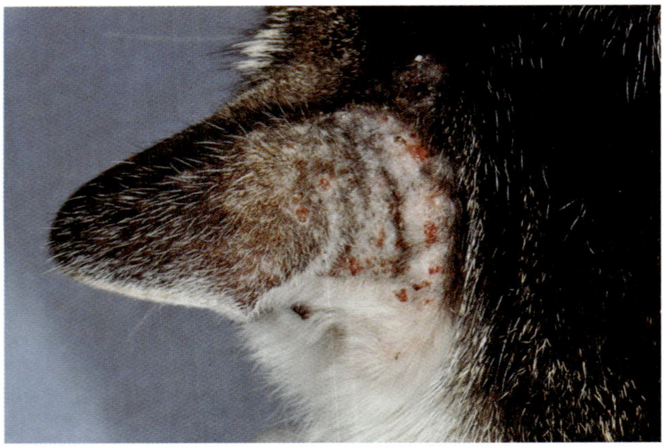

Figure 42.1 Clinical findings of mosquito bites in a cat. Note alopecia, papules, crusts, and erosions on the lateral aspect of the pinnae.

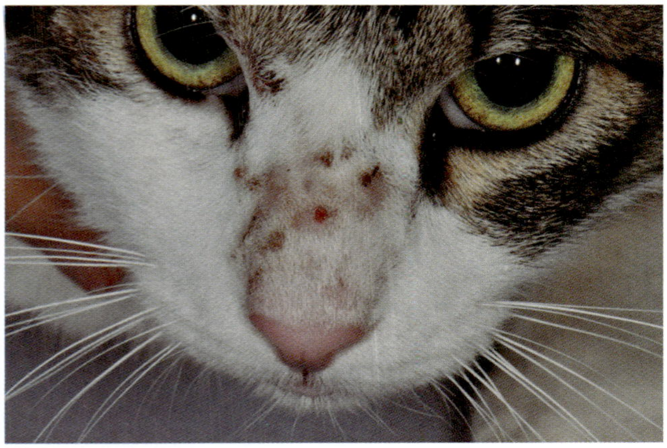

Figure 42.2 Clinical findings of mosquito bites in a cat. Note alopecia, papules, crusts, and erosions on the nasal bridge.

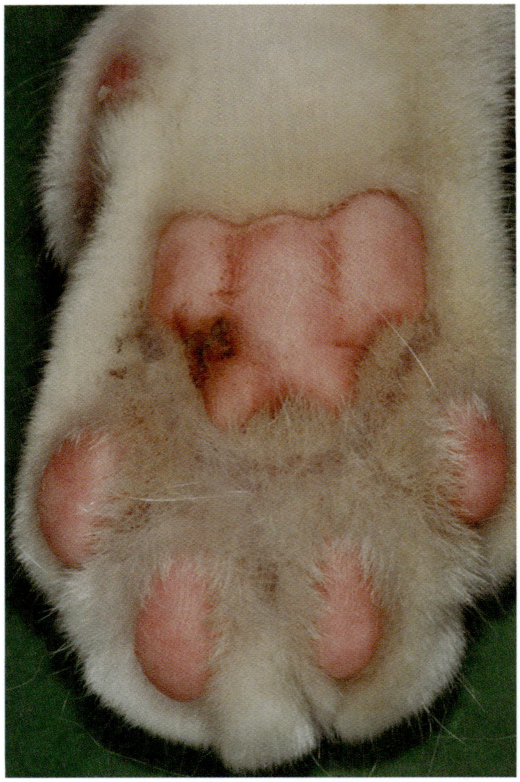

Figure 42.3 Clinical findings of mosquito bites in a cat. Note pigmented scaly crusts, and erythema on the outer margin of the main footpad.

with the frequency of mosquito attacks. The age at the initial onset of the disease varies from 8 months to 6 years, with a mean age of 3.0 years [5]. No sex and breed predisposition have been observed. Typical clinical features include summer seasonality.

Differential diagnoses include ear mite infestation, food allergy, herpes virus dermatitis, autoimmune disorders such as pemphigus foliaceus or cutaneous lupus erythematosus, and photo-induced dermatitis such as solar dermatitis and photosensitive dermatitis.

Diagnostic tests

Clinical features can suggest mosquito bites; however, most bites are not observed directly. Diagnosis can be confirmed using the challenge test with a live mosquito. Laboratory findings are not definitive but helpful in its diagnosis in everyday practice. An immunoassay has been developed to measure mosquito salivary specific IgE antibodies in humans. It is thought that in the future sensitive and specific *in vitro* immunoassays will be developed using recombinant mosquito salivary allergens for humans and hopefully for cats [11].

Challenge test

Mosquito bites can be confirmed by capturing one of the most common mosquitoes in each area and season. A female mosquito is placed in a tube with the open end of the tube placed on the lateral thorax or pinna until the mosquito is completely replenished (Figure 42.4). The wheal is grossly observed at the site within 20 minutes as a positive reaction. In some cases recurrence of the lesions on the pinnae, nasal bridge, or shaved dark-haired areas can be used to confirm the diagnosis.

Cytology

Cytology of the impression smears at the erosive lesions may show remarkable eosinophil infiltrations with mild to moderate numbers of lymphocytes, macrophages, basophils, and/or mast cells.

Histopathology

Histological findings include diffuse perivascular eosinophilic dermatitis with lymphocyte, macrophage,

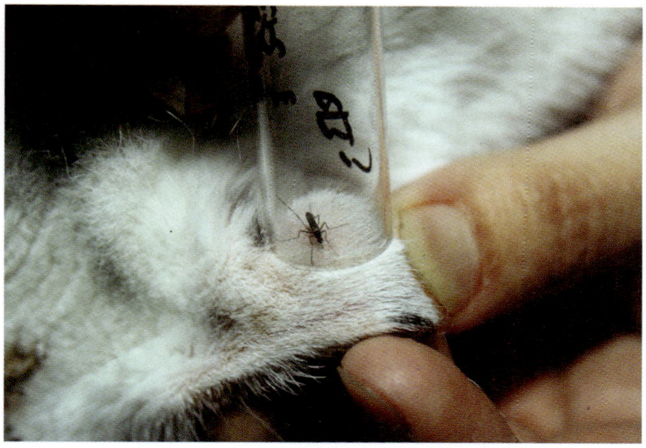

Figure 42.4 Challenge test. A female mosquito is placed in a tube, with the open end of the tube placed on the lateral pinna or thorax until the mosquito is completely replenished.

neutrophil, and/or mast cell infiltrations. Perifollicular and/or follicular eosinophil infiltrations and a superficial band of eosinophils are observed. In addition, some cases involve flame figures, which are small to moderately sized foci of degenerated eosinophils. In some cases there may also be eosinophilic furunculosis. In the epidermis, serocellular crusting, severe spongiosis, subcorneal pustules, erosion, ulceration, and/or moderate acanthosis may be observed.

Laboratory blood tests

Results of complete blood count tests may reveal eosinophilia and no apparent abnormality in serum chemistry parameters. Serum electrophoresis may reveal hypergammaglobulinaemia [5].

Treatment

There are several strategies that can be used to prevent mosquito bites. Mosquito bite avoidance is essential in areas such as tall grass, bush, wetlands, and swamps, particularly when mosquitoes are most active. Each species displays daily active rhythms in their living areas. In general, *Aedes* spp. are active during the daytime while house mosquitoes, including *Culex* and *Anopheles* spp., are active during the night time [12]. For instance, *A. albopictus*, one of the most prevalent mosquitoes in Japan, shows peak blood feeding at dusk in areas with water, such as ponds and puddles [12]. The owner must be instructed that affected cats should be kept indoors, particularly during the late afternoon.

Insect repellent is another strategy for preventing mosquito bites. The two principal categories of commercially available insect repellents include plant-derived essential oils and synthetic chemicals. The former group includes citronella, oil of eucalyptus, peppermint, tea-tree oil, lavender, soybean oil, and neem oil [13]. The synthetic chemical DEET (*N*, *N*-diethyl-*m*-toluamide) is the most widely used repellent in humans [13]; however, DEET may be toxic to cats; permethrin-based products can also be toxic unless specifically formulated for use on cats. To repel mosquitoes the cat owner should apply repellents topically to the affected area every day because the efficacy of many of the agents is low due to the short-lived duration of action. Generally, this procedure is not acceptable for cats and their owners. Aomori Hiba (*Thujopsis dolabrata* Sieb. et Zucc. var *hondai* Makino) derived acid oil, which is a repellent available in Japan, has persistent activity [14]. This long-acting agent can be applied as an oil-dipped cloth wrapped around the collar.

Glucocorticoids are the most reliable agents for controlling skin lesions. Continuous scratching behaviour can induce a vicious cycle of inflammation even for cats in a mosquito-free environment. Topical therapy is not sufficient in most cases. Systemic glucocorticoids are often effective for improving lesions rapidly. Some cases require treatment for a few months because of its seasonality. Injectable long-acting steroids may be convenient although oral products are preferred for safety. Oral prednisolone is commonly dispensed in general practice and the cats may require more than 2 mg/kg once or twice per day; alternatives include oral triamcinolone, 0.5 mg/kg once every day. Once the lesions have resolved, oral therapy should be tapered to the lowest dose and frequency. All cats receiving long-term glucocorticoid therapy should be monitored for metabolic effects and infections, including bacteria, fungus, and virus.

Immunotherapy with injections of gradually increasing doses of mosquito saliva proteins is expected to prevent reactions to mosquito bites. This therapy, however, is neither well studied nor widely used for mosquito allergy because commercial mosquito whole body extracts that are currently available contain few mosquito saliva proteins and many non-salivary proteins. Such extracts are ineffective in down-regulating specific immune responses to mosquito salivary allergens and may cause additional sensitization [15].

References

1. Wilkinson GT, Bate MJ. A possible further clinical manifestation of the feline eosinophilic granuloma complex. *Journal of the American Animal Hospital Association* 1984; **20**: 325–331.
2. Mason KV, Evans AG. Mosquito bite-caused eosinophilic dermatitis in cats. *Journal of the American Veterinary Medical Association* 1991; **198**: 2086–2088.
3. Johnstone AC, Graham DG, Andersen HJ. A seasonal eosinophilic dermatitis in cats. *New Zealand Veterinary Journal* 1992; **40**: 168–172.

4. Ihrke PJ, Gross TL. Conference in dermatology no.2 mosquito-bite hypersensitivity in a cat. *Veterinary Dermatology* 1994; **5**: 33–36.
5. Nagata M, Ishida T. Cutaneous reactivity to mosquito bites and its antigens. *Veterinary Dermatology* 1997; **8**: 19–26.
6. Scott DW, Miller WH Jr., Griffin CE. Feline mosquito bite hypersensitivity. *Muller and Kirk's Small Animal Dermatology*, 6th edn. Philadelphia: W.B. Saunders, 2001: 635–636.
7. Gross TL, Ihrke PJ, Walder EJ, *et al.* Feline mosquito-bite hypersensitivity. *Skin Diseases of the Dog and Cats: Clinical and Histological Diagnosis*, 2nd edn. Oxford: Blackwell Science Ltd, 2005: 122–126.
8. Mellanby K. Man's reaction to mosquito bites. *Nature* 1946; **158**: 554.
9. Maibach HI, Skinner WA, Strauss WG, *et al.* Factors that attract and repel mosquitoes in human skin. *Journal of the American Medical Association* 1966; **196**: 263–266.
10. Goma LKH. *The Mosquito*. London: Hutchinson & Co, Ltd., 1966: 75–83.
11. Peng Z, Simons FER. Advances in mosquito allergy. *Current Opinion in Allergy and Clinical Immunology* 2007; **7**: 350–354.
12. Sasa M. Mosquitoes' life. In: Sasa M, Kurihara T, Kamimura K., eds. *Science for Mosquito* [in Japanese]. Tokyo: Hokuryusha, 1976: 75–90.
13. Burns DA. Diseases caused by arthropods and other noxious animals. In: Burns T, Breathnach S, Cox N, *et al.*, eds. *Rook's Textbook of Dermatology*, 8th ed. Oxford: Wiley-Blackwell, 2010: 38.5–38.7.
14. Inamori Y, Morita Y, Sakagami Y, *et al.* The excellence of Aomori Hiba (Hinokiasunaro) in its use as building materials of Buddhist temples and Shinto shrines. *Biocontrol Science* 2006; **11**: 49–54.
15. Peng Z, Simons FER. Comparison of proteins, IgE, and IgG binding antigens, and skin reactivity in commercial and laboratory-made mosquito extracts. *Annals of Allergy Asthma and Immunology* 1996; **77**: 371–376.

Part 3

Equine Allergy

(Editor: Wayne Rosenkrantz)

Section 1

Culicoides Hypersensitivity and Other Insect Allergies

43

Pathogenesis and epidemiology of *Culicoides* hypersensitivity

Bettina Wagner
College of Veterinary Medicine, Cornell University, Ithaca, NY, USA

Conflict of interest: none declared.

Introduction

Culicoides hypersensitivity is a seasonal, recurrent immunoglobulin E (IgE)-mediated allergic dermatitis in horses. It is characterized by pruritus, alopecia, and excoriations occurring during the summer months. The disease is known by different names, such as summer eczema, summer seasonal recurrent dermatitis, sweet itch, Kasen, Queensland itch, or insect bite hypersensitivity. *Culicoides* hypersensitivity affects all horse breeds. It has been described in Icelandic horses, thoroughbreds, Arabians, warmbloods, draft horses, quarter horses, Friesian horses, and different pony breeds. *Culicoides* hypersensitivity occurs all over the world in countries where *Culicoides* midges are endemic [1–10]. Besides their aetiological role in the pathogenesis of hypersensitivity in horses, *Culicoides* also serves as a vector for transmission of infectious diseases such as bluetongue in sheep or African horse sickness [11].

Epidemiology

The prevalence of *Culicoides* hypersensitivity ranges worldwide from 3% in Great Britain [12], to 38% in Germany [6], and 60% in Queensland, Australia [13]. The disease has also been reported in many other parts of the world, including Scandinavia, Switzerland, the Netherlands, Israel, Japan, Canada, and the United States [1–5,7,9,10,14].

The large variation in prevalence in different countries can be explained by many different factors that influence the disease [15]. Prevalence of *Culicoides* hypersensitivity varies depending on the environment and exposure to the midges. Horses that are kept outside all of the time have a much higher chance to get bitten by *Culicoides* midges than stabled horses. Consequently, disease prevalence varies with climate and between different horse breeds. Typically, pleasure horses are more frequently affected with *Culicoides* hypersensitivity than race or competition horses. Other factors that influence clinical disease are age and genetic predisposition of the individual horse. Clinical signs of allergy are usually not observed before horses are 2–4 years of age. In addition, prevalence is influenced by the time horses first get exposed to *Culicoides*. The latter phenomenon was first observed in Icelandic horses. In Iceland, *Culicoides* midges do not occur and the allergic condition is not observed. Clinical signs only developed after export of the horses from Iceland [2]. Epidemiological studies confirmed that between 26 and 72% of the Icelandic horses exported to Europe developed the disease, while only 7–27% of Icelandic horses born in Europe became affected with *Culicoides* hypersensitivity [4,8,9,16].

Culicoides characteristics, life cycle, and breeding sites

Culicoides midges are biting, haematophagous insects of 1–3 mm in size, and belong to the family

Veterinary Allergy, First Edition. Edited by Chiara Noli, Aiden Foster, and Wayne Rosenkrantz.

Ceratopogonidae. They are commonly known as gnats, midges, punkies, or no-see-ums. More than 1400 species of *Culicoides* are described worldwide. They occur on all continents with the exception of the Antarctica, New Zealand, Iceland, and the Hawaiian Islands. *Culicoides* are found in tropical areas and regions with moderate temperatures. Around 96% of the adult *Culicoides* species are obligate blood suckers and attack mammals and birds.

The life cycle of *Culicoides* includes egg, four larval stages, pupa, and imago. The immature stages require free water or moisture. Breeding sites can be manifold, including streams, marshes, ponds, swamps, tree holes, saturated soil, animal dung, rotting fruit, and other vegetation. Eggs are laid in batches, adhere to a substrate, are sensitive to drying, and hatch within 2 to 7 days. Larvae swim with characteristic eel-like motion. Their development depends on temperature and takes from 4 to 5 days up to several weeks. In regions with moderate temperatures, larvae can overwinter. The brief pupal stage usually lasts for 2 to 3 days. Most adult *Culicoides* take blood meals mainly around sunrise and sunset. A few species are also active during the day. Only female *Culicoides* are haematophagous, while males are not. The flight range of *Culicoides* is within a few hundred meters for most species. Most midges survive for less than 10 to 20 days and only occasionally live for up to 90 days. Females take multiple blood meals during their life [11].

Pathogenesis

IgE-mediated allergic mechanisms were first implicated in the pathogenesis of *Culicoides* hypersensitivity about 30 years ago. This was based on observations of immediate skin reactions developing after intradermal testing with *Culicoides* extracts [1–4]. With the development of monoclonal antibodies to equine IgE [17,18], the IgE-mediated allergic aetiology was confirmed for *Culicoides* hypersensitivity. This was performed by transferring the allergic reaction from affected to healthy horses via IgE obtained from allergic horses (Prausnitz–Küstner reaction). After challenge with *Culicoides* extract, clinically healthy recipient horses developed immediate skin reactions only at the sites of the IgE transfer from affected donors but not at the transfer sites of IgE from healthy donors [19]. Today, various techniques are available to detect soluble IgE or the sensitization of mast cells or basophils with *Culicoides*-specific IgE [20]. See Chapters 44 and 46 for more information.

The immune pathogenesis of *Culicoides* hypersensitivity is not yet fully understood. However, it is likely that the major immune mechanisms are similar to those of IgE-mediated allergies in humans [15]. *Culicoides* hypersensitivity is a multifactorial disease and the development of clinical allergy depends on several parameters, such as genetic predisposition, environmental exposure, and the condition and immune status of the individual horse.

Sensitization of mast cells and basophils with *Culicoides*-specific IgE is a central event in the disease pathogenesis and always precedes the development of clinical disease. However, mast cell sensitization with allergen-specific IgE does not necessarily mean that a horse will also develop allergy since many clinically healthy horses are also sensitized to *Culicoides* [21]. Despite their sensitization status, these horses are well able to balance their immune reactions without becoming affected with allergy. The currently favoured hypothesis is that the onset of *Culicoides* hypersensitivity results from an immune imbalance characterized by increased numbers of allergen-specific T helper 2 (Th2)-cells combined with reduced numbers and functions of allergen-specific regulatory T cells in affected horses. The decreased ability to regulate immune reactions to *Culicoides* allergens may lead to increased allergen-specific effector cell responses, such as enhanced Th2-cell immunity and *Culicoides*-specific IgE production, and finally the development of clinical allergy.

Most of the cellular immune parameters involved in *Culicoides* hypersensitivity have been investigated in Icelandic horses. Increased numbers of Th cells and enhanced interleukin-13 (IL-13) mRNA expression were observed in tissues of local skin lessons from allergic horses [22]. Icelandic horses with clinical allergy had increased *Culicoides*-specific T helper 2 (Th2)-cell responses compared to clinically healthy horses. Furthermore, exported allergic horses from Iceland had higher allergen-specific Th2-cell numbers than allergic Icelandic horses born in continental Europe [23]. These findings suggest that the increased allergy prevalence in exported Icelandic horses could be influenced by the delayed first exposure to *Culicoides*.

The neonatal and young foal immune system reacts differently than that of adult horses [24]. Horses that are exposed to *Culicoides* early in life may have developed immune mechanisms as young horses that prevent the development of clinical allergy when they get older. In support of the reduced regulatory immune function in allergic horses are findings showing that regulatory cytokines such as IL-10 and transforming growth factor-β1 (TGF-β1) can reduce IL-4 production in Th2 cells from allergic horses *in vitro* [23]. Stimulation of peripheral blood cells from allergic horses with *Culicoides* resulted in lower numbers of regulatory T cells compared to clinically healthy horses [25]. These examples indicate the progress that has been made in recent years to

Table 43.1 Allergen candidates from the saliva of *Culicoides* midges

Origin (*Culicoides* species)	Putative allergen	Function	Accession numbers	Protein size (kDa)	References
C. sonorensis	Cul s 1	Maltase	AY603565	66	[29]
	D7	D7 family salivary proteins	AY603569 AY603607		[27]
C. nubeculosus	Cul n 1	Antigen 5 like protein	EU978899	25.4	[32]
	Cul n 2	Hyaluronidase	HM145950	46.7	[30,31]
	Cul n 3	Putative cysteine endopeptidase	HM145951	44.6	[31]
	Cul n 4	Secreted salivary protein	HM145952	17.5	
	Cul n 5	Secreted salivary protein	HM145953	45.7	
	Cul n 6	Secreted salivary protein	HM145954	16.9	
	Cul n 7	Unknown salivary protein	HM145955	20.9	
	Cul n 8	Maltase	HM145956	68.7	[28,30,31]
	Cul n 9	D7 family salivary protein	HM145957	15.5	
	Cul n 10	Secreted salivary protein	HM145958	47.8	[31]
	Cul n 11	Trypsin	HM145959	30.1	

understand the immune pathogenesis of *Culicoides* hypersensitivity in horses. Further investigations of the detailed immune mechanisms leading to development of, or prevention from, clinical disease will allow us to better understand, manage, and prevent *Culicoides* hypersensitivity in horses.

Culicoides allergens

Culicoides hypersensitivity is caused by allergens from the saliva of the midges. Allergens are injected into the horse's skin during the blood meal. *Culicoides* saliva contains various pharmacologically active substances that inhibit coagulation, support sugar meal digestion and help to overcome host tissue barriers and immunological defences [15]. The comparison of extracts from different *Culicoides* species by intradermal testing showed that horses reacted to all species of *Culicoides* even if they were previously just exposed to some of them [5]. This suggested that the inducing allergens are conserved between different *Culicoides* species. Initial western blot studies using *Culicoides* salivary gland extracts revealed several proteins that were detected by serum IgE from allergic horses [26]. More recently, different groups performed proteomic approaches on salivary gland extracts to identify the allergens causing *Culicoides* hypersensitivity. This revealed several allergen candidates (Table 43.1). The most frequently identified putative allergens of *Culicoides* are: (1) maltase, an enzyme involved in sugar meal digestion; (2) members of the D7 complex, a group of not yet classified, small salivary proteins; and (3) hyaluronidase [27–31]. However, several additional salivary proteins of *Culicoides* were identified and might be involved in the pathogenesis of *Culicoides* hypersensitivity [30,31]. Out of the putative allergens shown in Table 43.1, involvement in the pathogenesis of *Culicoides* hypersensitivity has been demonstrated for maltase (Cul s 1, Cul n 8) by intradermal and *in vitro* sensitization testing of allergic and clinically healthy horses [29,31]. In addition, positive intradermal testing results have been observed for Cul n1 to Cul n5, Cul n 7, Cul n 9, and Cul n 10 [31,32]. The putative allergens of *Culicoides* are valuable tools to improve our knowledge of the pathogenesis of *Culicoides* hypersensitivity, to generate better and diagnostic tests for allergic horses and possibly also for the development of new treatment options.

References

1. Braverman Y. Preferred landing sites of *Culicoides* species (Diptera: Ceratopogonidae) on a horse in Israel and its relevance to summer seasonal recurrent dermatitis (sweet itch). *Equine Veterinary Journal* 1988; **20**: 426–429.
2. Larsen HJ, Bakke SH, Mehl R. Intradermal challenge of Icelandic horses in Norway and Iceland with extracts of *Culicoides* spp. *Acta Veterinary Scandinavica* 1988; **29**: 311–314.
3. Greiner EC, Fadok VA, Rabin EB. Equine *Culicoides* hypersensitivity in Florida: biting midges aspirated from horses. *Journal of Medical Entomology* 1990; **4**: 375–381.
4. Halldordsottir S, Larsen HJ. An epidemiological study of summer eczema in Icelandic horses in Norway. *Equine Veterinary Journal* 1991; **23**: 296–299.

5. Anderson GS, Belton P, Kleider N. Hypersensitivity of horses in British Columbia to extracts of native and exotic species of *Culicoides* (Diptera: Ceratopogonidae). *Journal of Medical Entomology* 1993; **30**: 657–663.
6. Littlewood JD. Incidence of recurrent seasonal pruritus ('sweet itch') in British and German Shire horses. *Veterinary Research* 1998; **142**: 66–67.
7. Steinman A, Peer G, Klement E. Epidemiological study of *Culicoides* hypersensitivity in horses in Israel. *Veterinary Record* 2003; **152**: 748–751.
8. Lange S, Hamann H, Deegen E, *et al.* Investigation of the prevalence of summer eczema in Icelandic horses in northern Germany. *Berliner Munchener Tierarztliche Wochenschrift* 2005; **118**: 481–489.
9. Björnsdóttir S, Sigvaldadóttir J, Broström H, *et al.* Summer eczema in exported Icelandic horses: influence of environmental and genetic factors. *Acta Veterinary Scandinavica* 2006; **48**: 3.
10. Van Grevenhof EM, Ducro B, Heuven HC, *et al.* Identification of environmental factors affecting the prevalence of insect bite hypersensitivity in Shetland ponies and Friesian horses in The Netherlands. *Equine Veterinary Journal* 2007; **39**: 69–73.
11. Mellor PS, Boorman J, Baylis M. Culicoides biting midges: their role as arbovirus vectors. *Annual Reviews in Entomology* 2000; **45**: 307–340.
12. McCaig J. A survey to establish the incidence of sweet itch in ponies in the United Kingdom. *Veterinary Records* 1973; **93**: 444–446.
13. Riek RF. Studies on allergic dermatitis (Queensland Itch) of the horse I. Description, distribution, symptoms and pathology. *Australian Veterinary Journal* 1953; **29**: 177–184.
14. Greiner EC. Entomologic evaluation of insect hypersensitivity in horses. *Veterinary Clinics North America Equine Practice* 1995; **11**: 29–41.
15. Schaffartzik A, Hamza E, Janda J, *et al.* Equine insect bite hypersensitivity: What do we know? *Veterinary Immunology and Immunopathology* 2012; **147**: 113–126.
16. Brostrom H, Larsson A, Troedsson M. Allergic dermatitis (sweet itch) of Icelandic horses in Sweden: an epidemiological study. *Equine Veterinary Journal* 1987; **19**: 229–236.
17. Wagner B, Radbruch A, Rohwer J, *et al.* Monoclonal anti-equine IgE antibodies with specificity for different epitopes on the immunoglobulin heavy chain of native IgE. *Veterinary Immunology and Immunopathology* 2003; **92**: 45–60.
18. Wilson AD, Harwood L, Torsteinsdottir S, *et al.* Production of monoclonal antibodies specific for native equine IgE and their application to monitor total serum IgE responses in Icelandic and non-Icelandic horses with insect bite hypersensitivity. *Veterinary Immunology and Immunopathology* 2006; **112**: 156–170.
19. Wagner B, Miller WH, Morgan EE, *et al.* IgE and IgG antibodies in skin allergy of the horse. *Veterinary Research* 2006; **37**: 813–825.
20. Wagner B. IgE in horses: Occurrence in health and disease. *Veterinary Immunology and Immunopathology* 2009; **132**: 21–30.
21. Wagner B, Miller WH, Erb HN, *et al.* Sensitization of skin mast cells with IgE antibodies to *Culicoides* allergens occurs frequently in clinically healthy horses. *Veterinary Immunology and Immunopathology* 2009; **132**: 53–61.
22. Heimann M, Janda J, Sigurdardottir OG, *et al.* Skin-infiltrating T cells and cytokine expression in Icelandic horses affected with insect bite hypersensitivity: a possible role for regulatory T-cells. *Veterinary Immunology and Immunopathology* 2011; **140**: 63–74.
23. Hamza E, Wagner B, Jungi TW, *et al.* Reduced incidence of insect-bite hypersensitivity in Icelandic horses is associated with a down-regulation of interleukin-4 by interleukin-10 and transforming growth factor-β1. *Veterinary Immunology and Immunopathology* 2008; **122**: 65–75.
24. Wagner B, Burton A, Ainsworth DM. Interferon-gamma, interleukin-4 and interleukin-10 production by T helper cells reveals intact Th1 and regulatory T_R1 cell activation and a delay of the Th2 cell response in equine neonates and foals. *Veterinary Research* 2010; **41**: 47.
25. Hamza E, Steinbach F, Marti E. $CD4^+CD25^+$ T cells expressing FoxP3 in Icelandic horses affected with insect bite hypersensitivity. *Veterinary Immunology and Immunopathology* 2011; **148**: 139–144.
26. Hellberg W, Wilson AD, Mellor P, *et al.* Equine insect bite hypersensitivity: Immunoblot analysis of IgE and IgG subclass responses to *Culicoides nubeculosus* salivary gland extract. *Veterinary Immunology and Immunopathology* 2006; **113**: 99–112.
27. Langner KF, Darpel KE, Denison E, *et al.* Collection and analysis of salivary proteins from biting midge *Culicoides nubeculosus* (Diptera: Ceratopogonidae). *Journal of Medical Entomology* 2007; **44**: 238–248.
28. Wilson AD, Heesom KJ, Mawby WJ, *et al.* Identification of abundant proteins and potential allergens in *Culicoides nubeculosus* salivary glands. *Veterinary Immunology and Immunopathology* 2008; **122**: 94–103.
29. Langner KF, Jarvis DL, Nimtz M, *et al.* Identification, expression and characterisation of a major salivary allergen (Cul s 1) of the biting midge *Culicoides sonorensis* relevant for summer eczema in horses. *International Journal of Parasitology* 2009; **39**: 243–250.
30. Russell CL, Heesom KJ, Arthur CJ, *et al.* Identification and isolation of cDNA clones encoding the abundant secreted proteins in the saliva proteome of *Culicoides nubeculosus*. *Insect Molecular Biology* 2009; **18**: 383–393.
31. Schaffartzik A, Marti E, Torsteinsdottir S, *et al.* Selective cloning, characterization, and production of the *Culicoides nubeculosus* salivary gland allergen repertoire associated with equine insect bite hypersensitivity. *Veterinary Immunology and Immunopathology* 2011; **139**: 200–209.
32. Schaffartzik A, Marti E, Crameri R, *et al.* Cloning, production and characterization of antigen 5 like proteins from *Simulium vittatum* and *Culicoides nubeculosus*, the first cross-reactive allergen associated with equine insect bite hypersensitivity. *Veterinary Immunology and Immunopathology* 2010; **137**: 76–83.

44

Equine immunoglobulin E

Eliane Marti and Eman Hamza

Clinical Immunology Group, Department of Clinical Research and Veterinary Public Health, Vetsuisse Faculty, University of Bern, Bern, Switzerland

Conflict of interest: none declared.

Structure and function of IgE

Immunoglobulins (Ig), also called antibodies, are glycoproteins that mediate humoral immunity and are produced by B lymphocytes. Activated B cells differentiate into immunoglobulin-producing plasma cells. Immunoglobulins produced by one plasma cell are normally specific for a single antigen. The basic structure of all immunoglobulin molecules is a Y-like unit consisting of two identical light chains and two identical heavy chains linked together by disulphide bonds (Figure 44.1). Heavy and light chains have N-terminal variable (V) and C-terminal constant (C) regions. Each immunoglobulin molecule is bifunctional: the V region of the molecule binds to the antigen while the C region mediates binding of the immunoglobulin to host tissues. The class and subclass (also called isotype) of an immunoglobulin molecule is determined by its heavy chain type. The different immunoglobulin isotypes are associated with different functions. Mammals express some or all of the five known immunoglobulin classes: IgM, IgD, IgG, IgA, and IgE. Immunoglobulin E (IgE) has, compared to the other immunoglobulin classes, some characteristic features:

1. IgE, like IgM, has a higher molecular mass (200 kDa versus 150 kDa) than IgG because, like IgM, it consists of four instead of three constant region heavy chain domains.
2. IgE is found in extremely low concentrations in serum (in the ng/mL range in humans living in industrialized countries) compared to IgG (mg/mL range, reviewed in Dullaers *et al.* [1]). In domestic species, total serum IgE levels in the microgram per mL range have been described. These higher IgE levels compared to humans are most probably due to the often high degree of infection with endoparasites in domestic animals [2], which has practically disappeared in humans living in industrialized countries.
3. The half-life of free serum IgE is very short (2 days). However, upon antigen recall, memory B cells can rapidly give rise to antibody-secreting plasma cells. Furthermore, long-lived plasma cells provide long-term antibody titres [3,4].
4. Most of the IgE is bound on the surface of cells by the high-affinity (FcεRI) or low-affinity (FcεRII, CD23) receptor. FcεRII can be induced on a broad range of immune cells, including activated B cells, but also on structural cells such as airway epithelium [1]. Equine CD23 has recently been shown to be expressed by a subpopulation of B cells and a few T cells and monocytes using recently produced monoclonal antibodies to CD23 [5]. IgE is bound to mast cells and basophils through the high-affinity IgE receptor (FcεRI). It has been shown in horses that the recombinant equine FcεRIα binds equine IgE [6]. A rapid release of inflammatory agents from mast cells and basophils, such as histamine and

Veterinary Allergy, First Edition. Edited by Chiara Noli, Aiden Foster, and Wayne Rosenkrantz.

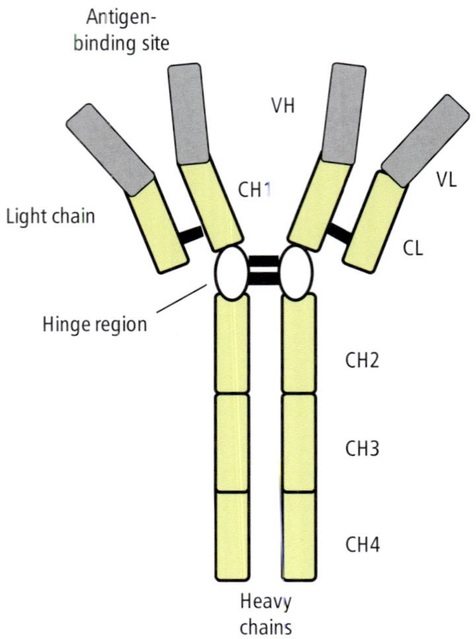

Figure 44.1 Immunoglobulin E structure: IgE consists of two identical light chains and two identical heavy chains linked together by disulphide bonds. Both the heavy (H) and light (L) chains have N-terminal variable (V) and C-terminal constant (C) regions. IgE, like IgM, has four constant region heavy chain domains (CH1–CH4). IgG has only three CH domains (CH1–CH3).

sulphidoleukotrienes (see section 'IgE in *Culicoides* hypersensitivity' and Table 44.1), but also of many other factors including cytokines, is triggered through cross-linking of FcεRI-bound IgE molecules. For this reason IgE was first called 'reagin' [7]. Allergic reactions can be transferred passively by injecting serum of sensitized patients into the skin of non-affected individuals followed by challenge of the skin sites with the specific antigen. Positive skin reactions can be induced in non-sensitized individuals by intradermal injection of the allergen up to 4 days after injection of serum from a sensitized patient. This is the so-called Prausnitz–Küstner reaction, which has also been described in horses (see section '*Culicoides*-specific IgE') [8,9]. Furthermore, IgE, in contrast to other immunoglobulin classes, is heat labile [10]; it loses the capacity for passive sensitization after heating and can no longer be precipitated with anti-IgE antibodies. The antigen binding site(s), however, remain functional after heating (at 56°C for 2 to 4 hours). The inactivation of IgE antibodies after heat treatment has been explained by conformational changes in the C-terminal region of the ε chains, which is the part binding to mast cells and basophils [11,12].

All of these characteristic features may be used to investigate whether immune reactions are mediated by IgE, and to characterize IgE-specific reagents.

The nucleotide sequence of the equine constant region of the IgE heavy chain gene (IGHE) has been determined by various groups [13–16] and, like in other mammals, consists of four exons (CH1 to CH4). It maps to equine chromosome 24 [17], between the genes coding for the constant regions of IgG5 and IgA [18]. Polymorphism of IgE has been described but has not been associated with equine allergic disease [18,19].

Antibodies for detection of equine IgE

The extremely low concentration of IgE in serum has hampered the isolation of pure IgE. The discovery of human myeloma IgE, immunocytoma rat IgE, and the construction of mouse and dog IgE hybridomas allowed the production of polyclonal and monoclonal antibodies specific for IgE of these species. In the horse, however, no IgE gammopathy has yet been discovered. Suter and Fey [20,21], as well as Halliwell and Hines [22], isolated IgE from horse sera using classical biochemical purification methods and immunized rabbits to produce anti-IgE antibodies. According to the authors, these antisera had to be absorbed with other immunoglobulin classes before they could be used as anti-IgE reagents and thus their specificity probably remained questionable. Consequently, molecular technologies were used to produce, first, a partial equine IgE in *E. coli* [23] and then the complete IgE [24]. These IgE molecules were used for the production of polyclonal [23] and monoclonal antibodies specific for equine IgE [25,26]. Another approach consisted of using the nucleotide sequence of equine IgE to prepare a peptide-based immunogen to elicit equine epsilon chain-specific antisera [27]. While the polyclonal antibodies were useful for some applications, the monoclonal antibodies to equine IgE, which are described in the review by Wagner *et al.* [18], have considerably improved the detection of equine IgE.

IgE in *Culicoides* hypersensitivity

It is now generally accepted that IgE-mediated reactions to allergens from insects, mainly of the genus *Culicoides* (midges), often play a key role in the pathogenesis of *Culicoides* hypersensitivity. However, it was not until recently that a direct correlation between IgE antibodies and *Culicoides* hypersensitivity could be demonstrated. A possible role for IgE-mediated reactions in *Culicoides*

Table 44.1 Published studies indicating that IgE-mediated reactions are involved in the pathogenesis of equine *Culicoides* hypersensitivity

Method [Reference]	Antigens used	Reagent used for IgE detection
Prausnitz–Küstner experiments		
Matthews *et al.* 1983 [8]	*C. pulicaris* extract*	na
Wagner *et al.* 2006 [9]	*Culicoides* spp. extract	Anti-equine IgEmAb for purification of serum IgE
Histamine release assays		
Marti *et al.* 1999 [34]	*C. nubeculosus* extract; *Simulium* spp. extract	na
Langner *et al.* 2008 [36]	*C. nubeculosus* extract and saliva *C. sonorensis* extract and saliva	na
Wagner *et al.* 2008 [37]	*Culicoides* spp. extract	na
Van der Meiden *et al.* 2012 [57]	*C. obsoletus, C. nubeculosus, C. sonorensis* extracts	Anti-equine IgEmAb
Sulphidoleukotriene release assays		
Marti *et al.* 1999 [34]	*C. nubeculosus* extract; *Simulium* spp. extract	na
Baselgia *et al.* 2006 [35]	*C. nubeculosus* extract; *Simulium vittatum* extract	na
Immunohistochemistry		
Van der Haegen *et al.* 2001 [38]	na	Affinity-purified chicken anti-recombinant equine IgEAb; *In situ* hybridization for equine IgE mRNA
Wilson *et al.* 2008 [56]	Native *Culicoides* spp.	Affinity purified chicken anti-recombinant equine IgEAb
Immunoblots following 1 or 2D-electrophoresis		
Hellberg *et al.* 2006 [42]	*C. nubeculosus* SGE	Anti-equine IgEmAb
Wilson *et al.* 2008 [56]	*C. nubeculosus* SGE; native *C. obsoletus* and *pulicaris* Group thorax extracts	Anti-equine IgEmAb
Hellberg *et al.* 2009 [52]	*C. nubeculosus and Simulium vitattum* SGE	Anti-equine IgEmAb
Langner *et al.* 2009 [49]	Recombinant *C. sonorensis* salivary allergen Cul s1	Anti-equine IgEmAb
ELISA		
Frey *et al.* 2008 [59]	*Culicoide*s spp. extract	Allercept™ (human high affinity IgE receptor)
Langner *et al.* 2008 [36]	*C. nubeculosus* extract and saliva *C. sonorensis* extract and saliva	Anti-equine IgEmAb
Schaffartzik *et al.* 2010 [50]	Recombinant antigen5-like proteins from *Simulium. vittatum* (Sim v 1) and *C. nubeculosus* (Cul n 1)	Anti-equine IgEmAb
Schaffartzik *et al.* 2011 [51]	Recombinant *C. nubeculosus* salivary gland proteins	Anti-equine IgEmAb
Van der Meide *et al.* 2012 [57]	*C. obsoletus, C. nubeculosus, C. sonorensis*	Anti-equine IgEmAb
Peeters *et al.* 2013 [58]	Recombinant *C. nubeculosus* and *C. obsoletus* salivary gland proteins; *C. nubeculosus* thorax extract; *C. obsoletus* Group extract	Anti-equine IgEmAb
Van der Meide *et al.* 2013 [60]	Recombinant *C. obsoletus* and *C. sonorensis* salivary gland proteins	Anti-equine IgEmAb

na, not applicable; Ab, antibody; mAb, monoclonal antibody; SGE, salivary gland extract.
*If not specified, extract was whole-body extract.

hypersensitivity was suggested many years ago indirectly, by intradermal tests with extracts of various *Culicoides* species and sometimes also other insect extracts [28–33] and, more recently, by *in vitro* histamine or sulphido-leukotriene release assays with *Culicoides* extracts (summarized in Table 44.1) [34–37].

IgE in skin

A further indication of the involvement of IgE in *Culicoides* hypersensitivity was given by an immunohistochemical study of skin biopsies [38] using a chicken antibody specific for an equine IgE fragment [23], which weakly recognizes native IgE but strongly reacts with denatured IgE. Significantly more IgE-protein-positive cells were found in the dermis and epidermis of lesional skin biopsies from horses with *Culicoides* hypersensitivity than in the skin of non-affected horses [38]. Double staining for IgE-protein and the mast cell enzyme tryptase revealed that the majority of the IgE-protein-bearing cells in the dermis are probably mast cells, whereas the cells in the epidermis are probably Langerhans cells, according to what is known from studies in the human field [39]. Unfortunately, this could not be confirmed because reagents for detection of equine Langerhans cells were not available. Strikingly, significantly more IgE-mRNA-positive cells were detected in the dermis of lesional skin biopsies of *Culicoides* hypersensitivity-affected horses than in skin from healthy horses, which suggests that IgE is also produced locally in *Culicoides* hypersensitivity. Interestingly, in human allergic diseases such as asthma or rhinitis, there is now growing evidence that IgE-secreting plasma cells are not only found in the bone marrow, but also in the draining lymph nodes and locally in the mucosa (reviewed in [1]).

Total serum IgE

In domestic animals, total serum IgE levels are usually not increased in allergic individuals compared to controls [40], as is the case in humans, because IgE levels are strongly influenced by the degree of parasitic infection [2,41]. However, surprisingly, total serum IgE levels were increased in *Culicoides* hypersensitivity-affected horses of the Icelandic breeds compared to controls [25] and in one study [26] this difference even reached the level of significance. This was not observed in horses belonging to other breeds [26], such as Kladruby horses[19]. The differences between healthy and allergic Icelandic horses might be due to the extremely strong Th2-type and IgE response against *Culicoides* allergens in *Culicoides* hypersensitivity-affected horses imported to Europe from Iceland, whereas this is not usually observed in horses born outside Iceland [42,43].

Culicoides-*specific IgE*

The first indication of the involvement of *Culicoides*-specific reaginic antibodies was reported by Matthews *et al.* [8]. They reported the presence of a reagin-like antibody against *Culicoides pulicaris* extract in the serum of horses affected with sweet itch (*Culicoides* hypersensitivity) and showed that this antibody could confer Prausnitz–Küstner sensitivity, is thermolabile, and susceptible to 2-mercaptoethanol reduction, all characteristic features of IgE (see section 'Structure and function of IgE'). Furthermore, this reagin-like antibody could be eluted on diethylaminoethyl dextran-52 anion exchange chromatography independently of IgG, IgG(T), and IgM. Taken together, these findings indicated that this reagin-like antibody was possibly equine IgE specific for *Culicoides* allergens.

A more recent study using immunohistochemistry with the chicken anti-equine IgE antibody described above [23], showed for the first time that sera from horses with *Culicoides* hypersensitivity, but not from healthy controls, contain IgE antibodies binding to salivary glands of *Culicoides* [44]. Sera from both *Culicoides* hypersensitivity-affected and healthy horses exposed to *Culicoides* contained salivary gland-specific IgG antibodies, probably reflecting a 'normal' immune response to *Culicoides* bites [44].

The *Culicoides*-specific IgE response could only be investigated in greater detail with the availability of monoclonal antibodies specific to equine IgE [25,26]. In 2006, Wagner *et al.* [9] elegantly confirmed the study by Mathews *et al.* [8]; they purified IgE from serum of horses affected with *Culicoides* hypersensitivity and performed a modified Prausnitz–Küstner experiment. They showed that the transfer of IgE purified from the serum of a horse with *Culicoides* hypersensitivity to the skin of a healthy horse induced classic type I allergic reactions upon allergen challenge at the site of IgE injection. Concurrently, Hellberg *et al.* [42] investigated IgE binding to *Culicoides nubeculosus* salivary gland extract by immunoblot. They identified 10 IgE-binding protein bands in this extract and found that sera from horses with *Culicoides* hypersensitivity contained IgE to *C. nubeculosus* salivary gland proteins significantly more often than sera from non-affected horses. Furthermore, *Culicoides* hypersensitivity-affected horses showed a large variety of IgE-binding patterns, suggesting that many different allergens are involved in *Culicoides* hypersensitivity and that the sensitization pattern is highly individual. Interestingly, *C. nubeculosus* salivary gland-specific IgE was transferred from the mare to the foal via the colostrum [45]. However, maternal IgE to *Culicoides* allergens is probably not relevant in *Culicoides* hypersensitivity, because *Culicoides* hypersensitivity does not usually develop before the second year of life and maternally derived cell-bound and serum IgE disappears within the first 2–4 months of age [45,46]. It is thus unlikely that maternally derived IgE plays a significant role in the pathogenesis of *Culicoides* hypersensitivity.

Beside the lack of monoclonal antibodies specific for equine IgE, the study of the *Culicoides* allergen-specific IgE response was hampered by the lack of pure allergens for *Culicoides* hypersensitivity. Only crude whole-body extracts were available and these, in addition to their lack of standardization, have various drawbacks, as with other crude allergen extracts: they are complex biological mixtures containing, beside the relevant allergenic proteins in unknown concentrations, many non-allergenic proteins, carbohydrates, and low-molecular-weight substances like histamine or immunosuppressive compounds [47]. Furthermore, false-positive reactions in intradermal tests with *Culicoides* extracts are relatively frequent, making intradermal testing (IDT) with crude *Culicoides* extract an unreliable method for diagnostic purposes (reviewed in [48]). Since 2009, *Culicoides* allergens have been characterized at the molecular level and expressed as recombinant proteins, either in insect cells [49] or in *E. coli* [50,51]. The first recombinant allergen described to be relevant for *Culicoides* hypersensitivity, a maltase of *Culicoides sonorensis* (Cul s 1), showed binding to serum IgE *in vitro* and skin test reactivity *in vivo* in horses with *Culicoides* hypersensitivity but not in healthy control horses [49]. Furthermore, 11 recombinant *C. nubeculosus* allergens have been identified and expressed. IgE sensitization to these allergens is associated with *Culicoides* hypersensitivity and ranges from 13 to 56.5%, depending on the allergen tested [50,51]. The recombinant *C. nubeculosus* allergens that were tested in IDT elicited immediate type skin reactions after intradermal application in *Culicoides* hypersensitivity-affected but not in non-affected horses, suggesting that these recombinant allergens are functionally relevant [50,51]. *Culicoides* hypersensitivity-affected horses had detectable serum IgE levels against a mean number of four r-allergens and the horses showed a large variety of IgE-binding patterns to these recombinant allergens. Interestingly, it was also shown that IgE binding to *Simulium vittatum* allergens, which has been associated with *Culicoides* hypersensitivity [52], is probably due to cross-reactive proteins present in both insect species (reviewed in [48]). This has been demonstrated by inhibition ELISA and western blots for one allergen, an antigen 5-like protein present in both *S. vittatum* (Sim v 1) and *C. nubeculosus* (Cul n 1) with a sequence identity of about 50% [50]. Cross-reactivity between antigens has been widely described in human allergic diseases [53,54].

There is currently sparse information regarding the conservation of IgE-binding epitopes between different *Culicoides* species. Whereas some studies using IDT or histamine release tests suggest that most horses with *Culicoides* hypersensitivity react to many different *Culicoides* species [31,36], even though they have not been exposed to their bites [33], others suggest that the use of *Culicoides* species present in the environment where the horse is living leads to a better performance of IDT [55] and stronger IgE-binding in western blots [56,57]. A study has shown that *Culicoides* hypersensitivity-affected horses in the Netherlands had significantly higher IgE titres against local *Culicoides* species (*C. obsoletus*) than against captive bred *C. nubeculosus* or against *C. sonorensis* not found in the wild in the Netherlands. Furthermore, at a low allergen extract concentration of 0.5 μg/mL but not at a ten-times higher concentration, *C. obsoletus* extract induced a significantly higher histamine release in whole blood of *Culicoides* hypersensitivity-affected horses than the other extracts [57]. In that study the IgE ELISA using *C. obsoletus* extract as allergen had a high sensitivity and specificity of 93.2% and 90%, respectively.

The performance of an IgE ELISA with different recombinant *C. nubeculosus* or *C. obsoletus* allergens, as well as *Culicoides* extracts, for the diagnosis of *Culicoides* hypersensitivity in Belgium warmblood horses was evaluated [58]. A combination of IgE levels against two recombinant *C. obsoletus* (Cul o 1 and Cul o 2) and one *C. nubeculosus* allergen (Cul n 4), together with *C. obsoletus* extract, resulted in the best performing test. Furthermore, the performance of the test improved with the increasing severity of clinical signs of *Culicoides* hypersensitivity. This IgE ELISA had a sensitivity of 70%, a specificity of 97%, and a total accuracy of 92% [58]. Further studies are needed to compare the performance of IgE ELISAs with *Culicoides* extracts or recombinant allergens. The lower sensitivity of an ELISA that uses a combination of IgE levels against recombinant allergens and *C. obsoletus* extract [58] compared to an ELISA with *C. obsoletus* extract only [57] may be due to different study populations, i.e. different degrees of *Culicoides* hypersensitivity severity or to different horse breeds tested; Peeters *et al.* [58] tested sera from warmblood horses, whereas van der Meide *et al.* [57] used sera from Icelandic horses and Shetland ponies. As mentioned in Section Total serum IgE, it has been shown that *Culicoides* hypersensitivity-affected Icelandic horses frequently display very strong IgE responses to *Culicoides* allergens.

Overall, these studies suggest that although *Culicoides* hypersensitivity-affected horses often show IgE-binding or IgE-mediated reactions to *Culicoides* species not present in their environment, indicating the presence of species-shared allergens, the use of local *Culicoides* species seems to result in stronger IgE binding. This suggests the presence of additional allergens in native species and/or of higher titres or affinity of IgE antibodies to partly conserved allergens from native *Culicoides* species. However, availability of such extracts may be a limiting factor in their use for diagnostic purposes.

IgE serology to confirm diagnosis of Culicoides hypersensitivity

Various tests for serological IgE testing in *Culicoides* hypersensitivity are commercially available. Unfortunately, the performance of these tests has usually not been published. The quality of the allergen extracts and/or the reagents used to detect equine IgE are often not known and questionable. The only test that has been evaluated for *Culicoides* hypersensitivity is Allercept™ (HESKA corporation) a non-competitive, solid-phase ELISA test, that uses the recombinant human high-affinity IgE receptor (FcεR1α), which has been tested in horses of the Icelandic breed; it was shown that serological testing with this ELISA was not suitable as a tool for establishing a diagnosis of *Culicoides* hypersensitivity [59], although, overall, horses with *Culicoides* hypersensitivity had higher serum IgE levels to *Culicoides* extract than healthy control horses. However, the 95% confidence overlap was too high between the groups to permit a reliable diagnosis. The studies by van der Meide *et al.* [57] and Peeters *et al.* [58] indicate that the serological diagnosis of *Culicoides* hypersensitivity may be improved through the use of reagents specific for equine IgE, such monoclonal antibodies to equine IgE combined with pure allergens such as recombinant allergens or good-quality *Culicoides* extracts preferably made from local *Culicoides* species. Importantly, commercially available diagnostic tests should be standardized and the performance of these tests evaluated and published.

Conclusion

Numerous studies have demonstrated that IgE-mediated reactions to *Culicoides* play an important role in the pathogenesis of *Culicoides* hypersensitivity. Our knowledge about the specific allergens involved in *Culicoides* hypersensitivity has vastly improved over recent years. Thirteen different IgE-binding antigens from *Culicoides* spp. have been characterized at the molecular level and expressed as recombinant proteins. We cannot, however, exclude that even more *Culicoides* allergens will be identified in the future. The highly individually variable reaction pattern to these allergens is a challenge for the study of the immune response to these specific allergens as well as for the development of allergen-specific immunotherapies with pure allergens. Future studies should aim at understanding why some horses produce IgE antibodies to *Culicoides* salivary allergens whereas the majority do not develop an allergic immune response to these antigens, although exposed to *Culicoides* bites to a similar degree. An understanding of these mechanisms would probably allow an improvement in the treatment of *Culicoides* hypersensitivity in the future.

Acknowledgements

We are grateful to Ruth Parham for her careful comments on the manuscript. Eman Hamza was supported by the Swiss National Science Foundation grant no. 310000-116803/1.

References

1. Dullaers M, De Bruyne R, Ramadani F, *et al.* The who, where, and when of IgE in allergic airway disease. *Journal of Allergy and Clinical Immunology* 2012; **129**: 635–645.
2. Pernthaner A, Shaw RJ, McNeill MM, *et al.* Total and nematode-specific IgE responses in intestinal lymph of genetically resistant and susceptible sheep during infection with *Trichostrongylus colubriformis*. *Veterinary Immunology and Immunopathology* 2005; **104**: 69–80.
3. Luger EO, Fokuhl V, Wegmann M, *et al.* Induction of long-lived allergen-specific plasma cells by mucosal allergen challenge. *Journal of Allergy and Clinical Immunology* 2009; **124**: 819–826.
4. Luger EO, Wegmann M, Achatz G, *et al.* Allergy for a lifetime? *Allergology International* 2010; **59**: 1–8.
5. Wagner B, Hillegas JM, Babasyan S. Monoclonal antibodies to equine CD23 identify the low-affinity receptor for IgE on subpopulations of IgM+ and IgG1+ B-cells in horses. *Veterinary Immunology and Immunopathology* 2012; **146**: 125–134.
6. McAleese SM, Brown JK, Macrae AI, *et al.* Cloning and expression of the extra-cellular part of the alpha chain of the equine high-affinity IgE receptor and its use in the detection of IgE. *Veterinary Immunology and Immunopathology* 2006; **110**: 187–191.
7. Prausnitz C, Küstner H. Studienüber die Uberempfindlichkeit. *Zentralblatt für Bakteriologie* 1921; **86**: 160–169.
8. Matthews AG, Imlah P, McPherson EA. A reagin-like antibody in horse serum: 1. Occurrence and some biological properties. *Veterinary Research Communications* 1983; **6**: 13–23.
9. Wagner B, Miller WH, Morgan EE, *et al.* IgE and IgG antibodies in skin allergy of the horse. *Veterinary Research* 2006; **37**: 813–825.
10. Ishizaka K, Ishizaka T, Menzel AE. Effect of heat on γE, γG and γA antibodies in sera of ragweed sensitive patients. *Journal of Immunology* 1967; **99**: 610–618.
11. Bennich H, von Bahr-Lindström H. Structure of immunoglobulin E. In: Brent L, Hoborow J, eds. *Progress in Immunology*, 2ndedn. New York: North-Holland American Elsevier Publishing, 1974: 49–58.
12. Takatsu K, Ishizaka T, Ishizaka K. Biological significance of disulfide bonds in human IgE molecules. *Journal of Immunology* 1975; **114**: 1838–1845.
13. Marti E, Szalai G, Bucher K, *et al.* Partial sequence of the equine immunoglobulin epsilon heavy chain cDNA. *Veterinary Immunology and Immunopathology* 1995; **47**: 363–367.

14. Navarro P, Barbis DP, Antczak D, *et al.* The complete cDNA and deduced amino acid sequence of equine IgE. *Molecular Immunology* 1995; **32**: 1–8.
15. Watson JL, Pettigrew HD, Wilson LK, *et al.* Isolation and partial expression of a cDNA encoding equine IgE heavy chain and production of polyclonal antibodies to the recombinant protein. *Journal of Veterinary Allergy and Clinical Immunology* 1997; **5**: 135–142.
16. Wagner B, Siebenkotten G, Radbruch A, *et al.* Nucleotide sequence and restriction fragment length polymorphisms of the equine Cvarepsilon gene. *Veterinary Immunology and Immunopathology* 2001; **82**: 193–202.
17. Wagner B, Miller DC, Lear TL, *et al.* The complete map of the Ig heavy chain constant gene region reveals evidence for seven IgG isotypes and for IgD in the horse. *Journal of Immunology* 2004; **173**: 3230–3242.
18. Wagner B. IgE in horses: occurrence in health and disease. *Veterinary Immunology and Immunopathology* 2009; **132**: 21–30.
19. Vychodilova L, Matiasovic J, Bobrova O, *et al.* Immunogenomic analysis of insect bite hypersensitivity in a model horse population. *Veterinary Immunology and Immunopathology* 2013;**152**:260–268.
20. Suter M, Fey H. Isolation and characterization of equine IgE. *Zentralblatt für Veterinärmedizin Reihe B Journal of Veterinary Medicine Series B* 1981; **28**: 414–420.
21. Suter M, Fey H. Further purification and characterisation of horse IgE. *Veterinary Immunology and Immunopathology* 1983; **4**: 545–553.
22. Halliwell RE, Hines MT. Studies on equine recurrent uveitis. I Levels of immunoglobulin and albumin in the aqueous humour of horses with and without intraocular disease. *Current Eye Research* 1985; **4**: 1023–1031.
23. Marti E, Peveri P, Griot-Wenk M, *et al.* Chicken antibodies to a recombinant fragment of the equine immunoglobulin epsilon heavy-chain recognising native horse IgE. *Veterinary Immunology and Immunopathology* 1997; **59**: 253–270.
24. Wagner B, Siebenkotten G, Leibold W, *et al.* Expression of a 4-(hydroxy-3-nitro-phenyl) acetyl (NP) specific equi-murine IgE antibody that mediates histamine release in vitro and a type I skin reaction in vivo. *Equine Veterinary Journal* 2002; **34**: 657–665.
25. Wagner B, Radbruch A, Rohwer J, *et al.* Monoclonal anti-equine IgE antibodies with specificity for different epitopes on the immunoglobulin heavy chain of native IgE. *Veterinary Immunology and Immunopathology* 2003; **92**: 45–60.
26. Wilson AD, Harwood LJ, Torsteinsdottir S, *et al.* Production of monoclonal antibodies specific for native equine IgE and their application to monitor total serum IgE responses in Icelandic and non-Icelandic horses with insect bite dermal hypersensitivity. *Veterinary Immunology and Immunopathology* 2006; **112**: 156–170.
27. Kalina WV, Pettigrew HD, Gershwin LJ. IgE ELISA using antisera derived from epsilon chain antigenic peptides detects allergen-specific IgE in allergic horses. *Veterinary Immunology and Immunopathology* 2003; **92**: 137–147.
28. Bravermann Y, UngarWaron H, Rith K, *et al.* Epidemiological and immunological studies of sweet itch in horses in Israel. *Veterinary Record* 1983; **112**: 521–524.
29. Quinn PJ, Baker KP, Morrow AN. Sweet itch: responses of clinically normal and affected horses to intradermal challenge with extracts of biting insects. *Equine Veterinary Journal* 1983; **15**: 266–272.
30. Larsen HJ, Bakke SH, Mehl R. Intradermal challenge of Icelandic horses in Norway and Iceland with extracts of Culicoides spp. *Acta Veterinaria Scandinavia* 1988; **29**: 311–314.
31. Halldorsdottir S, Larsen HJ, Mehl R. Intradermal challenge of Icelandic horses with extracts of four species of the genus *Culicoides*. *Research in Veterinary Science* 1989; **47**: 283–287.
32. Fadok VA, Greiner EC. Equine insect hypersensitivity: skin test and biopsy results correlated with clinical data. *Equine Veterinary Journal* 1990; **22**: 236–240.
33. Anderson GS, Belton P, Kleider N. Hypersensitivity of horses in British Columbia to extracts of native and exotic species of *Culicoides* (Diptera: Ceratopogonidae). *Journal of Medical Entomology* 1993; **30**: 657–663.
34. Marti E, Urwyler A, Neuenschwander M, *et al.* Sulfidoleukotriene generation from peripheral blood leukocytes of horses affected with insect bite dermal hypersensitivity. *Veterinary Immunology and Immunopathology* 1999; **71**: 307–320.
35. Baselgia S, Doherr MG, Mellor P, *et al.* Evaluation of an *in vitro* sulfidoleukotriene release test for diagnosis of insect bite hypersensitivity in horses. *Equine Veterinary Journal* 2006; **38**: 40–46.
36. Langner KF, Darpel KE, Drolet BS, *et al.* Comparison of cellular and humoral immunoassays for the assessment of summer eczema in horses. *Veterinary Immunology and Immunopathology* 2008; **122**: 126–137.
37. Wagner B, Childs BA, Erb HN. A histamine release assay to identify sensitization to *Culicoides* allergens in horses with skin hypersensitivity. *Veterinary Immunology and Immunopathology* 2008; **126**: 302–308.
38. van der Haegen A, Griot-Wenk M, Welle M *et al.* Immunoglobulin-E-bearing cells in skin biopsies of horses with insect bite hypersensitivity. *Equine Veterinary Journal* 2001; **33**: 699–706.
39. Bieber T, Ring J, Braun-Falco. Comparison of different methods for enumeration of Langerhans cells in vertical cryosections of human skin. *British Journal of Dermatology* 1988; **118**: 385–395.
40. Scharrenberg A, Gerber V, Swinburne JE, *et al.* IgE, IgGa, IgGb and IgG(T) serum antibody levels in offspring of two sires affected with equine recurrent airway obstruction. *Animal Genetics* 2010; **41**: 131–137.
41. Hamza E, Torsteinsdottir S, Eydal M, *et al.* Increased IL-4 and decreased regulatory cytokine production following relocation of Icelandic horses from a high to low endoparasite environment. *Veterinary Immunology and Immunopathology* 2010; **133**: 40–50.
42. Hellberg W, Wilson AD, Mellor P, *et al.* Equine insect bite hypersensitivity: immunoblot analysis of IgE and IgG subclass responses to *Culicoides nubeculosus* salivary gland extract. *Veterinary Immunology and Immunopathology* 2006; **113**: 99–112.
43. Hamza E, Doherr MG, Bertoni G, *et al.* Modulation of allergy incidence in Icelandic horses is associated with a change in IL-4-producing T cells. *International Archives of Allergy and Immunology* 2007; **144**: 325–337.
44. Wilson AD, Harwood LJ, Bjornsdottir S, *et al.* Detection of IgG and IgE serum antibodies to Culicoides salivary gland antigens in horses with insect dermal hypersensitivity (sweet itch). *Equine Veterinary Journal* 2001; **33**: 707–713.
45. Marti E, Ehrensperger F, Burger D, *et al.* Maternal transfer of IgE and subsequent development of IgE responses in the horse (*Equus callabus*). *Veterinary Immunology and Immunopathology* 2009; **127**: 203–211.
46. Wagner B, Flaminio JB, Hillegas J, *et al.* Occurrence of IgE in foals: evidence for transfer of maternal IgE by the colostrum and late onset of endogenous IgE production in the horse. *Veterinary Immunology and Immunopathology* 2006; **110**: 269–278.
47. Schmid-Grendelmeier P, Crameri R. Recombinant allergens for skin testing. *International Archives of Allergy and Immunology* 2001; **125**: 96–111.

48. Schaffartzik A, Hamza E, Janda J, *et al.* Equine insect bite hypersensitivity: what do we know? *Veterinary Immunology and Immunopathology* 2012; **147**: 113–126.
49. Langner KF, Jarvis DL, Nimtz M, *et al.* Identification, expression and characterisation of a major salivary allergen (Cul s 1) of the biting midge *Culicoides sonorensis* relevant for summer eczema in horses. *International Journal of Parasitology* 2009; **39**: 243–250.
50. Schaffartzik A, Marti E, Crameri R, *et al.* Cloning, production and characterization of antigen 5 like proteins from *Simulium vittatum* and *Culicoides nubeculosus*, the first cross-reactive allergen associated with equine insect bite hypersensitivity. *Veterinary Immunology and Immunopathology* 2010; **137**: 76–83.
51. Schaffartzik A, Marti E, Torsteinsdottir S, *et al.* Selective cloning, characterization and production of the *Culicoides nubeculosus* salivary gland allergen repertoire associated with equine insect bite hypersensitivity. *Veterinary Immunology and Immunopathology* 2011; **139**: 200–209.
52. Hellberg W, Mellor PS, Torsteinsdóttir S, *et al.* Insect bite hypersensitivity in the horse: comparison of IgE-binding proteins in salivary gland extracts from *Simulium vittatum* and *Culicoides nubeculosus*. *Veterinary Immunology and Immunopathology* 2009; **132**: 62–67.
53. Zeller S, Rhyner C, Meyer N, *et al.* Exploring the repertoire of IgE-binding self-antigens associated with atopic eczema. *Journal of Allergy and Clinical Immunology* 2009; **124**: 278–285, e1–7.
54. Pfiffner P, Stadler BM, Rasi C, *et al.* Cross-reactions vs co-sensitization evaluated by in silico motifs and in vitro IgE microarray testing. *Allergy* 2012; **67**: 210–216.
55. Sloet van Oldruitenborgh-Oosterbaan MM, van Poppel M, de Raat IJ, *et al.* Intradermal testing of horses with and without insect bite hypersensitivity in The Netherlands using an extract of native *Culicoides* species. *Veterinary Dermatology* 2009; **20**: 607–614.
56. Wilson AD, Heesom KJ, Mawby WJ, *et al.* Identification of abundant proteins and potential allergens in *Culicoides nubeculosus* salivary glands. *Veterinary Immunology and Immunopathology* 2008; **122**: 94–103.
57. van der Meide NM, Meulenbroeks C, van Altena C, *et al. Culicoides obsoletus* extract relevant for diagnostics of insect bite hypersensitivity in horses. *Veterinary Immunology and Immunopathology* 2012; **149**: 245–254.
58. Peeters LM, Janssens S, Goddeeris BM, *et al.* Evaluation of an IgE ELISA with *Culicoides* spp. extracts and recombinant salivary antigens for diagnosis of insect bite hypersensitivity in Warm-blood horses. *The Veterinary Journal* 2013 Jul 24. doi:pii: S1090-0233(13)00294-3. 10.1016/j.tvjl.2013.06.010. [Epub ahead of print]
59. Frey R, Bergvall K, Egenvall A. Allergen-specific IgE in Icelandic horses with insect bite hypersensitivity and healthy controls, assessed by Fcepsilon R1 alpha-based serology. *Veterinary Immunology and Immunopathology* 2008; **126**: 102–109.
60. van der Meide NM, Roders N, Sloet van Oldruitenborgh-Oosterbaan MM, *et al.* Cloning and expression of candidate allergens from *Culicoides obsoletus* for diagnosis of insect bite hypersensitivity in horses. *Veterinary Immunology and Immunopathology* 2013; **153**: 227–239.

45

Clinical manifestations of *Culicoides* hypersensitivity

Janet D. Littlewood

Veterinary Dermatology Referrals, Landbeach, Cambridge, UK

Conflict of interest: none declared.

Culicoides hypersensitivity is the commonest of the allergic skin diseases of equids with an almost worldwide distribution, and with many different colloquial names for the condition. The term 'sweet itch' is a corruption of 'sweat itch', reflecting that the disorder is usually seen in the summer months. The condition occurs in grazing animals with a definite seasonal pattern, from spring to autumn in temperate climates, when the adult biting gnats are on the wing. In tropical and subtropical climates affected animals may show clinical signs all year round, often with seasonal exacerbations, as different species of midges (gnats) tend to survive throughout the year in such regions. The condition does not occur in parts of the world where *Culicoides* insects are not found, such as Iceland.

Any breed of horse may be affected, but certain breeds have been reported to be at increased risk of developing the disease, including Icelandic ponies [1,2], shire horses in Germany [3], Friesians, Shetland ponies [4], Welsh ponies, Arabs, Connemaras, Swiss warmbloods, and quarter horses [5], although other studies have shown no breed predisposition amongst horses [6,7], but ponies were at increased risk [7]. An overall prevalence of 2.79% was recorded in a survey of pony clubs in the United Kingdom, with marked regional differences that could be accounted for by the geographical variations, lower incidence reported in higher parts of the country, and increased prevalence in lowland, valley, and coastal regions [8].

The disease can develop at any age, but onset of clinical signs is usually in young adult horses, 3–4 years of age. The severity of clinical signs tends to progress with age. There is no association with gender or coat colour [7], but a familial tendency to develop the disease is well recognized [9] and can be documented in about one-third of cases [3,5], with heritability associated with certain equine leucocyte antigen (ELA) haplotypes in some families [10,11].

As the condition is associated with hypersensitivity reactions to various salivary proteins of *Culicoides* species, the distribution of clinical lesions in affected animals correlates with the preferential feeding sites of the insects. Three clinical syndromes have been described [12]:

- syndrome I (dorsal distribution): horses show lesions on the mane and lateral neck, shoulders and withers, rump and tail, and also on the face and ears (Figure 45.1);
- syndrome II (ventral distribution): horses show lesions on the face, ears, intermandibular space, chest, belly, and groin (Figure 45.2);
- syndrome III (combination of dorsal and ventral distribution) (Figure 45.3).

In the report defining these presentations, which comprised affected horses from the south-eastern United States of America, the most commonly encountered was

Veterinary Allergy, First Edition. Edited by Chiara Noli, Aiden Foster, and Wayne Rosenkrantz.

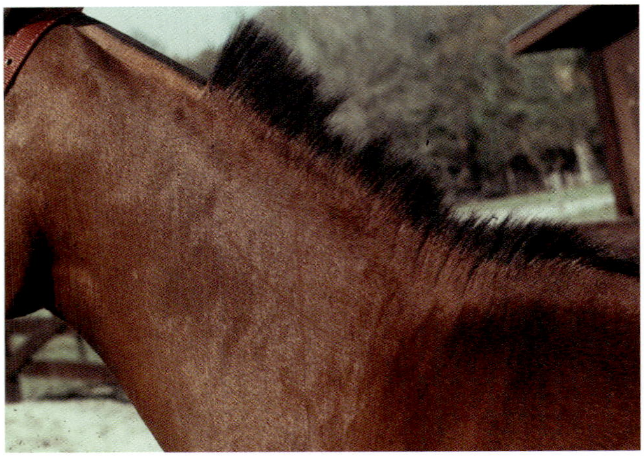

Figure 45.1 *Culicoides* hypersensitivity in a quarter horse showing partial loss of mane. (Reprinted with permission from Wayne Rosenkrantz.)

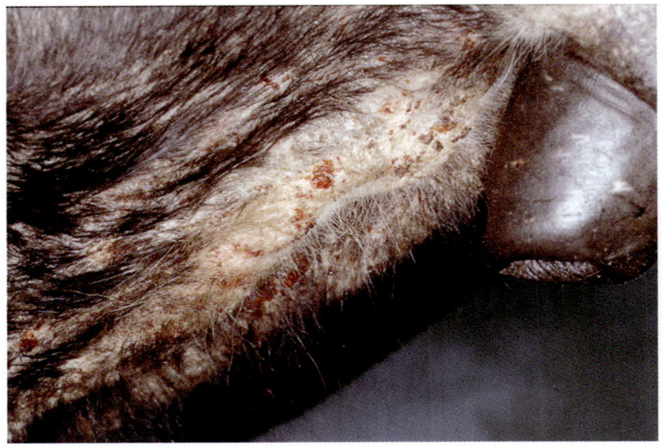

Figure 45.3 Welsh mountain pony with *Culicoides* hypersensitivity lesions affecting the ventral midline with alopecia, crusted papules, scaling, lichenification, thickening, and folding of skin. (Reprinted from [13]. © 2003, with the permission of John Wiley & Sons, Ltd.)

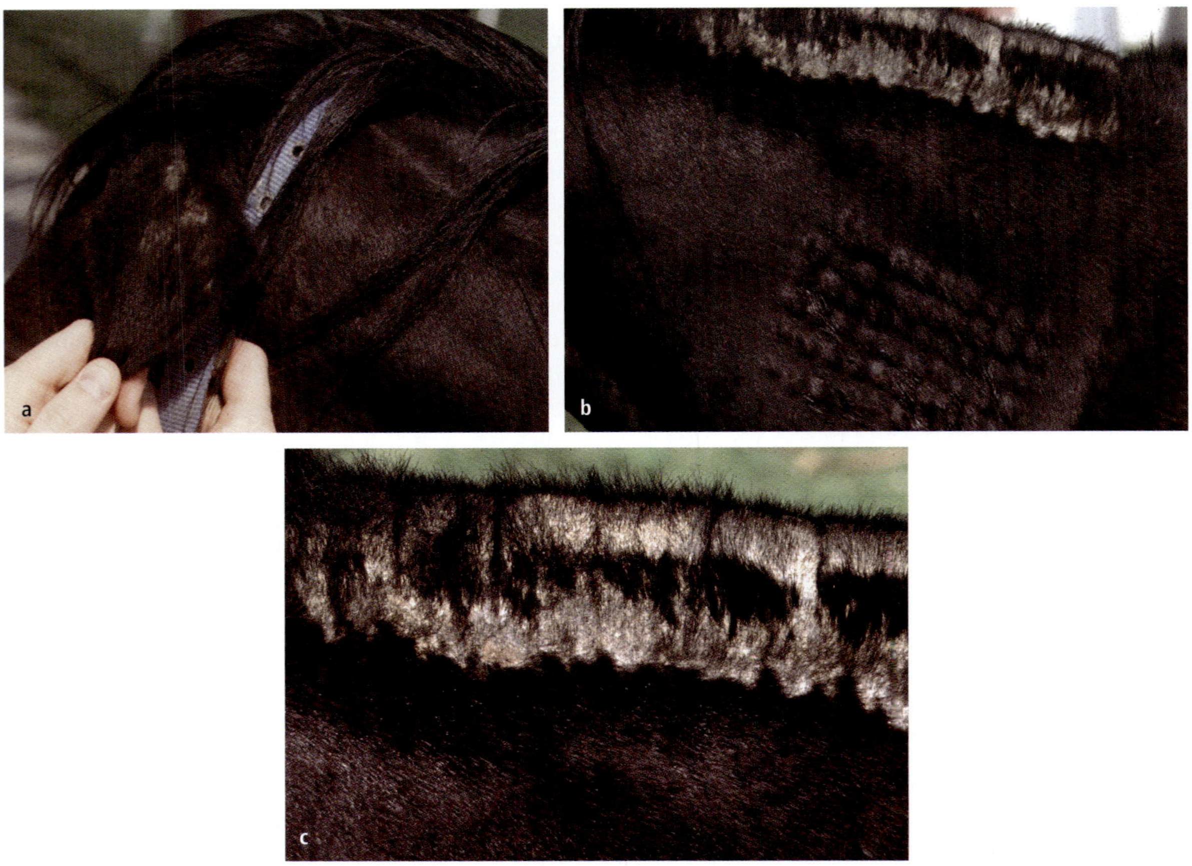

Figure 45.2 Thoroughbred horse with *Culicoides* hypersensitivity lesions affecting (a) the ears showing patchy alopecia, excoriations, and surface scaling; and (b) the mane with severe progressive alopecia, lichenification, and excoriations with intradermal testing (IDT) site also shown with positive *Culicoides* and other insect reactions. (c) Close up of mane. (Reprinted with permission from Wayne Rosenkrantz.)

syndrome III, with syndrome II being the least common presentation. The preferred landing sites of different species of *Culicoides* have been studied in various geographical locations and thus the species implicated in causing disease have been identified [14–16]. The prevalence of ventral compared to dorsal lesions may vary in different parts of the world, depending on the geographical distribution of ventrally feeding species of midges.

Of a group of 29 affected horses studied in the United Kingdom (UK), all showed involvement of the mane and tail, with 41% having head lesions, 31% rump lesions, 5% with lesions on the withers, 5% with lesions on the ventrum, 4% flanks, 3% shoulders, and one horse having medial hind limb involvement [17]. This was the first publication to document the occurrence of ventral lesions in horses with sweet itch in the UK.

The major clinical sign associated with *Culicoides* hypersensitivity is pruritus, which may be intense and severe. In early cases papular lesions may be seen with tufting of hair in affected regions and marked hyperaesthesia [18], but secondary lesions due to self-inflicted trauma soon supersede. Affected animals will rub on any convenient structure, including stables, shelters, fencing, trees, gate posts, and may be seen rolling or dragging their undersides on the ground. Manipulation or rubbing of the affected areas can often elicit 'nibbling', a positive itch reflex reaction. The severity of pruritus is often worse in the evenings, around the time of dusk, which is the preferred feeding time of the insects. Broken and damaged hairs are seen, progressing to localized areas of alopecia. Self-inflicted damage may cause erosions and excoriations, with serous oozing. Secondary bacterial infections may occur, with crusting lesions of superficial folliculitis or tail pyoderma, or more extensive areas of severe inflammation and oozing.

Chronically affected animals show more extensive partial to full alopecia, with thickening of the skin (lichenification) and scaling (Figure 45.4). The skin may develop transverse ridges, rugal folds, which fail to resolve in the winter months. Severely affected animals often lose all the hair on the proximal third of the tail and much of the mane, resulting in a 'buzzed-off' appearance, as a result of which owners often clip off the remaining mane hair, known as a 'hogged mane'. Disturbances of pigmentation may be seen, with melanoderma and melanotrichia at sites of insect bites and self trauma, although in chronic cases leucoderma and leukotrichia may be seen (Figures 45.5 and 45.6). Occasionally, animals with *Culicoides* hypersensitivity may develop nodular cutaneous lesions, which histologically may contain eosinophilic collagenolysis and/or granulomas.

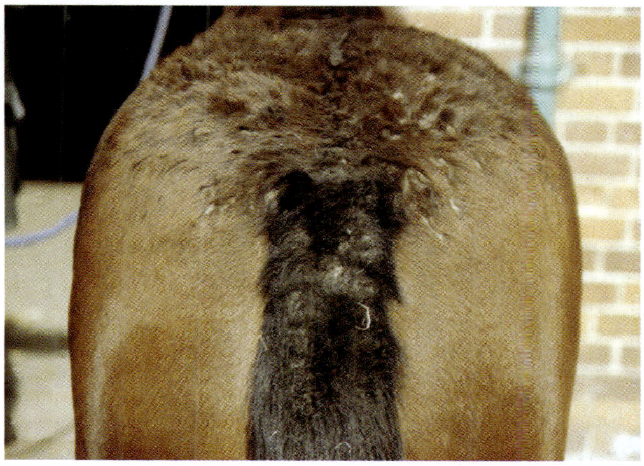

Figure 45.5 Pony with *Culicoides* hypersensitivity showing patchy melanotrichia on the rump in addition to focal patches of alopecia and partial alopecia of the tail base with broken, damaged hairs.

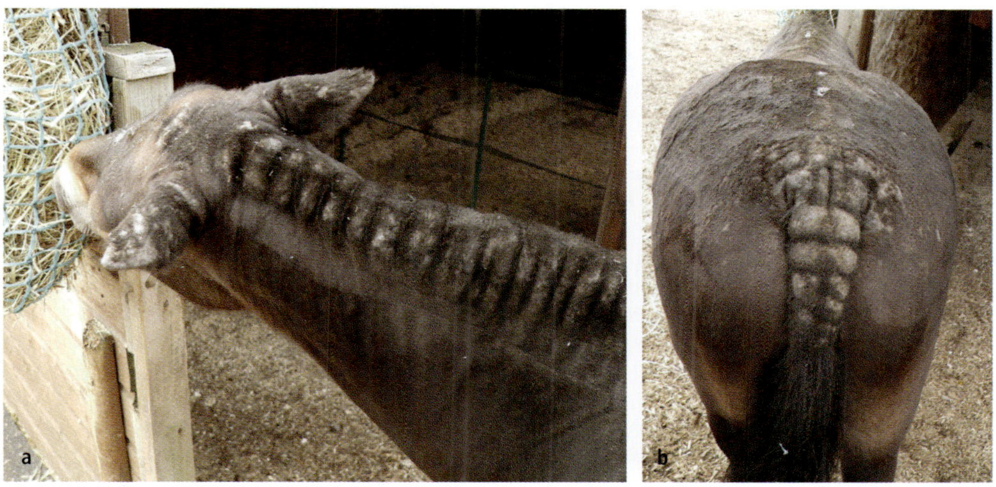

Figure 45.4 Pony with chronic, long-standing *Culicoides* hypersensitivity, showing (a) loss of all hair of mane with underlying prominent rugal folds and patches of alopecia affecting the ears, temporal region, poll, and crest regions; and (b) extensive partial to full alopecia of the proximal half of the tail with marked thickening and folding of the skin, with lesions of alopecia and damaged, disrupted hair extending to the dorsolateral rump region. (Reprinted with permission from Nicola Jarvis MRCVS.)

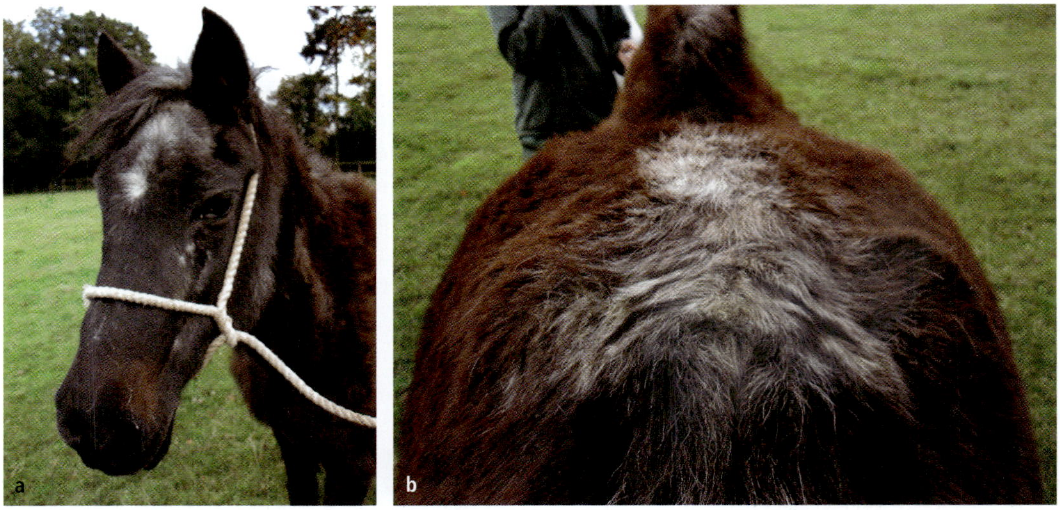

Figure 45.6 Welsh mountain pony with chronic lesions of *Culicoides* hypersensitivity, with patches of leucotrichia on (a) the face and (b) the caudal dorsolateral rump.

Affected horses may show a range of behavioural problems such as restlessness, anxiety, nervousness, and aggression. The constant irritation may interfere significantly with foraging and grazing, resulting in loss of bodyweight and condition. Severely affected animals may be unfit for riding or working. The welfare issues associated with *Culicoides* hypersensitivity should not be underestimated and in some cases the severity of pruritus and resulting skin lesions may force owners to consider euthanasia.

References

1. Broström H, Larsson, Å, Troedsson M. Allergic dermatitis (sweet itch) of Icelandic horses in Sweden: an epidemiological study. *Equine Veterinary Journal* 1987; **19**: 229–236.
2. Halldórdsóttir H, Larsen HJ. An epidemiological study of summer eczema in Icelandic horses in Norway. *Equine Veterinary Journal* 1991; **23**:296–299.
3. Littlewood JD. Incidence of recurrent seasonal pruritus ('sweet itch') in British and German shire horses. *Veterinary Record* 1998; **142**: 66–67.
4. van den Boom R, Ducro B, Sloet van Oldruitenborgh-Oosterbaan MM. Identification of factors associated with the development of insect-bite hypersensitivity in horses in the Netherlands. *Tijdschrift voor Diergeneeskunde* 2008; **133**: 554–559.
5. Scott DW, Miller WH Jr. *Equine Dermatology*, 2nd edn. Maryland Heights, Missouri: Elsevier Saunders, 2011: 303–311.
6. Anderson GS, Belton P, Kleider N. The hypersensitivity of horses to *Culicoides* bites in British Columbia. *Canadian Veterinary Journal* 1988; **29**: 718–723.
7. Steinman A, Peer G, Klement E. Epidemiological study of *Culicoides* hypersensitivity in horses in Israel. *Veterinary Record* 2003; **152**: 748–751.
8. McCaig J. A survey to establish the incidence of sweet itch in ponies in the United Kingdom. *Veterinary Record* 1973; **94**: 444–446.
9. Gerber H. The genetic basis of some equine diseases. *Equine Veterinary Journal* 1989; **21**: 244–248.
10. Halldórdsóttir S, Lazary S, Gunnarsson E, *et al.* Distribution of leucocyte antigens in Icelandic horses affected with summer eczema compared to non-affected horses. *Equine Veterinary Journal* 1991; **23**: 300–302.
11. Marti E, Berber H, Lazary S. On the genetic basis of equine allergic diseases: II. Insect bite dermal hypersensitivity. *Equine Veterinary Journal* 1992; **24**: 113–117.
12. Fadok VA, Greiner EC. Equine insect hypersensitivity: skin test and biopsy results correlated with clinical data. *Equine Veterinary Journal* 1990; **22**: 236–240.
13. Lloyd DH, Littlewood JD, Craig JM, Thomsett LR. *Practical Equine Dermatology*. Oxford: Wiley Blackwell, 2003: 19.
14. Mellor PS. The probable cause of 'sweet itch' in England. *Veterinary Record* 1974; **95**: 411–415.
15. Townley P, Baker KP, Quinn PJ. Preferential landing and engorging sites of *Culicoides* species landing on a horse in Ireland. *Equine Veterinary Journal* 1984; **16**: 117–120.
16. Braverman Y. Preferred landing sites of *Culicoides* species (Diptera: Ceratopogonidae) on a horse in Israel and its relevance to summer seasonal recurrent dermatitis (sweet itch). *Equine Veterinary Journal* 1988; **20**: 426–429.
17. Craig JM, Lloyd DH, Jones RG. A double-blind placebo-controlled trial of an evening primrose and fish oil combination vs. hydrogenated coconut oil in the management of recurrent seasonal pruritus in horses. *Veterinary Dermatology* 1997; **8**: 177–182.
18. Baker KP, Quinn PJ. A report on the clinical aspects and histopathology of sweet itch. *Equine Veterinary Journal* 1978; **10**: 243–248.

46

Culicoides hypersensitivity: diagnosis

Kerstin Bergvall

Swedish University of Agricultural Sciences, Department of Clinical Sciences, Uppsala, Sweden

Conflict of interest: none declared.

Introduction

The diagnosis of *Culicoides* hypersensitivity is primarily based on history and physical findings, and ruling out appropriate differentials. There is currently no simple diagnostic test that can readily and accurately discriminate *Culicoides* hypersensitivity from other insect bite hypersensitivities or other non-insect bite hypersensitivities in horses.

The clinical presentation of pruritus, a geographic location *Culicoides* are known to inhabit, correlation with seasonality, and lesional distribution are strongly supportive of the diagnosis. Clinical lesions are variable but typically include excoriations, broken hairs and alopecia, crusted papules, and lichenification involving the base of the mane and tail, ear pinnae, face, and ventral midline. Depending on the species and geographic location, there are different clinical patterns with dorsal, ventral, and combinations of lesion distribution (see Chapter 45). Although any horse can be affected, the signalment can be further suggestive of the diagnosis if the horse belongs to a predisposed breed (i.e. Icelandic, shire, Friesian, Arabian, and quarter horse and Shetland ponies [1–7]) and if additional risk factors are present (i.e. age over 2 years [6,8], Icelandic horse imported from Iceland [9–11], and family history [12,13]).

Where the history and clinical findings are compatible with *Culicoides* hypersensitivity, differential diagnoses with a potentially similar presentation should be excluded, e.g. ectoparasite infestation, forage mites, and oxyuriasis (if only the base of the tail and rump areas are affected). Other forms of hypersensitivity reactions (non-*Culicoides* insect hypersensitivities, atopic dermatitis, and adverse food reactions) need to be considered. These are discussed in Chapters 48 to 53. Adverse food reactions tend to be more year round and lack seasonality but can be intermittent if proteins are fed intermittently. Atopic dermatitis can be more difficult to distinguish because this is also commonly seasonal and may coexist with any insect bite hypersensitivity, and clinical distributions and signs can overlap. See Table 46.1 for key diagnostic features.

To exclude differential diagnoses, a complete clinical and dermatologic examination under good light is essential. A magnifying lens and a flea comb are useful tools when looking for lice. Skin scrapings and tape preparations aid in detection of chorioptic and psoroptic mange, trombicula larvae, forage mites, *Oxyuris* eggs, and poultry mites (*Dermanyssus gallinae*). If poultry mites are suspected then the environment of the horse should be examined because the mites are active at night and hide in cracks and crevices away from daylight, and thus can be difficult to find on the horse. Fungal cultures can be helpful to rule out dermatophyte infections. Cytology can be extremely beneficial to identify some infectious agents and can also be important in the initial diagnostic investigation depending upon the type of clinical lesions that are present.

Histopathology

The histology is not pathognomonic for *Culicoides* hypersensitivity; it is merely consistent with a hypersensitivity

Veterinary Allergy, First Edition. Edited by Chiara Noli, Aiden Foster, and Wayne Rosenkrantz.

Table 46.1 Key diagnostic features for *Culicoides* hypersensitivity

History	Living in *Culicoides* endemic area Seasonality compatible with insect season Imported from Iceland Family history Less common if living along coast line
Signalment	Breed at risk (Icelandic, Friesian, shire, Arabian, quarter horse, thoroughbred, Swiss warmblood, Shetland and Welsh ponies, Connemara) Age over 2 years
Clinical signs	Pruritus Base of mane and base of tail affected Ventral midline affected Pinnae affected Intermandibular space affected Broken hairs/hypotrichosis at base of mane and base of tail Oedema at base of mane/base of tail/along ventral midline Excoriations base of mane/base of tail/face/withers Scaling/crusting/crusted papules at base of mane and base of tail/ventral midline/ear pinnae/intermandibular space Lichenification at base of mane and base of tail/ventral midline/ear pinnae
Diagnostic tests	Ectoparasites not found Response to avoidance of biting midges (e.g. insect blanket, stabling from dusk to dawn, insect repellents, windy pasture)/lack of relapse after control of ongoing inflammation + avoidance of biting midges

reaction. A perivascular to diffuse infiltration of eosinophils and mononuclear cells is present; however, the predominance of eosinophils may help some clinicians to suspect that insect reactions are more likely. The inflammation can be present in the superficial dermis and/or in deeper dermis and subcutis. Increased numbers of mast cells positive for tryptase have been described in the upper dermis, hair follicle epithelia, and dermal papilla, and also increased numbers of antigen-presenting cells (MHCII-positive cells, likely Langerhans cells) at the dermoepidermal junction. Oedema is not uncommon in the subepidermal location and fibrosis can develop. The epidermis is hyperplastic with hyperkeratosis, sometimes with transverse ridges and folds. Spongiosis and exocytosis of lymphocytes and eosinophils are also common findings. Excoriations can cause erosions and ulcerations, and necrosis can be seen. Additionally, eosinophilic mural folliculitis, sometimes necrotizing, and focal eosinophilic granulomas have been reported. Immunohistochemistry has identified most infiltrating lymphocytes as CD4-positive, and to a lesser degree CD3-positive, T cells [3,12–17].

Allergy testing

Allergen-specific IgE levels can either be measured by quantification in serum (using of mono- or polyclonal antibodies that bind to various parts of the IgE antibody or capture with the high affinity FcεRI receptor [18–21]) or by dynamic tests. These tests (intradermal and basophil degranulation) measure histamine or sulphido-leukotriene release through allergen-mediated cross-linking of IgE on mast cells or basophils.

Serum testing

Total IgE

Although immediate, IgE-mediated type I hypersensitivity reactions to *Culicoides* salivary antigens have been shown to be important in the pathogenesis of *Culicoides* hypersensitivity, the measurement of total IgE is not considered to be a useful parameter for discrimination between allergic and non-allergic horses [22]. Serum IgE concentrations have been shown to be influenced by endoparasitism [23]; in two reports there was significantly higher levels of total serum IgE in imported Icelandic horses with *Culicoides* hypersensitivity compared to healthy controls [19,24]. Such a difference has not been demonstrated in other breeds or horses born outside Iceland [23,25].

Allergen-specific IgE

Serology testing for allergen-specific IgE is provided by several laboratories. Many serology companies claim that antihistamine therapy, and possibly low or moderate doses of prednisolone and dexamethasone, will not interfere with the test results; however, there are no studies to substantiate these claims. The possible pitfalls that need to be considered with these types of tests are whether the test method specifically detects IgE and not IgG and whether relevant allergens have been used (see section "Allergens sources"). The relatively high concentrations of IgG compared to IgE in serum may interfere with serum assays because IgG antibodies will also bind to allergens [26,27]. Test results with mono- and polyclonal antibodies to various parts of the IgE molecule have been shown to correlate poorly with intradermal testing, in comparison with tests performed using the high-affinity receptor [28]. It has been reported that monoclonal antibody reagents are more specific for IgE than polyclonal anti-IgE reagents [18,19]. Commercially available *Culicoides* allergen extracts have yielded numerous positive reactions in healthy horses [24,26], and poor specificity and sensitivity was reported in a 2008 study from Sweden [29]. In one small-scale study from the Netherlands [30], 7/10 horses with clinical disease reacted to *Culicoides* extracts, compared to only one of the ten healthy controls.

Other *in vitro* tests, not commercially available, are the dynamic tests where peripheral blood basophils are challenged with allergens and the release of histamine and sulphidoleukotrienes are measured [26,31,32]. Nonallergic and allergic horses have been shown to have equal amounts of IgE on basophils given that there was no significant difference in the concentration of histamine released after anti-IgE stimulation in both groups of horses. However, after incubation with allergens, especially *Culicoides* extract, allergic horses released significantly more histamine [26,32]. There was, however, histamine release also in clinically healthy horses, indicating either sensitization without disease [32], or that this test is not sufficiently specific to distinguish allergic from normal horses, or that other antibodies could affect histamine release such as IgG(T) [33]. Another group of investigators demonstrated that incubating peripheral blood lymphocytes from 147 insect bite-reactive horses and 153 healthy controls with *Culicoides nubeculosis* extract released leukotrienes at levels above the cut-off level in 78% of affected horses as compared to only 3% of the controls [34]. Dynamic testing in the form of *in vitro* histamine release test was, furthermore, considered more sensitive for diagnosis of *Culicoides* hypersensitivity as compared to measuring serum levels of IgE by ELISA in one study including 10 affected and 10 healthy Shetland ponies [30]. The authors also reported a high histamine response in some horses with low levels of IgE as measured by mouse monoclonal anti-IgE.

Intradermal testing

With the use of intradermal injections of allergens, the presence of allergen-specific IgE bound to mast cells in the skin can be detected. When an allergen cross-binds IgE on the mast cell surface, degranulation occurs and inflammatory mediators are released, resulting in a visible wheal and flare reaction, which can be palpated and measured. As horses with suspected *Culicoides* hypersensitivity are pruritic they can also be very sensitive to the touch, which can elicit a twisting reaction of the skin; therefore, sedation is commonly needed to perform intradermal testing. The author prefers premedication with detomidine hydrochloride in combination with butorphanol (intravenously); xylazine could also be used. The usual site for an intradermal test in horses is the lateral neck. A sedated horse may still occasionally move and this may make strict intradermal injections more difficult to perform. The author uses the shoulder area, which allows the horse to move the head or neck without disturbing the test procedure. The hair coat is shaved as for surgical preparation; the area should not be washed. A marking pen is used to indicate where allergens are to be injected, including negative and positive controls (saline and histamine 1 : 1000 w/v or 1 : 100 000 dilution). The same volume of each allergen is injected intradermally (approximately 0.05–0.1 mL) and the test area is inspected for immediate reactions after 15–30 minutes and late reactions after 4–6 hours [35–37]. In *Culicoides* hypersensitive horses, evaluation after 60 minutes was reported to be the most rewarding [38].

Delayed reactions (read after 24 hours) in severely affected horses were more common than in milder cases. The wheal formation of the tested allergen is compared to the saline (negative control) and the histamine reaction (positive control), by size and turgidity at palpation. Wheal diameter was reported as the most useful parameter, whereas turgidity or firmness did not contribute to test sensitivity and specificity in one study [38]. If the skin is unpigmented at the test area, erythema can also be noticed in positive reactions. Small areas of cutaneous haemorrhage may result from the intradermal injection and should not be confused with an erythema reaction. The reactions are subjectively graded from 0 to 4, comparing the injected allergens to the controls. The performance of intradermal testing requires practical training and the horse should ideally not be treated with antihistamines or corticosteroids for 7 and 14 days, respectively, prior to testing to avoid interference with test results (see Chapter 53). Furthermore, the allergen source and concentration can affect the skin reactivity (see section "Allergens sources").

Immediate-type reactions were significantly more common in insect hypersensitive horses compared with healthy controls [4,26,37–40]. One study involving 18 affected and 23 healthy horses reported a sensitivity and specificity of 100% if the wheal diameter at 24 hours was 1 cm or more and skin fold thickness increased by more than 10% [35]. However, positive reactions are also frequently recorded in healthy horses [28,41,42]. Intradermal testing with *Culicoides* extract in 43 affected and 38 controls could not discriminate between hypersensitive and healthy horses and the sensitivity was given as 52% [41].

Allergens sources

In both *in vitro* and *in vivo* testing the source of allergen is critical for a valid result. Horses with *Culicoides* hypersensitivity develop immediate (Type I) and delayed (Type IV) hypersensitivity reactions to *Culicoides* extracts [1–4,37,40]. Commercially available allergen sources for testing *Culicoides* hypersensitivity are usually made from a crude extract of the insect as a whole-body extract (WBE). These crude extracts contain not only the salivary antigens but also a variety of other proteins and substances that might be irritant or not relevant to the disease [42,43]. The commercial allergen extracts have not been standardized for allergen content [1,4,35,37,38] and have revealed substantial variation in detectable protein content [27]. Furthermore, some allergens may contain histamine [24]. Thus, there are many reasons why testing with insect allergens can have a poor sensitivity and specificity, with poor repeatability for the diagnosis of *Culicoides* hypersensitivity [41,42]. If the offending allergen is present at too low a concentration then the sensitivity of the test will be low. If irrelevant, potentially irritant substances or cross-reactive, non-specific proteins are present then the test specificity might be reduced [27,44]. Although intradermal injection with crude extract of *Culicoides* often induces wheal reactions in *Culicoides* hypersensitivity horses [35,38], and studies have recorded more Type I reactions in affected horses as compared to normal controls [4,38,40], other studies have described frequent positive reactions in non-affected horses with intradermal and *in vitro* testing [24,26,29]. The use of WBE for intradermal testing and basophil degranulation testing resulted in higher numbers of false-positive reactions compared with tests using only *Culicoides* saliva antigen, which yielded results with high specificity [26]. In this and also another study [29], poor specificity and sensitivity were recorded for *Culicoides* WBE specific serum IgE and IgG antibody levels.

Over 500 species of *Culicoides* are recorded and several have been demonstrated to be important in *Culicoides* hypersensitivity, including *C. sonorensis*, *C. nubeculosus*, *C. imicola*, *C. obsoletus*, *C. robertsi*, and *C. pulicaris* [38,40,45–47]. In one study where six affected horses were challenged intradermally with extracts from two native and four exotic *Culicoides* spp. (from other continents), the horses reacted to all extracts including the four to which they were not thought to have been exposed, thereby suggesting that the offending allergen(s) were present in all extracts [4]. Cross-reactivity among *Culicoides* species was assumed in a study [26] of nine affected horses, which showed equal positive reactions to both intradermal and basophil degranulation tests to native German and exotic *Culicoides* extracts. Furthermore, intradermal testing with non-endemic species in Florida [48] yielded positive reactions in affected horses. Studies from the Netherlands, Norway, and Austria [30,40,41] have not shown cross-reactivity to WBE with different *Culicoides* species, indicating that use of extracts from native species is needed for a reliable diagnosis. A high specificity and sensitivity was recorded in an early study when using extracts from regional *Culicoides* for intradermal testing in six affected and six control horses [45].

Culicoides salivary antigens with major importance in the pathogenesis of *Culicoides* hypersensitivity have been cloned and expressed as recombinant proteins [25,49]. Hopefully, in the future there will be standardized allergen sources without contamination of irrelevant or irritant proteins. This will likely improve the sensitivity and specificity of *in vitro* and *in vivo* tests for *Culicoides* hypersensitivity.

In conclusion, commercially available tests based on WBE allergen sources do not reliably discriminate between diseased and healthy horses and cannot be recommended for the diagnosis of *Culicoides* hypersensitivity. Until recombinant, standardized salivary antigens are available the diagnosis is best made based on signalment, history, clinical presentation, exclusion of differential diagnoses, and improvement (or lack of relapse) after measures to ensure avoidance of exposure to biting insects.

References

1. Braverman Y, Ungar-Waron H, Frith K, *et al.* Epidemiological and immunological studies of sweet itch in horses in Israel. *Veterinary Record* 1983; **112**: 521–524.
2. Larsen HJ, Bakke SH, Mehl R. Intradermal challenge of Icelandic horses in Norway and Iceland with extracts of *Culicoides* spp. *Acta Veterinaria Scandinavia* 1988; **29**: 311–314.
3. Fadok VA, Greiner EC. Equine insect hypersensitivity: skin test and biopsy results correlated with clinical data. *Equine Veterinary Journal* 1990; **22**:236–240.

4. Anderson SG, Belton P, Kleider N. Hypersensitivity of horses in British Columbia to extracts of native and exotic species of *Culicoides* (Diptera: Ceratopogonidae). *Journal of Medical Entomology* 1993; **30**: 657–663.
5. Littlewood JD. Incidence of recurrent seasonal pruritus ('sweet itch') in British and German shire horses. *Veterinary Record* 1998; **142**: 66–67.
6. Steinman, G. Peer, Klement E. Epidemiological study of *Culicoides* hypersensitivity in horses in Israel. *Veterinary Record* 2003; **152**: 748–751.
7. vanGrevenhof EM, Ducro B, Heuven HC, *et al.* Identification of environmental factors affecting the prevalence of insect bite hypersensitivity in Shetland ponies and Friesian horses in The Netherlands. *Equine Veterinary Journal* 2007; **39**: 69–73.
8. Wilson AD, Harwood LJ, Bjornsdottir S, *et al.* Detection of IgG and IgE serum antibodies to *Culicoides* salivary gland antigens in horses with insect dermal hypersensitivity (sweet itch). *Equine Veterinary Journal* 2001; **33**: 707–713.
9. Brostrom H, Larsson A, Troedsson M. Allergic dermatitis (sweet itch) of Icelandic horses in Sweden: an epidemiological study. *Equine Veterinary Journal* 1987; **19**: 229–236.
10. Lange S, Hamann H, Deegen E, *et al.* Investigation of the prevalence of summer eczema in Icelandic horses in northern Germany. *Berliner und Münchenertierärztliche Wochenschrift* 2005; **118**: 481–489.
11. Bjornsdottir S, Sigvaldadottir J, Brostrom H, *et al.* Summer eczema in exported Icelandic horses: influence of environmental and genetic factors. *Acta Veterinaria Scandinavia* 2006; **48**: 3.
12. Riek RF. Studies on allergic dermatitis of the horse II. Treatment and control. *Australian Veterinary Journal* 1953; **29**: 185–187.
13. Anderson GS, Belton P, Kleider N. The hypersensitivity of horses to *Culicoides* bites in British Columbia. *Canadian Veterinary Journal* 1988; **29**: 718–723.
14. van der Haegen A, Griot-Wenk M, Welle M, *et al.* Immunoglobulin-E-bearing cells in skin biopsies of horses with insect bite hypersensitivity. *Equine Veterinary Journal* 2001; **33**: 699–706.
15. Kurotaki T, Narayama K, Oyamada T, *et al.* Immunopathological study on equine insect hypersensitivity ('kasen') in Japan. *Journal of Comparative Pathology* 1994; **110**: 145–152.
16. Kleider N, Lees MJ. *Culicoides* hypersensitivity in the horse: 15 cases in Southwestern British Columbia. *Canadian Veterinary Journal* 1984; **25**: 26–32.
17. Scott DW. Histopathologiecutanée de l'hypersensibilité aux piqures de *Culicoides* chez le cheval. *Point Vétérinaire* 1990; **22**: 583–588.
18. Wagner B, Radbruch A, Rohwer J, *et al.* Monoclonal anti-equine IgE antibodies with specificity for different epitopes on the immunoglobulin heavy chain of native IgE. *Veterinary Immunology and Immunopathology* 2003; **92**: 45–60.
19. Wilson AD, Harwood L, Torsteinsdottir S, *et al.* Production of monoclonal antibodies specific for native equine IgE and their application to monitor total serum IgE responses in Icelandic and non-Icelandic horses with insect bite dermal hypersensitivity. *Veterinary Immunology and Immunopathology* 2006; **112**: 156–170.
20. Kalina WV, Pettigrew HD, Gershwin LJ. IgE ELISA using antisera derived from epsilon chain antigenic peptides detects allergen-specific IgE in allergic horses. *Veterinary Immunology and Immunopathology* 2003; **92**: 137–147.
21. Marti E, Peveri P, Griot-Wenk M, *et al.* Chicken antibodies to a recombinant fragment of the equine immunoglobulin epsilon heavy-chain recognising native horse IgE. *Veterinary Immunology and Immunopathology* 1997; **59**: 253–270.
22. Scharrenberg, Gerber V, Swinburne JE, *et al.* IgE, IgGa, IgGb and IgG(T) serum antibody levels in offspring of two sires affected with equine recurrent airway obstruction. *Animal Genetics* 2010; **41** (Suppl. 2): 131–137.
23. Hamza E, Torsteinsdottir S, Eydal M, *et al.* Increased IL-4 and decreased regulatory cytokine production following relocation of Icelandic horses from a high to low endoparasite environment. *Veterinary Immunology and Immunopathology* 2010; **133**: 40–50.
24. Wagner B. IgE in horses: occurrence in health and disease. *Veterinary Immunology and Immunopathology* 2009; **132**: 21–30.
25. Hellberg W, Wilson AD, Mellor P, *et al.* Equine insect bite hypersensitivity: immunoblot analysis of IgE and IgG subclass responses to Culicoides nubeculosus salivary gland extract. *Veterinary Immunology and Immunopathology* 2006; **113**: 99–112.
26. Langner KF, Darpel KE, Drolet BS, *et al.* Comparison of cellular and humoral immunoassays for the assessment of summer eczema in horses. *Veterinary Immunology and Immunopathology* 2008; **122**: 126–137.
27. Morgan EE, Miller WH Jr, Wagner B. A comparison of intradermal testing and detection of allergen-specific immunoglobulin E in serum by enzyme-linked immunosorbent assay in horses affected with skin hypersensitivity. *Veterinary Immunology and Immunopathology* 2007; **120**: 160–167.
28. Lorch G, Hillier A, Kwochka KW, *et al.* Results of intradermal tests in horses without atopy and horses with atopic dermatitis or recurrent urticaria. *American Journal of Veterinary Research* 2001; **62**: 1051–1059.
29. Frey R, Bergvall K, Egenvall A. Allergen-specific IgE in Icelandic horses with insect bite hypersensitivity and healthy controls, assessed by FcepsilonR1alpha-based serology. *Veterinary Immunology and Immunopathology* 2008; **126**: 102–109.
30. van der Meide NM, Meulenbroeks C, van Altena C, *et al.* *Culicoides obsoletus* extract relevant for diagnostics of insect bite hypersensitivity in horses. *Veterinary Immunology and Immunopathology* 2012; **149**: 245–254.
31. Marti E, Urwyler A, Neuenschwander M, *et al.* Sulfidoleukotriene generation from peripheral blood leukocytes of horses affected with insect bite dermal hypersensitivity. *Veterinary Immunology and Immunopathology* 1999; **71**: 307–320.
32. Wagner B, Childs BA, Erb HN. A histamine release assay to identify sensitization to Culicoides allergens in horses with skin hypersensitivity. *Veterinary Immunology and Immunopathology* 2008; **126**: 302–308.
33. Wagner B, Miller WH, Morgan EE, *et al.* IgE and IgG antibodies in skin allergy of the horse. *Veterinary Research* 2006; **37**: 813–825.
34. Baselgia S, Doherr MG, Mellor P, *et al.* Evaluation of an in vitro sulphidoleukotriene release test for diagnosis of insect bite hypersensitivity in horses. *Equine Veterinary Journal* 2006; **38**: 40–46.
35. Ferroglio E, Pregel P, Accossato A, *et al.* Equine *Culicoides* hypersensitivity: evaluation of a skin test and of humoral response. *Journal of Veterinary Medicine A Physiology, Pathology, Clinical Medicine* 2006; **53**: 30–33.
36. Quinn PJ, Baker KP, Morrow AN. Sweet itch: responses of clinically normal and affected horses to intradermal challenge with extracts of biting insects. *Equine Veterinary Journal* 1983; **15**: 266–272.
37. McKelvie J, Foster AP, Cunningham FM, *et al.* Characterisation of lymphocyte subpopulations in the skin and circulation of horses with sweet itch (Culicoides hypersensitivity). *Equine Veterinary Journal* 1999; **31**: 466–472.
38. Sloet van Oldruitenborgh-Oosterbaan MM, van Poppel M, de Raat IJ, *et al.* Intradermal testing of horses with and without insect

bite hypersensitivity in The Netherlands using an extract of native *Culicoides* species. *Veterinary Dermatology* 2009; **20:** 607–614.

39. Anderson GS, Belton P, Kleider N. *Culicoides obsoletus* (Diptera: *Ceratopogonidae*) as a causal agent of Culicoides hypersensitivity (sweet itch) in British Columbia. *Journal of Medical Entomology* 1991; **28**: 685–693.
40. Halldorsdottir S, Larsen HJ, Mehl R. Intradermal challenge of Icelandic horses with extracts of four species of the genus *Culicoides. Research in Veterinary Science* 1989; **47**: 283–287.
41. Kolm-Stark G, Wagner R. Intradermal skin testing in Icelandic horses in *Austria. Equine Veterinary Journal* 2002; **34**: 405–410.
42. Lebis C, Bourdeau P, Marzin-Keller F. Intradermal skin tests in equine dermatology: a study of 83 horses. *Equine Veterinary Journal* 2002; **34**: 666–672.
43. Morris DO, Lindborg S. Determination of 'irritant' threshold concentrations for intradermal testing with allergenic insect extracts in normal horses. *Veterinary Dermatology* 2003; **14**: 31–36.
44. Eder C, Crameri R, Mayer C, *et al.* Allergen-specific IgE levels against crude mould and storage mite extracts and recombinant mould allergens in sera from horses affected with chronic bronchitis. *Veterinary Immunology and Immunopathology* 2000; **73**: 241–253.
45. Riek RF. Studies on allergic dermatitis (Queensland itch) of the horse: the aetiology of the disease. *Australian Journal of Agricultural Research* 1954; **5**: 109–129.
46. Mellor PS, McCraig J. The probable cause of 'sweet itch' in England. *Veterinary Record* 1974; **95**: 411–415.
47. Mullens BA, Owen JP, Heft DE, *et al.* Culicoides and other biting flies on the Palos Verdes Peninsula of Southern California, and their possible relationship to equine dermatitis. *Journal of the American Mosquito Control Association* 2005; **21**: 90–95.
48. Fadok VA. Update on equine allergies. *Veterinary Allergy and Clinical Immunology* 1997; **5**: 68–76.
49. Schaffartzik A, Marti E, Torsteinsdottir S, *et al.* Selective cloning, characterization, and production of the Culicoides nubeculosus salivary gland allergen repertoire associated with equine insect bite hypersensitivity. *Veterinary Immunology and Immunopathology* 2011; **139**: 200–209.

47

Culicoides hypersensitivity: therapy

Anthony A. Yu
Yu of Guelph Veterinary Dermatology, Guelph Veterinary Specialty Hospital, Guelph, ON, Canada

Conflict of interest: none declared.

Horses, as well as humans, dogs, and cats, can manifest allergies in many ways (i.e. insect allergies, atopic disease, recurrent airway obstruction (RAO), inflammatory airway disease (IAD), drug and adverse food reactions) [1]. A trend that is coming to light in all species is the fact that combination allergies are more commonplace than once believed. It is therefore important to keep in mind key concepts such as 'allergic threshold' and 'summation of effect' when diagnosing and treating *Culicoides* hypersensitivity. That is, a successful therapeutic protocol must encompass addressing the patient's predisposing and environmental influences along with treating the secondary perpetuating factors (bacteria and *Malassezia*), all while specifically targeting the primary aetiology. Even if dealing primarily with a classic case of *Culicoides* hypersensitivity, addressing other contributory factors may lower the allergen load, such that the summation of effect is brought below the allergic threshold. Therefore it is incumbent on the clinician to discuss all methods of allergen reduction and treatment with the client, regardless of which specific allergic condition has been identified. The client must also be educated regarding the chronicity of *Culicoides* hypersensitivity, the workload involved in multimodal therapy, and realistic expectations for control of the condition.

Prevention of *Culicoides* hypersensitivity

Development of *Culicoides* hypersensitivity requires a genetic predisposition. There should be a careful evaluation of the horse's lineage to determine if other offspring are also affected, along with a detailed examination of the medical and therapeutic history for evidence of allergies or use of anti-inflammatory medications such as glucocorticoids or antihistamines. This may provide evidence to recommend against the purchase of either a horse with a severe allergic dermatitis already present or one that may be naïve to the *Culicoides* midge. In a study evaluating 582 horses with *Culicoides* hypersensitivity, it was concluded that naïve horses with allergic tendencies developed more severe reactions when exposed to the *Culicoides* antigen later on in life and that early exposure to *Culicoides* beyond the perinatal phase, longer than formerly proposed, increased the likelihood of successful immune tolerance [2]. Therefore, it is advisable to avoid purchasing a predisposed naïve horse for an environment with a significant *Culicoides* burden. Also, due to the high level of reported heritability (18.2–30%), breeding recommendations should include 'outcrossing' to dilute the presumed genetic predisposition toward developing *Culicoides* hypersensitivity, by mating a non-affected mare or sire with the allergic individual [3–7].

For owners of a horse with *Culicoides* hypersensitivity, maintaining ideal body condition scores for the breed of horse may decrease inflammation by decreasing the release of adipokines and cytokines, consequently moving away from a T-helper 2 cell allergic response and helping to increase immunologic tolerance to antigens [8,9].

Vaccinations

There is mounting evidence in dogs that routine vaccinations may result in the stimulation of an allergic

Veterinary Allergy, First Edition. Edited by Chiara Noli, Aiden Foster, and Wayne Rosenkrantz.

response and sensitization to a specific offending allergen the dog is exposed to at the time of inoculation [10–12].

One study evaluated 52 horses over a 5-year span and noted that vaccination of horses every 6 months with several viral vaccines enhanced the likelihood that a percentage of the horses developed an IgE-mediated type 1 hypersensitivity to non-target bovine serum albumin proteins shared among the vaccines [13]. Although the investigators did not evaluate environmental allergens throughout the study, it is not difficult to extrapolate that horses with a predisposition toward developing IgE could easily become sensitized to *Culicoides* allergens. Based on the above findings, the following are the author's recommended vaccine strategies for a *Culicoides*-hypersensitivity horse:

1 Vaccinate outside of the animal's allergy season (e.g. winter time = lowest allergen load).
2 Split up vaccine injections by 2–4 week intervals or greater.
3 Consider titres in horses with severe immune-mediated reactions to vaccine [14].
4 Consider pre-/postvaccination use of anti-inflammatory medication to prevent reactions in known reactors where vaccines must be given.

Environmental control

Regardless of the manifestation of allergic reaction in a horse (cutaneous, gastrointestinal, or respiratory), avoidance or, at a minimum, a reduction in allergen exposure is the best treatment. Moving the affected horse away from standing water, manure piles, compost piles, and sheep or cattle are recommended. In one study *Culicoides* midges were most active at sunset, less so at sunrise, and very few or no midges were trapped in the afternoon or at night [15]. Based on these observations, turn-out in the evening or afternoon and stabling before dusk to after dawn may be simple management procedures to decrease the exposure to *Culicoides*. In barns without stable managers, this may be difficult to incorporate into the establishment's daily routine. Although this option is often impractical, it must be offered as an adjunct to systemic therapy for the horse in lieu of lifelong anti-inflammatory therapy. One of the challenges is that there are over 4000 species of biting midges in the Ceratopogonidae family, over 1000 in just one genus, *Culicoides*, with 31 subgenera and 38 species groups of *Culicoides* throughout the world [16,17]. Each of them thrive in different environments, on different substrates, and have varying geographic and seasonal distribution.

Three studies have tried to identify and quantify risk factors for *Culicoides* hypersensitivity from representative, large equine populations. Data from 3453 Friesian horse mares and 7074 Shetland pony mares were documented by inspectors during obligatory foal inspections [9]; data from 3284 Shetland and 2824 Friesian mares (n = 6108) in the Netherlands were based on 90 regions according to postal codes [18]; and in the third study questionnaires were used with direct physical examination of 408 horses on 18 farms in Israel [19]. The overall prevalence of *Culicoides* hypersensitivity ranged from 0% to 71.4% globally and the reported risk factors were primarily related to breed and age; however, within different regions and seasons, environmental factors also played a role. Several studies evaluating *Culicoides* populations directly using hand-net collections, light traps, or suction traps baited with CO_2 and 1-octen-3-ol, all with their own inherent errors, have also contributed to identification of environmental alterations that should be considered as part of a therapeutic recommendation, as given in Table 47.1 [9,18–27].

Insect control

The use of environmental larvicides, systemic avermectin and biorational pesticides, have met with either unproven or unfavourable results [28]. Therefore, the main thrust of barrier, insecticide, and repellent use has been focused on direct applications to the horse. On-horse insect control can be accomplished by the use of impregnable blankets that cover the entire body and are breathable, flysheets and/or fly masks impregnated with permethrin repellent, halters and other equipment with pockets for repellent sticks, repellent sprays, and kairomones. The application frequency of topical insecticides or repellents will depend on the product selection, geographic insect distribution, season of the year, and severity of the condition.

There are several manufacturers of breathable impregnable blankets that envelop the horse's entire body from head to hoof, which create a barrier that is impenetrable by the *Culicoides* midges, hence minimizing salivary exposure and allergic reactions [29,30]. Other blankets are impregnated with permethrin-based insect repellent treatment, similar to that used in clothing for people. For example there is an EPA-registered product in the USA called Insect Shield® repellent gear technology, which is odourless, colourless, and maintains 100% efficacy against *Aedesa egypti* through 25 washings and 80% through 70 washes [31].

The use of plant-based natural terpinoids, such as D-limonene, citronella, lemon eucalyptus oil, and neem seed extracts, have gained increasing interest due to

Table 47.1 Environmental factors to help minimize *Culicoides* exposure (note that variations may occur based on *Culicoides* species located in the various geographic locations)

Geography	Stable	Paddocks
High altitudes >800 m above sea level	Dusk and dawn closed-door stabling with finely screened windows 0.9 mm^2 impregnated with pyrethroids, *N,N*-diethyl-meta-toluamide (DEET) or organophosphates (8% propoxur)	More arid environment
Colder environments limit flight range and reproduction	In-barn insecticide sprays, CO_2 and semiochemical-emitting insect traps using 500 mL/min CO_2 combined with 4.1 mg/h (R)-1-octen-3-ol	Lack of standing water Avoid ponds, large water troughs Consider adding fish to ponds to ingest *Culicoides* eggs and larvae
Low humidity	Clean environment/decreased odour Remove manure twice daily	Minimal shade
Fewer evergreen trees	Attach high velocity fans (not ceiling fans) to stalls to create a wind current >1–3 m/s	Keep manure away from paddocks and barn
Coastal regions or top of a hill with high wind speeds	Lack of presence of other livestock	Fly wasps/predators

supposed decreased impact on the environment and on the individual in comparison to synthetic pesticides. These essential oils are ingested, absorbed, or inhaled by the insects and then alter basic metabolic, biochemical, physiological, and behavioural functions of insects, including interference with the neuromodulator octopamine or GABA-gated chloride channels [32]. The oils have larvicidal activity and may suppress adult maturation. As different essential oils may either repel or attract insects, often a combination of essential oils is formulated to take advantage of their synergistic repellent effects.

One manufacturer has incorporated the essential oil technology into citronella and cedar wood oil strips that insert into specially designed Velcro straps, which can be attached to tack, halters, leg protection, and blankets or simply braided into either the mane or tail depending on clinical signs and distribution of biting gnats [33]. In a non-placebo controlled evaluation, heat generated from the horse and climate help to vaporize the active ingredients, increasing its efficacy and lasting up to 1 month depending on the climactic conditions [34]. Although promising, safety trials and global efficacy with various species of *Culicoides* are still required on horses before recommending widespread use as an alternative to synthetic pyrethroids.

The more traditional insect repellents originate from the pyrethroid family. Synthetic pyrethroids have been studied in a controlled manner at varying concentrations, such as 2–3.6% permethrin and 5% cypermethrin, with greater than 80% midge mortality after 7 days and residual activity of 50% at day 35, although the response varied between studies, possibly because susceptibility to the different products was species dependent [35–37]. Other off-label products that have anecdotal reports of efficacy include:

1 Cyfluthrin, a fourth-generation pyrethroid, that provides ten times the potency and extended residual activity (30 days) in comparison to third-generation products [38].
2 Topical high-concentration permethrin-containing canine flea products have been used off label, every 2–4 weeks, with success [39,40]. It is recommended to apply topical vitamin E 1000–2000 IU to the site of application to avoid adverse reactions such as paraesthesia [41].

In general, the author uses products with at least 2% permethrin concentrations or above at frequencies that vary from daily to monthly based on the severity of the patient's condition, the type of product (spray, spot-on), and an assessment of owner compliance.

Kairomones

A novel area of research focus is the use of kairomones or semiochemicals, which are olfactory cues emanating from the breath, skin, urine, and faeces of the host that may either act as attractants or repellents for biting insects [42]. Whereas pheromones typically attract only male insects, kairomones are indiscriminative of sex and thus have a greater potential to control an entire species of insects. By means of electroantennograms, researchers have characterized semiochemical responses of several *Culicoides* species, classifying them into repellents and attractants [43]. Using this information, researchers have developed a 'push–pull' control strategy whereby 7-octenoic acid, (E)- and (Z)-3-methyl-2-hexanoic acid, and 6-methyl-5-hepten-2-one have a repellent or 'push' effect and can be used on affected individuals, while attractants, including lactic acid, acetone, butanone, CO_2, and 1-octen-3-olare, are used in traps to 'pull' the insect in and destroy them. However, due to variable responses to the type, combination, and dose of kairomones amongst species of *Culicoides,* such as *C. nubeculosus* and *C. impunctatus*, further studies will be required to delineate an ideal recipe for a 'push–pull' control strategy for each specific geographic region [43].

Topical non-insecticide therapy

Shampoo therapy should not be overlooked in the treatment of *Culicoides* hypersensitivity. The simple act of bathing with cool water rehydrates the skin, improving the integrity of the epidermal barrier; results in vasoconstriction, hence decreasing delivery of inflammatory mediators to the skin; helps to minimize percutaneous absorption of allergens; and, finally, with appropriate ingredient selection, addresses secondary superficial infections. The selection of shampoos should be based on the patient's skin condition and may include: colloidal oatmeal products (shampoos, conditioners, and bath treatments) with or without a local anaesthetic (pramoxine HCl) or corticosteroids for pruritic dermatoses; sulphur/salicylic acid shampoos for horses with excess scale; antimicrobial shampoos (benzoyl peroxide, chlorhexidine, or imidazoles) if secondary infections have been identified; or a combination of one or more of the above.

As bacterial infections may exacerbate clinical signs of *Culicoides* hypersensitivity, topical antimicrobial agents may help to ameliorate pruritus. If environmental conditions are not conducive to shampoo therapy, topical leave-on sprays or dips such as oxychlorine, stannous fluoride (0.4%), or accelerated hydrogen peroxide are highly bactericidal and can be used daily on affected areas [44].

Lime sulphur also provides effective multimodal topical therapeutic as it provides not only ectoparasitic activity, but also antipruritic, antiseborrhoeic, antifungal, and antimicrobial effects in all animals at 2% concentrations or greater. Although most commercial lime sulphur products do not have specific labelling for horses, it is a safe and proven treatment option that can be applied as a dip or spray-on formulation and left to drip-dry. Applications as frequently as once daily and as little as once weekly can be used, based on the severity of the condition. Client education should emphasize that coat colour changes might occur at the site of application on the horse, especially in light-coloured horses, and also that lime sulphur may tarnish owners' gold jewellery and stain wood.

Topical steroids have also shown good efficacy when treating small animal cases. Unfortunately, most of these products are not labelled for use in equine medicine. Several veterinary topical steroid products that the author has used for the treatment of localized lesions include:

1 1% hydrocortisone, leave-on conditioner in a non-irritating base;
2 0.1% mometasone ointment combined with an antibiotic and antifungal agent;
3 0.015% triamcinolone spray in a 10% alcohol base;
4 0.584 mg/mL esterified hydrocortisone aceponate spray.

Anecdotal benefits have been reported when steroids are added to topical insecticide sprays in the treatment of *Culicoides* hypersensitivity [44]. Attaining pharmacologic knowledge of drug interactions prior to compounding products is advised. Also, when choosing a topical steroid, one must strive for products with minimal side effects; that is, minimal to no haematological and biochemical changes, suppression of the adrenal axis, and local cutaneous alterations (atrophy, alopecia, comedone formation, and secondary infections).

Systemic therapy

As *Culicoides* hypersensitivity has been characterized as an IgE-mediated reaction with an imbalance between T helper 2 (Th2) and T regulatory (Treg) cells shown both in the skin and with peripheral blood mononuclear cells, systemic treatment strategies should be directed at restoring this equilibrium. In addition, other conditions that may mimic *Culicoides* hypersensitivity such as onchocerciasis and oxyuriasis should be eliminated [45,46].

Other inflammatory mediators that have been investigated may also be potential targets for therapy, but thus far they are still in their experimental stages, such as platelet activating factor antagonists [47].

Allergen-specific immunotherapy

Allergen-specific immunotherapy (ASIT) has shown mixed results for the treatment of *Culicoides* hypersensitivity.

Immunotherapy using crude *Culicoides* antigens combined with mycobacterial cell wall extract revealed a 90% (9/10) positive response in severely affected *Culicoides* hypersensitivity horses after 1 year, with complete resolution of clinical signs in 37.5% (3/8) and good to excellent response in 63.5% (5/8) after 2 years of weekly immunotherapy [48]. On the other hand, a controlled, double-blind trial of 14 privately owned horses with varying degrees of *Culicoides* hypersensitivity revealed no statistical difference between control and treated groups using an aqueous extract of whole, unfed *Culicoides variipennis* (n = 6) after a 6-month trial [49]. Although the exact reasons for inconsistencies in response to ASIT may be due to individual responses, a number of factors may contribute to the variable responses, such as: a lack of allergen standardization; whether antigen selection was based on intradermal or serological test or both; incorporation of non-specific immunostimulants (e.g. mycobacterial cell wall); variety of immunotherapy induction and maintenance protocols; dose and route of allergen administration (i.e. subcutaneous, intradermal); postinduction immunotherapy aftercare; and lack of objective data in a controlled environment.

It was noted that when using whole-body extracts, it is important to use native *Culicoides* spp. to improve the intradermal or serologic testing methods [50]. Hence the selection of native *Culicoides* spp. is more likely to improve the response to ASIT [50]. It has also been demonstrated in a group of healthy horses with no skin diseases that 14% of horses aged 1–3 years and 38% of older horses showed skin reactions to *Culicoides* allergen extract [51]. Therefore, a positive reaction to a skin test does not necessarily denote a cause and affect; hence, it is imperative that clinical and historical findings with the likelihood of exposure are taken into account when formulating ASIT [51]. A homologous allergen (antigen 5-like protein: Sim v 1 and Cul n 1), has been detected in the salivary glands of both *Simulium* (black fly) and *Culicoides*, respectively [52]. There may be some cross-reactivity between these insect allergens and this may explain the anecdotal success reported with the use of *Ctenocephalides* (flea) antigens for immunotherapy in some horses with *Culicoides* hypersensitivity.

In an effort to standardize immunotherapy and improve success rates, research to identify antigenic proteins from *Culicoides* salivary gland extract (SGE) is underway. Currently, 11 SGEs have been identified for *Culicoides nubeculosus* (Cul n 1 to Cul n 11; 12–75 kDa) using PCR techniques [45,53,54]. Recombinant salivary gland allergens will potentially improve the diagnostic and therapeutic effects of immunotherapy because they will provide greater consistency, decrease adverse reactions, and minimize the diluting effects of non-antigenic components from whole crude extracts of *Culicoides* spp. With the current technology, there is an opportunity to not only duplicate but also improve upon the results of previous studies, such as that by Anderson *et al.* [48]. The future of immunotherapy for *Culicoides* hypersensitivity will most likely evolve to recombinant salivary gland extracts to promote isotype switching toward an IgG response, in combination with non-specific immunomodulators, such as CpG oligodeoxynucleotides or mycobacterial cell wall extracts, to shift the local immune defence system toward a Th1 response.

Regardless of how the immunotherapy is formulated, the client should be aware that it is not a 'light-switch' type of treatment. It can often take up to 12 months before the full benefits are noted and most horses require lifelong maintenance injections of 1.0 mL every 7 to 28 days, depending on the response and allergen exposure. Hence, implementation of multimodal therapy for *Culicoides* hypersensitivity (e.g. avoidance, insect control, fatty acids, antihistamines, phosphodiesterase inhibitors, and glucocorticoids) will provide symptomatic relief during the induction phase.

Polyunsaturated N-3 and N-6 fatty acids

The possible mechanisms by which polyunsaturated N-3 and N-6 fatty acids (PUFAs) exert their positive clinical benefit in *Culicoides* hypersensitivity are still under investigation, but include repair of the epidermal barrier. Fatty acid supplements have shown variable reported responses in horses with *Culicoides* hypersensitivity [55–58].

Six horses, positive to *Culicoides* spp. on intradermal test, were supplemented with flaxseed (*Linum usitatissimum*) in a 42-day, placebo-controlled, double-blind, cross-over trial [55]. Results revealed reduced mean skin test responses to *Culicoides* spp. concurrent with a significant decrease in long-chain saturated fatty acids (behenic acid (22 : 0), lignoceric acid (24 : 0)) in the hair of horses receiving flaxseed. There were no adverse reactions reported in the study. The author recommends administration of 60–120 mL of freshly ground flax seed to allergic horses for those owners interested in pursuing this avenue.

Another double-blinded, cross-over study evaluated the clinical efficacy of high-dose linseed oil (alpha-linolenic acid) for the treatment of *Culicoides* spp. hypersensitivity. There was no significant change in pruritus and lesional area of 17 privately owned horses from north Florida, USA [56]. The study horses were supplemented with either 200 mL of linseed oil (omega 3 fatty acid) or 200 mL of corn oil (omega 6 fatty acid) daily for 6 weeks, followed by a 6-week washout period, and then each horse was crossed over to the other supplement for an additional 6 weeks. Interestingly, despite the lack of significant statistical clinical data, most owners stated that horses improved while supplemented with linseed oil. Perhaps corn oil resulted in a positive clinical effect that closely equalled that of linseed oil, hence minimizing the statistical difference between the effects of the two oils. Alternatively, the duration of the study may not have been long enough to alter objective findings as compared to subjective evaluations.

One other commonly used seed-based oil supplement was evaluated in a placebo-controlled, double-blinded study. Sunflower oil was administered to 25 horses while another 25 received placebo for 30 days, after which all horses were placed on sunflower oil for an additional 30 days. The severity of the clinical signs of *Culicoides* hypersensitivity in all horses was scored based on clinical evaluation and digital photographs taken before and after the first 30 days of the trial, as well as owners' assessment of clinical severity prior to the investigation and after the first and second 30-day periods [57]. A positive clinical effect of the supplement was noted by investigators in comparison to those receiving placebo. However, there were no treatment-group differences noted by the horse owners in this study.

The difference in results is most likely attributable to the variability of the research parameters, namely the type of allergic reaction being evaluated—*Culicoides* hypersensitivity versus atopic dermatitis or a combination of parameters being evaluated. In two placebo-controlled studies evaluating the effect of fish oil alone or in combination with evening primrose oil, significant reductions in the production of proinflammatory mediators (PGE2) as well as changes in plasma phospholipid concentration between test and placebo groups were noted for dihomogammalinolenic acid and docosahexaenoic acid ($P < 0.01$) and alpha linolenic acid ($P < 0.05$), respectively [58,59]. Even with these significant objective alterations, no clinical difference between treated and placebo was noted during the short study period.

Hence, to make any conclusions on the efficacy of the essential fatty acids based on current equine studies is difficult. Our knowledge of clinical benefits of PUFAs in recent canine atopic dermatitis studies along with the lack of significant adverse reactions (mainly diarrhoea), would recommend prescribing its use in equine dermatology as adjunct to any long-term anti-inflammatory protocol or as a preventative prior to the development of clinical signs in predisposed individuals. Improvement in pruritus and/or skin condition should be not be expected for at least 8 weeks post initiation of PUFA supplementation. A variety of PUFAs exist on the veterinary market and are typically administered at their labelled dose or double dose during an inflammatory crisis.

Antihistamines and tricyclic antidepressants

Antihistamines and tricyclic antidepressants (TCA) provide a non-steroidal alternative for long-term control of allergic reactions in horses. The value of these drugs in *Culicoides* hypersensitivity remains to be determined. The H1 receptor antagonist activity of these drugs is sometimes complemented by other mechanisms of action, including antiserotonin/serotonin re-uptake inhibition. Exact dosing and recent pharmacokinetic studies are emerging in the horse [60–68]. Table 47.2 lists the antihistamines and TCAs that are prescribed to horses by the author, in order of preference.

Similar to humans and other domestic species, there is tremendous variation in the response to antihistamines/TCAs depending on the severity and lesion type. For instance, a 57–79% inhibition of histamine-induced wheal formation was noted after only 7 days of cetirizine administration [67]. However, no significant difference from placebo was noted after 0.4 mg/kg twice daily of cetirizine for 3 weeks in horses with *Culicoides* hypersensitivity [68]. In particular, when using antihistamines in *Culicoides* hypersensitivity they should either be used early in the disease process when clinical signs are easier to manage or later in the therapeutic regimen when attempting to taper glucocorticoids. Therefore, despite the paucity of synergism between antihistamines/TCAs and other anti-inflammatory therapies reported in the horse, it may still be worthwhile

Table 47.2 Antihistamines and tricyclic antidepressants that are prescribed to horses by the author, in order of preference

Antihistamine	Dose	Frequency
Cetirizine	0.2–0.4 mg/kg	Twice daily
Hydroxyzine hydrochloride or pamoate	0.5–1.0 mg/kg	Three times daily
Doxepin hydrochloride	0.5–0.75 mg/kg	Twice daily
Amitriptyline	1–2 mg/kg	Twice daily
Chlorpheniramine	0.25 mg/kg	Twice daily
Diphenhydramine	0.75–1 mg/kg	Twice daily
Fexofenadine	10 mg/kg	Three times daily
Pyrilamine maleate	1 mg/kg	Twice daily
Diethylcarbamazine syrup	6–12 mg/kg	Once to twice daily

to combine therapies as carried out in other species. Also, if a lack of response is noted to antihistamines, it is sometimes necessary to try several different classes of antihistamines at 2-week intervals before finding the most effective option. Lastly, topical administration of antihistamines is generally thought to be relatively ineffective, but in one report topical administration of chlorpheniramine was shown to block antigen-induced cutaneous responses in ponies with insect hypersensitivity [60].

Although antihistamines and TCAs have fewer reported side effects (light sedation, occasional personality changes) than do corticosteroids, one must always keep in mind the anticholinergic properties of these medications, in particular in patients with glaucoma, gastrointestinal atony, cardiac arrhythmias, or urinary retention problems. Lastly, advise owners to contact show authorities regarding drug restrictions/withdrawals at least 14 days prior to the event.

Phosphodiesterase inhibitors

Pentoxifylline (PTX) is a synthetic xanthine derivative related to caffeine and theophylline. Its phosphodiesterase inhibition imparts major therapeutic benefits, including improvement in wound healing and connective tissue disorders, rheologic activity, and immunomodulatory properties [69–77].

PTX potentiates the effectiveness of many medications, including glucocorticoids [77–83]. Because PTX has rheologic activity it has been used as a treatment for laminitis. Because many *Culicoides*-hypersensitive horses require long-term glucocorticoids, some practitioners utilize PTX as a concurrent therapy to not only have a glucocorticoid dosage sparing effect but also to minimize the risk of laminitis [84]. Dosages for PTX are 10–15 mg b.i.d (20–30 mg/kg per day), with or without glucocorticoids. PTX provides a non-steroidal alternative with minimal side effects (hyperexcitability, sweating) for the purpose of tapering or eliminating the need for glucocorticoids in *Culicoides* hypersensitivity cases [85]. This medication should *not* be used in conjunction with anticoagulants or in horses with haemorrhagic disorders.

Glucocorticoids

Glucocorticoids have long been a standard therapy for allergies in the horse. Nowhere do they play more of a primary role than in the control of clinical signs associated with *Culicoides* hypersensitivity. Glucocorticoids work primarily by gene repression and inhibition of nuclear factor-kappa B, which directly or indirectly prevents the production of cytokines, chemokines, cell adhesion molecules, complement factors, and prostaglandin and leukotriene synthesis involved in the allergic response. Unfortunately, aggressive use of glucocorticoids in horses may cause various adverse effects, including steroid hepatopathy, laminitis, and iatrogenic hyperadrenocorticism [86–88]. Individual sensitivity to glucocorticoids may be directly related to Type 1:Type 2 11-β-hydroxysteroid dehydrogenase ratio [88]. Judicious use, and appropriate amounts and intervals, are key to minimizing adverse reactions.

The following are the two most commonly used glucocorticoids for the short-term treatment of *Culicoides* hypersensitivity:

1 Prednisolone, available as tablets or a compounded syrup or powder, is typically dosed at 0.5–1.5 mg/kg/day for 7–14 days during the induction phase then tapered to 0.2–0.5 mg/kg every 48 hours over 2–5 weeks for maintenance. If cost is an issue, prednisone may be substituted for prednisolone; however, the latter has been shown to have greater bioavailability in horses [89].
2 Dexamethasone, available as a powder, tablets, injectable (per os, intravenous, i.v., or intramuscular, i.m.); injectable dexamethasone solution given orally is 60–70% bioavailable compared to the i.v. route [90]. The initial loading oral or i.v. pulse dose is 0.05–0.1 mg/kg daily for 3–7 days, and then tapered to 0.01–0.02 mg/kg every 48–72 hours for maintenance. This regimen is particularly helpful in more refractory cases of *Culicoides* hypersensitivity.

Nutraceuticals

In a randomized, double-blinded, placebo-controlled study, the efficacy of sterile heat-killed actinomycete (*Tsukamurella inchonensis*) preparation, administered by injection for the treatment of equine *Culicoides* hypersensitivity (CHS) in 88 horses and ponies and one donkey was evaluated [91]. An initial course of three injections of killed bacterial suspension or placebo was given intradermally into the skin of the neck at 2-week intervals prior to the allergy season followed by 7 monthly injections throughout the CHS season. Treatment resulted in a significantly higher number of horses showing improvement or marked improvement over the severity of disease in the previous year, a delay in onset of clinical signs, statistically significant reduction in clinical score between weeks 8 and 20, and fewer horses requiring specific anti-inflammatory treatment compared to placebo. Similar results to injections of *G. bronchialis* or *R. coprophilus* effectively reduced the extent and severity of canine flea allergy lesions ($p < 0.001$), pruritus, and eosinophil numbers ($p < 0.0001$) [92].

To minimize the incidence of localized injection site reactions, BioEos Ltd produced a suspension of the heat-killed *Tsukamurella inchonensis* absorbed onto a powder and filled into capsules. Each capsule contains 1 mg of the reagent, made up in a trehalose base administered weekly. The mechanism of action proposed is that the adjuvants in the cell walls of the organisms have immunomodulatory activity that down-regulate Th2 lymphocytes response to tissue stress proteins, which share part of their amino-acid sequences with the heat-shock proteins of the bacteria, allowing the Th1 lymphocyte arm to predominate.

Methylsulfonylmethane is another nutraceutical that can be used as an adjunct to other anti-inflammatory therapies for its antioxidant properties. Controlled studies are lacking regarding its efficacy in *Culicoides* hypersensitivity; however, due to the absence of significant side effects, it can be used in *Culicoides* hypersensitivity horses initially at 10–12 g/500 kg twice daily, then tapered to a once daily dose.

Conclusion

Moving horses to areas that do not have *Culicoides* is often impractical for most clients and due to the intensity of the pruritus associated with *Culicoides* hypersensitivity, coupled with the difficulty in control of the *Culicoides* midges in most environments, a comprehensive multimodal approach is often needed. A combination of environmental control, insecticide therapy, and topical and/or systemic anti-inflammatory therapy catered to the individual clientele will achieve control of the clinical signs and help to minimize the side effects associated with any one treatment, in particular glucocorticoids.

References

1. Fadok VA. Update on equine allergies. *Journal of Veterinary Allergy and Clinical Immunology* 1997; **5**: 68–76.
2. Sommer-Locher B, Endriss V, Fromm E. Various circumstances regarding initial allergen exposure and their influence on development of insect bite hypersensitivity in horses. *Journal of Equine Veterinary Science* 2012; **32**: 158–163.
3. Anderson LS, Swinbune JE, Meadows JRS, *et al.* The same ELA class II risk factors confer equine insect bite hypersensitivity in two distinct populations. *Immunogenetics* 2012; **64**: 201–208.
4. Schurink A, Ducro BJ, Heuven HCM, *et al.* Genetic parameters of insect bite hypersensitivity in Dutch Friesian broodmares. *Journal of Animal Science* 2011; **89**: 1286–1293.
5. Altin J, Shen C, Liston A. Understanding the genetic regulation of IgE production. *Blood Review* 2010; **24**: 163–169.
6. Schurink A, van Grevenhof EM, Ducro BJ, *et al.* Heritability and repeatability of insect bite hypersensitivity in Dutch Shetland breeding mares. *Journal of Animal Science* 2009; **87**: 484–490.
7. Frey R, Bergvall K, Egenvall A. Allergen-specific IgE in Icelandic horses with insect bite hypersensitivity and healthy controls, assessed by FcepsilonR1alpha-based serology. *Veterinary Immunology and Immunopathology* 2008; **126**: 102–109.
8. Hersoug LG, Linneberg A. The link between the epidemics of obesity and allergic diseases: does obesity induce decreased immune tolerance? *Allergy* 2007; **62**: 1205–1213.
9. Schurink A, Podesta SC, Ducro BJ, *et al.* Risk factors for insect bite hypersensitivity in Friesian horses and Shetland ponies in The Netherlands. *Veterinary Journal* 2013; **195**: 382–384.
10. Tater KC, Jackson HA, Paps J, *et al.* Effects of routine prophylactic vaccination or administration of aluminum adjuvant alone on allergen-specific serum IgE and IgG responses in allergic dogs. *American Journal of Veterinary Research* 2005; **66**: 1572–1577.
11. Hogen Esch H, Dunham AD, Scott-Moncrieff C, *et al.* Effect of vaccination on serum concentrations of total and antigen-specific immunoglobulin E in dogs. *American Journal of Veterinary Research* 2002; **63**: 611–616.
12. Frick OL, Brooks DL. Immunoglobulin E antibodies to pollens augmented in dogs by virus vaccines. *American Journal of Veterinary Research* 1983; **44**: 440–445.
13. Gershwin LJ, Netherwood KA, Norris MS, *et al.* Equine IgE responses to non-viral vaccine components. *Vaccine* 2012; **30**: 7615–7620.
14. Schultz RD, Ford RB, Olsen J, *et al.* Titer testing and vaccination: a new look at traditional practices. *Veterinary Medicine* 2002; **97**: 1–13.
15. van der Rijt R, van den Boom R, Jongema Y, *et al.* *Culicoides* species attracted to horses with and without insect hypersensitivity. *Veterinary Journal* 2008; **178**: 91–97.
16. Rutledge-Connelly CR. *Biting Midges/Culicoides*. University of Florida Institute of Food and Agricultural Sciences, Department of Entomology and Nematology. Available at: http://entnemdept.ufl.edu/creatures/aquatic/biting_midges.htm. Accessed Dec 20, 2012.
17. Borkent A. *The Subgeneric Classification of Species of Culicoides—Thoughts and a Warning*. Available at: http://www.inhs.illinois.edu/research/FLYTREE/CulicoidesSubgenera.pdf. Accessed February 28, 2012.
18. Van Grevenhof EM, Ducro B, Heuven HCM, *et al.* Identification of environmental factors affecting the prevalence of insect bite hypersensitivity in Shetland ponies and Friesian horses in the Netherlands. *Equine Veterinary Journal* 2007; **39**: 69–73.
19. Steinman A, Peer G, Klement E. Epidemiological study of *Culicoides* hypersensitivity in horses in Israel. *Veterinary Record* 2003; **152**: 748–751.
20. Takken W, Verhulst N, Scholte EJ, *et al.* The phenology and population dynamics of *Culicoides spp.* in different ecosystems in The Netherlands. *Preventive Veterinary Medicine* 2008; **87**: 41–54.
21. Meiswinkel R, Baylis M, Labuschagne K. Stabling and the protection of horses from *Culicoidesbolitinos* (Diptera: Ceratopogonidae), a recently identified vector of African horse sickness. *Bulletin of Entomological Research* 2000; **90**: 509–515.
22. Venter GJ, Nevill EM, Van Der Linde TC. Seasonal abundance and parity of stock-associated *Culicoides* species (Diptera: Ceratopogonidae) in different climatic regions in southern Africa in relation to their viral vector potential. *Onderstepoort Journal of Veterinary Research* 1997; **64**: 259–271.
23. Ortega MD, Mellor PS, Rawlings P, *et al.* The seasonal and geographical distribution of *Culicoides imicola, C. pulicaris* group and *C. obsoletus* group biting midges in central and southern Spain. *Archives of Virology Supplementum* 1998; **14**: 85–91.
24. Barnard BJ. Some factors governing the entry of *Culicoides* spp. (Diptera: Ceratopogonidae) into stables. *Onderstepoort Journal of Veterinary Research* 1997; **64**: 227–233.

25. Greiner EC, Fadok VA, Rabin EB. Equine *Culicoides* hypersensitivity in Florida: biting midges collected in light traps near horses. *Medical and Veterinary Entomology* 1988; **2**: 129–135.
26. Pagea PC, Labuschagneb K, Nurtonc JP, *et al.* Duration of repellency of N,N-diethyl-3-methylbenzamide, citronella oil and cypermethrin against *Culicoides* species when applied to polyester mesh. *Veterinary Parasitology* 2009; **163**: 105–109.
27. Harrup LE, Logan JG, Cook JI, *et al.* Collection of *Culicoides* (Diptera: Ceratopogonidae) Using CO2 and Enantiomers of 1-Octen-3-ol in the United Kingdom. *Journal of Medical Entomology* 2012; **49**: 112–121.
28. Carpenter S, Mellor PS, Torr SJ. Control techniques for *Culicoides* biting midges and their application in the U.K. and northwestern Palaearctic. *Medical and Veterinary Entomology* 2008; **22**: 175–187.
29. National Sweet Itch Centre. *Boett® Blanket*. Available at: http://www.sweet-itch.co.uk/boett.html. Accessed December 20, 2012.
30. Bucas. *Buzz-Off®* Available at: http://www.bucas.com/products/fly-sheets-and-speciality-rugs/buzz-off/. Accessed December 20, 2012.
31. Insect Shield Technology® Available at: http://insectshield.com/OurTechnology/Research.aspx. Accessed December 20, 2012.
32. Khater HF. Prospects of botanical biopesticides in insect pest management. *Journal of Applied Pharmaceutical Science* 2012; **2**: 244–259.
33. Fly Armor®. http://www.flyarmor.net. Accessed July, 2013.
34. Hyman B. Fly Armor stands up to the heat; the warmer it gets, the better it works. *Horse Journal* 2012; **19**: 12.
35. Bourdeau PJ, Beis C, Chouilly C. Evaluation of permethrin and containing spray in the treatment of sweet itch in 25 horses. In: *Proceedings of the 15th Annual Member's meeting American Academy of Veterinary Dermatology/American College of Veterinary Dermatology*, 1999: 13–14.
36. Papadopoulos E, Rowlinson M, Bartram D, *et al.* Treatment of horses with cypermethrin against the biting flies *Culicoides nubeculosus, Aedesa egypti* and *Culexquinque fasciatus. Veterinary Parasitology* 2010; **169**: 165–171.
37. deRaat IJ, van den Boom R, Van Poppel M, *et al.* The effect of a topical insecticide containing permethrin on the number of *Culicoides* midges caught near horses with and without insect bite hypersensitivity in the Netherlands. *Tijdschrift voor Diergeneeskunde* 2008; **133**: 838–842.
38. Bayer Inc. *CyLence® Product Information.* Available at: http://bayerlivestock.ca/en/cylence/product-information.html. Accessed December 20, 2012.
39. http://www.petparents.com/products.aspx/about/k9-advantix-ii?subId=science. Accessed September 20, 2013.
40. Ceva. Vectra 3D®. Available at: http://www.ceva.us/us/Products/Product-List/Vectra-3D-R. Accessed December 20, 2012.
41. Flannigan SA, Tucker SB, Key MM, *et al.* Synthetic pyrethroid insecticides: a dermatological evaluation. *British Journal of Industrial Medicine* 1985; **42**: 363–372.
42. Logan JG, Birkett MA. Review: Semiochemicals for biting fly control: their identification and exploitation *Pest Management Science* 2007; **63**: 647–657.
43. Bhasin A, Mordue AJ, Mordue W. Electrophysiological and behavioural identification of host kairomones as olfactory cues for *Culicoides impunctatus* and *C. nubeculosus. Physiological Entomology* 2000; **25**: 6–16.
44. Marsella R. Therapeutic approach to equine allergic diseases. In: *Proceedings of the 7th World Congress of Veterinary Dermatology*, 2012: 504–506.
45. Schaffartzik A, Hamza E, Janda J, *et al.* Equine insect bite hypersensitivity: what do we know? *Veterinary Immunology and Immunopathology* 2012; **147**: 113–126.
46. Gortel K. Equine parasitic hypersensitivity. *Equine Practice* 1998; **20**: 14–16.
47. Foster AP, Lees P, Cunningham FM. Actions of PAF receptor antagonists in horses with the allergic skin disease sweet itch. *Inflammation Research* 1995; **44**: 412–417.
48. Anderson GS, Belton P, Jahren E, *et al.* Immunotherapy trial for horses in British Columbia with *Culicoides* (Diptera: Ceratopogonidae) hypersensitivity. *Journal of Medical Entomology* 1996; **33**: 458–466.
49. Barbet JL, Bevier D, Greiner EC. Specific immunotherapy in the treatment of Culicoides hypersensitive horses: a double-blind study. *Equine Veterinary Journal* 1990; **22**: 232–235.
50. van der Meide NMA, Meulenbroeks C, van Altena C, *et al.* Culicoides obsoletus extract relevant for diagnostics of insect bite hypersensitivity in horses. *Veterinary Immunology and Immunopathology* 2012; **149**: 245–254.
51. Wagner B, Miller WH, Erb HN, *et al.* Sensitization of skin mast cells with IgE antibodies to *Culicoides* allergens occurs frequently in clinically healthy horses. *Veterinary Immunology and Immunopathology* 2009; **132**: 53–61.
52. Schaffartzik A, Marti E, Crameri R, *et al.* Cloning, production and characterization of antigen 5 like proteins from *Simulium vittatum* and *Culicoides nubeculosus*, the first cross-reactive allergen associated with equine insect bite hypersensitivity. *Veterinary Immunology and Immunopathology* 2010; **137**: 76–83.
53. Schaffartzik A, Marti E, Torsteinsdottir S, *et al.* Selective cloning, characterization and production of the *Culicoides nubeculosus* salivary gland allergen repertoire associated with equine insect bite hypersensitivity. *Veterinary Immunology and Immunopathology* 2011; **139**: 200–209.
54. Hellberg W, Wilson AD, Mellor P, *et al.* Equine insect bite hypersensitivity: Immunoblot analysis of IgE and IgG subclass responses to *Culicoides nubeculosus* salivary gland extract. *Veterinary Immunology and Immunopathology* 2006; **113**: 99–112.
55. O'Neill W, McKee S, Clarke AF. Flaxseed (*Linum usitatissimum*) supplementation associated with reduced skin test lesional area in horses with *Culicoides* hypersensitivity. *Canadian Journal of Veterinary Research* 2002; **66**: 272–277.
56. Friberg CA, Logas D. Treatment of *Culicoides* hypersensitive horses with high-dose n-3 fatty acids: a double-blinded cross over study. *Veterinary Dermatology* 1999; **10**: 117–122.
57. van den Boom R, Driessen F, Streumer SJ, *et al.* The effect of a supplement containing sunflower oil, vitamins, amino acids and peptides on the severity of symptoms in horses suffering insect bite hypersensitivity. *Tijdschrift voor Diergeneeskunde* 2010; **135**: 520–525.
58. Craig JM, Lloyd DH, Jones RD. A double-blind placebo-controlled trial of an evening primrose and fish oil combination vs. hydrogenated coconut oil in the management of recurrent seasonal pruritus in horses. *Veterinary Dermatology* 1997; **8**: 177–182.
59. Hall JA, Van Saun RJ, Tornquist SJ, *et al.* Effect of type of dietary polyunsaturated fatty acid supplement (corn oil or fish oil) on immune responses in healthy horses. *Journal of Veterinary Internal Medicine* 2004; **18**: 880–886.
60. Foster AP, McKelvie J, Cunningham FM. Inhibition of antigen-induced cutaneous responses of ponies with insect hypersensitivity by the histamine-1 receptor antagonist chlorpheniramine. *Veterinary Record* 1998; **143**: 189–193.

61. Wasfi IA, Abdel Hadi AA, Elghazali M, *et al.* Comparative pharmacokinetics of diphenhydramine in camels and horses after intravenous administration. *Veterinary Research Communications* 2003; **27**: 463–473.
62. Törneke K, Ingvast-Larsson C, Pettersson K, *et al.* Pharmacokinetics and pharmacodynamics of clemastine in healthy horses. *Journal of Veterinary Pharmacology and Therapeutics* 2003; **26**: 151–157.
63. Manohar M, Goetz TE, Humphrey S, *et al.* H1-receptor antagonist, tripelennamine, does not affect arterial hypoxemia in exercising Thoroughbreds. *Journal of Applied Physiology* 2002; **92**: 1515–1523.
64. Olsén L, Ingvast-Larsson C, Bondesson U, *et al.* Cetirizine in horses: pharmacokinetics and effect of ivermectin pretreatment. *Journal of Veterinary Pharmacology and Therapeutics* 2007; **30**: 194–200.
65. Olsén L, Ingvast-Larsson C, Larsson P, *et al.* Fexofenadine in horses: pharmacokinetics, pharmacodynamics and effect of ivermectin pretreatment. *Journal of Veterinary Pharmacology and Therapeutics* 2006; **29**: 129–135.
66. Yu AA. Equine urticaria: a diagnostic dilemma. *Compendium of Continuing Education for the Practicing Veterinarian* 2000; **22**: 277–280.
67. Olsén L, Bondesson U, Broström H, *et al.* Cetirizine in horses: pharmacokinetics and pharmacodynamics following repeated oral administration. *Veterinary Journal* 2008; **177**: 242–249.
68. Olsén L, Bondesson U, Broström H, *et al.* Pharmacokinetics and effects of cetirizine in horses with insect bite hypersensitivity. *Veterinary Journal* 2011; **187**: 347–351.
69. Schmidt-Choudhury A, Furuta GT, Lavigne JA, *et al.* The regulation of tumor necrosis factor-alpha production in murine mast cells: pentoxifylline or dexamethasone inhibits IgE-dependent production of TNF-alpha by distinct mechanisms. *Cellular Immunology* 1996; **171**: 140–146.
70. Rickards KJ, Page CP, Lees P, *et al.* In vitro and ex vivo effects of the phosphodiesterase 4 inhibitor rolipram on thromboxane production in equine blood. *Journal of Veterinary Pharmacology and Therapeutics* 2003; **26**: 123–130.
71. Sykes BW, Furr MO. Equine endotoxaemia-a state-of-the-art review of therapy. *Australian Veterinary Journal* 2005; **83**: 45–50.
72. Barton MH, Ferguson D, Davis PJ, *et al.* The effects of pentoxifylline infusion on plasma 6 ketoprostaglandin F1 alpha and ex vivo endotoxin-induced tumour necrosis factor activity in horses. *Journal of Veterinary Pharmacology and Therapeutics* 1997; **20**: 487–492.
73. Barton MH, Moore JN, Norton N. Effects of pentoxifylline infusion on response of horses to in vivo challenge exposure with endotoxin. *American Journal of Veterinary Research* 1997; **58**: 1300–1307.
74. Weiss DJ, Richwagen K, Evanson OA. Effects of hematocrit and erythrocyte deformability on pulmonary vascular pressures in perfused pony lungs. *American Journal of Veterinary Research* 1996; **57**: 346–350.
75. Chilcoat CD, Rowlingson KA, Jones SL. The effects of cAMP modulation upon the adhesion and respiratory burst activity of immune complex-stimulated equine neutrophils. *Veterinary Immunology and Immunopathology* 2002; **88**: 65–77.
76. Zabel P, Entzian P, Dalhoff K, *et al.* Pentoxifylline in treatment of sarcoidosis. *American Journal of Respiratory Critical Care Medicine* 1997; **15**: 1665–1669.
77. Leguillette R, Desevaux C, Lavoie JP. Effects of pentoxifylline on pulmonary function and results of cytologic examination of bronchoalveolar lavage fluid in horses with recurrent airway obstruction. *American Journal of Veterinary Research* 2002; **63**: 459–463.
78. Briggs WA, Eustace J, Mathew S, *et al.* Pentoxifylline potentiates in vitro lymphocyte suppression by glucocorticoids and immunosuppressive drugs. *Journal of Clinical Pharmacology* 1998; **38**: 561–566.
79. Entzian P, Zahringer U, Schlaak M, *et al.* Comparative study on effects of pentoxifylline, prednisolone and colchicine in experimental alveolitis. *International Journal of Immunopharmacology* 1998; **20**: 723–735.
80. Funk JO, Ernst M, Schonharting MM, *et al.* Pentoxifylline exerts synergistic immunomodulatory effects in combination with dexamethasone or cyclosporin A. *International Journal of Immunopharmacology* 1995; **17**: 1007–1016.
81. Baskett A, Barton MH, Norton N, *et al.* Effect of pentoxifylline, flunixinmeglumine, and their combination on a model of endotoxemia in horses. *American Journal of Veterinary Research* 1997; **58**: 1291–1299.
82. Kasahara E, Yamagishi N, Tanaka M, *et al.* A child with simple ulcer of the colon effectively treated with the combination of prednisolone, azathioprine, and pentoxifylline. *Journal of Gastroenterology* 2002; **37**: 745–749.
83. Kiku Y, Matsuzawa H, Ohtsuka H, *et al.* Effects of chlorpromazine, pentoxifylline and dexamethasone on mRNA expression of lipopolysaccharide-induced inflammatory cytokines in bovine peripheral blood mononuclear cells. *Journal of Veterinary Medical Science* 2002; **64**: 723–726.
84. Ingle-Fehr JE, Baxter GM. The effect of oral isoxsuprine and pentoxifylline on digital and laminar blood flow in healthy horses. *Veterinary Surgery* 1999; **28**: 154–160.
85. Crisman MV, Wilcke JR, Correll LS, *et al.* Pharmacokinetic disposition of intravenous and oral pentoxifylline in horses. *Journal of Veterinary Pharmacology and Therapeutics* 1993; **16**: 23–31.
86. Cohen ND, Carter GK. Steroid hepatopathy in a horse with glucocorticoid-induced hyperadrenocorticism. *Journal of the American Veterinary Medical Association* 1992; **200**: 1682–1684.
87. Vandenabeele SIJ, White SD, Affolter VK, *et al.* Pemphigus foliaceus in the horse: a retrospective study of 20 cases. *Veterinary Dermatology* 2004; **15**: 381–388.
88. Johnson PJ, Slight SH, Ganjam VK, *et al.* Glucocorticoids and laminitis in the horse. *Veterinary Clinics of North America: Equine Practice* 2002; **18**: 219–236.
89. Peroni DL, Stanley S, Kollias-Baker C, *et al.* Prednisone per os is likely to have limited efficacy in horses. *Equine Veterinary Journal* 2002; **34**: 283–287.
90. White SD. Advances in equine atopic dermatitis, serologic and intradermal allergy testing. *Clinical Techniques in Equine Practice* 2005; **4**: 311–313.
91. Littlewood JD, O'Brien JK, Stanford JL, *et al.* Management of Culicoides hypersensitivity (sweet-itch) in equids using killed bacterial preparation BE-T101: a randomised, double-blind, placebo-controlled study. Proceedings of the 17th World Association of Veterinary Dermatology Congress, Hong Kong, 2008: Abstract A71.
92. Marro A, Pirles M, Schiaffino L, *et al.* Successful immunotherapy of canine flea allergy with injected Actinomycetales preparations. *Immunotherapy* 2011; **3**: 971–978.

48

Other biting insect allergies

Gwendolen Lorch

The Ohio State University, College of Veterinary Medicine, Columbus, OH, USA

Conflict of interest: none declared.

Introduction

The term 'allergen' is used to describe any substance stimulating the production of immunoglobulin IgE in a genetically disposed individual and is often used synonymously with 'antigen', a term commonly used to describe a substance that generates immunoglobulin responses other than IgE, or a cellular immune response. An '*allergen*' must possess three distinct molecular properties: (1) the property to sensitize (i.e. induce the immune system to produce high-affinity antibodies, particularly of the IgE class); (2) the property to elicit an allergic reaction in a sensitized subject; and (3) it must have the ability to bind IgE antibodies. Complete allergens have all these properties [1]. Most allergens are proteins, ranging in molecular weight from 5 to 100 kDa. The number of proteins from any given source that may be allergenic will vary, but sensitized patients producing IgE to a source will usually recognize more than one allergenic protein [2]. In human medicine, allergens are classified as either a major or minor allergen. A major allergen is generally regarded as one to which >50% of allergic patients react but some of those considered 'minor' on a population basis may, of course, be of clinical significance at an individual level [3].

Equine insect hypersensitivity is characterized as a chronic, debilitating, pruritic cutaneous malady initiated by an IgE-mediated immediate hypersensitivity to allergens of the class *Insecta* (e.g. midges, black flies) and possibly the *Arachnida* (mites). The first known records of insect hypersensitivity were documented in a veterinary handbook from the Tang Dynasty in China. Currently, arthropod allergens are classified as parenteral. The role of arthropods as aeroallergens in the initiation of insect hypersensitivity has yet to be determined using provocative challenges in horses with seasonal insect hypersensitivity. Certainly in humans, the allergenic activity of aerosolized midge resides in the haemoglobin (erythrocruorin) molecules produced by the midge larvae and excreted by the adult flies while airborne [4]. Characterization of clinically significant allergens causing insect hypersensitivity is in its infancy, with several sequenced but many yet to have their exact biochemical activities and *in vivo* relevance determined. The theoretical importance of this is that if we want to understand allergy we need to understand the allergens. If we understand the allergens, we may find better ways of producing appropriate modified allergens for treatment. The impact of molecular biology and genomics on our understanding of insect allergen structure and function over the last decade has been enormous. The data obtained during this period has contributed significantly to our current understanding of the pathogenesis of insect hypersensitivity.

Allergen material sources and characterization

For biting insects, the optimal allergen source in insect hypersensitivity may be the salivary glands [5–7]; however, in humans a number of additional insect-derived proteins have also been shown to be clinically significant and may be derived from whole insect bodies or from faeces. Major allergenic components in insects include heat shock protein-70-cognate-3,

Veterinary Allergy, First Edition. Edited by Chiara Noli, Aiden Foster, and Wayne Rosenkrantz.

apyrase, an enzyme that catalyses the breakdown of ATP to release phosphate, hyaluronidase, and phospholipase, the cysteine-rich secretory proteins (CAP) superfamily protein, antigen 5 (AG5), as well as proteins of unknown function [8]. Direct recovery of saliva from mosquitoes has been possible in the laboratory but these processes have not yet been developed for commercial distribution. As such, the whole body is used as a source material [9]. Insect allergens used in veterinary medicine are derived from whole insect bodies, or faeces, or both, allowing for significant heterogeneity in the spectrum of contamination with other allergens and concentrations of specific allergens. The need for standardized extracts that contain the major allergens to enhance specificity of 'allergy' tests was initially demonstrated in veterinary medicine when gel electrophoresis was used to separate the proteins from either whole body crude black fly, *Simulium vittatum*, and from the salivary gland extracts only (SGE). The resulting immunoblot membranes were probed for IgE antibodies in sera derived from apparently clinically normal horses. The sera bound non-specific IgE-binding substances of the whole-body extract but did not recognize IgE-binding proteins from black fly SGE. Likewise, sera from horses with insect hypersensitivity showed six specific IgE-binding patterns to black fly SGE whereas none of the healthy horses showed individual IgE-binding patterns on immunoblots [6].

The salivary proteins of black flies and midges are in the incipient phase of characterization and have long been thought to be significant allergen sources that contribute to insect hypersensitivity. A considerable limitation to identifying the major allergens of insect hypersensitivity has been the acquisition of adequate amounts of female fly SGE to determine, purify, and characterize the allergens, although this has been accomplished for *S. vittatum* and *Culicoides nubeculosus* [6,10–12]. Potential IgE-binding black fly allergens from SGE were identified by probing a phage surface display cDNA library expressing recombinant *S. vittatum* SGE proteins with sera from horses with insect hypersensitivity that were sensitized to this fly. Seven cDNA encoding IgE-binding proteins were identified and had sequence similarities to AG5-like protein, serine protease inhibitor, α-amylases, and three erythema proteins. One of the identified recombinant proteins, referred to as r-Sim v 1, shares 48% sequence homology with AG5 and could bind IgE from 60% of insect hypersensitivity-affected horses, suggesting that this recombinant protein may represent a major allergen [13]. However, it must be remembered that a single recombinant allergen does not represent all the isoallergenic forms of the allergen and might not be sufficiently 'globally diagnostic' to be able to detect all clinically relevant IgE antibodies in order to provide allergen specificity. The major and minor candidate *Simulium* salivary allergens have been sequenced; synthesis of these proteins may allow the determination of their endogenous biological activity through intradermal and serological tests in affected and control horses. This approach is similar to that used to identify recombinant *Culicoides* allergens [11].

Currently, there is no information regarding putative allergenic peptides from stable fly, house fly, mosquito, or horse fly proteins for insect hypersensitivity. Conversely, three human IgE-binding horse fly allergens have recently been characterized. To characterize these major allergens the microdissection of salivary glands from 60 000 female horse flies was performed to produce enough SGE for the study [14]. The human horse fly allergens identified were from *Tabanus yao* and included Tab y 1, an apyrase of 70 kDa, Tab y 2, a hyaluronidase of 35 kDa, and Tab y 5, an antigen 5-related protein, and a CAP protein superfamily member of 26 kDa.

The clinically relevant phenomenon of immunologic cross reactivity occurs when IgE antibodies raised against a sensitizing allergen can react to structurally related proteins from other allergenic sources. This not only occurs in human allergy but it has also been documented in insect hypersensitivity [6,15–18]. Both *in vitro* and *in vivo* IgE cross-reactivity between *C. nubeculosus* (Cul n 1) and Sim v 1 [13] allergens has been established. This cross-reactivity is posited to exist because Cul n 1 exhibits 69.7% sequence homology and 47.7% sequence identity with Sim v 1 at the primary structure level. Although the sequence is not identical it is suspected that the three-dimensional structure is similar enough to bind the same IgE molecules. Further evidence of equine IgE shared epitopes to the same salivary gland proteins was confirmed by the binding of sera from horses diagnosed with insect hypersensitivity to a 70-kDa protein that was present in both *Culicoides* and *Simulium* SGEs and was further identified with mass spectrometry as heat shock protein-70-cognate-3 [6].

The current progress of identifying potential major allergens in insect hypersensitivity forms the foundation from which more sensitive and specific diagnostic assays for insect hypersensitivity can be developed, as well as of providing the potential to add individualized major and minor allergens to allergen-specific immunotherapy (ASIT), which may ultimately improve efficacy.

Pathogenesis of biting insect hypersensitivity

The detailed pathogenesis of *Culicoides* hypersensitivity is extensively described in Chapter 43. This section will provide a simplistic overview of the pathogenesis of insect hypersensitivity using *Culicoides* hypersensitivity as the model. As with human allergic disease, insect hypersensitivity is partly under genetic control and, for example, the heritability of *Culicoides* hypersensitivity in Icelandic horses is estimated at 0.3 [19]. The biological basis for antigen recognition is held within the major histocompatibility complexes (MHC), products of immune response genes. The generation of an effector immune response depends on helper T-cell function, usually mediated by $CD4^+$ T-cell receptor recognition of antigenic peptide presented in the groove of a class II MHC molecule. Horse MHC complexes, i.e. equine leukocyte antigen (ELA) class II specificities, have been shown to be linked to *Culicoides* hypersensitivity susceptibility, which is similar to the human leukocyte antigen (HLA) class II that is implicated in the pathogenesis of several allergic phenotypes. Most recently, DNA genotyping of the ELA class II region in horses was shown to be associated with *Culicoides* hypersensitivity susceptibility in two genetically distinct breeds, Exmoor ponies and Swedish-born Icelandic horses [20]. Homozygosity across the entire MHC class II region is associated with a higher risk factor for developing *Culicoides* hypersensitivity, which represents the first risk allele identified in any species suffering from allergic disease, including man [20].

The reagin in serum that mediates the immediate-type wheal and flare reaction was identified as IgE in 1966 [21,22], and has been confirmed as the reaginic antibody in the skin of horses with insect hypersensitivity. Evidence for the pivotal role of allergen-specific IgE, and therefore a classical Type I hypersensitivity reaction, in the pathogenesis of *Culicoides* hypersensitivity was documented by performing a modified Prausnitz–Küstner experiment in which allergic reactions to *Culicoides* can be passively transferred to healthy animals using IgE purified from the serum of IH-affected horses [23].

Environmental antigen exposure for insect hypersensitivity is presumed to occur by parenteral contact. The details on how the *Culicoides* antigen is taken up, processed, and bound with development of sensitization has been previously described in Chapters 43 and 44. Eosinophils are particularly important in equine insect hypersensitivity and, although not directly involved in the immediate reaction, eosinophils are also drawn to the site of the reaction by specific chemotactic factors. Eosinophils contain cationic proteins, the best-characterized being major basic proteins, which have the potential to contribute to ongoing inflammatory reaction by producing cytotoxic cellular injury and its ability to induce basophil and mast cell degranulation [24]. In addition to eosinophils, it is likely that neutrophils are drawn to the site of an immediate hypersensitivity reaction by chemotactic factors. Each of the four cell types (mast cell, basophil, eosinophil, and neutrophil) is programmed to secrete significant quantities of mediators, which contributes to the general state of inflammation. This elicits clinical signs as a result of mediator-induced physiologic and anatomic changes. In horses, an IgE-mediated multicomponent response is sufficient to explain the acute phases of insect hypersensitivity; however, this does not exclude that other immunologic mechanisms are also involved in chronic stages of the disease. For example, *de novo* synthesis of inflammatory lipid mediators and Th2 cytokines occurs upon activation, contributing to the clinical signs of the IgE-dependent late-phase hypersensitivity reactions, which occur at 4–8 hours after the commencement of the initial challenge [25].

Clinical signs

Insect hypersensitivity is seen worldwide and is presumably the most common cause of allergic disease in horses. Although it is widely regarded as a hypersensitivity to *Culicoides* spp., it is now recognized that insect hypersensitivity can be seen as a result of hypersensitivity to other biting flies such as *Simulium* spp., *Tabanus* spp., stable fly (i.e. *Stomoxys* spp.), and mosquitoes [26]. The prevalence of *Culicoides* hypersensitivity can be 5–60% depending on the geographic region and exposure to insect bites [27–29]. This may be an underestimate because many horse owners do not report this problem until the severity renders the horse unusable. Not surprisingly, the prevalence of insect hypersensitivity due to insects other than *Culicoides* is unknown.

In areas where there is a distinct climatic difference between spring, summer, autumn, and winter, insect hypersensitivity is a seasonal disorder. In temperate, subtropical, or tropical environments, clinical signs of insect hypersensitivity may be year round. The disease is characterized by recrudesce of pruritus during the spring and summer months when insect exposure is the greatest, with regression of the pruritus in the winter months. When pastured with other horses, many of the other animals will not show any degree of pruritus. Onset of clinically apparent signs may develop at any age, with most horses in the midwest United States showing their initial signs between 6 and 10 years of age. It is not unheard of for horses to develop clinical signs as early as 2 years of age or as late as 16 years of age. No breed predisposition has been reported for other biting insect hypersensitivities, unlike that documented for *Culicoides* hypersensitivity. Typically, the intensity of the pruritus progresses each season as the horse ages.

The most common clinical sign of insect hypersensitivity is pruritus, which varies in severity from mild to intense. The time of day in which the horse's pruritus is most severe is often tied to the offending insects' feeding habits. Additionally, the distribution of the pruritus is also coupled to the preferred body feeding sites of the biting insect. Typical defence reactions by which the horses try to drive away these insects from their bodies are shuddering of the skin, tail swishing, foot stomping, swinging of the head, biting at the larger blood-sucking flies on the coat, rolling about on the ground, and occasionally continual fence pacing and restlessness. Sustained daily exposure and the associated irritation can lead to rapid weight loss and signs of self-mutilation.

Clinical signs for other biting insect hypersensitivities may be indistinguishable from those of *Culicoides* hypersensitivity. In addition to pruritus, horses with acute insect hypersensitivity may have multifocal regions of tufted to crusted papules and scale as initial lesions. Crusted papules are commonly located on the convex surface of the ear pinnae, poll, crest, lateral aspects of the neck, withers, shoulders, medial aspect of the foreleg, distal extremities, lateral aspect of the thigh and gaskin, the croup and dock. Multifocal areas of patchy hypotrichosis to alopecia, with erythematous macules and moist exudation of serum with associated erosions, are common. As the disease progresses the forehead, periocular, and intermandibular sites are commonly involved. Either focal midline (near the umbilicus) or diffuse ventral midline dermatitis represented by alopecia, excoriations, ulcerations, or crusted papules are additional clinical manifestations of other biting insect hypersensitivities (Figure 48.1). Conventional, papular to giant urticaria can develop within minutes to hours after the cutaneous injection of vasoactive components from the salivary glands of mosquitoes, stable flies, deer flies, black flies, or horse flies. The urticaria may be painful as well as pruritic and may be limited to a single bite area, it may present as a more-generalized response. Acute clinical signs superimposed on chronic effects are commonly encountered.

Chronic pruritus leads to unresolving alopecia, lichenification, persistent secondary bacterial folliculitis and furunculosis, scarring, and pigmentary abnormalities (hypopigmentation or hyperpigmentation, melanotrichia) of the hair coat or skin or both. Horses may persistently rub their tail causing hypotrichosis of the tail base, with frayed shorted hair and underlying thickening of the skin (Figure 48.2). Severely thinned to

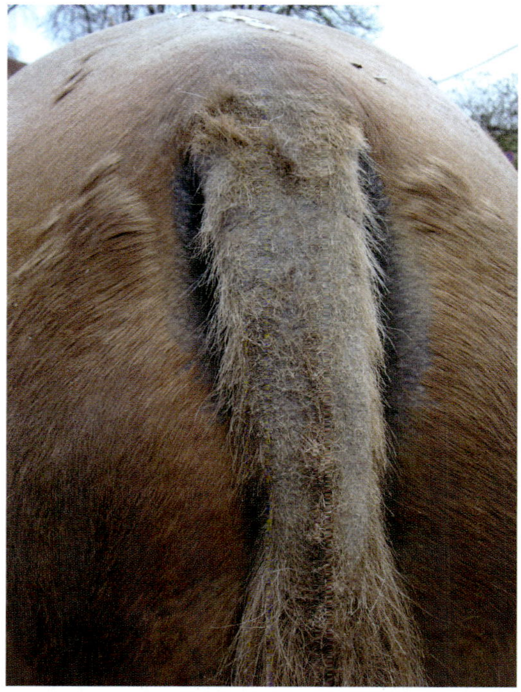

Figure 48.2 Horse with insect hypersensitivity and secondary tail pruritus. Hair shafts have become shorten, broken, and frayed on the lateral aspects of the tail while causing complete alopecia of the dorsomedial tail head.

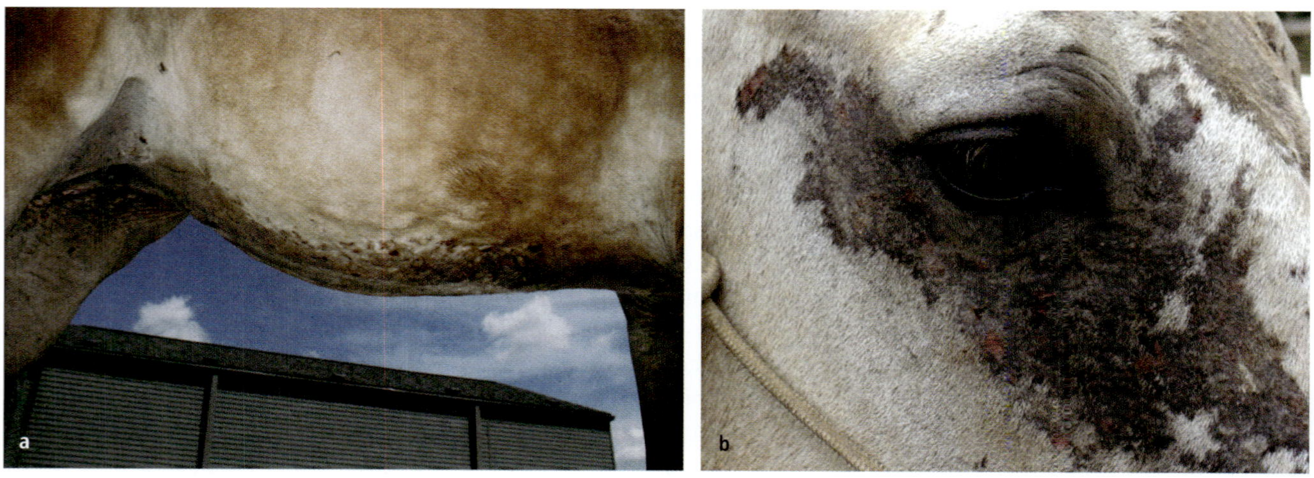

Figure 48.1 Horses with clinical signs of insect hypersensitivity. (a) Severe acute self-trauma of the ventral thorax and abdomen with alopecia, erythema, hyperpigmentation, erosion, and crusting. (b) Facial and periocular alopecia with adherent crusts and erosions.

nearly complete hair loss from the entire tail shaft, giving the appearance of a 'rat-tail', is common and hair regrowth resumes in the winter months, although hyperplasia of the skin may remain. The mane can also appear sparse, broken, and damaged.

An additional clinical presentation that may be mediated by an insect hypersensitivity but is not linked exclusively to this aetiology includes eosinophilic granulomas, which are non-painful, non-pruritic, well-circumscribed, firm, indurated, elevated papules to nodules that remain haired and occur anywhere on the body. Occasionally, the nodules will expel a whitish to gray caseous material that is likely necrotic or mineralized cellular debris.

Differential diagnosis

The list of differential diagnosis will vary according to geographic location, lesional distribution and number of horses affected. For a complete list of differentials see Chapter 46.

Diagnosis

The clinician should begin the diagnostic process with a through clinical history and physical examination. Clinical signs and seasonality that suggest a diagnosis of insect hypersensitivity are matched with suspected relevant allergen exposures and history. Once a clinician has a high degree of suspicion that the horse has insect hypersensitivity, then all other causes of equine seasonal pruritic disorders that correlate with the distribution must be ruled out. Once other differential diagnoses have been ruled out, improvement in pruritus with strict insect control and environmental modifications help to confirm the diagnosis of insect hypersensitivity.

Diagnostic confirmation

Diagnostic confirmation should include the identification of the suspected biting insect(s). The primary confirmatory tests for sensitization to detect allergen specific IgE for equine insect hypersensitivity are limited. The preferred test for detection of cutaneous IgE is the intradermal test (IDT) due to its ability to measure skin IgE and the practicality for the dermatologist in private practice. Current insect intradermal allergens are whole-body extracts and do not reliably provide the sensitivity needed to distinguish horses with insect hypersensitivity from clinically normal horses when read at the immediate-phase (15–30 minutes after injection) or late-phase reactions (4–8 hours). The value of the IDT for the diagnosis of insect hypersensitivity is still controversial; while earlier studies have shown the insect hypersensitivity horses have significantly more positive IDT reactions than controls [17,28,30], more recent findings have shown a low sensitivity and specificity of the IDT for insect allergens [31,32]. There is promising evidence that the use of recombinant insect allergens may be a more reliable source for intradermal testing once they become commercially available [11,12,15].

Laboratory-based *in vitro* tests include the cellular antigen stimulation test (CAST) for measurement of sulphidoleukotriene (sLT) release and an assay to measure histamine release from basophils after allergen-specific treatment of blood cells [5,33,34]. Further investigation showed that the histamine release assay could differentiate clinically affected from non-affected *Culicoides* hypersensitivity horses by the resulting histamine concentrations from peripheral blood cells. Likewise, the CAST had the highest diagnostic sensitivity (78%) and specificity (98%) levels for *C. nubeculosus* extracts. These tests may have clinical utility in the future with further optimization and are currently not commercially available. Serological methods for detection of soluble serum IgE are available and use anti-IgE detection reagents ranging from monoclonal to polyclonal antibodies and the human FcεRIα chain [35]. The unreliable specificities of the detection reagents for equine IgE and the use of crude allergen preparations in the assays results in poor performance and limited clinical utility for the diagnosis of insect hypersensitivity [36–38].

A skin biopsy collected for histopathological analysis of insect hypersensitivity is unlikely to have findings that are pathognomonic for insect hypersensitivity. In fact, the morphological diagnosis may be seen with adverse food reactions, atopic dermatitis, drug, or contact reactions. The major histological pattern is one of stereotypic eosinophilic-rich superficial and usually deep perivascular to interstitial or diffuse dermatitis. Some biopsy specimens may have numerous dermal lymphocytes but these are generally never the predominant leukocyte type. Mast cells are typically found in the superficial dermis or subepidermally, as well as in the hair follicle epithelium and in the dermal papilla [39,40]. The epidermis is mildly to moderately acanthotic, variably spongiotic with eosinophilic and lymphocytic exocytosis and orthokeratotic to limited areas of parakeratotic hyperkeratosis. The epidermis may have surface crusts with variable erosion and ulceration. Focal areas of infiltrative to necrotizing eosinophilic mural folliculitis and furunculosis may be present. Dermal edema and fibrosis can be prominent in chronic lesions. It is not uncommon to find small accumulations of degranulating eosinophils orientated around individual collagen fibres and coating them with eosinophilic material to form collagen flame figures of variable size and prominence, ranging from annular to oval, to a radiating configuration giving a 'starburst' appearance.

These tests are performed to strengthen the likelihood that the chosen allergy diagnosis is correct; however, they are not necessary for confirmation if all other potential causes of allergic disease can be exclusively ruled out; a feat that can be challenging in horses with a history and clinical signs consistent with both insect hypersensitivity and atopic dermatitis. A definitive diagnosis of allergic disease then permits a number of therapeutic interventions involving avoidance, environmental modifications, pharmacotherapy, or immunotherapy or both to be instituted.

Treatment

Clinical management for the horse with biting insect allergy is similar to that discussed in Chapter 47 for Culicoides hypersensitivity. Best practice management schemes should incorporate a detailed plan for allergen avoidance, i.e. insect control, as well as topical and systemic pharmacotherapy. These are accepted and marginally effective treatments for insect hypersensitivity.

Avoidance

Avoidance by separating the allergic horse from the allergen source is the least expensive and most effective mode of treatment for allergic disease; however, avoidance of insects in a rural environment is difficult to achieve. In order for avoidance and prevention strategies to be effective, not only should the characteristics, life cycle, breeding sites, and known control measures for the offending insects be taken into account but it is also necessary to identify and institute environmental management strategies. As insects are always present in the warmer months, use of protective fly gear as a physical barrier is mandatory for a horse with insect hypersensitivity. Complete coverage of the horse can be achieved with fly sheets that shield the front and hind legs as well as provide coverage of the tail and ventral abdomen with a bellyband. In addition, a fly mask with ear coverage as well as a neck cover and leg wraps should be used to ensure that all preferred feeding sites of flies are eliminated (Figure 48.3). The most useful fly sheets either have odourless permethrin-impregnated fibres or have pockets designed to hold insect-repellent inserts.

Pharmacotherapy

Pharmacotherapy improves but does not eliminate clinical signs and does not result in long-term improvement. It

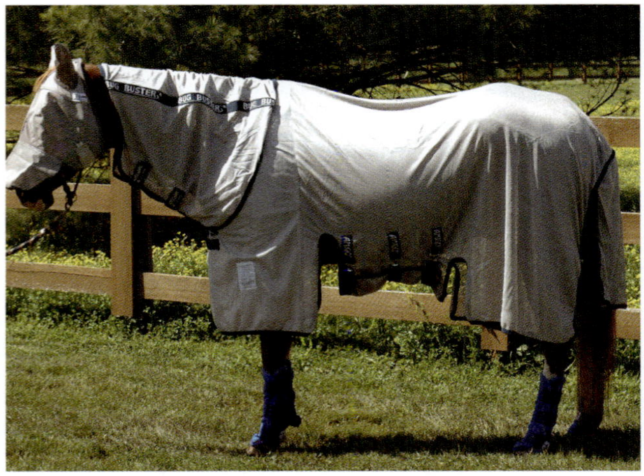

Figure 48.3 Horse wearing protective fly gear. The horse should be protected with a light-coloured, breathable, fine-mesh fabric that prevents the contact of flies with the horse's skin. Freely movable panels that cover the front and hind legs acts as 'fly swatters' when the horse moves so alighting of flies does not occur.

is unknown if, in some cases, natural desensitization occurs with frequent numerous bites. For *Culicoides* hypersensitivity the benefit of ASIT is controversial and it is generally ineffective [41]. As the accuracy of skin tests and *in vitro* determinations rely on the availability of well-characterized allergen extracts, so, too does effective ASIT. With the lack of allergen standardization and characterization of all the major allergens in insect hypersensitivity, these goals are clearly an unmet challenge in the field and would most likely serve to rapidly advance the effectiveness of immunotherapy for insect hypersensitivity.

Selected biting Diptera

Unique identifying features, life cycles, peak feeding, and preferred feeding sites of various other biting flies are presented in Table 48.1 and features seen in Figure 48.4.

Tabanidae (horse fly, deer fly)

Fly characteristics

There are 4200 species of blood-feeding tabanid flies (e.g. *Atylotus, Tabanus, Haematopota, Hybomitra, Chrysops*) in the world and around 350 species occur in North America, many of which exhibit different behaviour depending on the host [42]. Tabanids occur worldwide, being absent only at extreme northern and southern latitudes. These flies are among those known as gad flies, breeze flies, zimbs, or clegs. In Australia, they

Table 48.1 Selected characteristics and developmental times for various Diptera

Order	Family	Scientific name	Common name	Identifying characteristics	Sources	Adult occurrence	Life cycle	Peak feeding	Feeding sites
Cyclorrhapha **A subdivision of the Brachycera** **Flies have the shared trait of a circular aperture where the adult flies emerge from the pupal case**									
Diptera	Muscidae	*Musca domestica, Musca autumnalis* Linnaeus	House and face flies	Female bigger than male Sponging proboscis 6.4 mm in length Four narrow black stripes on thorax Grey or yellowish abdomen	Most commonly associated with decaying organic matter and/or manure from: humans horse farms poultry farms	Most abundant late summer and early autumn	From egg to adult in 9–25 days **Eggs** < 24 h **Larva** 5–14 days **Pupa** 3–10 days **Adults** live for 3–4 weeks Overwinter stage	Feed only on liquid from facial secretions and wounds and have ability to turn solids into liquids	Face, muzzle and in medial and lateral canthi of the eyes
Diptera	Muscidae	*Stomoxys calcitrans*	Stable flies	Bayonet-like proboscis 7–8 mm in length Pale bald spot behind head Checkerboard appearance due to dark spots on abdomen	Most commonly associated with decaying organic matter from horse, hog and poultry farms for egg laying, which occurs in: Damp hay/straw Animal manure Piles of lawn clippings	Most abundant in summer through to autumn	From egg to adult in 23–52 days **Eggs** 2–3 days **Larva** 1–3 weeks **Pupa** 2–4 weeks Overwinter in larval or pupal stage **Adults** live for 3–4 weeks	Early morning and again in late afternoon Prefer to feed outdoors Obligatory blood meal needed from warmblooded mammal, mainly horses and cattle	Horse: neck, lower legs, and underbelly Cattle: dorsum, lateral front legs, carpus, and to pastern

(Continued)

Table 48.1 (*Continued*)

Order	Family	Scientific name	Common name	Identifying characteristics	Sources	Adult occurrence	Life cycle	Peak feeding	Feeding sites
Diptera	Muscidae	*Haematobia irritans* or *Lyperosia irritans*	Horn flies	5 mm in length The palps are the same length as the proboscis Wings are set very flat	Mostly found on cattle but will feed on horses if cattle are not present Will not bite horses inside stable As flies emerge from pupa they immediately feed on cattle and remain on them their entire life Flies leave the host only to lay eggs in their fresh manure	Most abundant early summer Decline in summer but then increase in numbers again in late August and September when temperatures fall and rain increases	From egg to adult in 10–14 days **Eggs** 1–2 days **Larva** 4–8 days **Pupa** 6–8 days Overwintering stage **Adults** live for several weeks	Both female and males feed on blood and stay on host	Horse: feed in small or large groups that aggregate around the neck, shoulders, flanks, and abdomen and less commonly the lower legs Feed dorsally when cool but will feed ventrally during sunny hot weather

Brachycera **Many species are predators or scavengers or parasitoids as larvae** **Brachycera or 'shortened horn' refers to shortened antennae, often called stylate antennae** **Distal segments of antenna are annulated, giving the impression of many segments but 8 or fewer flagellomeres**									
Diptera	Tabanidae	*Chrysops* spp.	Deer flies	Zigzag patterned gold or green eyes Males have larger eyes that touch one another Mostly yellow or black with darker strips on abdomen Wings have dark markings 7–10 mm in size	Damp environments (marshes, beaches, wooded areas, wet meadows around ponds); vegetation, streams	Most abundant 4–5 weeks in June and July	From egg to adult 2 months to 3 years **Eggs** 2–3 days **Larva** 1–3 years **Pupa** 6 days–2 weeks **Adults** live for 1 month	Warm sunny days with little or no wind Attracted to moving objects and dark shapes Females feed on blood Males collect pollen	Anywhere on the body, but often feed on sites where the host will have difficulty dislodging them, such as the sides of face, neck ventrum, and lower legs Typically feed on moving animals
Diptera	Tabanidae	*Tabanus* spp.	Horse flies	8–25 mm in size Tarsi with 3 plantar pads and tarsal claws Some have striking colour patterns on their eyes Wing veins fork to form large 'Y' across the wing tip	Adults wide-ranging; larvae found in streams, ponds, and marshes, especially along the edges and on the sea shore	Most abundant 3–4 weeks in August in temperate climates	From egg to adult 2 months up to 3 years **Eggs** 2–3 days **Larva** 1 to several years Overwinter stage Develop through 6–13 instars, moults to pupa in spring **Pupa** 6 days–2 weeks **Adults** Males a few days Females 30–60 days	Warm sunny days with little or no wind Attracted to dark hair colour and motion Females feed on blood Males collect pollen	Feeding sites are the same as for *Chrysops* but prefer to bite stationary animals

(Continued)

Table 48.1 (*Continued*)

Order	Family	Scientific name	Common name	Identifying characteristics	Sources	Adult occurrence	Life cycle	Peak feeding	Feeding sites
Nematocera **Considered the most 'primitive' flies** **Delicate, slender bodies and long, narrow wings** **Distinctive feature is the antennae, which have 6 or more segments** **Larvae endowed with appendages for swimming, breathing, and gathering food in water**									
Diptera	Culicidae	*Aedes* spp. *Anopheles* spp. *Culex* spp.	Mosquitoes	Elongated cranial projecting proboscis with a bundle of stylets loosely encased in a sheath formed by the labium Wings with macrotrichiae (hairs) on veins and along the margins 3–15 mm in size Long antennae with 6 or more segments	Most commonly associated with stagnant, organic-rich water Distinct summer activity pattern in temperate zones and woodland with ponds	Most abundant in late spring and summer in temperate climates Activity may increase in tropical or subtropical zones after seasonal rains	From egg to adult in 5 days up to 1 year dependent on ambient temperature **Egg** from 48 h to 1 year or more May overwinter **Larva** 7–14 days **Pupa** 1–4 days **Adults** Males 1 week Females 1 week–5 months and can hibernate	Species-dependent and range from: dusk and dawn feeders daytime feeders night feeders Prefer low wind conditions Males feed on nectar and other sources of sugar	Species-dependent but generally head, neck, base of mane, axillae, upper medial limb regions, and ventral abdomen

Diptera	Simuliidae	*Simulium* spp.	Black flies	Small 2–5 mm in length Thorax is large and humped, resembles a buffalo Black to various shades of gray or yellow Strong fliers, will use wind current to travel up to 60 miles to feed	Prevalent wherever there is permanent or semipermanent running water Adults are wide ranging from savannah to forest	Active throughout the day but may increase in the morning and evening leading to a bimodal pattern of activity if in the heat of the tropical midday Do not emerge at night	From egg to adult species-dependent, generally 6–15 weeks **Egg** 3–7 days May enter diapause overwinter as egg or larva **Larva** 10–14 days to 7–10 weeks **Pupa** 2 days to 5 weeks, species-dependent **Adults** Males 2–10 weeks Females 3 weeks up to 85 days	Daytime feeders Prefer low wind conditions to still air Host choice based on visual, olfactory, and thermal cues	Feed on pinne, face, neck, ventrum, and legs

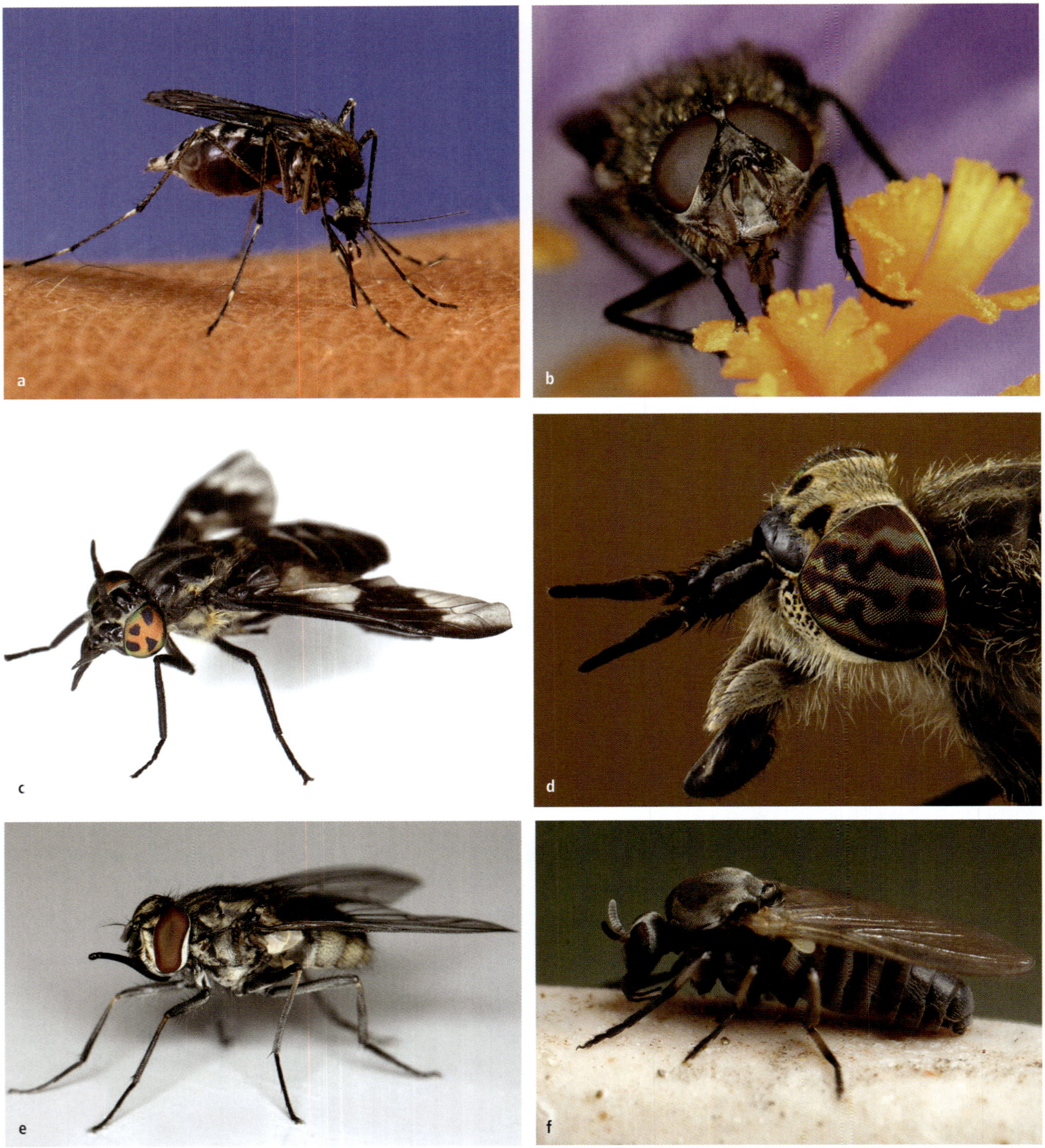

Figure 48.4 Biting insects of the order Diptera: (a) mosquito (*Aedes/Ochlerotatus sollicitans*); (b) house fly (*Musca domestica*); (c) deer fly (*Chrysops relictus*); (d) horse fly (*Haematopota crassicornis*); (e) stable fly (*Stomoxys calcitrans*) (courtesy of Håkon Haraldseide); (f) black fly (*Simulium*). (Reprinted with permission from Brian Valentine.)

are know as 'March flies'. The zimb, also known as *tsaltsalya* (Ethiopian) or *seriut* (Arabic), is any horse fly of the genus *Pangonia* found in Ethiopia. Adult horse and deer flies are most abundant in the midwest United States from early to late July but remain active year round in the southern environs. Different species have activity patterns that peak at different times of the day, which can vary from day to day and, are highly dependent on meteorological factors such as barometric pressure, cloud cover, wind speed, relative humidity, and an increase in evaporation [43,44]. The diversity of responses of the different species to meteorological factors makes it difficult to predict risk periods of high activity, and therefore recommendations for stabling, as most weather conditions in tropical, dry, and temperate climates will favour activity by at least one common species.

Adults are considered strong fliers and are very difficult to discourage. Tabanids are strongly attracted to all natural or artificial sources of horizontally polarized light, due to their polarization vision and positive polarotaxis [45]. For light to be attractive to tabanids, it must be reflected off horizontal surfaces to appeal to the polartactic senses located in the flies' ventral eye, an area that is specialized for horizontal polarization sensitivity. Female tabanid flies are telmophages (pool feeders), taking frequent, intermittent, and rapid bloodmeals from many different hosts, including horses, cattle, deer, and less commonly humans. This habit of interrupted feeding enables them to mechanically transmit pathogens of several diseases. It has been reported that horse flies need approximately ten landings on a host to obtain a complete meal [46]. Such multiple landings on a host provide an opportunity for the innate and adaptive immune defences to affect the horse flies.

Not surprisingly, horse flies have developed a number of countermeasures to overcome host immune responses. For example, immuoregulin TP1 peptide in horse fly salivary glands was found to suppress host IFN-γ and monocyte chemoattractant protein-1 and increase the secretion of IL-10 induced by lipopolysaccharide in mouse splenocytes [47]. The piercing stylets, developed from the maxilla and mandible, and are used to make an incision in the host's skin, which allows the fly to feed on the blood that wells up. Females of larger species are able to ingest up to 200 mg of blood (i.e. up to four times the weight of the fly) within only 1–3 minutes, suggesting that they possess potent anticoagulant proteins. Indeed, two different antihaemostatic strategies occur among Tabanidae: *Chrysops* inhibits platelet aggregation [48] whereas most other genera (e.g. *Tabanus* and *Hybomitra*) possess anticoagulant activities based mainly on the presence of a potent inhibitor of thrombin [49,50]. Potent antithrombin activity in the salivary glands of tabanids was noted during the discovery of tabanin, a thrombin inhibitor from *Tabanus bovis* [49]. Recently, a platelet aggregation inhibitor and a potent glycoprotein IIb/IIIa fibrinogen receptor antagonist have been isolated from the deer fly, *Chrysops* sp. [48].

Life cycle and breeding sites

Lifecycles of both the horse and deer fly are similar and are long; most species have only one generation per year. The first stage of development is the egg stage. They are laid in 'tiers' (masses) which contain a few 100 to 1000 eggs. Tabanid females usually lay their eggs on marsh plants or fresh vegetation next to freshwater bodies, because after egg hatching the larvae must drop down into water or mud where they develop. Immature larval tabanids are aquatic, semiaquatic, or terrestrial and the last-stage larva in a temperate region will overwinter in muddy soils, maturing in late spring.

When the horse fly larvae hatch from the eggs and drop to the water or soil during the third and later stages of larval development they become voracious predators of other invertebrates, plant tissues, and small vertebrates, such as insects and their larvae, young frogs, earthworms, small crustaceans, and other organisms. Deer fly larvae feed on organic debris and other small organisms. The larvae undergo several moults as they grow and move to drier soils to pupate. The pupal period varies between species, depending on the temperature.

Adult flies emerge from pupae and immediately begin mating and blood feeding. Females feed on blood to aid the development of their eggs but will also feed on nectar and plant juices for flight energy. Male tabanids survive on nectar, pollen, and aphid faeces.

Vector-borne diseases

Both haematophagous female horse and deer flies are either primary or secondary mechanical vectors of important animal and human diseases, including equine infectious anaemia, bovine leukaemia virus, anthrax (*Bacillus anthracis*), hog cholera, surra (*Trypanosom aevansi*), filariasis, tularaemia (*Francisella tularensis*), anaplasmosis, and Lyme disease [51–53]. They may also transmit papillomaviruses and dermatophyte infections. Transmission of disease is specific to the tabanid species.

Clinical features

Interestingly, horses with a white hair coat are less attractive to tabanids than horses with a brown or black hair coat [54]. The attraction of tabanids to a darker coloured hosts can be explained by the polarizing properties of the coat rather than by the darker colour or higher temperature [54]. The preferred alighting sites for tabanids sp. in descending order are: front legs >hind legs >belly >head and neck, and, finally, the back [55]. The bites produce painful oedematous wheals to nodules that may become pruritic. The blood left from the tabanid bite serves as an attractant milieu for other scavenger flies. Upon close examination of the resultant wheal, a central area of blood-tinged serum may be evident. Ventral midline dermatitis starting as cranial as the ventral thorax, extending caudally to the udder or prepuce, may provide evidence for tabanid-related hypersensitivity. Lesions may be particularly severe around the umbilicus. Because tabanid bites are painful, horses may become restless and unmanageable when they attempt to ward off attacks by these flies. With intense tabanid attacks, horses grazing in a sunny field may seek a shady forest or wooded area for refuge or completely forgo grazing if the attacks are intense, thus significant weight loss can occur.

Control measures: environmental

At present, no satisfactory methods have been developed for reducing tabanid populations [56]. It is difficult to impossible to locate or eliminate breeding sites of horse and deer flies. They breed in environmentally sensitive wetlands so effects of drainage or insecticide application on non-target organisms or water supplies is a concern. Breeding sites may be very extensive or some distance away from where the problem is occurring and as tabanids are strong fliers they have no reservations about obtaining a meal some distance from their breeding site. Larval control is equally impractical, especially in recreation areas or reservoirs. Application of adulticides is not practical because it requires the use of broad-spectrum insecticides, which can be toxic to fish, birds, and mammals. Researchers throughout the world continue to study the efficacy of tabanid traps with chemicals that mimic natural host odours as a method of control strategy, although species differences are known to occur. An effective environmentally friendly biting fly trap commonly used to capture tabinads is the NZI trap. This trap is a passive killing device that works through the attraction of flies to large blue and black objects. Flies die from exposure after entering the innovative configuration of cloth and netting [57]. Traps baited with a mixture of 1-octen-3-ol, acetone, and ammonia solution collect 14.5 times more tabanids compared to unbaited traps, whereas using aged donkey urine, lactic acid, and fresh human urine–baited traps will collect 12, 3.9, and 2.5 times as many tabanids as unbaited traps [58]. 1-Octen-3-ol a common attractant emitted by vertebrates, when presented with carbon dioxide (CO_2) attracts haematophagous arthropods, including mosquitoes and tabanids. Collaboration with the regional entomologists and extension agents in some countries may provide a viable option for arthropod management and vector control.

Horse

Prevention of hypersensitivity reactions commences with providing protective housing to shield the horses from the majority of tabanid attacks, which are most likely to occur during daylight hours.

Simulium *(black fly)*

Fly characteristics

More than 2100 species of black flies in the family Simuliidae have been described, in which the females of about 98% of the species feed on vertebrate blood. Black flies are found from arctic to tropical ecosystems, with the most abundant populations in northern USA, eastern Europe, and Canada. Black flies can have a significant impact on livestock fitness. The black fly is considered a pool feeder, which creates a subdermal haematoma from which it imbibes instead of piercing a blood vessel and feeding from the lumen, as a mosquito would feed.

The ability of the saliva to modulate components of the host immune system provides an opportunity for enhancing transmission of infectious agents. Haematophagous arthropods secrete a variety of molecules in their saliva to counteract the host haemostatic response of pathogens during bloodfeeding. These secretions prevent platelet aggregation, inhibit coagulation, and induce vasodilation. Black fly saliva is different from other haematophagous insects described as their salivary secretions have antihaemostatic effects against factor Xa [59], thrombin, factor V [60,61], and platelet aggregation mediated by apyrase, to prevent fibrin clot formation and create vasodilation [62]. Apyrase provides enzymatic activity that degrades ATP and ADP and is a potent stimulant of platelet aggregation. Black flies have evolved species-specific differences in the amount and repertoire of antihaemostatic and antithrombotic agents to account for the clotting time of their preferred host species.

The salivary components from black flies have been shown to have immunomodulatory effects such that pretreatment of murine splenocytes with salivary gland soluble products suppressed proliferation of both $CD4^+$ and $CD8^+$ T cells in response to IL-2 and IL-4 cytokines. The factor responsible for the inhibition was determined to be a protein or protein complex of a size greater than 50 kDa [63]. Additionally, splenocytes exposed to SGE produced lower levels of IL-5 and IL-10 when challenged with globulin-free ovalbumin and exposure resulted in the activation of caspase-3, suggesting that morphologic changes observed in the T cells was likely to be the result of induction of apoptosis [63,64].

Life cycle and breeding sites

The length of the life cycle from egg to adult is variable, depending on the black fly species and water temperature. Large populations are caused by extreme rainfall. Black flies are sexually dimorphic. Black flies only breed in running water. The number of broods produced per year depends on the species. Some produce multiple broods per year while other species produce only one clutch in which the eggs will remain in a protracted state of metabolic quiescence until they hatch the following year.

In general, a female can deposit 200–800 eggs in a gelatinous aggregation. The female deposits her eggs on the water's surface or on partly submerged stones, vegetation, or logs in rapid flowing water currents. Immature stages develop in oxygenated water sources that are moving at an average velocity of 1.5 feet per second. Larvae pass through six stages before reaching the pupae stage. Larvae cling to rocks by small hooklets on the short proleg and a sucker-like disc at the tip of the abdomen, which allows these filter feeders to feed on organic matter and detritus from flowing water. When ready to pupate, the larvae spin silken cocoons that secure them to the substrate in the stream. Adults emerge from the pupal case through a slit and float to the water surface on a bubble of air and females fly off in search of a blood meal and males in search of nectar. Some species mate as soon as adults emerge. Black flies prefer non-polluted water.

Diseases

The structural composition of the mouthparts, the chemical quality of the salivary molecules, the mechanism of mouthpart insertion and the resulting feeding lesion during blood feeding are important factors in the successful transmission of the cutaneous filariid nematode (*Onchocerca* spp.). Discovery of the *Wolbachia* bacterium in the filarial worms and its proinflammatory role in the human eye may present a novel method for treatment of this parasite [65]. Black flies are competent biological vectors of vesicular stomatitis virus [66]. As black flies are direct vectors of arboviruses, these flies have been implicated as a probable agent for papovaviruses and resultant equine ear papillomas or 'aural plaques' but direct evidence for this incrimination has not been documented.

Clinical features

Black fly swarm attacks can be fatal, which can be attributable to shock and sustained anticoagulant activity. Black fly bites inflict pain. Preferred biting sites are thinly haired areas and are species dependent. These include the pinnae, ventrum, legs, face, intermandibular space, and throatlatch region. The clinical appearance of black fly bites are wheals with evidence of a central pinpoint haemorrhagic crust, papules, focal areas of hypotrichosis to alopecia, with leukoderma. Pinnal aural plaques may commence as small, 2–3 mm, alopecic, shiny, depigmented papules on the inner concave surface of the pinnae. These lesions enlarge to well-demarcated, 1–3 cm raised, white to pale gray, hyperkeratotic plaques, which may have a surface characterized by tiny frond-like projections. Individual plaques may eventually coalesce to form a mass. These lesions do not spontaneously regress but may decrease in size when they are not irritated by fly bites.

Control measures: environmental

The history of simuliid pests and vector control is also the history of resistance due to the use of multiple pesticides to try and limit the transmission of human onchocerciasis and mansonellosis. Control of black flies is difficult because of the number of potential breeding sites. Biological larvacides developed for fly control include *Bacillus thuringiensis*, a naturally occurring, Gram-positive, rod-shaped, spore-forming bacterium, which is pathogenic to the larvae of a number of insect species when ingested by the larvae. *Bacillus thuringiensis* var. *israelensis* Serotype H14 *(Bti)* is a biological insecticide produced during sporulation of this bacterium. The protein product of the H14 serotype is used to selectively control the larvae of mosquitoes and black flies. It alters the permeability of the flies gut, allowing salts to enter under alkaline conditions. This in turn decreases feeding, development, and eventually causes death by starvation. *Bti* has been used against black flies for more than 30 years with mortality rates often around 95%. This high rate of efficacy in return results in intense selection and resistance should be of concern. Unfortunately, with the heady success of *Bti*, virtually all other research on biological control agents has been shut down since the 1980s. Most recently, a gender influence on microbial biodiversity of the black fly cuticle, haemolymph, haemocoel, gut tissue, and leg cavity has been demonstrated. In general, female flies harbour a less diverse bacterial community than do males. Understanding the physiological function of the associated bacterial community could provide clues for developing novel pest-management strategies [67].

Horse

Horses should be stabled at sunrise and sunset during seasons of particularly heavy black fly attacks. Black flies can travel up to 150 miles aided by wind migration but more typically travel 7–15 miles for a meal. The flies are particularly active in the early morning and evening. Due to their small size, black flies are capable of passing through a screened stall; however, they prefer to feed on their hosts outdoors. Frequent use of permethrin-based repellents and fly wear is helpful for control. Applying an occlusive emollient to the inside of the pinnae may help prevent black fly bites. Severe reactions may need to be controlled with short courses of systemic glucocorticoids.

Culicoidae (mosquitoes)

Characteristics

There are over 3500 species of mosquitoes in the world, which are arranged into approximately 41 genera. The most common genera of mosquitoes include *Culex*, *Aedes*, and *Anopheles*. The flight habits are species dependent. Often, wind is a factor in dispersal or migration of mosquitoes. Most mosquitoes stay within a mile or two of their source but some have been recorded as far as 75 miles from their breeding source. In general, *Aedes* are strong fliers and are known to fly miles from their breeding sources. Conversely, *Culex* are generally weak fliers and do not move more than 2 miles from their breeding source. They are persistent and painful biters and prefer to attack at dusk and after dark, and will readily enter dwellings for blood meals; domestic and wild birds are preferred over man and horses. *Culex* mosquitoes usually live only a few weeks during the warm summer months. Most *Anopheles* mosquitoes are crepuscular (active at dusk or dawn) or nocturnal. Some *Anopheles* feed indoors (endophagic) while others feed outdoors (endophilic). *Aedes* mosquitoes attack during daylight hours and prefer to bite mammals. The process of a mosquito questing for a blood meal involves a complex, interconnected cascade of behaviours, each probably having its own clues, be they visual, thermal, or olfactory. Mosquito populations are largest during warm humid weather.

Life cycle and breeding sites

All mosquitoes go through four stages in their life cycle: egg, larva, pupa, and adult. The lifecycle of the mosquito is strongly influenced by ambient temperature. The first three stages are aquatic and last 5–14 days, depending on the species and temperature. The duration from egg to adult occurs in as little as 5 days but usually takes 10–14 days in tropical conditions. Water is a necessary part of the mosquito's habitat. The ideal breeding site for mosquitoes are various kinds of temporary stagnant water, ranging from small lakes to a collection of rain water in rain barrels, horse troughs, puddles, ditches, or old tires. Many mosquitoes do not need a large amount or pollution-free water for breeding; even a small tin can filled with rain water can be an ideal breeding place. Mosquitoes prefer water sheltered from the wind by grass and weeds.

Fecundity is related to the size of the blood meal. An adult female will feed every few days. Protein from the blood meal is necessary for ovarian maturation and subsequent egg maturation. Once the eggs are fully developed, the female lays them and resumes host seeking. This cycle is repeated until the female dies. Most females can survive up to a month in captivity but most probably do not live longer than 1–2 weeks in nature.

Aedes and *Anopheles* mosquitoes lay their eggs one at a time or attached to form 'rafts', which consists of up to 200 eggs, as noted with *Culex* mosquitoes. A mosquito may lay a raft of eggs every third night during its lifespan. Regardless of how the eggs are laid, they all have the capability to float on the water surface. Certain species of *Aedes* deposit their eggs on damp soil that will be flooded by water (salt water high tides, irrigated pastures, sewage effluent ponds, and rain water ponds). Floods result in synchronous development of a vast number of eggs, which may produce enormous swarms with the capacity to exsanguinate mature livestock within 24 hours [68]. Most eggs hatch into larvae within 48 hours; while others might withstand subzero temperatures during the winter before hatching.

Mosquito larvae are commonly called 'wigglers' and must live in water for 7 to 14 days depending on the water temperature. *Culex* larvae must come to the surface at frequent intervals to obtain oxygen through their siphon, whereas *Aedes* do not have a breathing tube and must lie parallel to the water surface to obtain their oxygen supply. The larvae feed on micro-organisms and particulate organic matter, including algae and small organisms that live in water. The larvae moult four times within 2 weeks and the stage between a moult is called an instar. At the end of each instar the larvae moult, shedding their exoskeleton to allow for further growth. When the larva has acquired enough energy and size, metamorphosis is triggered after the fourth instar changing the larva into a pupa.

Mosquito pupae are considered to be in the resting, non-feeding stage. The pupa is comma-shaped when viewed from the side. The head and thorax are merged into a cephalothorax, with the abdomen curving around underneath. The pupa must also come to the surface frequently to breathe through a pair of respiratory trumpets on the cephalothorax. After a few days as a pupa, the dorsal surface of the cephalothorax splits and the adult mosquito emerges.

Adult mosquitoes usually mate within a few days after emerging from the pupal stage. Adult mosquitoes have a slender body with three sections: head, thorax, and abdomen. The head is specialized for acquiring sensory information and for feeding. It contains eyes and a pair of long, many-segmented antennae. The antennae are important for detecting host odours as well as odours of breeding sites where females lay eggs. The head also has an elongate, forward-projecting proboscis used for feeding and two sensory palps. The detection of octenol is accomplished by receptor neurons housed within the sensilla of the maxillary palps [69]. Adult *Anopheles* can be identified by their typical resting position, that is with their abdomen sticking up in the air rather than parallel to the surface on which they are resting. Mosquito body size, as measured by wing size, is an important determinant of blood meal size and blood feeding tendency. An average-sized mosquito removes 3.9 µL of blood per meal.

Diseases

The repeated feeding of female mosquito on different hosts makes them efficient vectors of many pathogens. There role in transmitting equine zoonotic disease is most pertinent as they severe as intermediate hosts for zoonotic viral encephalitides, including eastern, western, and Venezuelan encephalomyelitis viruses, West Nile virus, and vesicular stomatitis.

Clinical features

When climatic conditions are favourable horses may be attacked by swarms of mosquitoes, resulting in visible distress followed by a multifocal papular to urticarial response. The urticaria is generally followed by short-term pruritus or pain, which generally resolves within 48 hours. Feeding site predilection for mosquitoes depends on the species. Considering the widespread exposure of horses to mosquitoes and the frequency of mosquito bites, owners do not commonly report irritation from mosquitoes as a presenting complaint to the veterinarian. Perhaps this is because cutaneous reactions resolve quickly and anaphylaxis due to mosquito bites has never been reported to occur in horses.

Control measures: environmental

Effective mosquito management requires the integration of a variety of available control strategies, i.e. surveillance, source reduction, biological control methods, traps, environmentally friendly larvicides, and, when necessary, the use of insecticides. It is impractical in most regions to completely eliminate mosquito breeding areas. Control is directed against both larval and adult stages.

Traps

The general idea of traps is to reduce the number of questing mosquitoes that would otherwise be affecting the horse. Many products claim to significantly reduce or even collapse local mosquito populations by decreasing the number of egg-laying females through their capture. Traps are designed to desiccate or electrocute the captured mosquitoes. All of the traps utilize some form of attractant that lures the host-seeking females to a capture or killing device. There may be seasonal and circadian variables that affect mosquito responses to certain attractants. Most traps use CO_2, either through combustion of propane or from a CO_2 cylinder, as the primary attractant. The release rate of the plume of CO_2 mimics human exhalation, thus making the trap specific for haematophagous insects seeking mammalian hosts. CO_2 synergized with octenol increases the attractiveness by several orders of magnitude. These devices will trap and kill measureable numbers of mosquitoes. Whether this will produce a noticeable reduction in the mosquito population in each case will depend on a number of factors, such as absolute mosquito population size, size and type of breeding habitat producing re-infestation, wind velocity and direction, as well as the species of mosquito present, just to name a few.

The BG-Sentinel (Biogents, Regensburg, Germany) mosquito trap is used by mosquito professionals worldwide and is considered to be one of the most effective traps on the market. The BG trap mimics ascending convection currents created by a human host and employs attractive visual cues. An added feature of this trap is that it does not need to use CO_2 to catch *Aedes* or *Culex* spp.; with the addition of CO_2 it can catch a broader range of blood-seeking species. A special, non-toxic BG-Lure (Biogents, Regensburg, Germany) emits artificial skin emanations, consisting of ammonia, lactic acid, and caproic acid, in finely tuned rations through a large surface area, for up to 5 months. The BG-trap is unable to reduce populations of millions of mosquitoes, which occur after floods, nor is it able to eliminate the mosquito problem over night, and finally it cannot capture mosquitoes if insecticides or pesticides are sprayed in or around the trap. These traps are left running 24 hours a day, 7 days a week for as long as possible, and should be kept running even if the mosquito population has decreased to ensure that newly hatched mosquitoes or migrating mosquitoes can still be captured. It is important to note that traps alone should not be used as a sole means of mosquito control. For more information about mosquito control the reader is referred to the website of the American Mosquito Control Association http://www.mosquito.org/.

Horse

Avoid outdoor areas during twilight. Some mosquitoes are active at night and *Aedes* spp. feed during the day. Use of protective fly wear and repellents are mandatory for control of mosquito insect hypersensitivity.

References

1. Aalberse RC. Structural biology of allergens. *Journal of Allergy and Clinical Immunology* 2000; **106**: 228–238.
2. Lorch G, Hillier A, Kwochka KW, *et al.* Results of intradermal tests in horses without atopy and horses with atopic dermatitis or

recurrent urticaria. *American Journal of Veterinary Research* 2001; **62**: 1051–1059.
3. Lowenstein H. Purification and characterization of allergens. Summing-up. *Allergy* 1980; **35**: 210–211.
4. Baur X, Aschauer H, Mazur G, *et al.* Structure, antigenic determinants of some clinically important insect allergens: chironomid hemoglobins. *Science* 1986; **233**: 351–354.
5. Langner KF, Darpel KE, Drolet BS, *et al.* Comparison of cellular and humoral immunoassays for the assessment of summer eczema in horses. *Veterinary Immunology and Immunopathology* 2008; **122**: 126–137.
6. Hellberg W, Mellor PS, Torsteinsdottir S, *et al.* Insect bite hypersensitivity in the horse: Comparison of IgE-binding proteins in salivary gland extracts from *Simulium vittatum* and *Culicoides nubeculosus*. *Veterinary Immunology and Immunopathology* 2009; **132**: 62–67.
7. Hellberg W, Wilson AD, Mellor P, *et al.* Equine insect bite hypersensitivity: Immunoblot analysis of IgE and IgG subclass responses to Culicoides nubeculosus salivary gland extract. *Veterinary Immunology and Immunopathology* 2006; **113**: 99–112.
8. Gibbs GM, Roelants K, O'Bryan MK. The CAP superfamily: cysteine-rich secretory proteins, antigen 5, and pathogenesis-related 1 proteins—roles in reproduction, cancer, and immune defense. *Endocrine Reviews* 2008; **29**: 865–897.
9. Peng Z, Simons FE. Comparison of proteins, IgE, and IgG binding antigens, and skin reactivity in commercial and laboratory-made mosquito extracts. *Annals of Allergy, Asthma and Immunology* 1996; **77**: 371–376.
10. Russell CL, Heesom KJ, Arthur CJ, *et al.* Identification and isolation of cDNA clones encoding the abundant secreted proteins in the saliva proteome of *Culicoides nubeculosus*. *Insect Molecular Biology* 2009; **18**: 383–393.
11. Schaffartzik A, Marti E, Torsteinsdottir S, *et al.* Selective cloning, characterization, and production of the Culicoides nubeculosus salivary gland allergen repertoire associated with equine insect bite hypersensitivity. *Veterinary Immunology and Immunopathology* 2011; **139**: 200–209.
12. Langner KF, Jarvis DL, Nimtz M, *et al.* Identification, expression and characterisation of a major salivary allergen (Cul s 1) of the biting midge Culicoides sonorensis relevant for summer eczema in horses. *International Journal of Parasitology* 2009; **39**: 243–250.
13. Schaffartzik A, Weichel M, Crameri R, *et al.* Cloning of IgE-binding proteins from *Simulium vittatum* and their potential significance as allergens for equine insect bite hypersensitivity. *Veterinary Immunology and Immunopathology* 2009; **132**: 68–77.
14. Ma D, Li Y, Dong J, *et al.* Purification and characterization of two new allergens from the salivary glands of the horsefly, *Tabanus yao*. *Allergy* 2011; **66**: 101–109.
15. Schaffartzik A, Marti E, Crameri R, *et al.* Cloning, production and characterization of antigen 5 like proteins from *Simulium vittatum* and *Culicoides nubeculosus*, the first cross-reactive allergen associated with equine insect bite hypersensitivity. *Veterinary Immunology and Immunopathology* 2010; **137**: 76–83.
16. Zeller S, Glaser AG, Vilhelmsson M, *et al.* Immunoglobulin-E-mediated reactivity to self antigens: a controversial issue. *International Archives of Allergy and Immunology* 2008; **145**: 87–93.
17. Fadok VA, Greiner EC. Equine insect hypersensitivity: skin test and biopsy results correlated with clinical data. *Equine Veterinary Journal* 1990; **22**: 236–240.
18. Quinn PJ, Baker KP, Morrow AN. Sweet itch: responses of clinically normal and affected horses to intradermal challenge with extracts of biting insects. *Equine Veterinary Journal* 1983; **15**: 266–272.
19. Eriksson S, Grandinson K, Fikse WF, *et al.* Genetic analysis of insect bite hypersensitivity (summer eczema) in Icelandic horses. *Animal* 2008; **2**: 360–365.
20. Andersson LS, Swinbune JE, Meadows JRS, *et al.* The same ELA class II risk factors confer equine insect bite hypersensitivity in two distinct populations. *Immunogenetics* 2012; **64**: 201–208.
21. Ishizaka K, Ishizaka T, Hornbrook MM. Physicochemical properties of reaginic antibody. V. Correlation of reaginic activity with gamma-E-globulin antibody. *Journal of Immunology* 1996; **97**: 840–853.
22. Johansson SG, Bennich H. Immunological studies of an atypical (myeloma) immunoglobulin. *Immunology* 1967; **13**: 381–394.
23. Wagner B, Miller WH, Morgan EE, *et al.* IgE and IgG antibodies in skin allergy of the horse. *Veterinary Research* 2006; **37**: 813–825.
24. Gleich GJ, Adolphson CR, Leiferman KM. The biology of the eosinophilic leukocyte. *Annual Reviews in Medicine* 1993; **44**: 85–101.
25. Rivera J, Gilfillan AM. Molecular regulation of mast cell activation. *Journal of Allergy and Clinical Immunology* 2006; **117**: 1214–1225; quiz 1226.
26. Fadok VA, Foil L. Equine insect hypersensitivity workshop report. In: von Tscharner C, Halliwell REW, eds. *Advances in Veterinary Dermatology, Vol. 2*. London: Bailliere-Tindall, 1992: 390–394.
27. Anderson GS, Belton P, Kleider N. The hypersensitivity of horses to culicoides bites in British Columbia. *Canadian Veterinary Journal* 1998; **29**: 718–723.
28. Halldorsdottir S, Larsen HJ. An epidemiological study of summer eczema in Icelandic horses in Norway. *Equine Veterinary Journal* 1991;**23**: 296–299.
29. Riek RF. Studies on allergic dermatitis (Queensland itch) of the horse I and II. *Australian Veterinary Journal* 1953; **29**: 177–184.
30. Anderson GS, Belton P, Kleider N. Hypersensitivity of horses in British Columbia to extracts of native and exotic species of Culicoides (Diptera: Ceratopogonidae). *Journal of Medical Entomology* 1993; **30**: 657–663.
31. Kolm-Stark G, Wagner R. Intradermal skin testing in Icelandic horses in Austria. *Equine Veterinary Journal* 2002; **34**: 405–410.
32. Morris DO, Lindborg S. Determination of 'irritant' threshold concentrations for intradermal testing with allergenic insect extracts in normal horses. *Veterinary Dermatology* 2003; **14**: 31–36.
33. Wagner B, Childs BA, Erb HN. A histamine release assay to identify sensitization to *Culicoides* allergens in horses with skin hypersensitivity. *Veterinary Immunology and Immunopathology* 2008; **126**: 302–308.
34. Baselgia S, Doherr MG, Mellor R, *et al.* Evaluation of an in vitro sulphidoleukotriene release test for diagnosis of insect bite hypersensitivity in horses. *Equine Veterinary Journal* 2006; **38**: 40–46.
35. Frey R, Bergvall K, Egenvall A. Allergen-specific IgE in Icelandic horses with insect bite hypersensitivity and healthy controls, assessed by Fcepsilon R1 alpha-based serology. *Veterinary Immunology and Immunopathology* 2008; **126**: 102–109.
36. Eder C, Crameri R, Mayer C, *et al.* Allergen-specific IgE levels against crude mould and storage mite extracts and recombinant mould allergens in sera from horses affected with chronic bronchitis. *Veterinary Immunology and Immunopathology* 2000; **73**: 241–253.
37. Lorch G, Hillier A, Kwochka KW, *et al.* Comparison of immediate intradermal test reactivity with serum IgE quantitation by use of a radioallergosorbent test and two ELISA in horses with and

without atopy. *Journal of the American Veterinary Medical Association* 2001; **218**: 1314–1322.

38. Morgan EE, Miller WH, Wagner B. A comparison of intradermal testing and detection of allergen-specific immunoglobulin E in serum by enzyme-linked immunosorbent assay in horses affected with skin hypersensitivity. *Veterinary Immunology and Immunopathology* 2007; **120**: 160–167.
39. Rufenacht S, Marti E, von Tscharner C, *et al.* Immunoglobulin E-bearing cells and mast cells in skin biopsies of horses with urticaria. *Veterinary Dermatology* 2005; **16**: 94–101.
40. van der Haegen A, Griot-Wenk M, Welle M, *et al.* Immunoglobulin-E-bearing cells in skin biopsies of horses with insect bite hypersensitivity. *Equine Veterinary Journal* 2001; **33**: 699–706.
41. Barbet JL, Bevier D, Greiner EC. Specific immunotherapy in the treatment of *Culicoides* hypersensitive horses: a double-blind study. *Equine Veterinary Journal* 1990; **22**: 232–235.
42. Fairchild GB. A catalog of the Tabanidade (Diptera) of the Americas south of the United States. *Memoirs of the American Entomology Institute,* 1994: 249.
43. Okiwelu SN. Seasonal distribution and variations in diurnal activity of tabanidae in Republic-of-Zambia. *Mosquitoe News* 1975; **35**: 551–554.
44. Roberts RH. Diurnal activity of Tabanidae based on collections in malaise traps. *Mosquitoe News* 1974; **34**: 220–223.
45. Horvath G, Majer J, Horvath L, *et al.* Ventral polarization vision in tabanids: horseflies and deerflies (Diptera: Tabanidae) are attracted to horizontally polarized light. *Naturwissenschaften* 2008; **95**: 1093–1100.
46. Hollander AL, Wright RE. Impact of tabanids on cattle: blood meal size and preferred feeding sites. *Journal of Economic Entomology* 1980; **73**: 431–433.
47. Zhao R, Yu X, Yu H, *et al.* Immunoregulatory peptides from salivary glands of the horsefly, Tabanuspleskei. *Comparative Biochemistry and Physiology, Part B* 2009; **154**: 1–5.
48. Grevelink SA, Youssef DE, Loscalzo J, *et al.* Salivary gland extracts from the deerfly contain a potent inhibitor of platelet aggregation. *Proceedings of the National Academy of Sciences USA* 1993; **90**: 9155–9158.
49. Markwardt F, Schulz E. On the mechanism of the inhibitory effect of tabanine on blood coagulation. *Naunyn Schmiedebergs Archiv fur Pharmakologie und Experimentelle Pathologie* 1960; **238**: 320–328.
50. Markwardt F. Coagulation inhibitors from blood-sucking animals. A new line of developing antithrombotic drugs. *Pharmazie* 1994; **49**: 313–316.
51. Krinsky WL. Animal disease agents transmitted by horse flies and deer flies (Diptera: Tabanidae). *Journal of Medical Entomology* 1976; **13**: 225–275.
52. Foil LD. Tabanids as vectors of disease agents. *Parasitology Today* 1989; **5**: 88–96.
53. Luger SW. Lyme disease transmitted by a biting fly. *New England Journal of Medicine* 1990; **322**: 1752.
54. Horvath G, Blaho M, Kriska G, *et al.* An unexpected advantage of whiteness in horses: the most horsefly-proof horse has a depolarizing white coat. *Proceedings of the Royal Society B-Biological Sciences* 2010; **277**: 1643–1650.
55. Muzari MO, Skerratt LF, Jones RE, *et al.* Alighting and feeding behaviour of tabanid flies on horses, kangaroos and pigs. *Veterinary Parasitology* 2010; **170**: 104–111.
56. Barros AT, Foil LD. The influence of distance on movement of tabanids (Diptera: Tabanidae) between horses. *Veterinary Parasitology* 2007; **144**: 380–384.
57. Mihok S, Mulye H. Responses of tabanids to Nzi traps baited with octenol, cow urine and phenols in Canada. *Medical and Veterinary Entomology* 2010; **24**: 266–272.
58. Krčmar S, Mikuška A, Radolić V. Comparison of sampling tabanids (Diptera: Tabanidae) by four different potential attractants. *Journal of Applied Entomology* 2010; **134**: 608–613.
59. Jacobs JW, Cupp EW, Sardana M, *et al.* Isolation and characterization of a coagulation factor Xa inhibitor from black fly salivary glands. *Thrombosis and Haemostasis* 1990; **64**: 235–238.
60. Abebe M, Ribeiro JM, Cupp MS, *et al.* Novel anticoagulant from salivary glands of *Simuliumvittatum* (Diptera: Simuliidae) inhibits activity of coagulation factor V. *Journal of Medical Entomology* 1996; **33**: 173–176.
61. Abebe M, Cupp MS, Ramberg FB, *et al.* Anticoagulant activity in salivary gland extracts of black flies (Diptera: Simuliidae). *Journal of Medical Entomology* 1994; **31**: 908–911.
62. Cupp MS, Ribeiro JM, Cupp EW. Vasodilative activity in black fly salivary glands. *American Journal of Tropical Medicine and Hygiene* 1994; **50**: 241–246.
63. Tsujimoto H, Gray EW, Champagne DE. Black fly salivary gland extract inhibits proliferation and induces apoptosis in murine splenocytes. *Parasite Immunology* 2010; **32**: 275–284.
64. Cross ML, Cupp MS, Cupp EW, *et al.* Modulation of murine immunological responses by salivary gland extract of *Simulium vittatum* (Diptera: Simuliidae). *Journal of Medical Entomology* 1993; **30**: 928–935.
65. Saint Andre A, Blackwell NM, Hall LR, *et al.* The role of endosymbiotic *Wolbachia* bacteria in the pathogenesis of river blindness. *Science* 2002; **295**: 1892–1895.
66. Cupp EW, Mare CJ, Cupp MS, *et al.* Biological transmission of vesicular stomatitis virus (New Jersey) by Simulium vittatum (Diptera: Simuliidae). *Journal of Medical Entomology* 1992; **29**: 137–140.
67. Tang X, Adler PH, Vogel H, *et al.* Gender-specific bacterial composition of black flies (Diptera: Simuliidae). *Federation of European Microbiological Societies* 2012; **80**: 659–670.
68. Abbitt B, Abbitt LG. Fatal exsanguination of cattle attributed to an attack of salt marsh mosquitoes (*Aedes sollicitans*). *Journal of the American Veterinary Medical Association* 1981; **179**: 1397–1400.
69. Grant AJ, Dickens JC. Functional characterization of the octenol receptor neuron on the maxillary palps of the yellow fever mosquito, *Aedesa egypti. PLos One* 2011; **6**: e21785.

Website

American Mosquito Control Association(AMCA)http://www.mosquito.org/(accessed 29 May, 2012).

Section 2

Atopic Disease in Horses—Atopic Dermatitis and Food Hypersensitivity

49

Equine atopic dermatitis: pathogenesis

Valerie A. Fadok

North Houston Veterinary Specialists, Spring, TX, USA

Conflict of interest: none declared.

Horses develop a number of skin and respiratory disorders that have been attributed to allergy. These include pruritic skin diseases, recurrent urticaria, allergic rhinoconjunctivitis, and reactive airway disease. Allergen-specific IgE has been detected in these horses and allergen-specific immunotherapy used to ameliorate clinical signs [1–4].

Defining atopic dermatitis

The term 'atopy' describes an inherited predisposition to a constellation of diseases characterized by hyper-reactivity to environmental allergens, including foods. These diseases in humans include allergic rhinitis and conjunctivitis, asthma, and atopic dermatitis. Production of IgE in response to the offending allergens is part of the disease process; the production of allergen-specific IgE is the basis of intradermal testing and serum testing used to select allergens for immunotherapy. In the past, the production of IgE and its binding to the high-affinity Fc epsilon receptor on mast cells and basophils was the centrepiece of our understanding of atopy. Allergenic proteins were believed to be inhaled and somehow transported to the skin and mucous membranes, where they bound to and cross-linked cell-bound IgE. The rapid release of histamine and other preformed inflammatory mediators within minutes (Type I hypersensitivity reaction) was followed by the later release of lipid mediators, such as leukotrienes and cytokines that mediated inflammation (the late-phase IgE response). While we know that these pathways occur, we have learned that the pathogenesis of atopic dermatitis is much more complex.

Most of what we know about atopic dermatitis has come from studies of the spontaneous human disease and experimental models in mice [5–13]. Many of the features described for the human disease have also been verified in the canine disease, as least preliminarily [14–17]. The familial predisposition to atopy is associated with the potential inheritance of a large number of polymorphic genes that affect the function of the innate and acquired immune responses, as well as the structure and function of the skin barrier [18–19]. Abnormalities in the skin barrier are believed to allow for cutaneous absorption of allergenic proteins, which are taken up by dendritic cells and carried to the lymph node. Naïve T lymphocytes are activated and because the immune response is skewed toward a T helper 2 response, IgE production is induced and a variety of cytokines, including IL-4, IL-5, IL-6, IL-13, and IL-31, are released (Figures 49.1 and 49.2). An eosinophilic inflammatory infiltrate and itch are significant features of the atopic response in the skin. Allergen-specific IgE binds not only to mast cells and basophils, but also to Langerhans cells and other dendritic cells within the skin and mucous membranes and serves to capture allergen very efficiently. Subsequent exposure to the allergen results in amplification of the allergic response locally. Lack of suppression by T regulatory cells is part of the disease process, although it is not clear whether decreased T regulatory cell function is a cause or result of the disease process.

There is a complex interplay between the immune system and the nervous system, which promotes the

Veterinary Allergy, First Edition. Edited by Chiara Noli, Aiden Foster, and Wayne Rosenkrantz.

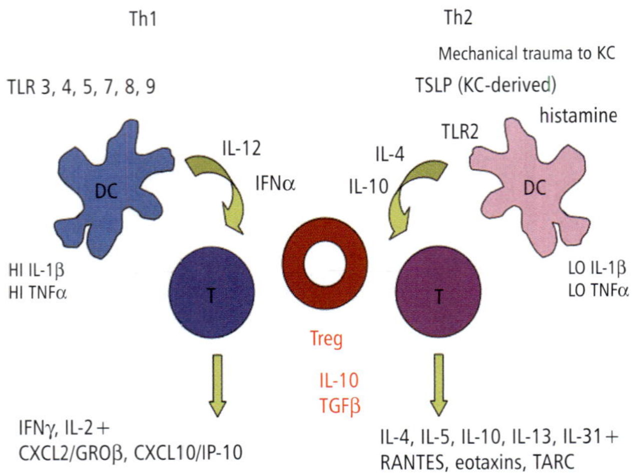

Figure 49.1 Simplified diagram of T helper 1 (Th1) and T helper 2 (Th2) pathways. Stimulation of toll-like receptors (TLR) on dendritic cells promotes the Th1 response in the presence of high levels of interleukin beta (IL-1β) and tumour necrosis factor alpha (TNF-α). Following stimulation of these TLR, interleukin-12 (IL-12) and interferon-alpha (IFN-α) are produced, driving the production of Th1 from naïve T cells. Th1 produce interferon gamma (IFN-γ), interleukin-2 (IL-2), as well as the chemokines listed. By contrast, in the presence of low levels of IL-1 and TNF-α, stimulation of dendritic cells by keratinocyte-derived cytokines, including thymic stromal lymphopoietin (TSLP), as well as histamine and TLR2 ligands, result in induction of the Th2 pathway. Cytokines including IL-4, IL-5, IL-10, IL-13, and IL-31 are produced. Multiple gene polymorphisms contribute to the determination of which pathway will predominate. T regulatory cells (Treg), producing interleukin-10 (IL-10) and transforming growth factor-beta (TGF-β), can down-modulate either pathway. KC, keratinocyte; HI, high; LO, low; DC, dendritic cell; T, T cell; CXCL, chemokine (C-X-C motif) ligand; RANTES, regulated on activation normal T cell expressed and secreted; TARC, thymus and activation regulated chemokine.

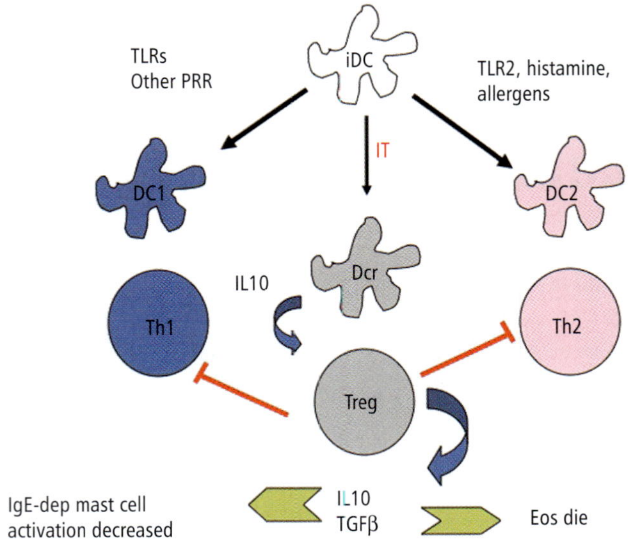

Figure 49.2 Proposed mechanisms of allergen-specific immunotherapy. It has been hypothesized that specific subsets of dendritic cells (DC) drive the T helper response. Immunotherapy is believed to activate the regulatory DC (DCr) that activates regulatory T cells. Production of IL-10 can decrease the IgE-dependent mast cell degranulation; TGF-β can induce eosinophil apoptosis. Treg inhibit both Th1 and Th2 responses. PRR, pattern recognition receptors; iDC, immature dendritic cell; IT, immunotherapy; Eos, eosinophil, TLR, toll-like receptor.

sensation of itch [10,20–23]. Th2 cytokines, particularly IL-31, directly stimulate itch by binding to their receptors on nerve fibres. Other pruritogenic mediators, including histamine, proteases, substance P, opioids, neurotrophins, and other neuroactive peptides, enhance the itch. Secondary infections with staphylococci and *Malassezia* yeast are frequent and further aggravate the level of itch. Inflammatory proteins from these microbes are absorbed more readily through the impaired skin barrier and contribute further to its breakdown. Staphylococci promote a Th2 response, and many patients can develop IgE against bacterial and yeast proteins, resulting in bacterial and yeast hypersensitivity. Over time, as the disease becomes chronic, there is a shift toward the T helper 1 cytokine response, with TNF alpha playing a more prominent role.

We have known for some time that the model of Th2/Th1 imbalance can be used to explain the immunological abnormalities associated with respiratory allergies, but recent studies have shown that an epithelial barrier defect likely contributes to these diseases as well. Using biopsies from human patients with and without chronic rhinosinusitis, investigators measured trans-tissue resistance and found it reduced in samples from affected patients [24]. Furthermore, they showed that the components of tight junctions, occluden and zonula occudens 1, were patchy, irregular, and decreased in diseased tissue. By culturing respiratory epithelial cells in an air–liquid interface, these finding could be replicated *in vitro*. Addition of IFNγ and IL-4 could mimic these changes when applied to epithelial cultures from normal individuals. Interestingly, a polymorphism in SPINK5 (serine protease inhibitor Kazal type 5), identified in human patients with atopic dermatitis, has also been incriminated in human patients with asthma and chronic sinusitis [19,25,26]. This polymorphism is believed to be a marker for atopy in general. SPINK5 is expressed in all epithelial tissues and is believed to inhibit the function of serine proteases. Another epithelial product central to atopy is the cytokine TSLP (thymic stromal lymphopoietin) [27]. This cytokine is produced by damaged epithelial cells and it is known to induce the Th2 phenotype in atopic dermatitis, allergic rhinoconjunctivitis, and asthma.

The evidence for atopic dermatitis in horses

It makes sense to hypothesize that similar mechanisms mediate atopic diseases in horses and evidence is slowly accumulating. The disease most like atopic dermatitis is the pruritus and dermatitis associated with *Culicoides* hypersensitivity (see Chapter 43) and, in some horses, associated with intradermal or serum test reactions to environmental allergens. In order to call the disease atopic dermatitis, we must verify that horses make IgE in response to environmental allergens, that they have an imbalance between Th2 and Th1 cells, that they absorb allergens through the skin, and that they have an impaired skin barrier. It is very clear that horses make IgE [28–34] and that allergen-specific IgE can be detected using intradermal and/or serum testing [35–39]. Based on what we know about mammalian IgE, we can make the assumption that horses, like other allergic mammals, use the same immunologic mechanisms. While we lack evidence with regard to pollens, moulds, dusts, or danders, there is good evidence that a Th2/Th1 imbalance is involved in horses with Culicoides hypersensitivity and that this insect bite hypersensitivity shares many features with atopic dermatitis (see Chapters 45 and 50).

Heimann *et al.* [40] used immunohistochemical staining to compare the distribution of $CD4^+$, $CD8^+$, and $FoxP3^+$ T regulatory cells between normal horses and those with insect hypersensitivity. As one would predict, there were increased numbers of T cells in the affected horses, but ratios of $FoxP^+$ T cells/$CD4^+$ were significantly lower in affected horses compared to normal horses [40]. Cytokine expression was assessed by real-time quantitative RT-PCR. Affected horses showed elevated mRNA levels for IL-13 in lesional and non-lesional skin, and lower mRNA levels for IL-10 in lesional skin. These data could support the hypothesis that insect hypersensitivity in horses is associated with imbalances in the ratio of T helper 2 cytokines and those produced by regulatory T cells. However, until the expression and function of the cytokine proteins have been demonstrated, we can come to no firm conclusions.

Hamza *et al.* [41] took a different approach by culturing equine peripheral blood mononuclear cells (PBMC) in the presence of mitogen, insect allergens, or irrelevant allergens. The cells were subsequently examined by flow cytometry for cytokine production and total cytokine measured by ELISA. There were seasonal differences in cytokine production from horses with insect hypersensitivity. Increased production of total IL-4, increased numbers of IL-4 producing cells and decreased production of IFN-gamma was seen in the summer, when lesions were active [41]. Subsequent studies showed that reduced incidence of insect hypersensitivity was associated with down-regulation of IL-4 producing cells and increased expression of IL-10 and TGF-beta [42]. Equine PBMC from affected Icelandic horses, when stimulated with *Culicoides* allergen, produced lower numbers of $FoxP3^+$ T regulatory cells than did those from healthy horses [43]. Addition of IL-4 to the cells of healthy horses was able to reduce the number of T regulatory cells. These data suggested that the decrease in T regulatory cells was secondary, rather than a primary cause of susceptibility to insect hypersensitivity. Last, equine TSLP has been cloned, expressed, and antibodies against it developed, which will allow for study of the role of this cytokine in skin and respiratory allergies [44].

Information about the genetic factors associated with insect hypersensitivities is slowly accumulating [45]. Differential gene expression in equine asthma is revealing potential new targets for therapy [46]. As these data accumulate, we should be able to discover commonalities between horses and other animals with atopic disease, but also interesting differences that will teach us about the complex interplay between environment and genetics in allergic disease.

Barrier dysfunction is considered an integral part of the pathogenesis of atopic dermatitis. In fact, the skin barrier and the immune response are believed to be tightly linked [47]. We know very little about the skin barrier of horses. An abstract presented at the World Congress of Veterinary Dermatology (2012) established that some of the ultrastructural changes associated with barrier defects in humans and dogs were seen in the skin of one atopic horse [48]. This finding supports continued study into the barrier function of horses and whether barrier repair will become part of a multimodal approach to the management of atopic dermatitis in horses.

Food allergy in horses as part of atopic diathesis

The role of food allergy in equine skin disease remains a mystery. While food allergy is believed to occur, there is very little in peer-reviewed literature about its prevalence, its causes, or its pathogenesis. Anecdotal reports that chronic urticaria can be caused by food allergy suggests a role for IgE, but there is no hard evidence. We have absolutely no information about the pathophysiology of food allergy in horses.

Mechanisms mediating food allergy in humans can be humoral or cell mediated. IgE-mediated disease results in the rapid onset of clinical signs after exposure to the food; cellular mechanisms may have a more delayed onset. Food allergy manifestations in humans include urticaria and angioedema, but also eosinophilic oesophagitis, and gastroenteritis. Many of the mechanisms mediating atopic disease in skin and the respiratory tract have been demonstrated in the gut. Memory T cells specific for gut-associated allergens home preferentially to the gut upon re-exposure [49] and dendritic cells have been shown to induce the Th2 response to food allergens [50,51]. Immunologic tolerance in the gut is actively mediated by regulatory T cells, which are induced by dendritic cells residing in the gut [52]. Experimental induction of food allergy requires genetic predisposition, adjuvants, and bypassing oral tolerance by exposure through other routes. Likely these requirements are needed in the clinical disease as well; disruption of the gut barrier by immunologic and non-immunologic mechanisms, along with increased food allergen load set the gut up for an allergic reaction [53]. Of interest is the fact that newer evidence suggests that food allergy may be induced by exposure through a disrupted skin barrier and that early oral exposure actually leads to tolerance [54]. Because the gut microflora are believed to play a critical role in the establishment of oral tolerance, the use of probiotics has been studied and shown to have beneficial results in the management of food allergy [55].

The only reports of food allergy in peer-reviewed literature relate to horses with recurrent urticaria; the implication would be that these are mediated by allergen-specific IgE [56–59]. Popular opinion suggests that pruritic skin disease might also have food allergy as a cause. The role of a Th2 helper response in equine food allergy remains to be determined.

References

1. Tallarico NJ, Tallarico CM. Results of intradermal allergy testing and treatment by hyposensitization of 53 horses with chronic obstructive pulmonary disease, urticaria, headshaking, and/or reactive airway disease. *Journal of Veterinary Allergy and Clinical Immunology* 1998; **6**: 25–35.
2. Rees CA. Response to immunotherapy in six related horses with urticaria secondary to atopy. *Journal of the American Veterinary Medical Association* 2001; **218**: 753–755.
3. Loewenstein C, Mueller RS. A review of allergen-specific immunotherapy in human and veterinary medicine. *Veterinary Dermatology* 2009; **20**: 84–98.
4. Stepnik CT, Outerbridge CA, White SD, *et al.* Equine atopic skin disease and response to allergen-specific immunotherapy: A retrospective study at the University of California-Davis (1991–2008). *Veterinary Dermatology* 2012; **23**: 29–35, e7.
5. Novak N, Leung DY. Advances in atopic dermatitis. *Current Opinion in Immunology* 2011; **23**: 778–783.
6. Moniaga CS, Kabashima K. Filaggrin in atopic dermatitis: Flaky tail mice as a novel model for developing drug targets in atopic dermatitis. *Inflammation and Allergy Drug Targets* 2011; **10**: 477–485.
7. Simon D, Kernland Lang K. Atopic dermatitis: From new pathogenic insights toward a barrier-restoring and anti-inflammatory therapy. *Current Opinion in Pediatrics* 2011; **23**: 647–652.
8. Rahman S, Collins M, Williams CM, *et al.* The pathology and immunology of atopic dermatitis. *Inflammation and Allergy Drug Targets* 2011; **10**: 486–496.
9. Boguniewicz M, Leung DY. Atopic dermatitis: A disease of altered skin barrier and immune dysregulation. *Immunology Reviews* 2011; **242**: 233–246.
10. Tanaka A, Matsuda H. Evaluation of itch by using NC/ngaTnd mice: A model of human atopic dermatitis. *Journal of Biomedicine and Biotechnology* 2011; **2011**: 790436.
11. Takeda K, Gelfand EW. Mouse models of allergic diseases. *Current Opinion in Immunology* 2009; **21**: 660–665.
12. Jin H, He R, Oyoshi M, *et al.* Animal models of atopic dermatitis. *Journal of Investigative Dermatology* 2009; **129**: 31–40.
13. Scharschmidt TC, Segre JA. Modeling atopic dermatitis with increasingly complex mouse models. *Journal of Investigative Dermatology* 2008; **128**: 1061–1064.
14. Marsella R, Sousa CA, Gonzales AJ, *et al.* Current understanding of the pathophysiologic mechanisms of canine atopic dermatitis. *Journal of the American Veterinary Medical Association* 2012; **241**: 194–207.
15. Olivry T. Is the skin barrier abnormal in dogs with atopic dermatitis? *Veterinary Immunology and Immunopathology* 2011; **144**: 11–16.
16. Marsella R, Olivry T, Carlotti DN, International Task Force on Canine Atopic Dermatitis. Current evidence of skin barrier dysfunction in human and canine atopic dermatitis. *Veterinary Dermatology* 2011; **22**: 239–248.
17. Marsella R, Girolomoni G. Canine models of atopic dermatitis: A useful tool with untapped potential. *Journal of Investigative Dermatology* 2009; **129**: 2351–2357.
18. Grammatikos AP. The genetic and environmental basis of atopic diseases. *Annals of Medicine* 2008; **40**: 482–495.
19. Brown SJ, McLean WH. Eczema genetics: current state of knowledge and future goals. *Journal of Investigative Dermatology* 2009; **129**: 543–552.
20. Suárez AL, Feramisco JD, Koo J, *et al.* Psychoneuroimmunology of psychological stress and atopic dermatitis: pathophysiologic and therapeutic updates. *Actadermato-venereologica* 2012; **92**: 7–15.
21. Hong J, Buddenkotte J, Berger TG, *et al.* Management of itch in atopic dermatitis. *Seminars in Cutaneous Medicine and Surgery* 2011; **30**: 71–86.
22. Lee CH, Yu HS. Biomarkers for itch and disease severity in atopic dermatitis. *Current Problems in Dermatology* 2011; **41**: 136–148.
23. Darsow U, Pfab F, Valet M, *et al.* Pruritus and atopic dermatitis. *Clinical Reviews in Allergy and Immunology* 2011; **41**: 237–244.
24. Soyka MB, Wawrzyniak P, Eiwegger T, *et al.* Defective epithelial barrier in chronic rhinosinusitis: the regulation of tight junctions by IFN-γ and IL-4. *Journal of Allergy and Clinical Immunology* 2012; **130**: 1087–1096, e10.
25. Liu Q, Xia Y, Zhang W, *et al.* A functional polymorphism in the SPINK5 gene is associated with asthma in a Chinese han population. *BMC Medical Genetics* 2009; **10**: 59.
26. Zhao LP, Di Z, Zhang L, *et al.* Association of SPINK5 gene polymorphisms with atopic dermatitis in northeast china. *Journal of the European Academy of Dermatology and Venereology* 2012; **26**: 572–577.
27. Ito T, Liu YJ, Arima K. Cellular and molecular mechanisms of TSLP function in human allergic disorders-TSLP programs the "TH2 code" in dendritic cells. *Allergology International* 2012; **61**: 35–43.
28. Suter M, Fey H. Isolation and characterization of equine IgE. *Zentralbl Veterinarmed B Journal of Veterinary Medicine Series B* 1981; **28**: 414–420.

29. Matthews AG, Imlah P, McPherson EA. A reagin-like antibody in horse serum: 1. Occurrence and some biological properties. *Veterinary Research Communications* 1983; **6**: 13–23.
30. Suter M, Fey H. Further purification and characterisation of horse IgE. *Veterinary Immunology and Immunopathology* 1983; **4**: 545–553.
31. Marti E, Peveri P, Griot-Wenk M, *et al.* Chicken antibodies to a recombinant fragment of the equine immunoglobulin epsilon heavy-chain recognising native horse IgE. *Veterinary Immunology and Immunopathology* 1997; **59**: 253–270.
32. Wagner B, Radbruch A, Rohwer J, *et al.* Monoclonal anti-equine IgE antibodies with specificity for different epitopes on the immunoglobulin heavy chain of native IgE. *Veterinary Immunology and Immunopathology* 2003; **92**: 45–60.
33. Wagner B, Miller WH, Morgan EE, *et al.* IgE and IgG antibodies in skin allergy of the horse. *Veterinary Research* 2006; **37**: 813–825.
34. Wagner B. IgE in horses: Occurrence in health and disease. *Veterinary Immunology and Immunopathology* 2009; **132**: 21–30.
35. Lorch G, Hillier A, Kwochka KW, *et al.* Results of intradermal tests in horses without atopy and horses with atopic dermatitis or recurrent urticaria. *American Journal of Veterinary Research* 2001; **62**: 1051–1059.
36. Lorch G, Hillier A, Kwochka KW, *et al.* Comparison of immediate intradermal test reactivity with serum IgE quantitation by use of a radioallergosorbent test and two ELISA in horses with and without atopy. *Journal of the American Veterinary Medical Association* 2001; **218**: 1314–1322.
37. Kalina WV, Pettigrew HD, Gershwin LJ. IgE ELISA using antisera derived from epsilon chain antigenic peptides detects allergen-specific IgEin allergic horses. *Veterinary Immunology and Immunopathology* 2003; **92**: 137–147.
38. Morgan EE, Miller WH, Wagner B. A comparison of intradermal testing and detection of allergen-specific immunoglobulin E in serum by enzyme-linked immunosorbent assay in horses affected with skin hypersensitivity. *Veterinary Immunology and Immunopathology* 2007; **120**: 160–167.
39. Petersen A, Schott HC. Effects of dexamethasone and hydroxyzine treatment on intradermal testing and allergen-specific IgE serum testing results in horses. *Veterinary Dermatology* 2009; **20**: 615–622.
40. Heimann M, Janda J, Sigurdardottir OG, *et al.* Skin-infiltrating T cells and cytokine expression in icelandic horses affected with insect bite hypersensitivity: A possible role for regulatory T cells. *Veterinary Immunology and Immunopathology* 2011; **140**: 63–74.
41. Hamza E, Doherr MG, Bertoni G, *et al.* Modulation of allergy incidence in Icelandic horses is associated with a change in IL-4-producing T cells. *International Archives of Allergy and Immunology* 2007; **144**: 325–337.
42. Hamza E, Wagner B, Jungi TW, *et al.* Reduced incidence of insect-bite hypersensitivity in Icelandic horses is associated with a down-regulation of interleukin-4 by interleukin-10 and transforming growth factor-beta1. *Veterinary Immunology and Immunopathology* 2008; **122**: 65–75.
43. Hamza E, Steinbach F, Marti E. CD4(+)CD25(+) T cells expressing foxp3 in Icelandic horses affected with insect bite hypersensitivity. *Veterinary Immunology and Immunopathology* 2012; **148**: 139–144.
44. Janda J, Plattet P, Torsteinsdottir S, *et al.* Generation of equine TSLP-specific antibodies and their use for detection of TSLP produced by equine keratinocytes and leukocytes. *Veterinary Immunology and Immunopathology* 2012; **147**: 180–186.
45. Andersson LS, Swinburne JE, Meadows JR, *et al.* The same ELA class II risk factors confer equine insect bite hypersensitivity in two distinct populations. *Immunogenetics* 2012; **64**: 201–208.
46. Lavoie JP, Lefebvre-Lavoie J, Leclere M, *et al.* Profiling of differentially expressed genes using suppression subtractive hybridization in an equine model of chronic asthma. *PLoS One* 2012; **7**: e29440.
47. De Benedetto A, Kubo A, Beck LA. Skin barrier disruption: a requirement for allergen sensitization? *Journal of Investigative Dermatology* 2012; **132**: 949–963.
48. Marsella R, Samuelson D, Johnson C, *et al.* Pilot investigation on skin barrier in equine atopic dermatitis: observations on electron microscopy and measurements of transepidermal water loss. *Veterinary Dermatology* 2012; **23** (Suppl. 1): 77
49. Islam SA, Luster AD. T cell homing to epithelial barriers in allergic disease. *Nature Medicine* 2012; **18**: 705–715.
50. Ruiter B, Shreffler WG. The role of dendritic cells in food allergy. *Journal of Allergy and Clinical Immunology* 2012; **129**: 921–928.
51. Kim JS, Sampson HA. Food allergy: a glimpse into the inner workings of gut immunology. *Current Opinion in Gastroenterology* 2012; **28**: 99–103.
52. Berin MC. Mechanisms of allergic sensitization to foods: bypassing immune tolerance pathways. *Immunology and Allergy Clinics of North America* 2012; **32**: 1–10.
53. Kunisawa J, Kiyono H. Aberrant interaction of the gut immune system with environmental factors in the development of food allergies. *Current Allergy and Asthma Reports* 2010; **10**: 215–221.
54. Lack G. Update on risk factors for food allergy. *Journal of Allergy and Clinical Immunology* 2012; **129**: 1187–1197.
55. Gigante G, Tortora A, Ianiro G, *et al.* Role of gut microbiota in food tolerance and allergies. *Digestive Diseases* 2011; **29**: 540–549.
56. Miyazawa K, Ito M, Ohsaki K. An equine case of urticaria associated with dry garlic feeding. *Journal of Veterinary Medical Science* 1991; **53**: 747–748.
57. Hallebeek AJ, Sloet van Oldruitenborgh-Oosterbaan MM. Oat bumps' in horses. Differential diagnosis and nutritional aspects. *Tijdschrift voor Diergeneeskunde* (In Dutch) 1995; **120**: 588–591.
58. Francqueville M, Sabbah A. Chronic urticaria in sports horses. *Allergieet Immunologie (Paris)* (In French) 1999; **31**: 212–213.
59. Volland-Francqueville M, Sabbah A. Recurrent or chronic urticaria in thoroughbred race-horses: Clinical observations. *European Annals of Allergy and Clinical Immunology* 2004; **36**: 9–12.

50

Clinical aspects of equine atopic disease

Wayne Rosenkrantz[1] and Stephen White[2]

[1]Animal Dermatology Clinic, Tustin, CA, USA
[2]School of Veterinary Medicine, University of California, Davis, CA, USA

Conflict of interest: Wayne Rosenkrantz: Medical Advisory boards and/or speaking: Pinnaclife Animal Health; Novartis Animal Health; Zoetis Animal Health; Elanco Animal Health; Veterinary Allergy Reference Lab (VARL) and Merck Animal Health.

Introduction

As discussed in Chapter 49, this condition is not as well defined and characterized in horses as it is in other species. While pruritus is typically considered the main clinical sign of atopic skin disease in most species [1–3], it has been reported that in the horse clinical signs may also include urticaria with or without pruritus [4–6]. It has also been implicated in recurrent airway obstruction (RAO) or inflammatory airway disease (IAD) [7,8]. Other ill-defined conditions that may be presented with and associated with atopic disease are eosinophilic granulomas, laminitis, and head tossing or shaking [9] (see section 'Concurrent diseases').

History and signalment

The disease may be seasonal or non-seasonal, depending on the allergen(s) involved. Similar to other species, the disease may start off more seasonal but progress to more year round disease with seasonal intensity. In a review of recurrent urticaria in 20 horses in the United Kingdom, the recurrent urticaria was more common in the autumn and early winter than in the summer. Seventy-five percent of the horses were thoroughbreds or thoroughbred crosses and the mean age of onset of the urticaria was 10.1 years with a range of 4–15 years [10]. In a retrospective study of cases seen at the School of Veterinary Medicine, University of California, Davis (SVM-UCD), the median age at onset was 9.4 years, with a range from 1 year (two horses) to 22 years (one horse). Although it has been commonly thought that thoroughbreds, quarter horses, warmbloods, Arabians, and Morgans, and males (usually geldings) are twice as likely as mares to have atopic disease, the SVM-UCD study did not support this. In their review of 54 horses with atopic disease, age, breed, and sex predilections were not seen [6]. It should be emphasized that this study was performed in California and that its findings may not relate to other parts of North America or beyond.

Clinical lesions

Pruritus, often directed against the face, distal legs, or trunk, is the most common clinical sign (Figures 50.1 and 50.2). However pruritus can be more generalized and mimic insect hypersensitivity distribution patterns (Figure 50.3). Alopecia, erythema, urticaria, and papules may all be present. Urticarial lesions may be quite severe, yet non-pruritic (Figure 50.4). In some cases, the urticaria lesions are associated with pitting oedema, most typically seen over the ventral thorax (Figure 50.5). There may be a familial predisposition for urticarial atopic dermatitis in the horse. Horses may have a secondary pyoderma, typified by excess scaling, small epidermal collarettes, or encrusted papules ('miliary dermatitis') (Figure 50.6). At the SVM-UCD, of 54 atopic horses, 28 (52%) presented with urticaria as the primary complaint, 18 (33%) with both pruritus and urticaria,

Veterinary Allergy, First Edition. Edited by Chiara Noli, Aiden Foster, and Wayne Rosenkrantz.

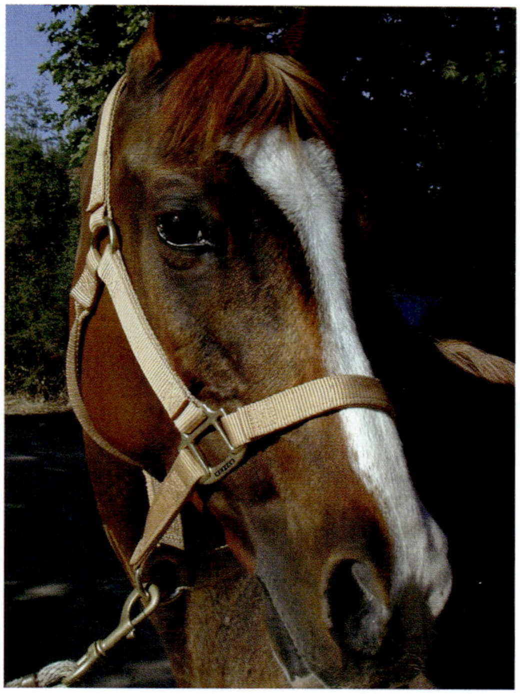

Figure 50.1 Atopic dermatitis with facial pruritus and alopecia.

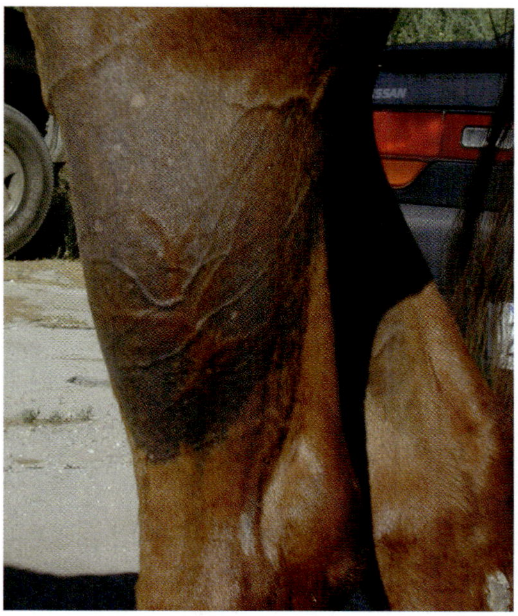

Figure 50.2 Atopic dermatitis with pruritus over rear legs and alopecia.

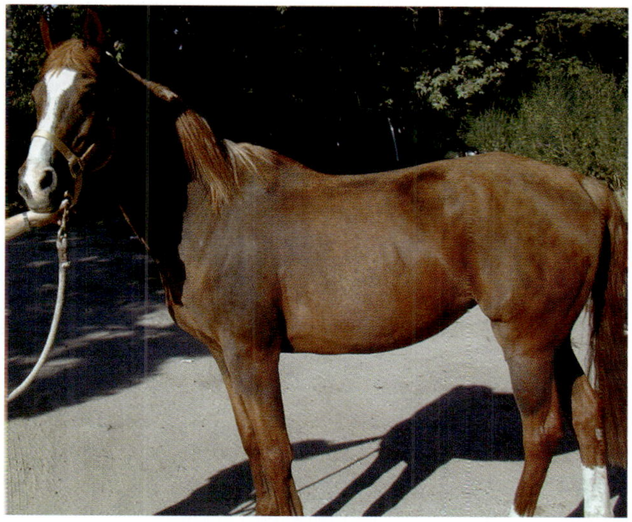

Figure 50.3 Atopic dermatitis showing classic distribution of pruritus over face, legs and trunk.

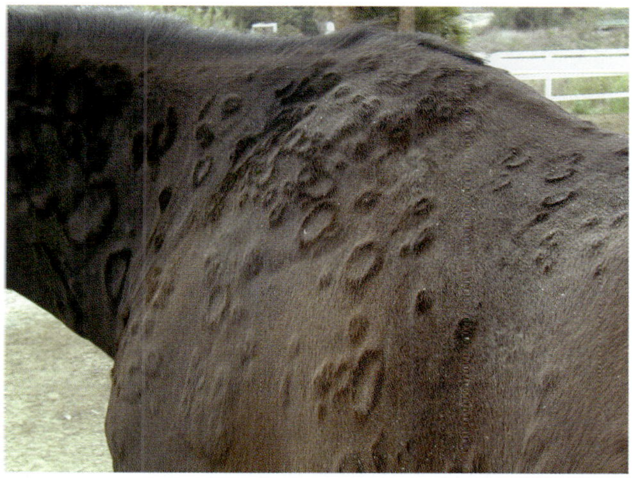

Figure 50.4 'Donut' urticarial lesions in association with atopic dermatitis.

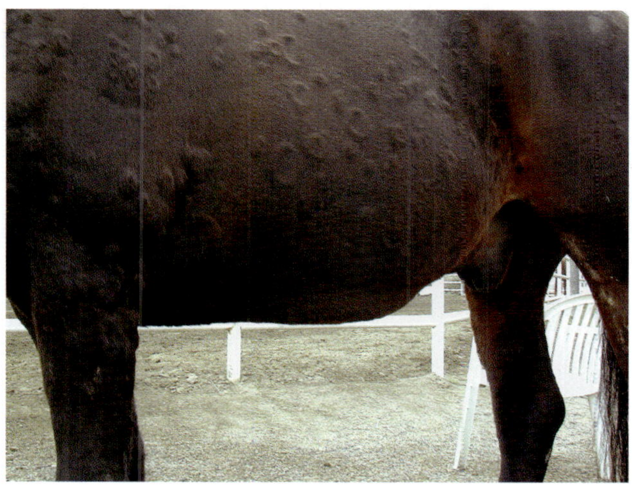

Figure 50.5 Ventral pitting oedema in severe urticaria from atopic dermatitis.

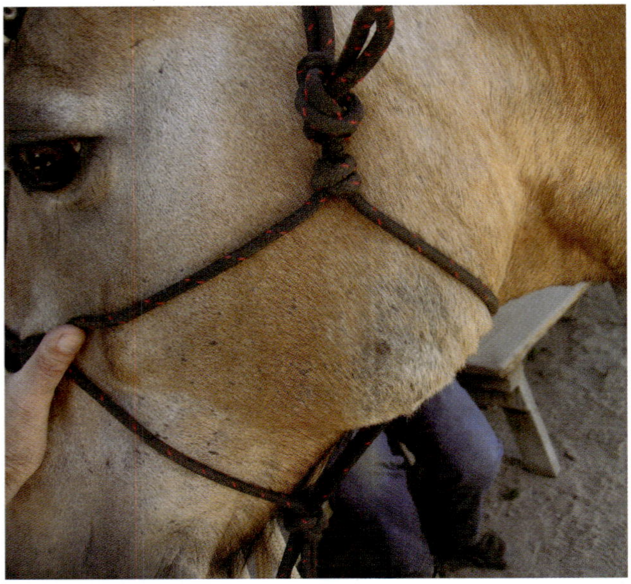

Figure 50.6 Crusted papules and excoriations on the lateral aspect of the face in atopic dermatitis case.

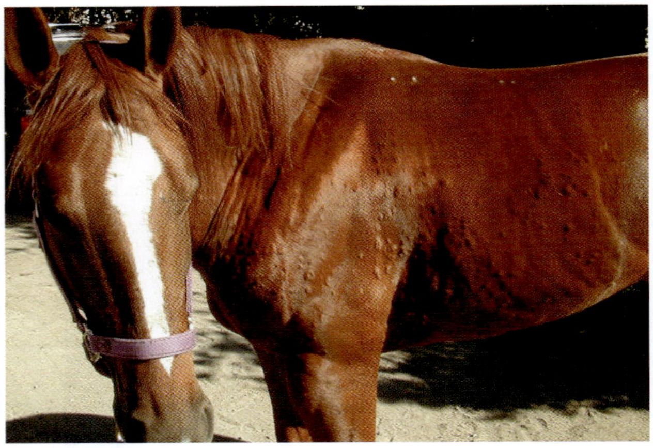

Figure 50.7 Concurrent eosinophilic granulomas with papular eruptions in atopic dermatitis.

and eight (15%) with pruritus alone. The average length of time horses were reported to have clinical signs prior to presenting to the SVM-UCD was 24.9 months (range 4 months to 5 years) for pruritus, 16 months (range 1 month to 10 years) for pruritus and urticaria, and 14.7 months (range 1 month to 5 years) for urticaria. Twelve of the 54 horses were reported to experience their clinical signs seasonally (urticaria ($n = 4$), pruritus ($n = 2$), both ($n = 6$)) [6].

Concurrent diseases

In the authors' experience, hypersensitivity to insect and environmental allergens commonly co-exist in atopic dermatitis in the horse [6]. In the SVM-UCD study, 10/54 cases were diagnosed with concurrent insect bite hypersensitivity. In addition to biting insects, other environmental insects may also play a role either through inhalation or percutaneous absorption. Black ants, house fly, caddis fly, and mayfly, and dust and storage mites are arthropods that that may induce this type of hypersensitivity. It is also possible that concurrent adverse food reactions may play a role in the clinical presentation of the atopic horse. Most food-allergic horses would classically be considered when presented with non-seasonal pruritic disease or urticarial signs. Pruritus and urticaria may be seen on parts of the body less likely to be affected by an insect hypersensitivity (but not always) and would include the lateral caudal thorax and flanks. Pruritus limited to the base of the tail would also increase the consideration of an adverse food reaction. Similar to other species with adverse food reactions, one author (WR) has also seen concurrent gastrointestinal symptoms in the form of diarrhoea or soft stools. Concurrent eosinophilic granulomas have been reported in some atopic dermatitis cases (Figure 50.7) and, although many other aetiologies more commonly create such lesions, atopic dermatitis with concurrent insect hypersensitivities should also be considered [11].

At the SVM-UCD, in addition to the 10 horses with concurrent insect hypersensitivities, additional concurrent diagnoses included: four with concurrent pyoderma, two with vasculitis, one with *Malassezia* dermatitis and superficial pyoderma, and one with alopecia areata [6].

References

1. Fadok VA. Overview of equine pruritus. *Veterinary Clinics of North America: Equine Practice* 1995; **11**: 1–10.
2. Scott DW, Miller WH. *Equine Dermatology*. Philadelphia, PA: WB Saunders, 2003: 433–436.
3. Lorch G, Hillier A, Kwochka KW, *et al.* Results of intradermal tests in horses without atopy and horses with atopic dermatitis or recurrent urticaria. *American Journal of Veterinary Research* 2001; **62**: 1051–1059.
4. White S. Advances in equine atopic dermatitis, serologic and intradermal allergy testing. *Clinical Techniques in Equine Practice* 2005; **4**: 311–313.
5. Rees CA. Response to immunotherapy in six related horses with urticaria secondary to atopy. *Journal of the American Veterinary Medical Association* 2001; **218**: 753–755.
6. Stepnik CT, Outerbridge CA, White SD, *et al.* Equine atopic skin disease and response to allergen-specific immunotherapy: a retrospective study at the University of California-Davis (1991–2008). *Veterinary Dermatology* 2011; **23**: 29–35, e7.
7. van der Haegen A, Kunzle F, Gerber V, *et al.* Mast cells and IgE-bearing cells in lungs of RAO-affected horses. *Veterinary Immunology and Immunopathology* 2005; **108**: 325–334.

8. Cordeau ME, Joubert P, Dewachi O, *et al.* IL-4, IL-5 and IFN-gamma mRNA expression in pulmonary lymphocytes in equine heaves. *Veterinary Immunology and Immunopathology* 2004; **97**: 87–96.
9. Tallarico NJ, Tallarico C. Results of intradermal allergy testing and treatment by hyposensitization of 64 horses with chronic obstructive pulmonary disease, urticaria, headshaking, and/or reactive airway disease. *Veterinary Allergy and Clinical Immunology* 1998; **6**: 25–35.
10. Paterson S. A retrospective study into the causes and incidence of recurrent urticaria in the horse. *Veterinary Dermatology* 2012; **23** (Suppl. 1): 42.
11. Mathison PT. Eosinophilic nodular dermatoses. *Veterinary Clinics of North America: Equine Practice* 1995; **11**: 75–89.

51

Equine urticaria

Valerie A. Fadok

North Houston Veterinary Specialists, Spring, TX, USA

Conflict of interest: none declared.

Overview

Most veterinarians will agree that the occurrence of urticaria is most common in horses, compared to other species we treat. In spite of that fact, the peer-reviewed veterinary literature is sparse with regard to aetiology, pathogenesis, rational diagnostic approaches, and effective treatment [1–14]. A number of review articles have been written, sharing the experiences of each of the authors, but hard evidence is lacking [15–19]. For example, it has been suggested that thoroughbred and Arab horse breeds may be predisposed, but without large numbers and comparison to general hospital or outpatient presentations, it is difficult to know breed incidence. Usually, the history and the location and appearance of the hives will help determine what diagnostics will be indicated. While urticarial lesions are intensely pruritic in humans, many horses with hives are non-pruritic. In some horses, localized angioedema will also occur and result in the seepage of serum through the skin (Figure 51.1). In addition, urticaria lesions can take on interesting shapes, such as target lesions, serpiginous, and circinate forms (Figure 51.2), and even long linear forms, which occur in a parallel banding pattern on the sides of the trunk ('zebra' or 'striped' urticaria) (Figure 51.3). With the more unusual forms it may be necessary to collect a skin biopsy of the lesions because erythema multiforme in the horse can mimic the circular and target forms of urticaria.

Mast cell degranulation

Mast cells, as the bearers of the high-affinity IgE receptor, are the major cells involved in the development of urticarial lesions, although basophils, macrophages, and other cells may also contribute. Mast cells contain a variety of preformed inflammatory mediators (histamines, proteases, proteoglycans) within their granules, but they are also capable of quickly manufacturing lipid mediators (arachidonic acid metabolites, platelet activating factor), as well as synthesizing a number of cytokines and chemokines. Under normal circumstances, mast cell activity is critical in wound healing as well as protection against pathogens. The major trigger for mast cell degranulation is the cross-linking of IgE tightly bound to the high affinity FcεR receptor on the cell surface. Mast cells will also degranulate in response to physical injury and chemical stimuli (opioids, alcohol, polymyxin B), as well as by activated complement proteins (C3a, C5a). Other hormones and mediators, including corticotrophin releasing hormone, substance P, and neurotensin, can also trigger mast cell degranulation [20–22].

Mast cells have been studied in the skin of 32 horses with urticaria [23]. While IgE-positive cells were found in greater numbers in the skin of horses with urticaria lesions, compared to normal horses, tryptase positivity and toluidine blue positivity were lower, which supports the notion that mast cells had degranulated during the disease process. More recently, the inflammatory infiltrate and cytokine production were studied in the skin of eight horses with recurrent urticaria [24].

Veterinary Allergy, First Edition. Edited by Chiara Noli, Aiden Foster, and Wayne Rosenkrantz.

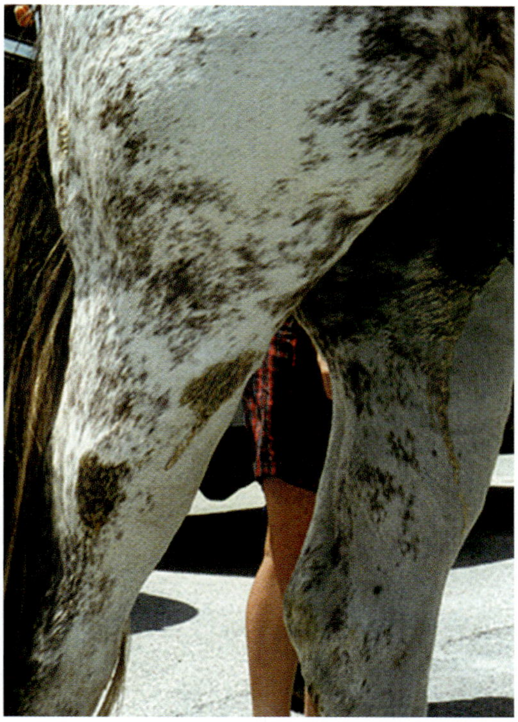

Figure 51.1 Focal angioedema with serum leakage, cause unknown.

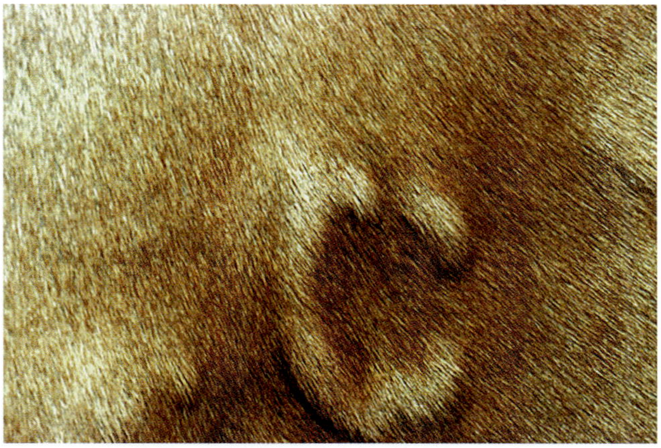

Figure 51.2 Circinate urticaria, cause unknown.

Histopathological findings included dermal oedema associated with variable eosinophilic and lymphocytic perivascular infiltrates. Immunohistochemical staining showed increased numbers of eosinophils and macrophages, as well as mast cells, in lesional skin. Expression of cytokine mRNA was analysed, and increased amounts for IL-4, IL-4 receptor, IL-13, and thymic stromal lymphopoietin (TSLP) were found in lesional skin. Given that the first three cytokines are expressed by mast cells and that mast cells have been implicated in the regulation of epithelial-derived TSLP,

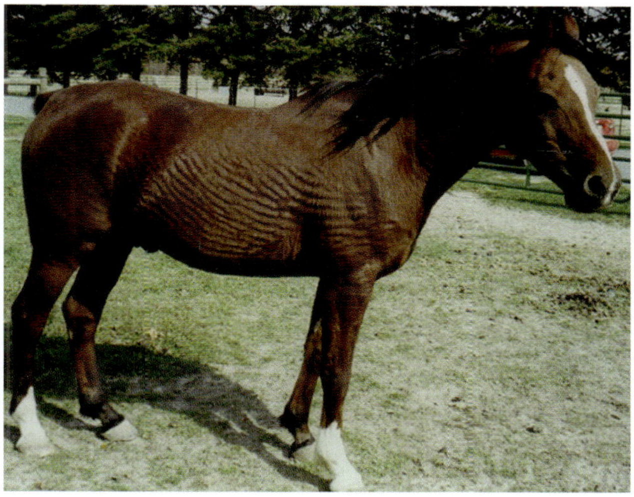

Figure 51.3 Linear urticaria, idiopathic. (Reprinted with permission from Hal Schott.)

these findings are not a surprise. What is of interest is that these same cytokines are involved in atopic dermatitis, a disease with very different clinical signs. Perhaps it is the barrier defect of atopic dermatitis that determines whether a horse will have hives or atopic dermatitis in response to environmental stimuli?

Acute versus chronic urticaria

To develop a rational approach to urticaria, it is important to separate acute urticaria from chronic and/or recurrent urticaria. In human medicine, physicians designate acute urticaria as those lasting 6 weeks or less [25–27]. It seems reasonable to use 6–8 weeks for horses as well. Acute urticaria can often be attributed to drugs (Figure 51.4), vaccines, blood transfusions, viral infections, insects (papular urticaria) (Figure 51.5), or exposure to nettles [16]; treatment with antihistamines is recommended, although many veterinarians will use glucocorticoids as well. While not well studied in horses, urticarial reactions in humans can accompany bacterial or fungal infections and treatment would address these infections specifically. It makes no sense to spend a lot of time and resources on initial or short-lasting outbreaks of urticaria if the cause is not immediately apparent. Many animals will do well if medicated consistently with an antihistamine such as hydroxyzine, used two to three times a day for 2–3 months. It is important to keep in mind that antihistamines work best to prevent future outbreaks of urticaria rather than as a treatment for active urticaria. For outbreaks of short duration and mild severity (e.g. seasonal urticarial lasting 3–4 months), antihistamines could be used as sole therapy.

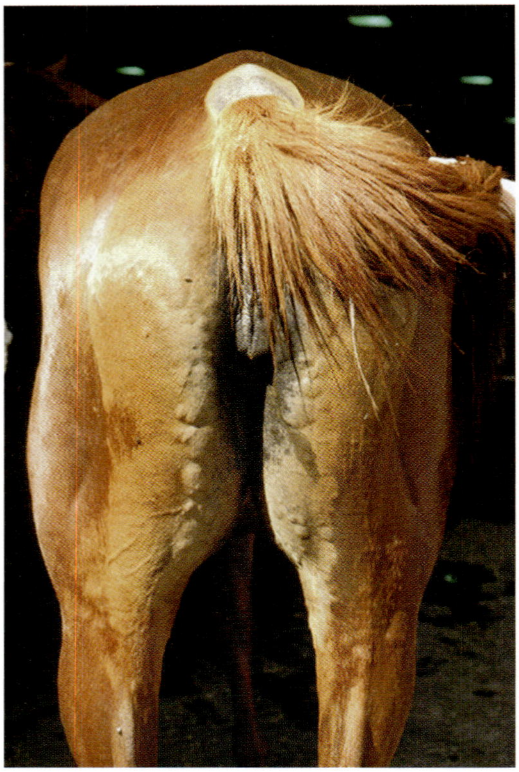

Figure 51.4 Acute urticaria associated with administration of phenylbutazone.

Potential causes for and recommended approach to chronic or recurrent urticaria

The causes of chronic and/or recurrent urticaria in horses can be quite difficult to determine. If drugs or supplements can be ruled out then searching for an allergic underlying cause is advocated. Clues in the history can be used to decide whether to consider food allergy or environmental allergies, such as those to pollens, moulds, dusts, danders, mites, and insects. Continual outbreaks of urticaria lesions could support embarking on an elimination diet trial to rule out food allergy, whereas intermittent outbreaks of hives would be more compatible with an environmental allergy.

Food allergy has been implicated as a cause of urticaria in horses (Figure 51.6) [3,12,13] but elimination diet testing in horses is difficult. We know very little about food allergy and food intolerance in horses, particularly how long a hypoallergenic diet should be fed. In general, it has been recommended to change the source of grass hay (e.g. from alfalfa to timothy) and stop grain supplements. Stopping grain works well for easy keeping pony breeds, but may not be a good plan for performance horses. In those cases, changing the source of the grain or changing from a sweet feed mix to a pure grain is

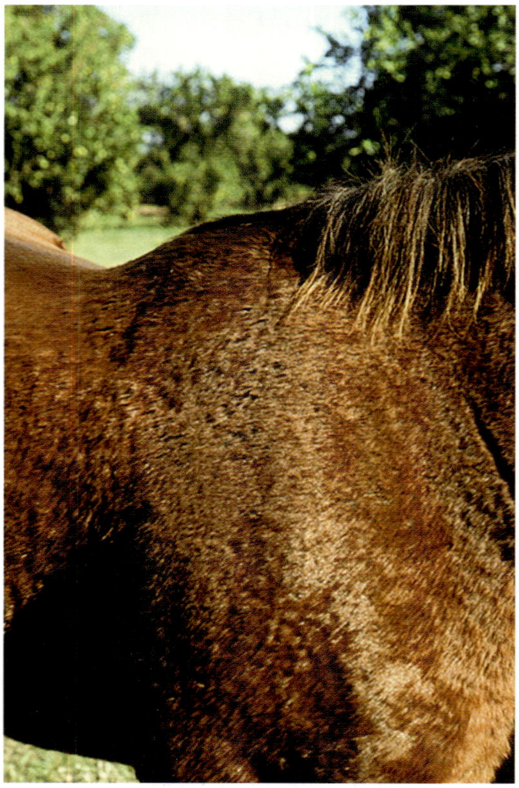

Figure 51.5 Papular urticaria associated with mosquito bite hypersensitivity.

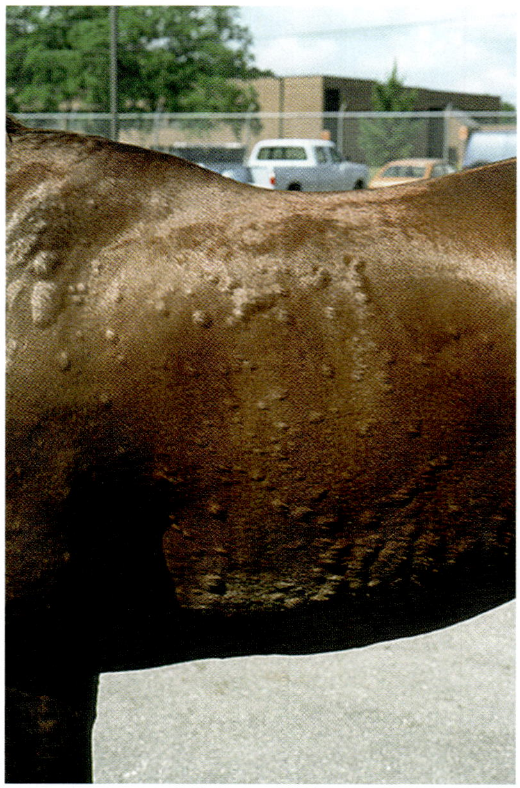

Figure 51.6 Chronic urticaria associated with food allergy (alfalfa).

advocated. Unfortunately, many horses are given a wide variety of supplements without veterinary knowledge. It is very useful to have the owners keep a food diary for 5–7 days in which they list everything that horse ingests. It is anyone's guess as to how long to feed the elimination diet; most authors have empirically suggested a minimum of 4 weeks and up to 8 weeks in some cases.

Immunotherapy (ASIT)

The intradermal test can be used to select allergens for allergen-specific immunotherapy (ASIT) for those horses who experience urticaria as a result of environmental allergies [16,28–30]. As for dogs, there has been no standardization of extracts, testing protocols, or assessment of response to treatment. Nevertheless, those who test horses can provide testimonial evidence of ASIT efficacy and there are at least two studies that support ASIT for the treatment of atopic urticaria [4,6]. The major problem with the intradermal test is that so few veterinarians are able to do the procedure. In many cases, it is reasonable to suggest serum testing instead. It is better that horses be tested and put on immunotherapy than not, and testimonial evidence supports the efficacy of ASIT based on serum testing (see Chapter 54 for more details).

Drug allergy, food allergy, and environmental allergies account for the majority of immunological urticaria; however, contact urticaria represents an interesting immunologic variant. In such cases the urticaria lesions result from direct application of topical medications, plants, leather conditioners, or soaps, and the lesions are restricted to the areas to which the allergen is applied [16,18].

Non-immunological urticaria includes those induced by physical causes, including pressure, heat, cold, water (aquagenic), solar exposure, and exercise. Of these, dermatographism (a type of pressure urticaria) and cholinergic urticaria/pruritus have been demonstrated in horses in the peer-reviewed literature [2,11]. There are anecdotal reports of cold-induced urticaria in horses as well.

Dermatographism, a pressure urticaria, clinically presents as urticaria lesions or more diffuse swelling at sites at which tack are used, such as the saddle, bridle, or harness areas. Diagnosis is made by drawing patterns on the skin with a blunt instrument and observing the developing wheals over the following 15–20 minutes. Dermatographism, like other forms of physical urticaria, may sometimes only be manifested when allergenic foods have been eaten prior to the pressure being applied. Combined food/physical urticarias can present diagnostic challenges, but may be easier to treat, because avoidance of the food, at least before riding or driving, should solve the problem.

Cholinergic urticaria (CU)/pruritus was diagnosed in an 8-year gelding with a history of intense itch following exercise [11]. The diagnosis was made by inducing the itch in response to vigorous exercise or a hot water bath to increase the core body temperature. In humans, this disease remains incompletely understood, and it is believed that there are four subtypes: cholinergic urticaria with poral occlusion, cholinergic urticaria with sweat allergy, cholinergic urticaria with acquired generalized hypohidrosis, and idiopathic cholinergic urticaria [31,32]. The disease is characterized by pinpoint urticaria lesions that are intensely pruritic, and acetylcholine appears to be a major mediator. The poral occlusion variant is associated with lymphocytic infiltrates around the pores and some horse owners believe that this variant can contribute to eventual hypohidrosis or anhidrosis. The sweat hypersensitivity form is poorly understood but has been documented by intradermal injection of diluted autologous sweat as well as acetylcholine. Interestingly, desensitization with autologous sweat has been reported as efficacious in some affected humans, and the observation that omalizumab (anti-human IgE) has been effective in some (but not all) patients supports the notion that this type of CU is mediated by IgE [33,34]. The hypohidrosis and anhidrosis in people develop as a result of down-regulation of acetylcholine receptors. These receptors can be up-regulated with high doses of glucocorticoids, and high-dose pulse glucocorticoids are recommended as the primary treatment choice. Given the occurrence of hypohydrosis and anhidrosis in horses, it is tempting to speculate that cholinergic urticarial may play a larger role than our literature would suggest.

Non-cholinergic exercise-induced urticaria cases differ from those with cholinergic urticaria by the fact that they are induced by exercise only; hot baths will not stimulate an attack [35]. One of the more interesting facts about the physical urticaria, particularly those associated with exercise, is their combination with other allergens, particularly those associated with foods [36,37]. In people, shellfish or wheat proteins such as gliadin or glutenin are the most common foods, and the reaction is made even more complex by the observation that aspirin seems to contribute to the severity of the reactions. Food-dependent exercise-induced urticaria most often occur in recreational and competitive athletes. It is tempting to speculate that some of the 'stress-induced' urticaria seen in racing thoroughbreds might be food-dependent exercise-induced. Consuming the offending food within 4–5 hours of exercise induces the reaction. Diagnosis is made by feeding the suspected foods then exercising vigorously. It would be critical to be prepared for emergency treatment of anaphylaxis. Once the diagnosis is established, simply avoiding feeding the offending food prior to exercise prevents the outbreak.

Cold-induced urticaria in humans are usually acquired, and follow viral infections such as Epstein–Barr virus (infectious mononucleosis), hepatitis, and HIV, bacterial infections such as *Helicobacter pyloris* and borreliosis, and parasitic infections such as toxoplasmosis or leishmaniasis [38,39]. How these infections induce the response remains to be seen, but it is a long-lasting change. Diagnosis is made by using the ice cube test. In humans, an ice cube is placed on the skin of the forearm until the skin is well chilled. The urticaria and itch develop as the skin is warmed. This test is difficult to standardize; recently, an electronic device that allows application of specific temperatures to the skin has been developed. Prevention is best, as in humans exposure to cold can induce anaphylaxis, particularly when cold drinks contact the larynx and pharynx. Treatment requires high doses of antihistamines and patients should have access to epinephrine. This author has demonstrated cold-induced urticaria in one horse in Colorado, USA; it appeared to be acquired, and seemed to follow an upper respiratory infection. Diagnosis was based on using the ice cube test as described above. The horse was subsequently sold and moved to the southern parts of Arizona where exposure to cold was much less likely.

Other potential causes for urticaria might defy categorization as immunologic or physical. Stress is known to exacerbate urticaria and in some cases induce outbreaks without other known stimuli. It has been demonstrated recently in humans that corticotrophin-releasing hormone (CRH) can stimulate mast cell degranulation, in conjunction with neurotensin and substance P [20–22]. Stress has been incriminated as a potential cause for urticaria in racehorses [16].

Treatment of urticaria

The treatment of urticaria involves addressing the underlying cause and antihistamines remain the mainstay. As mentioned above, hydroxyzine has been found to be very effective to repress the development of new lesions. It can be used at 1–2 mg/kg (usually 400 to 600 mg) two to three times a day. Sedation is the most common side effect, but passes within a few days. It has been noted that for human patients, doses four times that used for allergic rhinitis may be required. Other advocated treatments include fatty acid therapy (usually flaxseed oil-based products), and corticosteroids (e.g. 1 mg/kg/day of prednisolone or 0.1 mg/kg/day dexamethasone). In human patients with intractable urticaria, ciclosporin may be effective [40]. For many urticarias, including some physical ones, omalizumab (anti-human IgE) has been very effective, supporting the notion that even the physical urticarias may, in fact, be mediated by IgE [41,42].

References

1. Bathe AP. An unusual manifestation of nettle rash in three horses. *Veterinary Record* 1994; **134**: 11–12.
2. Cornick JL, Brumbaugh GW. Dermatographism in a horse. *Cornell Vet* 1989; **79**: 109–116.
3. Volland-Francqueville M, Sabbah A. Recurrent or chronic urticaria in thoroughbred race-horses: clinical observations. *European Annals of Allergy and Clinical Immunology* 2004; **36**: 9–12 (In French).
4. Stepnik CT, Outerbridge CA, White SD, *et al.* Equine atopic skin disease and response to allergen-specific immunotherapy: A retrospective study at the university of California-Davis (1991–2008). *Veterinary Dermatology* 2012; **23**: 29–35, e7.
5. Rodriguez-Palacios A, Quesada R, Baird J, *et al.* Presumptive fluphenazine-induced hepatitis and urticaria in a horse. *Journal of Veterinary Internal Medicine* 2007; **21**: 336–339.
6. Rees CA. Response to immunotherapy in six related horses with urticaria secondary to atopy. *Journal of the American Veterinary Medical Association* 2001; **218**: 753–755.
7. Nielsen IL, Jacobs KA, Huntington PJ, *et al.* Adverse reaction to procaine penicillin G in horses. *Australian Veterinary Journal* 1988; **65**: 181–185.
8. Miyazawa K, Ito M, Ohsaki K. An equine case of urticaria associated with dry garlic feeding. *Journal of Veterinary Medical Science* 1991; **53**: 747–748.
9. Matthews NS, Light GS, Sanders EA, *et al.* Urticarial response during anesthesia in a horse. *Equine Veterinary Journal* 1993; **25**: 555–556.
10. Maplesden DC, Cote JF, Mitchell D. Allergy in a horse. *Journal of the American Veterinary Medical Association* 1956; **128**: 152.
11. Logas D, Kunkle G, Calderwood-Mays M, *et al.* Cholinergic pruritus in a horse. *Journal of the American Veterinary Medical Association* 1992; **201**: 90–91.
12. Hallebeek AJ, Sloet van Oldruitenborgh-Oosterbaan MM. 'Oat bumps' in horses. Differential diagnosis and nutritional aspects. *Tijdschr Diergeneeskd* 1995; **120**: 588–591 (In Dutch).
13. Francqueville M, Sabbah A. Chronic urticaria in sports horses. *Allergie et Immunologie (Paris)* 1999; **31**: 212–213 (In French).
14. Farmer CG. Penicillin: Adverse reaction in horses. *Veterinary Record* 1980; **106**: 298.
15. Yu AA. Equine urticaria: A diagnostic dilemma. *Compendium On Continuing Education For The Practicing Veterinarian* 2000; **22**: 277–280.
16. Scott DW, Miller WH. *Equine Dermatology*. St. Louis, MO: Saunders, 2003: 422–449.
17. Paterson S. Investigation of skin disease and urticaria in the horse. *In Practice* 2000; **22**: 446–455.
18. Fadok VA. Of horses and men: Urticaria. *Veterinary Dermatology* 1990; **1**: 103–112.
19. Akucewich LH, Kunkle GA. Urticaria. *Compendium Equine Edition* 2007; **2**: 100–111.
20. Lytinas M, Kempuraj D, Huang M, *et al.* Acute stress results in skin corticotropin-releasing hormone secretion, mast cell activation and vascular permeability, an effect mimicked by intradermal corticotropin-releasing hormone and inhibited by histamine-1 receptor antagonists. *International Archives of Allergy and Immunology* 2003; **130**: 224–231.

21. Singh LK, Pang X, Alexacos N, *et al.* Acute immobilization stress triggers skin mast cell degranulation via corticotropin releasing hormone, neurotensin, and substance P: A link to neurogenic skin disorders. *Brain Behavior and Immunity* 1999; **13**: 225–239.
22. Theoharides TC, Donelan JM, Papadopoulou N, *et al.* Mast cells as targets of corticotropin-releasing factor and related peptides. *Trends in Pharmacological Sciences* 2004; **25**: 563–568.
23. Rüfenacht S, Marti E, von Tscharner C, *et al.* Immunoglobulin E-bearing cells and mast cells in skin biopsies of horses with urticaria. *Veterinary Dermatology* 2005; **16**: 94–101.
24. Hinden S, Klukowska-Rötzler J, Janda J, *et al.* Characterization of the inflammatory infiltrate and cytokine expression in the skin of horses with recurrent urticaria. *Veterinary Dermatology* 2012; **23**: 503–e99.
25. Fromer L. Treatment options for the relief of chronic idiopathic urticaria symptoms. *Southern Medical Journal* 2008; **101**: 186–192.
26. Maurer M, Grabbe J. Urticaria: Its history-based diagnosis and etiologically oriented treatment. *Deutsches Ärzteblatt International* 2008; **105**: 458–465.
27. Zuberbier T, Maurer M. Urticaria: Current opinions about etiology, diagnosis and therapy. *Acta Dermato-Venereologica* 2007; **87**: 196–205.
28. Jose-Cunilleras E, Kohn CW, Hillier A, *et al.* Intradermal testing in healthy horses and horses with chronic obstructive pulmonary disease, recurrent urticaria, or allergic dermatitis. *Journal of the American Veterinary Medical Association* 2001; **219**: 1115–1121.
29. Evans AG, Paradis MR, O'Callaghan M. Intradermal testing of horses with chronic obstructive pulmonary disease and recurrent urticaria. *American Journal of Veterinary Research* 1992: **53**: 203–208.
30. Delger JM. Intradermal testing and immunotherapy in horses. *Veterinary Medicine* 1997; **92**: 635–639.
31. Bito T, Sawada Y, Tokura Y. Pathogenesis of cholinergic urticaria in relation to sweating. *Allergology International* 2012; **61**: 539–544.
32. Nakamizo S, Egawa G, Miyachi Y, *et al.* Cholinergic urticaria: Pathogenesis-based categorization and its treatment options. *Journal of the European Academy of Dermatology and Venereology* 2012; **26**: 114–116.
33. Metz M, Bergmann P, Zuberbier T, *et al.* Successful treatment of cholinergic urticaria with anti-immunoglobulin E therapy. *Allergy* 2008; **63**: 247–249.
34. Sabroe RA. Failure of omalizumab in cholinergic urticaria. *Clinical and Experimental Dermatology* 2010; **35**: e127–129.
35. Schwartz LB, Delgado L, Craig T, *et al.* Exercise-induced hypersensitivity syndromes in recreational and competitive athletes: A PRACTALL consensus report (what the general practitioner should know about sports and allergy). *Allergy* 2008; **63**: 953–961.
36. Beaudouin E, Renaudin JM, Morisset M, *et al.* Food-dependent exercise-induced anaphylaxis—update and current data. *European Annals of Allergy and Clinical Immunolology* 2006; **38**: 45–51.
37. Kidd JM, Cohen SH, Sosman AJ, *et al.* Food-dependent exercise-induced anaphylaxis. *Journal of Allergy and Clinical Immunology* 1983; **71**: 407–411.
38. Siebenhaar F, Weller K, Mlynek A, *et al.* Acquired cold urticaria: Clinical picture and update on diagnosis and treatment. *Clinical Experimental Dermatology* 2007; **32**: 241–245.
39. Morais-Almeida M, Marinho S, Gaspar A, *et al.* Cold urticaria and infectious mononucleosis in children. *Allergologia et Immunopathologia* 2004; **32**: 368–371 (in Spanish).
40. Trojan TD, Khan DA. Calcineurin inhibitors in chronic urticaria. *Current Opinion in Allergy and Clinical Immunology* 2012; **12**: 412–420.
41. Nam YH, Kim JH, Jin HJ, *et al.* Effects of omalizumab treatment in patients with refractory chronic urticaria. *Allergy, Asthma Immunology and Research* 2012; **4**: 357–361.
42. Mauro M, Incorvaia C, Formigoni C, *et al.* The anti-IgE antibody omalizumab as a probe to investigate the role of IgE in pathology. *Panminerva Medica* 2012; **54**: 305–312.

52

Equine headshaking syndrome

Harold C. Schott II[1] and Annette D. Petersen[2]

[1] Department of Large Animal Clinical Sciences, College of Veterinary Medicine, Michigan State University, East Lansing, MI, USA
[2] Department of Small Animal Clinical Sciences, College of Veterinary Medicine, Michigan State University, East Lansing, MI, USA

Conflict of interest: none declared.

Clinical syndrome

Headshaking can be a normal, voluntary behaviour of equids. However, when this behaviour becomes more frequent or severe, often without apparent stimulus, it is also recognized as the headshaking or head-tossing syndrome. This syndrome is a medical problem that is most commonly manifested as repetitive, rapid tic-like head-tossing in a vertical plane, although side-to-side or rotary movements of the head can also be observed [1–5]. Owners may initially suspect that their horse is reacting to an insect flying up a nostril, but they subsequently seek veterinary evaluation as the syndrome becomes recurrent and interferes with work or well-being.

Headshaking syndrome is most commonly observed during exercise, usually at a trot during which the head is held more stationary, but it can also occur at rest or during exercise at other gaits. Additional signs include excessive snorting or lacrimation, flipping the upper lip, an anxious facial expression, nasal discharge, rubbing the nares or side of the face (on the inside of a lower forelimb, a post or the ground), and striking out at the nose with a foreleg [1–5]. Headshaking can be so severe that riding and, at times, even handling the horse can be unsafe. If poorly responsive to treatment and management changes, some affected horses become unsuitable for use and their owners may ultimately request euthanasia [6].

Clinical evaluation of 100 horses [2] and two owner-completed surveys of 109 [4] and 254 horses [5] with headshaking syndrome reported mean ages at onset (or recognition) of 7.3, 7.5, and 9 years. Geldings were over-represented (63–78%) but no breed predilection was found. Horses that are overweight have also been suggested to be at greater risk for development of headshaking syndrome [7]. Affected horses in these reports were mostly used for pleasure riding and more than 80% had the characteristic headshaking or head-tossing in a vertical plane. From 59 to 64% of affected horses in these studies had seasonal exacerbation, starting in spring and abating in the late summer or autumn. Further, up to 50% of horses also had a history of being acquired by the current owner in late autumn or winter months when the problem was not apparent [2,4]. Seasonal occurrence could suggest that photoperiod and associated neurohumoral changes, ambient temperature and humidity, as well as exposure to allergens or other environmental triggers, may play a role in headshaking syndrome.

Causes of headshaking syndrome

There are many causes of headshaking syndrome in horses, including disorders of the upper airway, oral cavity, ears, eyes, and other soft tissues of the head and neck [1,7–15]. Further, neurological and musculoskeletal disorders may also present with headshaking as the primary complaint [16,17] (Table 52.1). A comprehen-

Veterinary Allergy, First Edition. Edited by Chiara Noli, Aiden Foster, and Wayne Rosenkrantz.

Table 52.1 Possible causes of headshaking in horses (adapted from Scott D and Miller W: *Equine Dermatology*, 2nd edn. Philadelphia: Elsevier Saunders, 2011: 465, © 2011, with permission of Elsevier)

Diseases of the upper airway	Allergic rhinitis or non-allergic (vasomotor) rhinopathy Nasal foreign body Harvest mites (*Trombicula* spp.) in false nostril Nasal or sinus tumours Sinusitis Paranasal sinus cyst Ethmoid haematoma Guttural pouch infection ± chondroids Pharyngeal or laryngeal mass
Diseases of the oral cavity	Oral ulcers or lacerations Bit problems (pain with bars) Dental and periodontal disease Foreign body
Diseases of the ear	Trombiculosis (chiggers) Ear mites (*Psoroptes* spp.) Otic foreign bodies (grass awns, hard wax, spinose ear tick) Otitis externa/media/interna ± temporohyoid osteoarthropathy Aural plaques Neoplasia of the auditory canal Trauma from application of ear twitch, aural haematoma Dentigerous or dermoid cyst ± aural fistula
Diseases of the eye	Melanotic iris cyst Uveal or retinal lesions *Habronema* spp., *Onchocerca* spp. (larva migrans) Lens luxation Ocular foreign body
Diseases of the nervous system	Encephalopathy (hepatic, viral) Cervical instability (subclinical wobbler) Traumatic cranial/cervical injuries Equine protozoal myeloencephalitis Trigeminal neuralgia
Diseases of the skeletal system	Exostosis of the occipital protuberance Nuchal crest fractures Subtle lameness
Diseases of the soft tissues of the head	Bridle fit problems Parotid gland disease
Miscellaneous	Stereotypic behaviour Behavioural difficulties exacerbated by rider head and neck flexion Neck pain Photo optic–trigeminal nerve summation Inappropriate response to noise Partial asphyxia Idiopathic

sive review of headshaking syndrome by Cook postulated 58 causes of headshaking [1,8–10]; thus, it should not be surprising that evaluation and management of headshaking syndrome is frustrating for both owners and veterinarians. The diagnostic approach is one of exclusion of potential causes combined with 'trial and error' drug treatment and management changes. As an example, despite an exhaustive diagnostic evaluation, Lane and Mair [2] were able to identify suspected causes of headshaking in only 11 of 100 horses. Problems found included ear mite infestation, otitis interna, cranial nerve dysfunction, neck injury, ocular disease, guttural pouch mycosis, dental and sinus disorders, and suspected vasomotor rhinitis. However, confirmation of a cause by correction of the abnormality resulted in resolution of headshaking in only two horses. As a consequence, these authors coined the term 'idiopathic headshaker' to describe the clinical syndrome of headshaking for which no cause can be determined. Despite the long list of potential causes of headshaking, temporohyoid osteoarthropathy, trigeminal neuralgia/neuropathy, and allergy warrant more detailed discussion as recent work supports a potentially important role for these disorders in headshaking syndrome. Further, they may be amenable to medical or surgical treatment.

Temporohyoid osteoarthropathy

A syndrome of headshaking with or without deficits of the facial and/or vestibular nerves has been attributed to otitis media/interna [18–20]. However, rather than typical signs of a middle/inner ear infection (i.e. accumulation of purulent debris in the guttural pouch) this disorder is associated with bony proliferation of the temporohyoid joint and proximal shaft of the stylohyoid bone that separates the medial and lateral compartments of the guttural pouch (Figure 52.1). Early descriptions of this disorder implicated an infectious aetiology by recovery of bacteria via tympanocentesis or at post-mortem examination [18–20]; however, this has not been confirmed by others [21] and the term temporohyoid osteoarthropathy (THO) is now the preferred name for this disease. A breed predilection for stock-type horses (e.g. quarter horses, paints and appaloosas) further calls into question an infectious aetiology.

Affected horses are most commonly presented when neurological deficits develop, as bony proliferation leads to impingement of the facial and/or vestibular nerves in the area of the acoustic meatus. Neurologic signs may develop acutely in some horses (e.g. sudden onset of ear droop or vestibular ataxia) while in others refractory corneal ulcers (due to loss of eyelid muscle tone and decreased lacrimation) or a subtle, intermittent head tilt may be more gradually recognized by horse owners [20,22]. Further questioning often reveals that affected horses may have had a much longer history (months to years) of headshaking, playing with their tongue or bit, or chewing irregularly [19,20,22]. Consequently, endoscopic examination of both guttural pouches to assess for THO is indicated in the evaluation of horses with headshaking syndrome [23]. Although conservative medical management has had fair success in management of THO [22], surgical removal of the ceratohyoid bone has recently been advocated as the treatment of choice [24]. In theory, this surgical procedure removes the mechanical stress and pain associated with the arthritic or fused temporohyoid joint. Ideally, surgery should be performed early in the course of THO to alleviate headshaking before neurological signs may develop.

Trigeminal neuralgia/neuropathy

Over the past couple of decades, trigeminal neuralgia/neuropathy (TN) has received progressively greater attention as one of the major causes of idiopathic headshaking in horses [3,15,25–28]. Support for TN as a cause of headshaking syndrome was initially provided more than a century ago by Williams (1899) who described infraorbital neurectomy as a successful treatment for headshaking [29]. More recently, temporary improvement following perineural anaesthesia of various branches of the trigeminal nerve and lasting improvement by neurectomy, chemical sclerosis, or coil compression of the infraorbital or maxillary nerves has provided convincing evidence that TN plays an important role in headshaking syndrome in horses [3,25,26,28,30,31].

Interest in TN as a cause of headshaking in horses largely developed as an extension of knowledge about this condition in people, in whom it can cause a sudden, shooting or burning sensation across the face. This syndrome, also known as *tic douloureux*, has been recognized since the first century and the superficial, sharp and intense pain has been termed 'lancinating' because it extends along one or more paths of the trigeminal nerve [32]. The maxillary branch is most commonly affected and, curiously, the right side is more commonly affected than the left, possibly due to a narrower right foramen rotundum and foramen ovale through which the nerve passes. In people, the syndrome can be debilitating and is associated with a high suicide rate [32]. In contrast to horses, TN is relatively simple to diagnose in humans because patients can clearly describe the facial pain and path along which it radiates, as well as suspected triggers (e.g. talking, chewing, teeth brushing, shaving, or even light touch or a cool breeze). In horses, stimuli that appear to trigger TN include exposure to bright light or sunshine (photic headshaking), noise, smell, and touch [4,5,15]. Additional stimuli that accompany exercise include increases in airflow through the nasal passages, blood flow to nasal and turbinate mucosa, and rate and intensity of the maxillary arterial pulse, adjacent to the maxillary nerve [3,28].

In people, TN is separated into two syndromes by the International Headache Society: (1) classical TN, in which no specific cause can be determined other than vascular compression; and (2) symptomatic TN, for which a causative lesion can be detected [33]. This classification parallels the findings of Lane and Mair [2] in horses, in which a causative lesion was suspected in 11 cases (symptomatic TN) while the remainder were

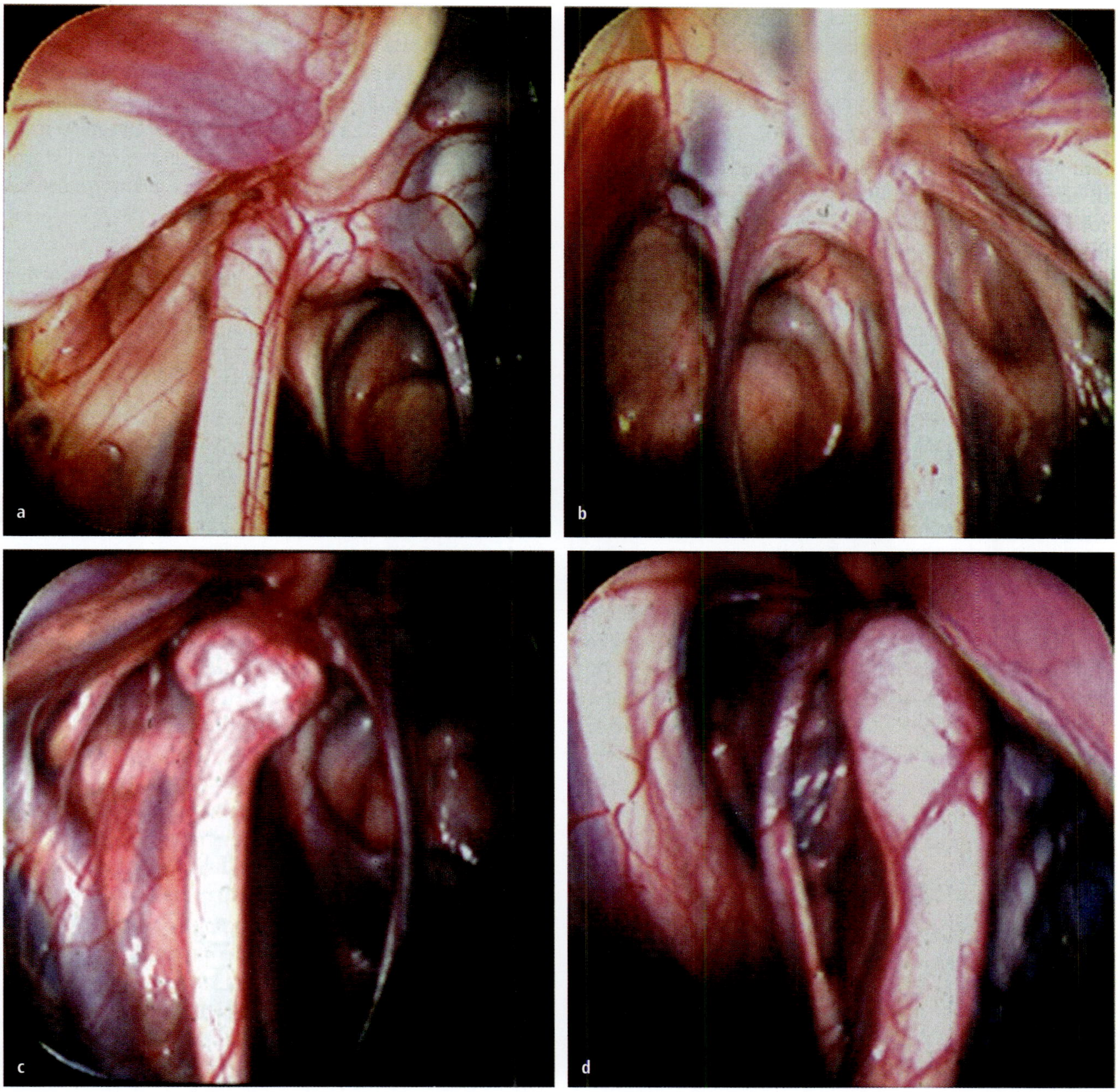

Figure 52.1 Endoscopic images of the right (a and c) and left (b and d) stylohyoid bones and temporohyoid joints within the guttural pouches; (a and b) normal stylohyoid bones and temporohyoid articulations; (c and d) marked bony proliferation at the temporohyoid joint (c) and marked thickening of the entire proximal aspect of the stylohyoid bone in a horse with bilateral temporohyoid osteoarthropathy and headshaking.

considered idiopathic headshakers (classical TN). The only pathological finding in people with classical TN is partial demyelination of the trigeminal nerve, apparently associated with vascular compression. The working hypothesis is that demyelination alters trigeminal nerve electrophysiology, allowing generation of ectopic impulses that summate to cause facial pain [32]. In horses, histopathological investigation of trigeminal nerves collected from horses with headshaking syndrome, including the ganglion and several of its branches, has failed to identify demyelination or other pathology [7,34]. However, a recent report documented decreased latencies of somatosensory evoked potentials following stimulation of the trigeminal nerve in four horses with headshaking syndrome, when compared with normal horses [35]. This finding was consistent with increased excitability of the nerve. Latent equine herpes virus 1 (EHV-1) infection of the trigeminal ganglion has been suggested as a potential cause of altered trigeminal nerve function. However, a recent study failed to support this hypothesis as latent EHV-1 infection, as detected by real-time PCR, was found in the trigeminal ganglia of only one of eight geldings with headshaking syndrome [36].

Because headshaking syndrome is more frequently observed in geldings and is often seasonal, Pickles and others [37] advanced a novel hypothesis that increased activity of gonadotropin releasing hormone (GnRH), leading to increased circulating concentrations of luteinizing hormone (LH) and follicle-stimulating hormone (FSH), could lead to seasonal changes in trigeminal nerve excitability in affected geldings. To test this hypothesis, a GnRH vaccine was administered to 19 geldings with headshaking syndrome. Although the vaccine was effective in decreasing LH and FSH concentrations, there was no improvement in seven headshaking signs recorded serially by owners using a visual analogue scale [37].

Medication with carbamazepine, an anticonvulsant and mood-stabilizing drug, is the initial treatment approach to managing classical TN in people, with doses ranging from 100 to 2400 mg/day (or 1.5–35 mg/kg, per os (p.o.), divided into two or three doses). Other medications that have been used alone or in combination when carbamazepine is unsuccessful or provides only partial relief include baclofen, gabapentin, and phenytoin [32]. Many patients respond, at least temporarily, to single or combination therapy with these drugs. Unfortunately, medication is often only partly successful in controlling pain or may only work for a few weeks; consequently, percutaneous or open surgical treatments involving partial trigeminal rhizotomy (by injection, compression, or transection) and microvascular decompression are often pursued [32]. Over time, open microvascular decompression has proven to be the most successful technique, with persistent relief for more than 10 years after the procedure in more than 70% of patients treated by this method [38].

Cyproheptadine (0.3 mg/kg, p.o., twice daily), an antihistamine with antiserotonergic properties, was one of the initial drugs advocated for treatment of headshaking syndrome in horses [15,39]. In a report of seven horses with photic headshaking, treatment with cyproheptadine resulted in improvement in five horses [15] and 43/61 (70%) of owners surveyed reported improvement in headshaking when their horses were treated with this drug [4]. In contrast, a subsequent report by Newton and others [3] did not find this medication helpful in TN-associated headshaking, but few of the cases in this report were considered photic headshakers. However, when carbamazepine (4–8 mg/kg, p.o., four times a day) was combined with cyproheptadine (0.2–0.3 mg/kg, p.o., twice daily), seven horses had dramatic improvement in clinical signs within 3–4 days of starting these medications [3]. A variety of other medications, including non-steroidal anti-inflammatory drugs, antihistamines, various systemic and inhaled corticosteroids, gabapentin, alpha-2-agonists, fluphenazine, phenytoin and phenobarbitol, melatonin, and even sodium cromoglycate eye drops, have also been used to treat headshaking syndrome in horses [2–4,7,15,30,39–41]. Unfortunately, as in people, improvement with medical therapy tends to either be incomplete or may be short-lived.

Because medical treatment alone does not produce satisfactory improvement in many cases, other approaches to managing TN have been pursued. When a photic stimulus is apparent, tinted contact lenses have been helpful for some horses [4] but results have been inconsistent [3]. Similarly, application of a 'nose net' (Figure 52.2) resulted in substantial improvement in 25% of cases [42]. Nose nets are thought to help by providing continual sensory stimulation to the face and muzzle. Repetitive action potentials within the sensory branches of the trigeminal nerve may result in inhibition of nociceptive input (gate-control theory) or a dampening (tachyphylaxis) of the response [3,42]. Other conservative management strategies, supported only by anecdotal reports, have included intranasal corticosteroid administration, topical application of sunscreen and other lotions over the muzzle and nares, acupuncture or chiropractic manipulation, and dietary supplementation with magnesium (a natural sedative) [7].

Of interest, a recent randomized controlled study comparing a nutritional supplement to a placebo did not show any alleviation of headshaking signs assessed by blinded analysis of video recordings of the horses. However, a favourable placebo effect was evident when outcome was based on subjective owner reporting of clinical signs [43]. This finding emphasizes the importance of critical evaluation of clinical signs when various medications, alternative therapies, or diet and management changes are implemented. This is best accomplished by having the owner keep a daily diary of ambient conditions and frequency and severity of clinical signs, utilizing an available scoring system [3] and/or visual analogue scales [37]. A final factor that complicates assessment of efficacy of conservative treatments for headshaking syndrome is the observation that as many as 20–30% of affected horses may spontaneously stop headshaking after several years of exhibiting the syndrome [7].

When the trigger for TN-associated headshaking remains unidentified or cannot be avoided and

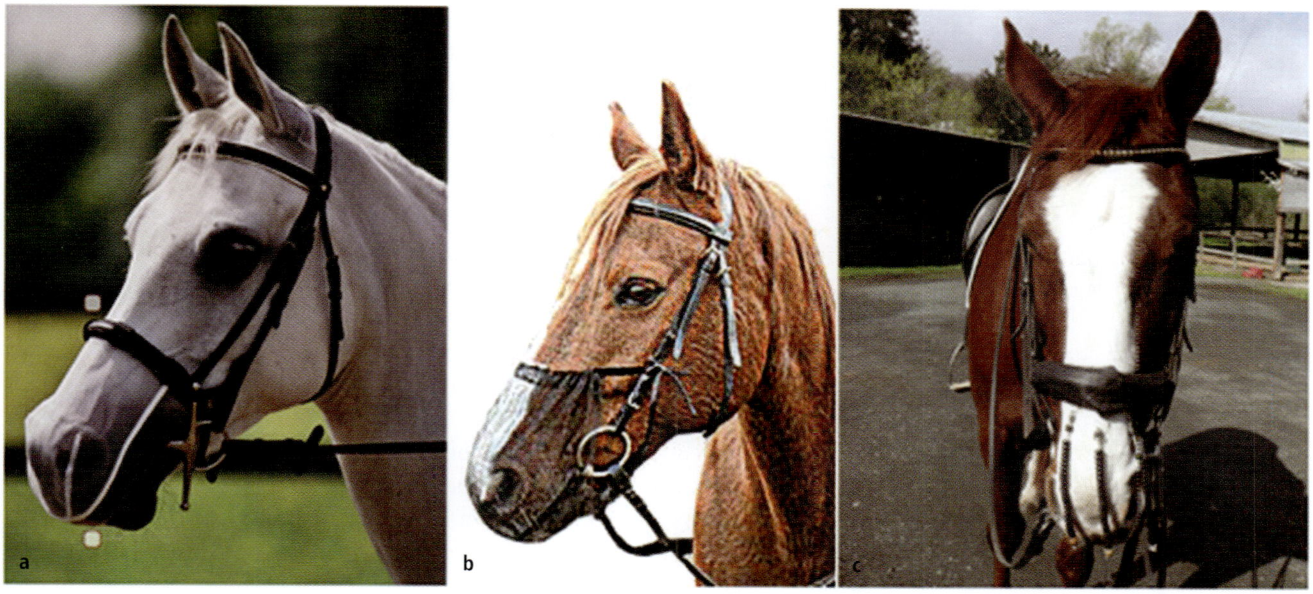

Figure 52.2 Examples of nose nets that can be used to manage headshaking syndrome associated with trigeminal neuralgia/neuropathy: (a) net covers the nares and maxilla; while that in (b) extends over the lips as well. The device shown in (c) is comprised of several strands of beads that stimulate the nares and skin over the nose, rather than a fine mesh screen material. These various types of nose nets can be used on a 'trial and error' basis to see if this continual stimulation attenuates headshaking during exercise. (Reprinted with permission from http://www.headshakingsyndrome.com/treartments/html)

conservative treatment is no longer helpful, interruption of transmission in the affected branch of the trigeminal nerve may be the only remaining treatment option. Ideally, evidence to support a diagnosis of TN should be made by perineural maxillary nerve anaesthesia before an invasive procedure is pursued; however, this is not always possible because nearly a third of horses presented for evaluation of headshaking in one study failed to display the syndrome, perhaps due to lack of the appropriate stimulus at the time of examination or excitement that can override the usual trigger [3]. Bilateral infraorbital neurectomy, performed where the nerve exits the infraorbital foramen, was the initial surgical procedure reported [29]; however, improvement in only a limited number of horses was reported in subsequent case series and headshaking worsened considerably in a few horses [25,30,31]. Further, operated horses frequently traumatized their nostrils and face due to either lack of sensation or suspected hyperaesthesia. Consequently, infraorbital neurectomy is no longer a recommended treatment for idiopathic headshaking syndrome, unless repeated infraorbital perineural anaesthesia demonstrates consistent improvement.

The next invasive treatment attempted to correct headshaking syndrome associated with TN involved chemical sclerosis of the maxillary nerve, after perineural anaesthesia of the nerve near its entry into the infraorbital canal (at the maxillary foramen below the orbit) produced improvement in clinical signs. This procedure involved passing a needle up the infraorbital canal, under radiographic or fluoroscopic guidance, to a level near the maxillary foramen and depositing 5 mL of 10% phenol in almond oil. Although outcome was successful in five horses, headshaking returned within 6 weeks to 9 months [3]. Most recently, compression of the maxillary nerve by placing platinum vascular embolization coils in a similar location in the caudal part of the infraorbital canal near the maxillary foramen (Figure 52.3) has been pursued in an attempt to produce long-term resolution of headshaking [26]. Although unproven, the coils have been suggested to cause pressure degeneration of the nerve. Because degeneration may take several weeks, medication with cyproheptadine, carbamazepine, and/or gabapentin may be necessary for 2–4 weeks following the procedure. Reported success after at least 6 months of follow up approached 60% and increased to 85% in horses in which the procedure was repeated a second time [28]. A final procedure worthy of consideration in an occasional horse with exercise-associated headshaking is diversion of airflow via a permanent tracheostomy. Because increased airflow through the nasal passages during exercise can be a stimulus for headshaking, a tracheostomy is a reasonable consideration (on a 'trial and error' basis) and did result in long-term success in two horses with TN-associated headshaking refractory to other treatments [3].

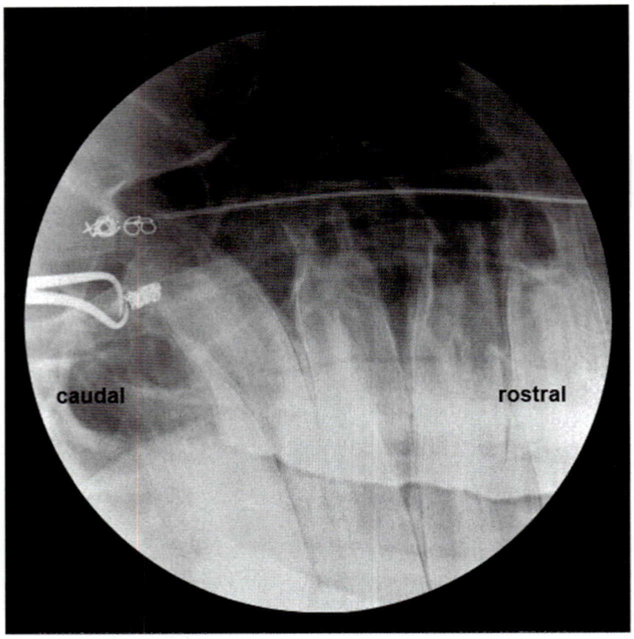

Figure 52.3 Intraoperative radiographic image during placement of platinum coils to compress the maxillary nerve near the maxillary opening of the infraorbital canal above the most caudal molar in a horse with headshaking syndrome. The clump of radiopacity adjacent to the tips of the towel clamp is a group of four coils that have already been placed. The stylet used to place the coils can be seen within the infraorbital canal side as well as several coils that have been placed on the contralateral side.

Allergy

The seasonal occurrence of signs in many idiopathic headshakers led Lane and Mair [2] to suggest that headshaking syndrome may be a clinical manifestation of allergy. These investigators found a number of idiopathic headshakers to have a recurrent cough (27% of cases evaluated) and 32% of horses examined by airway endoscopy had excessive mucus in the trachea, consistent with recurrent airway obstruction (RAO or 'heaves'). Along with RAO, these authors further suggested that allergic rhinitis may be an important trigger for headshaking syndrome because it is a common problem in humans, affecting up to 30% of adults and 40% of children [44]. Of interest, in addition to increased serous nasal secretions, congestion, sneezing, and airflow obstruction, a further sign of allergic rhinitis in people can be facial pain.

To investigate a potential role for allergic rhinitis in headshaking syndrome in horses, nasal mucosal biopsies, as well as detailed gross and microscopic examination of the head and nasal passages, have been performed in a number of headshakers but little pathologic evidence of underlying allergic disease has been found [34]. Nevertheless, some horses with headshaking syndrome do appear to respond to treatment with antihistamines, locally or systemically administered corticosteroids, and sodium cromolyn (by inhalation or eye drops). Because a favourable response to these medications would be consistent with an inflammatory, possibly allergic, trigger, the potential role of allergic rhinitis in headshaking syndrome in horses remains to be fully elucidated. Finally, it is important to recognize that allergy and TN are not mutually exclusive disorders, because inflammation associated with allergy could, in theory, be another factor contributing to altered trigeminal nerve excitability.

In contrast to the uncertain role of allergic rhinitis, non-allergic rhinopathy (previously termed vasomotor rhinitis) has been documented to cause headshaking syndrome in a horse and a pony [2,13]. Although the cause of vasomotor rhinitis is not fully understood, it is a non-seasonal and non-allergic rhinitis thought to be a consequence of altered autonomic control of nasal mucosal blood flow and secretions [44]. With increased airflow during exercise, patients with non-allergic rhinopathy can develop clinical signs that are indistinguishable from allergic rhinitis. Signs can be alleviated by use of both vasoactive drugs (i.e. decongestants) and intranasal corticosteroids. To add further confusion, it also warrants mention that not all allergic rhinitis is seasonal, depending on the offending allergen. For example, dust mites, animal dander, and mould spores can be present year round and lead to perennial allergic rhinitis in people [44].

Another approach to investigate a potential role for allergy in headshaking syndrome in horses has been 'trial and error' allergen-specific immunotherapy (ASIT) following intradermal testing (IDT). However, owners wanting to pursue testing need to be well informed that it may take a year or longer to determine whether or not ASIT will be helpful in control of headshaking. In a report by Madigan and others [15], one horse with headshaking syndrome tested for atopy by IDT was treated with both environmental changes and hyposensitization with no improvement. Similarly, in the owner survey reported by Madigan and Bell [4], most headshakers failed to respond to treatment with antihistamines or corticosteroids prescribed for possible allergies. In contrast, a subsequent report of ASIT guided by results of IDT in 64 horses included five with headshaking syndrome (tested because of additional signs consistent with allergic diseases including conjunctivitis, serous nasal discharge, lip swelling) [6]. Four of these horses had long-term follow up with one excellent response (slow improvement over a 3-year period), one good response (significant improvement but adjunct medical therapy occasionally required), and two poor responses. One of the poor responders also had a paranasal sinus cyst that likely contributed to headshaking, making the true response to ASIT difficult to evaluate. All in all, these authors concluded that ASIT may be a useful adjunctive therapy in management of headshaking syndrome but stated that more horses needed to be evaluated to determine the true value of ASIT. For example, in their one excellent response that slowly improved over 3 years, it is difficult to determine whether improvement occurred spontaneously or in response to ASIT. The authors of this chapter have also performed IDT in a single case of headshaking and this horse responded favourably to ASIT as the only treatment and was able to return to performance after several years during which severe headshaking had precluded competition.

In on-line discussions within a veterinary dermatology list server, eight veterinary dermatologists from the United States and Europe further reported one or more horses with headshaking syndrome that responded favourably to ASIT following IDT. Most of these cases had a history of seasonal headshaking and an extensive diagnostic evaluation to exclude other possible causes. These reports, albeit anecdotal, lead to support of including IDT and possible ASIT in the diagnostic evaluation of headshaking syndrome. However, to accurately evaluate the therapeutic efficacy of ASIT in management of headshaking syndrome, a larger number of horses would need to be studied in a randomized, placebo-controlled clinical trial over several years. Unfortunately, this would be a daunting study to complete and is unlikely to be forthcoming in the next few years. As a consequence, use of IDT and ASIT in evaluation and management of headshaking syndrome is likely to remain difficult to validate and will remain biased by subjective evaluation of patients' clinical response.

References

1. Cook WR. Headshaking in horses: part 1. *Equine Practice* 1979; **1**: 9–17.
2. Lane JG, Mair TS. Observations on headshaking in the horse. *Equine Veterinary Journal* 1987; **19**: 331–336.
3. Newton SA, Knottenbelt DC, Eldridge PR. Headshaking in horses: possible aetiopathogenesis suggested by the results of diagnostic tests and several treatment regimes used in 20 cases. *Equine Veterinary Journal* 2000; **32**: 208–216.
4. Madigan JE, Bell SA. Owner survey of headshaking in horses. *Journal of the American Veterinary Medical Association* 2001; **219**: 334–337.
5. Mills DS, Cook S, Taylor K, *et al.* Analysis of the variations in clinical signs shown by 254 cases of equine headshaking. *Veterinary Record* 2002; **150**: 236–240.
6. Tallarico NJ, Tallarico CM. Results of intradermal allergy testing and treatment by hyposensitization of 64 horses with chronic obstructive pulmonary disease, urticaria, headshaking, and/or reactive airway disease. *Veterinary Allergy and Clinical Immunology* 1998; **6**: 25–35.
7. Headshakerinfo.org. Available at: http://www.headshakerinfo.org/ (accessed 12 December, 2012).
8. Cook WR. Headshaking in horses: part 2. History and management. *Equine Practice* 1979; **1**: 36–39.
9. Cook WR. Headshaking in horses: part 3. Diagnostic tests. *Equine Practice* 1980; **2**: 31–40.
10. Cook WR. Headshaking in horses: part 4. Special diagnostic procedures. *Equine Practice* 1980; **2**: 7–15.
11. Tuft JFD. Headshaking in horses. *Veterinary Record* 1946; **58**: 359.
12. Kold SE, Ostblom LC, Philipsen HP. Headshaking caused by a maxillary osteoma in a horse. *Equine Veterinary Journal* 1982; **14**: 167–169.
13. McGorum BC, Dixon PM. Vasomotor rhinitis with headshaking in a pony. *Equine Veterinary Journal* 1990; **22**: 220–222.
14. Mair TS. Headshaking associated with *Trombicula autumnalis* larval infestation in two horses. *Equine Veterinary Journal* 1994; **26**: 244–245.
15. Madigan JE, Kortz G, Murphy C, *et al.* Photic headshaking in the horse: 7 cases. *Equine Veterinary Journal* 1995; **27**: 306–311.
16. Moore LA, Johnson PJ, Messer NT, *et al.* Management of headshaking in three horses by treatment for protozoal myeloencephalitis. *Veterinary Record* 1997; **141**: 264–267.
17. Voigt A, Saulez MN, Donnellan CM. Nuchal crest avulsion fracture in 2 horses: a cause of headshaking. *Journal of the South African Veterinary Association* 2009; **80**: 111–113.
18. Power HT, Watrous BJ, de Lahunta A. Facial and vestibulocochlear nerve disease in six horses. *Journal of the American Veterinary Medical Association* 1983; **183**: 1076–1080.
19. Blythe LL, Watrous BJ. Pearson EA, *et al.* Otitis media/interna in the horse—a cause of headshaking and skull fractures. *Proceedings of the American Association of Equine Practitioners* 1990; **36**: 517–527.
20. Blythe LL. Otitis media and interna and temporohyoid osteoarthropathy. *Veterinary Clinics of North America: Equine Practice* 1997; **13**: 21–42.
21. Naylor RJ, Perkins JD, Allen S, *et al.* Histopathology and computed tomography of age-associated degeneration of the equine temporohyoid joint. *Equine Veterinary Journal* 2010; **42**: 425–430.
22. Walker AM, Sellon DC, Cornelisse CJ, *et al.* Temporohyoid osteoarthropathy in 33 horses (1993–2000). *Journal of Veterinary Internal Medicine* 2002; **16**: 697–703.
23. Hassel DM, Schott HC 2nd, Tucker RL, *et al.* Endoscopy of the auditory tube diverticula in four horses with otitis media/interna. *Journal of the American Veterinary Medical Association* 1995; **207**: 1081–1084.
24. Pease AP, van Biervliet J, Dykes NL, *et al.* Complication of partial stylohyoidectomy for treatment of temporohyoid osteoarthropathy and an alternative surgical technique in three cases. *Equine Veterinary Journal* 2004; **36**: 46–550.
25. Mair TS. Assessment of bilateral infra-orbital nerve blockade and bilateral infra-orbital neurectomy in the investigation and treatment of idiopathic headshaking. *Equine Veterinary Journal* 1999; **31**: 262–264.
26. Roberts VLH, McKane SA, Williams A, *et al.* Caudal compression of the infraorbital nerve: A novel surgical technique for treatment of idiopathic headshaking and assessment of its efficacy in 24 horses. *Equine Veterinary Journal* 2009; **41**: 165–170.
27. Roberts V. Idiopathic headshaking in horses: understanding the pathophysiology. *Veterinary Journal* 2011; **168**: 17–18.
28. Roberts VLH, Perkins JD, Skärlina E, *et al.* Caudal anesthesia of the infraorbital nerve for diagnosis of idiopathic headshaking and caudal compression of the infraorbital nerve for its treatment, in 58 horses. *Equine Veterinary Journal* 2013; **45**: 107–110.

29. Williams LW. Involuntary shaking of the head and its treatment by trifacial neurectomy. *American Veterinary Review* 1899; **23**: 321–326.
30. Mair TS, Howarth S, Lane JG. Evaluation of some prophylactic therapies for the idiopathic headshaker syndrome. *Equine Veterinary Journal* 1992; **24** (Suppl. 11): 10–12.
31. Wilkins PA, Ducharme NG, Lesser FR. Headshakers: A diagnostic dilemma. *Proceedings of the American Association of Equine Practitioners* 1993; **39**: 263–264.
32. Krafft RM. Trigeminal neuralgia. *American Family Physician* 2008; **77**: 1291–1296.
33. Anon. Headache Classification Subcommittee of the International Headache Society. The international classification of headache disorders: 2nd edn. *Cephalalgia* 2004; **24** (Suppl. 1): 9–160.
34. Newton SA. *The Functional Anatomy of the Trigeminal Nerve of the Horse*. PhD thesis. University of Liverpool, UK, 2001.
35. Pickles KJ, Gibson TJ, Johnson CB, *et al.* Preliminary investigation of somatosensory evoked potentials in equine headshaking. *Veterinary Record* 2011; **168**: 511–514.
36. Aleman M, Pickles KJ, Simonek G, *et al.* Latent equine herpesvirus-1 in trigeminal ganglia and equine idiopathic headshaking. *Journal of Veterinary Internal Medicine* 2012; **26**: 192–194.
37. Pickles KJ, Berger J Davies R, *et al.* Use of gonadotrophin-releasing hormone in headshaking horses. *Veterinary Record* 2011; **168**: 19–23.
38. Barker FG, Janetta PJ, Bissonette DJ, *et al.* The long term outcome of microvascular decompression for trigeminal neuralgia. *New England Journal of Medicine* 1996; **334**: 1077–1083.
39. Wilkins PA. Cyproheptadine: Medical treatment for photic headshakers. *Compendium of Continuing Education for the Practicing Veterinarian* 1997; **19**: 98–111.
40. Mills DS, Cook S, Taylor K, *et al.* Reported response among 254 cases of equine headshaking. *Veterinary Record* 2002; **150**: 311–313.
41. Stalin CE, Boydell IP, Pike RE. Treatment of seasonal headshaking in three horses with sodium cromoglycate eye drops. *Veterinary Record* 2008; **163**: 305–306.
42. Mills DS, Cook S, Taylor K, *et al.* Field study of the efficacy of three types of nose net for the treatment of headshaking in horses. *Veterinary Record* 2003; **152**: 41–44.
43. Talbot WA, Pinchbeck GL, Knottenbelt DC, *et al.* A randomized, blinded, crossover study to assess the efficacy of a feed supplement in alleviating the clinical sign of head shaking in 32 horses. *Equine Veterinary Journal* 2013; **45**: 293–297.
44. Tran NP, Vickery J, Blaiss MS. Management of rhinitis: allergic and non-allergic. *Allergy, Asthma and Immunology Research* 2011; **3**: 148–156.

53

Diagnostic workup of equine atopic disease

Wayne Rosenkrantz[1] and Stephen White[2]

[1] Animal Dermatology Clinic, Tustin, CA, USA
[2] School of Veterinary Medicine, University of California, Davis, CA, USA

Conflict of interest: Wayne Rosenkrantz: Medical Advisory boards and/or speaking: Pinnaclife Animal Health; Novartis Animal Health; Zoetis Animal Health; Elanco Animal Health; Veterinary Allergy Reference Lab (VARL) and Merck Animal Health.

Introduction

Diagnosis of atopic dermatitis is based on history, clinical signs, and the exclusion of other differential diagnoses. A seasonal history is often seen initially, particularly with atopic disease and insect hypersensitivities. Food allergy typically has more of a year-round history but can be a concurrent problem in some atopic disease cases. Clinical signs are listed in Chapter 50. Testing for allergen-specific IgE may include intradermal testing (IDT) and serum *in vitro* testing (SIVT); such tests can not be used to diagnose atopic disease but rather are used in the selection of allergens for allergen-specific immunotherapy (ASIT) and for avoidance of identifiable allergens. Careful historical evaluation and correlation with reactions will improve avoidance and ASIT success rates. Another diagnostic tool that may be helpful is dermatohistopathology.

Dermatopathology

Dermatopathology may not be particularly rewarding in the diagnosis of atopic dermatitis because it is relatively non-specific; but it can rule out other infectious, neoplastic, and autoimmune disorders. Many cases will exhibit mixed eosinophilic perivascular infiltrates with variable degrees of surface crusting, erosions, and ulcerations. Other features seen could include spongiosis, exocytosis, and patchy areas of ortho- and para-hyperkeratosis. Focal areas of eosinophilic folliculitis and eosinophilic granulomas can be seen, more often in insect hypersensitivity.

In a study carried out at the SVM-UCD, 11 horses (urticaria ($n = 6$), pruritus ($n = 2$) and both ($n = 3$)) had skin biopsies performed. Six horses were diagnosed with eosinophilic dermatitis consistent with urticaria, two horses were diagnosed with vasculitis, one horse was diagnosed with perivascular dermatitis consistent with hypersensitivity, one horse was diagnosed with eosinophilic, histiocytic, lymphoplasmacytic dermatitis consistent with hypersensitivity, and one horse was diagnosed with pyotraumatic dermatitis [1].

IgE testing

Testing for IgE using intradermal testing (IDT) has been investigated extensively in the past decade. It has been utilized for the selection of allergens for ASIT, rather than as a diagnostic tool, in humans, dogs, cats, horses, and other mammalian species. IDT is an *in vivo* test that requires intradermal injection of allergens that, in theory, bind and bridge reaginic IgE antibodies on the surface of mast cells and result in mast cell degranulation, and giving rise to wheal and flare reactions. An alternative to IDT is serum *in vitro* testing (SIVT); however, the efficacy of this test compared to IDT is controversial. A series of excellent articles investigating IDT in horses with atopic dermatitis, recurrent urticaria, chronic obstructive pulmonary disease (COPD), and healthy

Veterinary Allergy, First Edition. Edited by Chiara Noli, Aiden Foster, and Wayne Rosenkrantz.

horses as controls, have been published from research performed at the Ohio State University, USA [2–5]. The interpretive conclusion is that horses with these diseases (at least in the USA) generally have a higher incidence of positive reactions than healthy horses, but that the diagnosis (as in other species) can not be made solely on the basis of the results of IDT or SIVT alone; rather, these tests should be interpreted in light of the history of the disease (i.e. a horse with seasonal signs is more likely to have an allergic response to allergens it is exposed to seasonally—pollens in the summer, barn dust in the winter). This interpretation thus will increase the clinician's ability to determine which allergens might be relevant for ASIT, should the owners elect to choose that route of treatment.

Serum *in vitro* testing

The controversy over these tests relates to problems of technique, non-specific binding, lack of standardization between laboratories, allergen preparation, and sample processing. Most laboratories use a polyclonal anti-IgE reagent; the specificity and the affinity of the reagents may vary between laboratories. One study found a sensitivity of 47.3% and a specificity of 81.7%, with a positive predictive value of 68.7% and a negative predictive value of 64.7%, in horses with atopic disease and horses without atopic disease using IDT as the standard. This study used three different allergen-specific assays and found that none produced results similar to those obtained by IDT; however, an ELISA based on the Fc-epsilon-R1-alpha performed significantly better overall than the others [4]. Another study also showed a poor correlation between IDT and an ELISA using a monoclonal antibody specific for horse IgE, with only 2/61 allergens (timothy and quack) having substantial agreement between IDT and IgE ELISA. In this study, it was concluded that commercial allergen extracts contained a high variation in detectable protein and that high concentrations of allergen-specific IgG in the horse serum competed with IgE for binding to the plates [6].

Another study used an ELISA method to evaluate and compared levels of allergen-specific IgE in Icelandic horses, with and without *Culicoides* hypersensitivity, from Iceland and Sweden. The investigators also looked at patterns of allergen-specific IgE to insects, pollens, moulds, and mites in those groups of horses and examined the clinical significance of employing two different cut-off levels for the ELISA. The study comprised a total number of 99 horses and sera from the horses was analysed blindly with the use of a non-competitive, solid-phase ELISA-test, designed to detect the presence of allergen-specific IgE in sera using the recombinant alpha chain of the high-affinity IgE receptor (Fc-epsilon-R1-alpha). Even with the use of two cut-off levels of 150 and 300 EA, this study showed that serological testing with the high-affinity IgE receptor is at present not suitable as a tool for establishing a diagnosis of *Culicoides* hypersensitivity or equine atopy [7].

An *in vitro* bioassay has also been reported to study the role of allergens in horses with recurrent airway obstruction (RAO). This assay measures the calcium release from rat basophilic leukaemia 2H3 (RBL-2H3) cells preincubated with horse sera and then stimulated with the allergen being tested. The RBL-2H3 cell line is a commonly used histamine-releasing cell line used in inflammation, allergy, and immunological research. In this particular study, the assay was able to discriminate between normal and horses with RAO for two allergens involved in RAO, *Aspergillus fumigatus* and *Faenia rectivirgula* [8]. It is possible that such an assay could be developed into a diagnostic test for other environmental allergens involved with atopic dermatitis.

Further supporting value for SIVT were two studies. The first was a study reported from the SVM-UCD. In 27 horses that were reported to benefit from ASIT, 13 horses had their ASIT formulated based on the results of IDT, nine had their ASIT based on a serum test, and five had both an IDT and a serum test. A chi-square analysis used to compare the success proportions of ASIT between skin tests, serum tests, and both showed no statistical difference between the three groups ($P = 0.53$) [1]. These results likely reflect the impact of how well the clinician correlates positive reactions with the history of exposure to positive allergens and clinical symptoms. The second study was a prospective 2-year evaluation of ASIT in horses based on IDT, SIVT, or a combination of IDT and SIVT demonstrated a decrease in a visual analogue score of 1.2 for each 12-month period of ASIT therapy and no significant differences among treatment groups [9]. In addition there was excellent agreement between initial allergen-specific IgE concentrations and both immediate and delayed IDT results, and between immediate IDT and IgG results. Specific concentration of serum IgE and IgG decreased significantly for allergens that were included in ASIT.

Several laboratories offer equine SIVT throughout the United States and abroad. The reader should check with their local laboratory before considering this option. It should be emphasized that the accuracy, reproducibility, and standardization of such labs has not been validated in any studies. Results of SIVT should be carefully correlated with appropriate history and physical findings for allergen selection for ASIT and not used for diagnostic purposes.

Intradermal testing

Intradermal testing is not without its share of problems but has generally shown that allergic horses react more frequently to IDT then healthy horses [2–5,10]. However one report from Austria compared IDT results between 38 normal horses and 43 horses with 'summer seasonal recurrent dermatitis' using 22 allergens (pollens, moulds, mites and insects, including *Culicoides variipennis*). Differences between the two groups of horses were found only in the reactions to deer fly, horse fly and *C. variipennis*; in the latter differences were only noted at a 1 : 10 000 w/v dilution and the normal horses had more reactions [11]. Such problems may reflect the concentrations at which allergens are used because irritant threshold concentrations will vary from allergen to allergen and by not testing at correct concentrations both false-positive and false-negative reactions can occur [12].

Some studies have attempted to determine optimum testing concentrations. Threshold concentrations (TC) of allergens in 41 normal horses, using three to five serial dilutions of 27 allergens, were the focus of one study. The TC was determined for nine pollens (2000 to >6000 PNU/mL), four moulds (4000 to >6000 PNU/mL), seven insects (ant, horse fly 125 PNU/mL; house fly, cockroach 250 PNU/mL; moth 60 PNU/mL; mosquito 1000 PNU/mL; *Culicoides nubeculosus* 1 : 5000 w/v), and three of four storage mites (1 : 10 000 w/v). The TC was not determined due to excessive reactivity at the lowest concentrations tested for dust mites (*Dermatophagoides farinae*, <1 : 12 000 w/v; *D. pteronyssinus*, <1 : 30 000 w/v, and *Acarussiro*, <1 : 10 000 w/v). This study suggested testing concentrations for IDT in atopic horses may be > or =1000 PNU/mL for pollens and moulds, 60 to 250 PNU/mL for most insects and <1 : 12 000 w/v for dust mites [13].

One other major problem with IDT is that it is not readily available to all practitioners because it is often not financially practical to maintain the extracts to perform testing themselves nor are specialists always available to do the testing. In addition to knowing the correct testing concentrations, the allergen selection depends upon the geographical region, although many allergens are found world wide. Most specialists utilize similar allergens to what is used in small animals in their area, with the addition of more insects and moulds. Tables 53.1 and 53.2 include the tests and allergen concentrations that the authors utilize at their respective locations in northern and southern California. In Table 53.1 all allergens are tested at 1000 PNUs/mL unless listed differently, which for many of the insects is typical. A few of the insects are listed in weight to volume (w/v) concentrations. In a study that was performed in southern California in horses with both insect and environmental allergies the following allergens were found to be the most prevalent: house fly, horse fly, black fly, *Culicoides variipennis*, *Culicoides nubeculosus*, *Curvularia*, pepper tree, eucalyptus, western juniper, red mulberry, box elder, English plantain, western ragweed, and smooth brome [9]. In the same study there was no difference between normal and affected horses when it came to reactivity to deer fly, yellow dock, Russian thistle, and fireweed.

The most common allergens implicated on IDT and serologic tests at the UCD were the house dust mites *Dermatophagoides farinae* and *D. pteronyssinus*, olive tree, Bermuda grass, sage, and the mould *Penicillium notatum* [1]. In a study from France of presumed atopic horses, the most common positive allergens were *Culicoides* spp. and the house dust mites [14]. It appears that house dust mite allergens are very important in atopic dermatitis in the horse. Additionally, the presence of house dust mite allergens in horse blankets has been demonstrated [15]. It is also likely that some dust mite reactions in horse may be detecting cross-reactivity with storage mites because this is a very prevalent allergen in horse feeds, hay, and shavings.

Once antigen selection for testing has been made, these need to be obtained and prepared. Allergenic extracts should be from a reputable supply company. As mentioned above in this section, standard concentration of pollen and mould allergens for testing is variable, but allergen companies will typically supply basic testing concentrations. Solutions for skin testing should be refrigerated and made up fresh every 4 weeks to maintain appropriate potency.

In order to obtain optimal results with IDT, the horse should be withdrawn from antihistamine therapy for several days (5–10 days) and oral glucocorticoids for 10–14 days prior to testing. Longer withdrawal periods may be needed if oral glucocorticoids have been used for extended periods of time or if long-acting injectable glucocorticoids have been used. One study evaluated intradermal testing and withdrawal times for hydroxyzine (after 500 mg twice daily for 7 days) and dexamethasone (after 20 mg once daily for 7 days) in five horses without allergic symptoms before and after treatment with these drugs. Testing was repeated in 3–4 hours, 7 days, and 14 days after drug withdrawal. No differences were found between pre- and post-treatment subjective IDT scores for either drug. However, wheal diameter for histamine and house dust, dust mite mix, and black ant extracts decreased ($P < 0.05$) at all times post injection for IDT performed 3–4 hours after the final dose of both medications. Wheal diameter returned to pretreatment levels 14 days after discontinuation of dexamethasone and 7 days after discontinuation of hydroxyzine. This

Table 53.1 Veterinary Medical Teaching Hospital, University of California, Davis, Dermatology and Allergy Service Intradermal Skin Testing (Reprinted with permission from University of California, Davis)

Clinician:

Date:

Controls

201 Saline ______

202 Histamine (1 : 100 000) ______

Inhalants

203 House dust (500) ______

204 Cat epithelia ______

205 Pyrethrum ______

206 Sheep epithelia ______

Trees and shrubs

207 Acacia ______

208 Alder, White ______

209 Ash, Arizona ______

210 Birch, White ______

211 Box Elder (500) ______

212 Cedar, Red ______

213 Cypress, Arizona (1 : 1000) ______

214 Elm, Chinese ______

215 Maple, Red ______

216 Mulberry, White ______

217 Oak, Calif. White ______

218 Olive ______

219 Orange Tree ______

220 Privet ______

221 Western Sycamore ______

222 Walnut, English ______

Grasses

223 Bermuda ______

224 Johnson ______

225 Kentucky Blue ______

Weeds

226 Dandelion ______

227 Dock, Yellow ______

228 Lambs Quarter ______

229 Pigweed, R/R _____

230 Plantain, English ______

231 Ragweed, Western ______

232 Russian Thistle ______

233 Sorrel, Red/Sheep

Cultivated plants

234 Alfalfa ______

235 Corn (250) ______

236 Oat, Cultivated _____

237 Mustard ______

238 Rye, Perennial ______

230 Sugar Beets ______

240 Wheat, Cultivated _____

Moulds

241 *Alternaria tenius* ______

242 *Aspergillus niger* ______

243 *Curvularia spicifera* ______

244 *Fusarium moniliforme* ______

245 *Hormodendrum hordei* ______

246 *Mucor plumbeus* ______

247 *Penicillium notatum* ______

248 *Pullularia pullulans* ______

Insects

249 Flea (1 : 1000) ______

250 *D. farinae* (1 : 1000) ______

251 *D. pteronyssinus* (1 : 1000) _

252 Ant, Black (1 : 1000) ______

253 Cockroach, American ______

254 Deerfly ______

255 Housefly ______

256 Mosquito ______

257 *Culicoides* (1 : 1000) ______

258 Horsefly ______

Additional allergens

259 Grain Mill Dust (1 : 5000) ______

260 Grain Smut (1 : 5000) ______

261 Eucalyptus ______

262 Tobacco ______

263 Sage ______

264 Feathers ______

265 *Malassezia* ______

266 *Tyrophagus putrescentiae*______

All antigens tested at 1000 PNU unless otherwise indicated.

Table 53.2 Animal Dermatology Clinic Southern California Equine Skin Test (Reprinted from www.animaldermatology.com, with permission of Animal Dermatology Clinic)

Date:	Dr.:	Patient:	Client:
Controls		**Grasses**	
1. Saline		32. Bermuda *Cynodon dactylon*	
2. Histamine		33. Seven grass mix	
Insects		34. Brome *Bromus inermis*	
3. Mosquito *Culicidae*, 1000		35. Perennial rye *Lolium perenne*	
4. Mosquito *Culicidae*, 250		36. Orchard *Dactylis glomerata*	
5. Deer fly *Chrysops* sp., 1000		37. Timothy *Phleum pratense*	
6. Deer fly *Chrysops* sp., 250		38. Alfalfa *Medicago sativa*	
7. Black ant *Camponotus pennsylvanicus*, 125		**Trees**	
8. Flea *Ctenocephalides canis/felis* 1000, w/v		39. Box elder *Acer negundo*	
9. Flea *Ctenocephalides canis/felis* 400, w/v		40. Palm *Arecastrum romanzoffianum*	
10. Storage mite *Acarus siro*		41. Western juniper *Juniperus occidentalis*	
11. Storage mite *Tyrophagus putrescentiae*		42. *Acacia* spp.	
12. *Culicoides variipennis*, 1:1000		43. Western oak mix *Quercus* spp.	
13. *Culicoides variipennis*, 1 : 10 000		44. Western walnut mix *Juglans* spp.	
14. Horse fly *Tabanus* spp., 1000		45. Olive *Olea europaea*	
15. Horse fly *Tabanus* spp., 250		46. *Melaleuca quinquenervia*	
16. House fly *Musca domistica*, 1000		47. *Eucalyptus globulus*	
17. House fly *Musca domistica*, 250		48. Orange *Citrus sinensis*	
18. Moth Lepidoptera		49. California cottonwood *Populus fremontii*	
19. Dust mite *Dermatophagoides farinae*, 250		50. Arroyo willow *Salix lasiolepis*	
20. Dust mite *Dermatophagoides farinae*, 62.5		51. White mulberry *Morus alba*	
21. Caddis fly *Trichoptera*		52. Pepper tree *Schinus* spp.	
22. May fly *Ephemeroptera*		53. Salt cedar *Tamarix gallica*	
Epithelia		**Weeds**	
23. Cat dander *Felis catus*		54. Pigweed mix *Amaranthus* spp.	
24. Feather chicken, duck, goose		55. Lambs quarter *Chenopodium album*	
25. Mouse *Mus musculus*		56. Russian thistle *Salsola kali*	
26. Rat *Rattus norvegicus*		57. Firebrush *Kochia scoparia*	
27. Pyrethrum *Chrysanthemum cinerariifolium*		58. Western ragweed *Ambrosia* spp.	
Moulds		59. Sage mix *Artemisia* spp.	
28. *Curvularia spicifera*		60. Dandelion *Taraxacum officinale*	
29. *Fusarium* mix		61. *Baccharis* spp.	
30. *Mucor* mix		62. Mustard *Brassica* spp.	
31. *Penicillium* mix		63. Dock/sorrel *Rumex* spp.	
		64. English plantain *Plantago lanceolata*	
		65. Nettle *Urtica dioca*	

Scoring legend: 0 or left blank, no reaction: 1, low reaction; 2, moderate reaction; 3, strong reaction; 4, very strong reaction.
If a '+' is beside a score, slightly larger than the score/number.

study concluded that treatment of horses with dexamethasone or hydroxyzine for 7 days had no effect on testing results but did decrease IDT wheal diameters. Based on the findings of this study, withdrawal times of 14 and 7 days for dexamethasone and hydroxyzine, respectively, prior to IDT could be recommended [16]. Skin testing usually requires sedation and shaving. The authors and other specialists have had good success utilizing xylazine hydrochloride, butorphanol, and detomidine intravenously. Phenothiazine tranquilizers should be avoided as they may inhibit IDT reactions.

The best site for testing is the lateral cervical region above the jugular furrow, between the jaw and the shoulder (Figure 53.1). The skin just below the mane should be avoided because it is thicker and more difficult to inject. The site should be clipped with a number 40 blade and sites ink-marked for reference of antigen identification. Approximately 0.05 to 0.1 mL of the antigen is injected intradermally. Injections should be made 2 cm apart to avoid overlapping of reactions and misinterpretation of results. Reactions should be evaluated at 15–30 minutes and if possible at 45 minutes, 4–6 hours, and at 24 to 48 hours (Figure 53.2). It may be impractical to do 24–48 hour assessment in many clinical situations. Owners can be advised to observe for late-onset or delayed reactions (swellings) and can measure and report these via the phone. Reactions are subjectively interpreted as with small animals, scoring reactions 0, 1, 2, 3, and 4. Grading is based upon size, demarcations, depth, and turgor of the wheals compared to a positive control (histamine 1:100 000 dilution) and a negative control (saline). Reactions greater than 2 are considered positive.

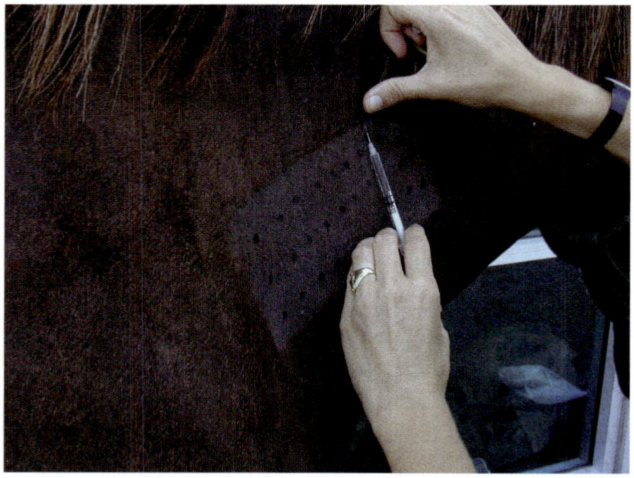

Figure 53.1 Intradermal testing injection technique showing standard site for testing at the lateral cervical region above the jugular furrow.

Adverse food reaction testing

Although available, there is no accurate *in vitro* or *in vivo* test for food allergies. The only accurate way to diagnose an adverse food reaction or intolerance is food avoidance. In small animals it is known that a restricted diet takes between 6 and 8 weeks or longer to document food allergy; however, such time limits have not been confirmed in the horse. The 4 weeks that is currently recommended may be too short and the author currently recommends 6 weeks in the horse. It can be difficult to convince an owner to do an elimination diet in a horse. Selection of a protein source that is foreign or not commonly fed is recommended. The authors have had

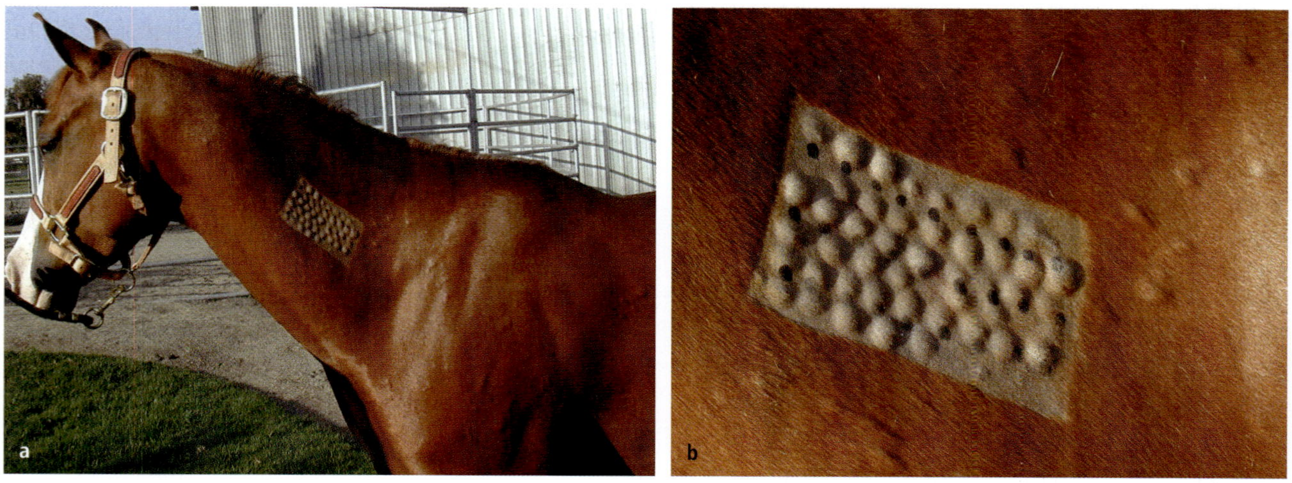

Figure 53.2 Positive intradermal reactions in an atopic dermatitis case with both urticarial and pruritic skin disease at 45 minutes post injections.

success with timothy or barley hay if these are not routinely fed. In addition, unnecessary supplements, vitamins, and other drugs should be discontinued during the diet period. At the end of the dietary trial the horse should be rechallenged with the previous diet and/or supplements. Generally, adding back one item every 5–7 days is recommended to determine which food group or protein is responsible.

References

1. Stepnik CT, Outerbridge CA, White SD, *et al.* Equine atopic skin disease and response to allergen-specific immunotherapy: a retrospective study at the University of California-Davis (1991–2008). *Veterinary Dermatology* 2011; **23**: 29–35, e7.
2. Jose-Cunilleras E, Kohn CW, Hillier A, *et al.* Intradermal testing in healthy horses and horses with chronic obstructive pulmonary disease, recurrent urticaria, or allergic dermatitis. *Journal of the American Veterinary Medical Association* 2001; **219**: 1115–1121.
3. Lorch G, Hillier A, Kwochka KW, *et al.* Results of intradermal tests in horses without atopy and horses with atopic dermatitis or recurrent urticaria. *American Journal of Veterinary Research* 2001; **62**: 1051–1059.
4. Lorch G, Hillier A, Kwochka KW, *et al.* Comparison of immediate intradermal test reactivity with serum IgE quantitation by use of a radioallergosorbent test and two ELISA in horses with and without atopy. *Journal of the American Veterinary Medical Association* 2001; **218**: 1314–1322.
5. Lorch G, Hillier A, Kwochka KW, *et al.* Results of intradermal tests in horses without atopy and horses with chronic obstructive pulmonary disease. *American Journal of Veterinary Research* 2001; **62**: 389–397.
6. Morgan EE, Miller WH, Jr., Wagner B. A comparison of intradermal testing and detection of allergen-specific immunoglobulin E in serum by enzyme-linked immunosorbent assay in horses affected with skin hypersensitivity. *Veterinary Immunology and Immunopathology* 2007; **120**: 160–167.
7. Frey R, Bergvall K, Egenvall A. Allergen-specific IgE in Icelandic horses with insect bite hypersensitivity and healthy controls, assessed by FcepsilonR1alpha-based serology. *Veterinary Immunology and Immunopathology* 2008; **126**: 102–109.
8. Moran G, Burgos R, Araya O, *et al.* In vitro bioassay to detect reaginic antibodies from the serum of horses affected with recurrent airway obstruction. *Veterinary Research Communications* 2010; **34**: 91–99.
9. Radwanski N, Morris D, Boston R, *et al.* A prospective evaluation of clinical and immunological responses to allergen-specific immunotherapy in horses with atopic dermatitis. *Veterinary Dermatology* 2012; **23** (Suppl. 1): 42.
10. Rosenkrantz W, Griffin C, Esch R, *et al.* Responses in horses to intradermal challenge of insects and environmental allergens with specific immunotherapy. In: Hillier A, Foster AP, Kwochka KW, eds. *Advances in Veterinary Dermatology*, vol. 5. Oxford: Blackwell Publishing, 2005: 191–200.
11. Kolm-Stark G, Wagner R. Intradermal skin testing in Icelandic horses in Austria. *Equine Veterinary Journal* 2002; **34**: 405–410.
12. Morris DO, Lindborg S. Determination of 'irritant' threshold concentrations for intradermal testing with allergenic insect extracts in normal horses. *Veterinary Dermatology* 2003; **14**: 31–36.
13. Baxter CG, Vogelnest LJ. Determination of threshold concentrations of multiple allergenic extracts for equine intradermal testing using normal horses in three seasons. *Veterinary Dermatology* 2008; **19**: 305–313.
14. Lebis C, Bourdeau P, Marzin-Keller F. Intradermal skin tests in equine dermatology: a study of 83 horses. *Equine Veterinary Journal* 2002; **34**: 666–671.
15. Wallace JC, Vogelnest LJ. Evaluation of the presence of house dust mites in horse rugs. *Veterinary Dermatology* 2010; **21**: 602–607.
16. Petersen A, Schott HC, 2nd. Effects of dexamethasone and hydroxyzine treatment on intradermal testing and allergen-specific IgE serum testing results in horses. *Veterinary Dermatology* 2009; **20**: 615–622.

54

Equine atopic disease symptomatic therapy and allergen-specific immunotherapy

Wayne Rosenkrantz[1] and Stephen White[2]

[1] Animal Dermatology Clinic, Tustin, CA, USA
[2] School of Veterinary Medicine, University of California, Davis, CA, USA

Conflict of interest: Wayne Rosenkrantz: Medical Advisory boards and/or speaking: Pinnaclife Animal Health; Novartis Animal Health; Zoetis Animal Health; Elanco Animal Health; Veterinary Allergy Reference Lab (VARL) and Merck Animal Health.

Introduction

Equine atopic skin disease is typically considered a lifelong disease that requires chronic management. Management strategies include allergen avoidance, topical therapy, systemic medications, such as antihistamines, glucocorticoids, and tricyclic antidepressants, or a combination of all of these [1]. Some of these options have undesirable adverse effects and limitations on usage in competition sporting events and avoidance of allergens is often impractical. Allergen-specific immunotherapy (ASIT) is therefore a practical option for many cases [2,3]. ASIT has been used successfully in the management of atopic skin disease in horses [2–4]. Intradermal and serum tests have been utilized for identification of allergens to be used in ASIT in horses [1].

The concepts of allergic threshold and summation of effect are just as important in treating equine atopic disease as they are in other species. The allergic threshold is a theoretic level above which clinical signs occur and this is due to not only the primary allergens but also other secondary factors such as bacterial infection and bacterial and yeast overgrowth. Other factors that may also contribute include dryness to the skin from the primary atopic disease or environmental humidity as well as psychogenic components. All of these variables have a 'summation effect' that can push cases above their allergic threshold, resulting in clinical disease. Therefore it is also important to address all predisposing horse and environmental factors to achieve a successful therapeutic protocol.

Avoidance

Although avoidance of allergens is an optimal way of preventing hypersensitivity reactions it is highly impractical in horses. However, there are certain allergens that may be reduced in the environment with subsequent reduction of clinical signs. In some situations a complete change in environment can be helpful to avoid regionally active allergens.

Dust, storage mite, and mould control

Dust and moulds can be reduced but rarely eliminated. They are found in high concentrations in a variety of feeds and bedding materials (Table 54.1). There are a few considerations that can help. To minimize dust in barns, switch to rubber mats, peat, or pelleted bedding instead of shavings or straw bedding [5–8] and switch to grass silage, hydroponic, or wet down hay and/or pelleted rations.

House dust mites (*Dermatophagoides farinae* and *D. pteronyssinus*) can be found on horse blankets [9] and storage mites (*Tyrophagus, Blomina, Acarus*) that feed on mouldy bedding or hay are impossible to completely eliminate from the barn. However, measures to reduce

Veterinary Allergy, First Edition. Edited by Chiara Noli, Aiden Foster, and Wayne Rosenkrantz.

Table 54.1 Respirable dust and mould spores in a variety of feed and bedding

Feed/bedding	Respirable dust (particles× 10^3/L)	*A. fumigatus* (CFU/L)	*F. rectivirgula* (CFU/L)	*T. vulgaris* (CFU/L)
Good hay	63.0 (30.0)	20.1 (5.6)	3.1 (1.2)	3.3 (1.2)
Silage 78% DM	8.8 (2.5)	11.5 (6.5)	1.7 (1.2)	2.2 (0.7)
Silage ± 50% DM	4.5 (1.9)	4.5 (4.2)	0.4 (0.2)	1.2 (0.8)
Alfalfa pellets	9.5 (4.4)	2.6 (2.5)	0.1 (0.0)	0.4 (0.2)
Wood shavings	31.5 (12.9)	16.7 (2.9)	1.2 (0.7)	1.9 (1.4)
Cleanbox wood shavings	6.2 (0.1)	0.04 (0.05)	0.02 (0.04)	0.15 (0.09)
Good straw	11.6 (4.9)	9.5 (5.0)	0.4 (0.4)	0.8 (0.4)
Flax straw	9.3 (1.8)	2.4 (0.5)	0.2 (0.2)	1.4 (0.3)
Ecobed cardboard	5.7 (1.6)	0.03 (0.05)	0 (0)	0 (0.01)
Rolled grains	120.3 (30.6)	10.2 (0.6)	1.8 (1.6)	1.1 (1.1)
Whole grains	4.1 (0.9)	4.5 (1.5)	0.1 (0.0)	1.0 (0.1)
Molasses concentrates	2.1 (0.6)	0.8 (0.3)	0.3 (0.2)	3.0 (1.8)

Material was agitated in an air stream and particulates expressed per litre of air. CFU, colony-forming unit; DM, dry matter.
Adapted from Robinson NE. Recurrent airway obstruction (heaves). In: Lekeux P, ed. *Equine Respiratory Diseases*. Ithaca: International Veterinary Information Service. Available at: www.ivis.org, 30-Nov-2001.

these allergens may be attempted. Common suggestions for house dust mite reduction include washing horse blankets in hot water (<55°C/130°F) to reduce house dust allergen and to use house dust mite miticidal agents (borates, Ecology Works® DustMite Control) in the barn before new bedding is placed in stalls every 4–6 months. For storage mite control, the same measures for house dust mites may be helpful and, if possible, the utilization of feeds that are less likely to become mouldy. Simply moving a horse from an indoor barn situation to a pasture can also help for dust, mite, and mould allergies.

The positive effects of environment versus environment and anti-inflammatory therapy were evaluated in one study that showed changing to wood shavings and a pelleted diet in place of straw bedding and hay for 2 weeks resulted in improvement of recurrent airway obstruction (RAO) in 12 horses within 3 days and continued for 7 days [5]. The addition of steroids in this study induced a more rapid reduction in airway inflammation. Overall, airway function was best after 30 days at pasture. The notable improvement in lung function within 3 days of an environmental modification emphasized the need for allergen reduction [5,10]. An investigation of various peat–moss composites revealed fungi in sphagnum peat, various levels of endotoxin, and the presence of thermophilic actinomycetes and *Aspergillus fumigatus* in few-flowered peat materials [6]. The concentrations of inhalable dust were smaller in the few-flowered peats than in the sphagnum peats. It was concluded that there are differences in the dustiness and hygienic quality of peat bedding. In another study, shredded cardboard was evaluated as an appropriate bedding to minimize dust in bedding. Pulmonary function tests, arterial blood gases, airway inflammation scoring, and bronchoalveolar cytology were significantly different from those recorded in poor hygienic conditions, and it was concluded that cardboard bedding, used in conjunction with low-dust forage, might be appropriate to minimize dust exposure in horses with heaves [8].

Insect control

Similar to canine allergic dermatitis, both inhalation and percutaneous absorption of insect allergens most likely occurs. Black ants, house fly, caddis fly and mayfly, dust and storage mites are non-biting arthropods that may induce this type of hypersensitivity. As listed in Chapters 47 and 48, both repellents and environmental insecticides are often needed. In particular, in regards to controlling non-biting arthropods that may also contribute to allergic reactions via inhalation or percutaneous absorption, environmental insecticides can be helpful in reducing the levels of such allergens.

Elimination diet trials

In the authors' experience there is no accurate *in vitro* or *in vivo* test for diagnosing food allergies and the only accurate way to diagnose an adverse food reaction or intolerance is food avoidance. However, there is one report of 22 cases of recurrent or chronic urticaria in thoroughbred racehorses where positive intradermal tests with fresh allergenic foods were used to correlate with clinical signs, and the elimination of the suspect allergen brought about resolution of clinical signs such as urticaria and enteritis [11]. Such testing in both humans and in small animals has been highly controversial and it is currently best to rely on dietary elimination trials.

In dogs and cats, it may take between 6 and 8 weeks or longer of an elimination diet to document food allergies; however, similar time limits have not been confirmed in the horse. The 4 weeks that is currently recommended by many veterinarians may be too short and the authors currently recommend 6–8 weeks in the horse. It can be difficult to convince an owner to do an elimination diet in a horse. Selection of a protein source that is foreign or not commonly fed is recommended. The authors have had success with timothy, oats, or barley if not routinely fed. In addition, unnecessary supplements, vitamins, and other drugs should be discontinued for this time period. At the end of the dietary trial, the horse should be rechallenged with the previous diet and/or supplements. Generally, adding back one item every 5–7 days is recommended to determine which food group or protein is responsible.

Topical therapy

There are a variety of different topical repellents and insecticides available to use to control insect allergens, which have been previously discussed in Chapters 47 and 48. However, many practitioners fail to utilize other forms of topical therapy in atopic disease in the horse. As seen in other species with atopic dermatitis, topical therapy in the horse can provide emollient, moisturizing, and antipruritic effects and may improve epidermal barrier function. There is no evidence that the epidermal barrier function in atopic dermatitis horses is impaired. However, a pilot study did look at this ultrastructurally, using transmission electron microscopy, and functionally, by measuring transepidermal water loss, in two normal and two atopic horses. No differences were found for transepidermal water loss between normal and atopic horses. However, transmission electron microscopy showed that the stratum corneum had irregularities and abnormal amorphous lipids in the atopic horses, and that these changes were most prominent in atopic dermatitis sites [12]. More studies are needed but the simple process of bathing can remove or reduce surface allergens on the skin, minimizing percutaneous absorption and increasing skin hydration. Bathing with cool water in particular can reduce pruritus.

Bathing when combined with emollients and moisturizing agents may improve the integrity of the epidermal barrier and, when combined with antimicrobial agents, control secondary infections. The selection of shampoos should be based on the skin condition and may include colloidal oatmeal products (shampoos, conditioners, and bath treatments) with or without a local anaesthetic (pramoxine HCl) or glucocorticoids for more potent control of pruritus, sulphur/salicylic acid shampoos for excess scale, antimicrobial shampoos (benzoyl peroxide, ethyl lactate, chlorhexidine, or imidazoles) if secondary infections have been identified, or a combination of one or more of the above. The authors prefer products that typically are used in small animals rather than for humans when specific dermatological products are not readily available for horses. Topical glucocorticoids can be valuable for localized areas of pruritus but most of these products are not labelled for use in equine medicine. The authors have used several topical glucocorticoid-containing products. Some of the more effective and practical products include a mild 1% hydrocortisone, leave-on conditioner in a non-irritating base (Resicort®, Virbac) and a 0.015% triamcinolone spray (Genesis Topical Spray®, Virbac). These products tend to be safer for daily use and have fewer side effects than other more potent concentrations of triamcinolone, betamethasone, or dexamethasone creams and ointments.

When choosing a topical glucocorticoid, the goal is to select products with minimal side effects topically (local cutaneous atrophy, alopecia, comedone formation, and secondary infections) and systemically (minimal to no haematological and biochemical changes, suppression of the adrenal axis). Another product that is available in Europe which would be a good choice for localized pruritus control in the horse is a newer topical glucocorticoid, hydrocortisone aceponate (HCA; Cortavance®, Virbac SA, Carros, France), available as a 0.0584% spray formulation. It has been used successfully for the short-term treatment of pyotraumatic dermatitis and allergic dermatitis in dogs [13]. As a non-halogenated, di-ester topical glucocorticoid it is associated with better local and systemic tolerance compared to conventional topical glucocorticoids [14]. One author (WR) has used this product in one case of localized mane and tail pruritus with a good short-term response.

One study looked at cutaneous atrophy in horses comparing several topical glucocorticoids (hydrocortisone, diflorasone diacetate, mometasone furoate, and clobetasol propionate). The thoracic skin was treated daily for 12 days and the skin thickness was measured by the CT (compression thickness) method. The skin-thinning effect of diflorasone diacetate, mometasone furoate, and clobetasol propionate was quite similar. Hydrocortisone showed only a weak skin-thinning effect [15]. The study confirmed that atrophy can occur with some of the more potent glucocorticoids. In addition, the authors feel that the lower limbs of horses are particular sensitive to this side effect and special care needs to taken when using potent glucocorticoids in that location.

Systemic therapy

Antihistamines and tricyclic antidepressants

Antihistamines and tricyclic antidepressants (TCAs) can provide a non-steroidal alternative for long-term control of allergic reactions in horses. Antihistamines and some of the TCAs have classically been defined as chemicals that block the action of histamines at receptor sites. However, antihistamines and in particular the TCAs may also have antipruritic effects and reduce urticarial reactions by stabilizing mast cells and having antiserotonin properties. Although exact dosing based on pharmacokinetics is lacking in the horse, many practitioners use these drugs [16–19]. Antihistamines and TCAs typically have fewer side effects than glucocorticoids, although they are not nearly as effective.

One antihistamine used by many practitioners is pyrilamine maleate. It is given parenterally at a dose of 1 mg/kg. A study showed pyrilamine is poorly bioavailable orally in the horse (18%) and can be detected by sensitive enzyme-linked immunosorbent assay tests in urine for up to 1 week after a single administration. Care should be taken because the data suggest that the withdrawal time for pyrilamine after repeated oral administrations is likely to be at least 1 week or longer [20]. The authors' do not recommend its use because of this data and the limited success seen in cases referred where it has been previously used. The authors' favourite antihistamine is hydroxyzine pamoate at a dose of 1–1.5 mg/kg, three times a day. In our experience it has been more effective for urticaria than pruritus. Other antihistamines and TCAs used with limited success, on a twice-daily basis, include diphenhydramine 0.75–1 mg/kg, chlorpheniramine 0.25 mg/kg, amitriptyline 1–2 mg/kg, cetirizine 0.2–0.4 mg/kg, fexofenadine 10 mg/kg, and doxepin hydrochloride 0.5–0.75 mg/kg. Trying one or more of these products at 2-week intervals is often needed to give the drugs an adequate trial. Side effects are minimal and include light sedation, although occasional personality changes may be seen, which may require reduction of dosages or discontinuation of the drug. The American Quarter Horse Association recommends a 10-day withdrawal prior to any shows or competition.

Phosphodiesterase (PDE) inhibitors

Phosphodiesterase (PDE) inhibitors have been looked at as a group of drugs to help control allergic dermatitis in many species. Pentoxifylline (PTX) is a synthetic xanthine derivative that has phosphodiesterase inhibition activity, resulting in a variety of dermatologic therapeutic and anti-inflammatory effects in both animals and humans [21,22]. It has been used extensively in the canine for vasculitis and ischaemic dermatitis and has been empirically used for laminitis and airway disease in horses with conflicting results [21,23–28]. Details of the pentoxifylline mechanism of action in animals has not been determined. Its proposed benefit in vasculitic diseases is due to its rheological effects of increasing red cell deformability and decreasing platelet aggregation and adhesion, vasoconstriction, plasmin, antithrombin III, fibrinogen, alpha2 antiplasmin, alpha1 antitrypsin, and alpha2 macroglobulin [26,28]. It can improve wound healing by increasing fibroblast collagenases, decreasing fibroblast collagen, fibronectin, and glycosaminoglycans, and decreasing tumour necrosis factor (TNF) alpha [29–31]. The indication for pentoxifylline in allergic skin conditions is due to its ability to inhibit T- and B-cell activation and proliferation, to increase leukocyte deformability and chemotaxis, as well as production of IL-10 and PGE2, and to decrease: leukocyte adhesion and aggregation, neutrophil superoxide release, neutrophil degranulation, monocyte TNF-alpha production, leukocyte response to TNF alpha, lymphotoxin, and interferon-gamma, production and leukocyte response to IL-1 and IL-12, and natural killer cell activity [22,32–34].

The current proposed dose is 10–15 mg/kg twice daily. However, controversy exists about the pharmacokinetics of the drug in the horse and exact dosing is not known. Results indicate PTX is rapidly absorbed and metabolized. Higher serum PTX concentrations, area under the curve, and bioavailability were observed after the first oral dose, compared with the last dose. Serum concentrations of both PTX and metabolite 1 M1 reach serum concentrations considered to be therapeutic in humans and therapeutic in horses with endotoxaemia. Drug exposure appears to decrease by 30% with multiple dosages and thus the therapeutic efficacy may wane, at that point one may consider increasing the dose rate to 30 mg/kg/day by either increasing the dosage with twice-daily administration or by increasing the dosing frequency to three times daily [35]. The authors have had success in some cases of atopic dermatitis, urticaria (Figures 54.1 and 54.2), and contact allergies. In addition to using the drug as a sole therapy, it may have synergistic effects with glucocorticoids and/or have a steroid-sparing effect and thus may be combined with glucocorticoids and other anti-inflammatory drugs [32,36,37].

Fatty acid supplementation

Fatty acid supplementation has also increased in popularity as an option for atopic dermatitis in the horse. Most mammalian cell membranes incorporate

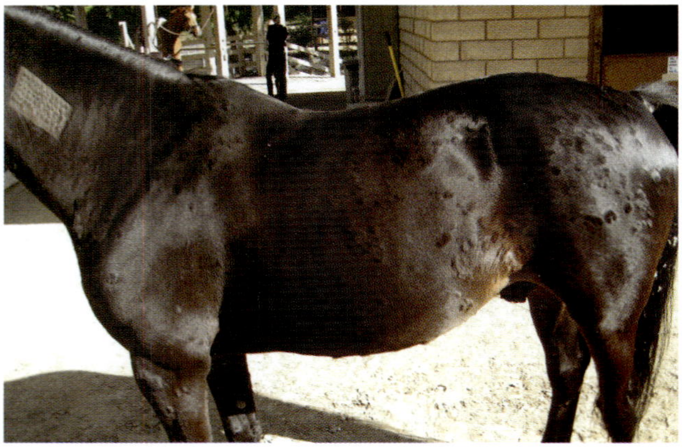

Figure 54.1 Urticarial lesions in atopic dermatitis before pentoxifylline treatment.

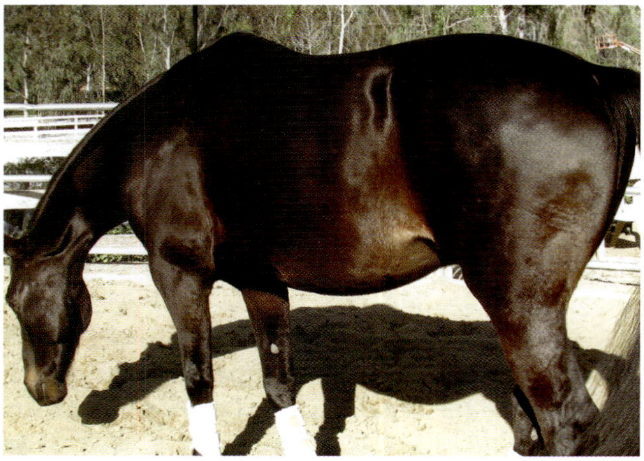

Figure 54.2 Same horse as in Figure 54.1, 1 month after pentoxifylline treatment.

polyunsaturated N-3 and N-6 fatty acids (PUFAs) and theoretically in atopic skin diseases there is a higher amount of proinflammatory mediators that are released and contribute to the clinical signs. The assumption is that by supplementing with PUFAs there is a modification of the arachidonic acid cascade, reducing proinflammatory mediators and resulting in a reduction of pruritus and urticaria. The exact mechanism of how PUFAs work in atopic dermatitis is not completely understood and there are variable reports on their efficacy in the horse.

In one study the circulating fatty acid profile and the acquisition and washout of fatty acids in response to n-3 supplementation was evaluated. A fatty acid supplement high in eicosapentaenoic (EPA) and docosahexaenoic (DHA) acid was fed to deliver EPA plus DHA at 0 (control), 10, 20, or 40 g/day to 16 mares (n = 4/group) for 28 days. Plasma was analysed before and multiple times throughout an 87-day period for the presence of 35 fatty acids by gas chromatography. Plasma EPA and DHA increased ($P < 0.05$) in a dose-responsive manner by day 3 of feeding and reached peak concentrations by day 7. Peak EPA and DHA concentrations of the 40 g/day supplement group were approximately 13 times and 10 times those of controls, respectively. Plasma EPA and DHA demonstrated a steep decline ($P < 0.05$) from peak values by 9 days after cessation of supplementation and were near presupplementation values by day 42. These results indicate that the circulating fatty acid milieu in horses can be influenced through targeted supplementation [38].

A few studies looked at the value of EFA supplementation in seasonally pruritic horses. At the University of Florida, 17 horses fed 200 mL of linseed per day for a 6-week period, showed no significant change in pruritus or lesional surface areas. However, this time frame may have been too short to completely evaluate the potential benefits of n-3 fatty acids [39]. In an open study of EFA supplementation, evidence of clinical improvement was noted in 10 out of 14 seasonally pruritic horses receiving an evening primrose oil and fish oil combination (approximate dose of one 5-g capsule per 100 kg body weight) [40]. However, the same authors followed up with a controlled placebo trial using double the original doses of fatty acid supplementation in 33 horses with seasonal pruritus. Even though significant differences in the change in plasma phospholipid concentration between test and placebo groups were seen for dihomogammalinolenic acid and docosahexaenoic acid ($P < 0.01$) and for alpha linolenic acid ($P < 0.05$), there was no difference in the seasonal pruritus control between the treated and placebo groups. This suggested that the open study result may have resulted from placebo effects [41].

Despite controversy, the authors will often combine fatty acid supplementation with other forms of therapy for its potentially synergistic benefits. A variety of supplements are available and range from using simple flax seed [42] to commercially enhanced supplements.

Allergen-specific immunotherapy

One of the most progressive areas for the treatment of equine allergic skin is allergen-specific immunotherapy (ASIT). There are now numerous studies demonstrating value for immunotherapy targeting both insect and environmental allergens. However, most studies have not been controlled and included only small numbers of horses. One study of *Culicoides* (Diptera: Ceratopogonidae) hypersensitivity evaluated ASIT in a double-blinded control fashion with poor results [43]. However, in another trial, all 10 horses with *Culicoides* hypersensitivity improved during immunotherapy and seven of these horses deteriorated again after cessation of therapy [44].

Differences in climate and study protocols make a comparison of the study results difficult. Most authors reported a 60 to 71%, good to excellent, response to ASIT based on the results of intradermal testing [2–4,45–47]. Reports evaluating the influence of multiple concurrent positive reactions to insects on the outcome of ASIT show conflicting results [4,46]. It may require a longer period of treatment to see improvement. In a placebo-controlled study in horses with insect and environmental hypersensitivities (n = 28), 64% of the horses treated with ASIT showed a 50% or greater improvement compared to only 23% with placebo [46].

In a large retrospective study at the Veterinary Medical Teaching Hospital, University of California at Davis (VMTH-UCD), USA, 41 horses seen over a 17-year period were treated with ASIT and, according to the owners surveyed, the overall response rate to ASIT was 84% [48](Figures 54.3 and 54.4). This percentage of success, as well as that in one other report of 92% in the management of equine urticaria [4], appear to overestimate the benefit of ASIT compared to what is reported in other studies. It is likely that owner assessment was skewed by placebo effect or because of concurrent medications. In the VMTH-UCD study, if the success of ASIT was evaluated as a sole therapy used in managing clinical signs of equine atopic skin, 59% of the cases were well controlled with a further small percentage (9%) of horses being considered partial responders (i.e. concurrent medications administered with ASIT but glucocorticoids were able to be discontinued). This would give a total response rate of 69% (22 of 32 horses), putting the success rate closer to previous reports. Also of interest was that of the 30 owners who reported using antipruritic medications prior to beginning ASIT, 57% (17 of 30) reported being able to discontinue those medications with the addition of ASIT [48].

Another study looked at the benefits of ASIT over an extended period of time in a prospective clinical and immunological study. Nineteen horses received ASIT for up to 24 months. Horses were randomized to one of three treatment groups: ASIT based upon intradermal test (IDT) results (n = 7); allergen-specific IgE results by ELISA (n = 6); or a combination based on IDT and ELISA results (n = 6). Serum concentrations of allergen-specific IgE and IgG were measured at initial evaluation (time 0) and every 4 months thereafter. Horse owners recorded visual analogue scale (VAS) scores at times 0, 12 months, and 24 months. There were no significant differences in VAS scores according to seasonality of signs. There was excellent agreement between allergen-specific IgE concentrations (time 0) and both immediate and delayed IDT results ($P < 0.00001$), and between immediate IDT and IgG results ($P = 0.003$). Specific concentration of serum IgE and IgG decreased significantly ($P < 0.05$) for 13% and 38% of allergens, respectively, that were included in ASIT [49]. These results suggest that ASIT provides significant clinical benefit and supports roles for both allergen-specific IgE and IgG in the pathogenesis of equine AD. These data also suggests that the clinical benefits from ASIT may result from reduction of allergen-specific IgE and IgG concentrations in serum.

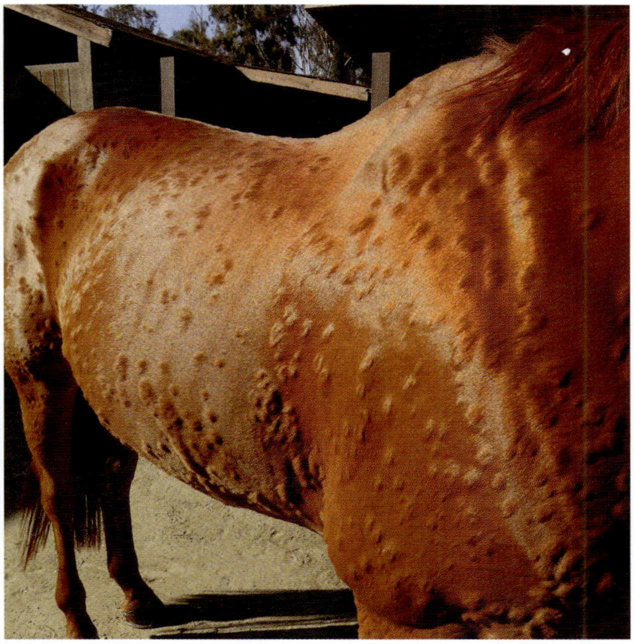

Figure 54.3 Urticaria before allergen-specific immunotherapy.

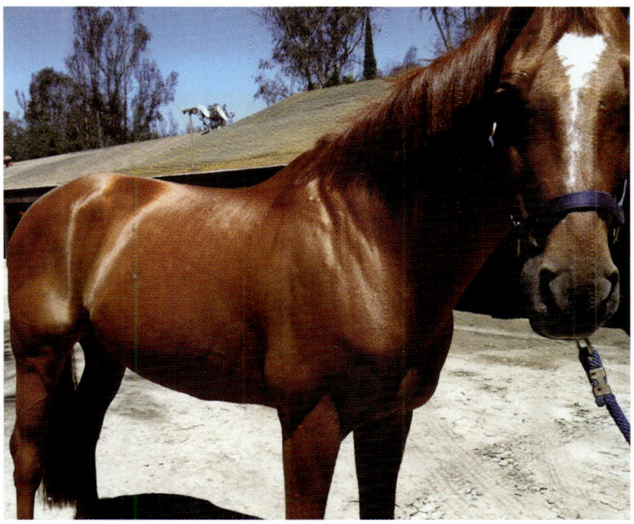

Figure 54.4 Urticaria 8 weeks after initiation of allergen-specific immunotherapy.

Most horses that show a response to ASIT will do so within the first 6 months of therapy [1,4,46,47]. The authors prefer ASIT based on IDT, although there are reports that immunotherapy based on serum *in vitro* testing (SIVT) may also have value and that ASIT based on SIVT is comparable to that of IDT [48,49]. In the VMTH-UCD study, of the 27 horses reported to have benefitted from ASIT, 13 horses had their ASIT formulated based on the results of IDT, nine had their ASIT based on a serum test, and five had both an IDT and a serum test. A chi-square analysis used to compare the success proportions of ASIT between skin tests, serum tests, and both showed no statistical difference between the three groups ($P = 0.53$) [48], and, as mentioned in the study above, some investigators do combine the results of IDT and SIVT and have ASIT success using combinations of the two testing methodologies [49].

The technique used for ASIT in horses is similar to that used in small animals (see Box 54.1). As in small animals, antigen volume and injection interval adjustments need

Box 54.1 Allergen specific immunotherapy (ASIT)—client information

ASIT is one type of treatment for allergies in horses. The major benefit is its relative lack of side effects. Theoretically, it helps by creating tolerance, which allows your horse to be exposed to higher levels of allergens without developing symptoms such as hives, itching, rubbing, chewing, etc.

ASIT is not always effective. Approximately 60% of the horses will be controlled. Of this 60%, approximately 50% will be controlled without the use of other drugs. The additional 10% are helped, though they are not totally controlled and may require the use of other medications.

The response to ASIT can be slow and gradual. Most horses do not respond until they have been on the injections for 3–6 months. Some may take as long as 9 months.

Once they have responded, treatment will usually be needed for life. Your horse must be re-evaluated after 4–5 months and some adjustments may need to be made in his/her treatment.

Side effects are rare. If swelling, itchiness, or hives appear within an hour of giving an injection, call the clinic. More serious side effects, which are even rarer, would include colic, diarrhoea, respiratory difficulties, or collapse associated with the injection. Call our clinic or an emergency clinic at once if this occurs. More serious side effects generally occur within the first few months of therapy; therefore, you should give these injections when you will be with your horse for an hour.

Important

- Antigens must be refrigerated.
- Your horse must be re-evaluated during the 10-day injection intervals, after 4–6 weeks, and again in 6 months.
- It may take 6–9 months to show a response to antigens.
- In most cases, antigen injections will be life-long.

Equine ASIT schedule

Day	Date/symptoms†	Amount	Day	Date/symptoms†	Amount
VIAL #1			25		1.0 cc
1		0.1 cc	10 day-intervals (recheck)‡		
3		0.2 cc	35		1.0 cc
5		0.3 cc	45		1.0 cc
7		0.4 cc	55		1.0 cc
9		0.6 cc	14-day intervals		
11		0.8 cc	69		1.0 cc
13		1.0 cc	83		1.0 cc
VIAL #2			97		1.0 cc
15		0.2 cc	111		1.0 cc
17		0.3 cc	20-day intervals		
19		0.4 cc	131		1.0 cc
21		0.6 cc	151		1.0 cc
23		0.8 cc	171	Recheck‡	1.0 cc

†Record date and any increase or reduction in clinical signs.
‡Call for a recheck appointment prior during 10-day cycle, some horses require volume and interval adjustments. A 6-month recheck should also be scheduled.

Do not stop injections without notifying your veterinarian.

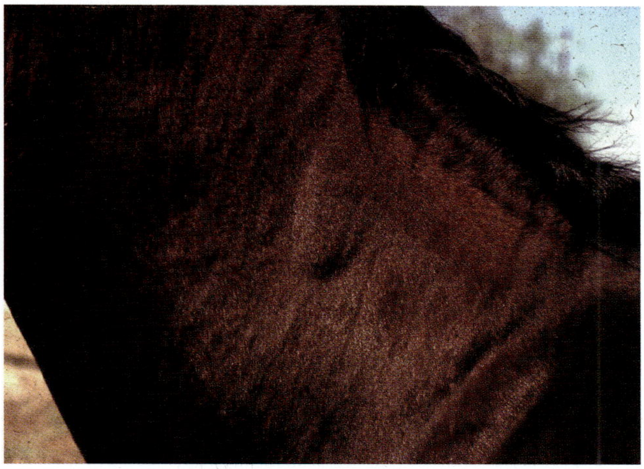

Figure 54.5 Localized antigen site reaction.

to be made for each case based upon clinical response. Clients should be given a detailed tutorial on how to give injections and what to look for regarding clinical response and possible reactions. Follow-up telephone calls and rechecks will increase the success of this therapy. Most horses required antigen booster injections at 7 to 14-day intervals, with volumes ranging from 0.5 to 1.0 mL. Shots are given subcutaneously over the lateral cervical area. Antigen reactions are uncommon, with swelling at injection sites being the most common (Figure 54.5), which generally resolve within 1–2 days. In the VMTH-UCD study only five owners reported an adverse effect of the ASIT (swelling at the injection site), which is consistent with a previous report and the authors' experiences [4]. Anaphylaxis is extremely rare with only anecdotal reports and no reports cited in the literature.

Glucocorticoids

Systemic glucocorticoids are often required in many atopic dermatitis cases. They are very frequently prescribed and certainly need to be used judiciously and in appropriate dosing and intervals. It is essential to make an accurate diagnosis before using glucocorticoid therapy to decide on the type, duration, and the dose of therapy required. Therapeutic dosages are not determined for any glucocorticoid in any equine dermatoses and each case needs to be treated individually. Recommended dosages are merely guidelines to follow.

The authors rely primarily on two glucocorticoids in practice, prednisolone and dexamethasone. Prednisone and prednisolone do not appear to be equal in terms of efficacy in the horse. Possible reasons why horses do not respond as well to oral prednisone are poor absorption, rapid excretion, failure of hepatic conversion to prednisolone, or a combination of all of these [50]. In one study of horses with COPD, it was found that neither prednisone or prednisolone could be detected after oral administration of prednisone [50].

Depending on the severity of the case, dosages may need to be at the high or low end of anti-inflammatory levels to control most allergic hypersensitivity conditions. Most induction periods range from 7 to 14 days followed by a tapering period of 2–5 weeks and then a maintenance period, which may be used for as short a time as a few months or indefinitely, depending on the severity of the case and the seasonality. Induction dosages for prednisolone are 0.5–1.5 mg/kg once daily with maintenance dosages at 0.2–0.5 mg/kg every other day. Some cases will be resistant to prednisolone and may respond to either injectable or oral dexamethasone. Often an initial loading dose of dexamethasone is needed at 0.02–0.1 mg/kg once daily, which may be followed by an oral maintenance dosage of 0.01–0.02 mg/kg every 2–3 days. This regimen is particularly helpful in more refractory cases.

When using oral glucocorticoids, writing out the induction, tapering, and maintenance dosages on a day-to-day basis is extremely helpful (see Box 54.2 for an example of a client handout schedule). Such a schedule allows safer administration at a 'threshold dose' so that the case remains disease free. Side effects from glucocorticoids do occur in horses but are not common,

Box 54.2 Glucocorticoid schedule—client information

Prednisolone and dexamethasone are glucocorticoid drugs. They have many effects on your horse's body—some are beneficial while some are not. We will attempt to use these medications so that we can minimize the undesirable effects. Common side effects include increased thirst, urination, and appetite. Food intake should be regulated so that your horse does not gain weight. Occasionally, these medications may potentiate colic, laminitis, and increase risk for infections. If you have any concerns regarding these side effects discontinue the medication and call your primary veterinarian. The following schedule should be followed in administering the medication. When given once daily, the medicine should always be given in the morning (7 to 9:00 AM). The number indicates how many tablets to give at that time and day. If the problem we are trying to control returns, give the previous effective dose and call your primary veterinarian.

(Continued)

Client name: Horse's name:

Medication/mg: Starting date (Day 1):

Day	AM	PM	†	Day	AM	†	Day	AM	†	Day	AM	†	Day	AM	†
1				13			25			37			49		
2				14			26			38			50		
3				15			27			39			51		
4				16			28			40			52		
5				17			29			41			53		
6				18			30			42			54		
7				19			31			43			55		
8				20			32			44			56		
9				21			33			45			57		
10				22			34			46			58		
11				23			35			47			59		
12				24			36			48			60		

† Record signs (itching, scratching, rubbing, or hives) as a level from 1–10 (1 best to 10 worse).

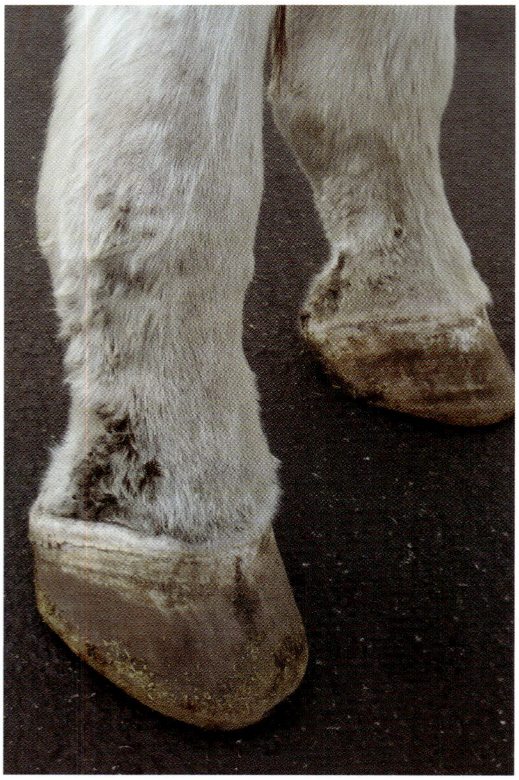

Figure 54.6 Suspected glucocorticoid-induced laminitis in a horse with pastern leukocytoclastic vasculitis (rear legs).

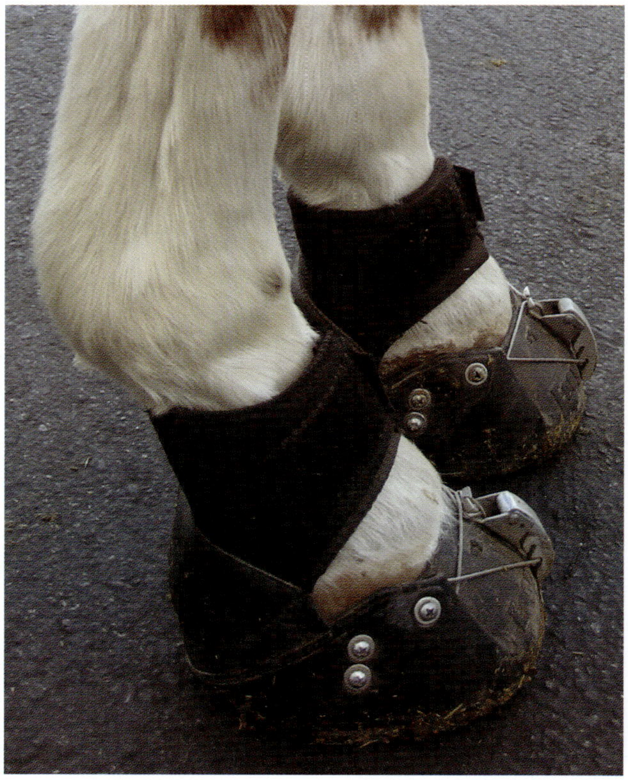

Figure 54.7 Same horse as in Figure 54.6, after discontinuation of glucocorticoids and with corrective boots (front legs).

especially when lower dosing and shorter intervals are utilized. They can create steroid hepatopathy, laminitis (Figures 54.6 and 54.7), increased susceptibility to infections, and iatrogenic hyperglucocorticoidism [51–53]. Local tissue activity of glucocorticoids is regulated by the steroid converting enzyme, 11-beta-hydroxysteroid dehydrogenase-1 (11-beta-HSD-1). There are studies to suggest that the individual sensitivity to glucocorticoids may be directly related to the ratio of Type 1:Type 2 11-hydroxysteroid dehydrogenase [53,54].

References

1. White S. Advances in equine atopic dermatitis, serologic and intradermal allergy testing. *Clinical Techniques in Equine Practice* 2005; **4**: 311–313.
2. Fadok VA. Overview of equine pruritus. *Veterinary Clinics of North America: Equine Practice* 1995; **11**: 1–10.
3. Scott DW, Miller WH. *Equine Dermatology*. Philadelphia, PA: WB Saunders, 2003: 427–449.
4. Tallarico NJ, Tallarico C. Results of intradermal allergy testing and treatment by hyposensitization of 64 horses with chronic obstructive pulmonary disease, urticaria, headshaking, and/or reactive airway disease. *Veterinary Allergy and Clinical Immunology* 1998; **6**: 25–35.
5. Jackson CA, Berney C, Jefcoat AM, *et al.* Environment and prednisone interactions in the treatment of recurrent airway obstruction (heaves). *Equine Veterinary Journal* 2000; **32**: 432–438.
6. Airaksinen S, Heiskanen ML, Heinonen-Tanski H, *et al.* Variety in dustiness and hygiene quality of peat bedding. *Annals of Agricultural and Environmental Medicine* 2005; **12**: 53–59.
7. Fleming K, Hessel EF, Van den Weghe HFA. Generation of airborne particles from different bedding materials used for horse keeping. *Journal of Equine Veterinary Science* 2008; **28**: 408–418.
8. Kirschvink N, Di Silvestro F, Sbai I, *et al.* The use of cardboard bedding material as part of an environmental control regime for heaves-affected horses: in vitro assessment of airborne dust and aeroallergen concentration and in vivo effects on lung function. *Veterinary Journal* 2002; **163**: 319–325.
9. Wallace JC, Vogelnest LJ. Evaluation of the presence of house dust mites in horse rugs. *Veterinary Dermatology* 2010; **21**: 602–607.
10. Leguillette R. Recurrent airway obstruction—heaves. *Veterinary Clinics of North America: Equine Practice* 2003; **19**: 63–86.
11. Volland-Francqueville M, Sabbah A. Recurrent or chronic urticaria in Thoroughbred racehorses: clinical observations. *Allergy and Immunology (Paris)* 2004; **36**: 9–12.
12. Marsella R, Sameulson D, Johnson C, *et al.* Pilot investigation on skin barrier in equine atopic dermatitis: observations on electron microscopy and measurements of transepidermal water loss. *Veterinary Dermatology* 2012; **23**: 78.
13. Nuttall T, Mueller R, Bensignor E, *et al.* Efficacy of a 0.0584% hydrocortisone aceponate spray in the management of canine atopic dermatitis: a randomised, double blind, placebo-controlled trial. *Veterinary Dermatology* 2009; **20**: 191–198.
14. Brazzini B, Pimpinelli N. New and established topical corticosteroids in dermatology: clinical pharmacology and therapeutic use. *American Journal of Clinical Dermatology* 2002; **3**: 47–58.
15. Kietzmann M, Kemmet S. Skin thinning effects of topically administered glucocorticoids in dogs and horses. *Veterinary Dermatology* 2012; **23** (Suppl.1): 42.
16. Manohar M, Goetz TE, Humphrey S, *et al.* H1-receptor antagonist, tripelennamine, does not affect arterial hypoxemia in exercising Thoroughbreds. *Journal of Applied Physiology* 2002; **92**: 1515–1523.
17. Torneke K, Ingvast-Larsson C, Pettersson K, *et al.* Pharmacokinetics and pharmacodynamics of clemastine in healthy horses. *Journal of Veterinary Pharmacology and Therapeutics* 2003; **26**: 151–157.
18. Wasfi IA, Abdel Hadi AA, Elghazali M, *et al.* Comparative pharmacokinetics of diphenhydramine in camels and horses after intravenous administration. *Veterinary Research Communications* 2003; **27**: 463–473.
19. Foster AP, McKelvie J, Cunningham FM. Inhibition of antigen-induced cutaneous responses of ponies with insect hypersensitivity by the histamine-1 receptor antagonist chlorpheniramine. *Veterinary Record* 1998; **143**: 189–193.
20. Dirikolu L, Lehner AF, Harkins JD, *et al.* Pyrilamine in the horse: detection and pharmacokinetics of pyrilamine and its major urinary metabolite O-desmethylpyrilamine. *Journal of Veterinary Pharmacology and Therapeutics* 2009; **32**: 66–78.
21. Marks SL, Merchant S, Foil C. Pentoxifylline: wonder drug? *Journal of the American Animal Hospital Association* 2001; **37**: 218–219.
22. Zargari O. Pentoxifylline: a drug with wide spectrum applications in dermatology. *Dermatology Online Journal* 2008; **14**: 2. Available at: http://dermatology-s10.cdlib.org/1411/reviews/pentoxy/zargari.html (accessed October, 2012).
23. Vitale C, Gross T, Magro C. Vaccine-induced ischemic dermatopathy in the dog. *Veterinary Dermatology* 1999; **10**: 131–142.
24. Rees CA, Boothe DM. Therapeutic response to pentoxifylline and its active metabolites in dogs with familial canine dermatomyositis. *Veterinary Therapeutics* 2003; **4**: 234–241.
25. Ingle-Fehr JE, Baxter GM. The effect of oral isoxsuprine and pentoxifylline on digital and laminar blood flow in healthy horses. *Veterinary Surgery* 1999; **28**: 154–160.
26. Weiss DJ, Richwagen K, Evanson OA. Effects of hematocrit and erythrocyte deformability on pulmonary vascular pressures in perfused pony lungs. *American Journal of Veterinary Research* 1996; **57**: 346–350.
27. Leguillette R, Desevaux C, Lavoie JP. Effects of pentoxifylline on pulmonary function and results of cytologic examination of bronchoalveolar lavage fluid in horses with recurrent airway obstruction. *American Journal of Veterinary Research* 2002; **63**: 459–463.
28. Kornreich B, Enyeart M, Jesty SA, *et al.* The effects of pentoxifylline on equine platelet aggregation. *Journal of Veterinary Internal Medicine* 2010; **24**: 1196–1202.
29. Schmidt-Choudhury A, Furuta GT, Lavigne JA, *et al.* The regulation of tumor necrosis factor-alpha production in murine mast cells: pentoxifylline or dexamethasone inhibits IgE-dependent production of TNF-alpha by distinct mechanisms. *Cellular Immunology* 1996; **171**: 140–146.
30. Barton MH, Ferguson D, Davis PJ, *et al.* The effects of pentoxifylline infusion on plasma 6-keto-prostaglandin F1 alpha and ex vivo endotoxin-induced tumour necrosis factor activity in horses. *Journal of Veterinary Pharmacology and Therapeutics* 1997; **20**: 487–492.
31. Chartier M, Falanga V. Healing of ulcers due to cryofibrinogenemia with colchicine and high-dose pentoxifylline. *American Journal of Clinical Dermatology* 2009; **10**: 39–42.
32. Briggs WA, Eustace J, Mathew S, *et al.* Pentoxifylline potentiates in vitro lymphocyte suppression by glucocorticoids and immunosuppressive drugs. *Journal of Clinical Pharmacology* 1998; **38**: 561–566.
33. Marsella R, Nicklin CF. Double-blinded cross-over study on the efficacy of pentoxifylline for canine atopy. *Veterinary Dermatology* 2000; **11**: 255–60.
34. Samlaska CP, Winfield EA. Pentoxifylline. *Journal of the American Academy of Dermatology* 1994; **30**: 603–621.
35. Liska DA, Akucewich LH, Marsella R, *et al.* Pharmacokinetics of pentoxifylline and its 5-hydroxyhexyl metabolite after oral and intravenous administration of pentoxifylline to healthy adult horses. *American Journal of Veterinary Research* 2006; **67**: 1621–1627.
36. Funk JO, Ernst M, Schonharting MM, *et al.* Pentoxifylline exerts synergistic immunomodulatory effects in combination with dexamethasone or cyclosporin A. *International Journal of Immunopharmacology* 1995; **17**: 1007–1016.
37. Baskett A, Barton MH, Norton N, *et al.* Effect of pentoxifylline, flunixinmeglumine, and their combination on a model of

endotoxemia in horses. *American Journal of Veterinary Research* 1997; **58**: 1291–1299.
38. King SS, Abughazaleh AA, Webel SK, *et al.* Circulating fatty acid profiles in response to three levels of dietary omega-3 fatty acid supplementation in horses. *Journal of Animal Science* 2008; **86**: 1114–1123.
39. Friberg C, Logas D. Treatment of *Culicoides* hypersensitive horses with high-dose n-3 fatty acids: a double-blinded crossover study. *Veterinary Dermatology* 1999; **10**: 117–122.
40. Craig JM, Lloyd DH. Use of an evening primrose oil and fish oil mixture in the management of sweet-itch in horses. In: Ihrke PJ, Mason IS, White SD, eds. *Advances in Veterinary Dermatology*, vol. 2. Oxford: Pergamon Press, 1992: 436.
41. Craig JM, Lloyd DH, Roger D, *et al.* A double-blind placebo-controlled trial of an evening primrose and fish oil combination vs. hydrogenated coconut oil in the management of recurrent seasonal pruritus in horses. *Veterinary Dermatology* 1997; **8**: 177–182.
42. O'Neill W, McKee S, Clarke AF. Flaxseed (*Linum usitatissimum*) supplementation associated with reduced skin test lesional area in horses with *Culicoides* hypersensitivity. *Canadian Journal of Veterinary Research* 2002; **66**: 272–277.
43. Barbet JL, Bevier D, Greiner EC. Specific immunotherapy in the treatment of Culicoides hypersensitive horses: a double-blind study. *Equine Veterinary Journal* 1990; **22**: 232–235.
44. Anderson GS, Belton P, Jahren E, *et al.* Immunotherapy trial for horses in British Columbia with *Culicoides (Diptera: Ceratopogonidae)* hypersensitivity. *Journal of Medical Entomology* 1996; **33**: 458–466.
45. Delger J. Intradermal testing and immunotherapy in horses. *Veterinary Medicine* 1997; **92**: 635–639.
46. Rosenkrantz W, Griffin C, Esch R, *et al.* Responses in horses to intradermal challenge of insects and environmental allergens with specific immunotherapy. In: Hillier A, Foster AP, Kwochka KW, eds. *Advances in Veterinary Dermatology*, Vol. 3. Oxford: Blackwell Publishing, 1998: 191–200.
47. Rees CA. Response to immunotherapy in six related horses with urticaria secondary to atopy. *Journal of the American Veterinary Medical Association* 2001; **218**: 753–755.
48. Stepnik CT, Outerbridge CA, White SD, *et al.* Equine atopic skin disease and response to allergen-specific immunotherapy: a retrospective study at the University of California-Davis (1991–2008). *Veterinary Dermatology* 2011; **23**: 29–35, e7.
49. Radwanski N, Morris DO, Boston R, *et al.* A prospective evaluation of clinical and immunological responses to allergen-specific immunotherapy in horses with atopic dermatitis. *Veterinary Dermatology* 2011; **23** (Suppl.1):42.
50. Peroni DL, Stanley S, Kollias-Baker C, *et al.* Prednisone per os is likely to have limited efficacy in horses. *Equine Veterinary Journal* 2002; **34**: 283–287.
51. Cohen ND, Carter GK. Steroid hepatopathy in a horse with glucocorticoid-induced hyperadrenocorticism. *Journal of the American Veterinary Medical Association* 1992; **200**: 1682–1684.
52. Ryu SH, Kim BS, Lee CW, *et al.* Glucocorticoid-induced laminitis with hepatopathy in a Thoroughbred filly. *Journal of Veterinary Science* 2004; **5**: 271–274.
53. Johnson PJ, Slight SH, Ganjam VK, *et al.* Glucocorticoids and laminitis in the horse. *Veterinary Clinics of North America: Equine Practice* 2002; **18**: 219–236.
54. Johnson PJ, Ganjam VK, Slight SH, *et al.* Tissue-specific dysregulation of cortisol metabolism in equine laminitis. *Equine Veterinary Journal* 2004; **36**: 41–45.

Section 3

Recurrent Airway Obstruction and Inflammatory Airway Disease

55

Recurrent airway obstruction and inflammatory airway disease

Vinzenz Gerber

Swiss Institute of Equine Medicine (ISME), Vetsuisse Faculty, University of Bern and ALP-Haras Avenches, Switzerland

Conflict of interest: none declared.

Pathogenesis

Classification and terminology

The focus of this chapter is on inflammatory airway disease (IAD) and recurrent airway obstruction (RAO) or heaves. According to consensus reports on RAO [1] and IAD [2], we are not using the previous umbrella term 'chronic obstructive pulmonary disease' (COPD), or terms such as chronic obstructive bronchitis/bronchiolitis, small-airway inflammatory disease, or small-airway disease.

Chronic lower airway disease is a major health problem of stabled mature horses. IAD and RAO are mainly associated with conventional indoor stable environments with hay feeding and straw bedding. Under these conditions, the air in the breathing zone of horses contains very high levels of organic dust with allergens and non-specific irritants [3–6]. It is thus not surprising that horses in conventional stable environments show a high incidence of mild to severe, non-infectious, lower airway disease [7].

Clinically, IAD and RAO present themselves as a continuum of increasing severity (see section 'Clinical aspects and diagnosis'). Horses with less-severe forms of chronic airway disease are said to have IAD, while those with moderate to severe signs of non-infectious lower airway disease generally suffer from RAO. While the latter is a well-defined disease entity (e.g. increased respiratory effort due to airway obstruction, coughing, and neutrophilic airway inflammation; see section 'Clinical aspects and diagnosis'), IAD is much less-well characterized, its definition relaying on the demonstration of lower airway inflammation and/or mild lung function deficits (see also sections 'Clinical aspects and diagnosis' and 'Guidelines'). Moreover, different, but as yet poorly defined, subtypes of IAD have been described, which currently complicates rather than helps clarify the definition of IAD.

Pathogenesis of inflammatory airway disease

Clinical signs of IAD (see also section 'Clinical signs of inflammatory airway disease') appear to be caused by a combination of airway inflammation, excessive mucus accumulation, and hyper-reactivity. The latter is often associated with increased eosinophils and mast cells in bronchial alveolar lavage fluid (BALF) [8,9]. The aetiopathogenesis of IAD is still poorly defined. The exact identities and potential interactions of causative agents have not been investigated in IAD, but are likely to vary between individuals and populations due to differences in management practices, age, and individual susceptibility.

IAD in young racehorses (mainly defined by the presence of excessive airway mucus) appears to be associated with increased isolation of common bacteria from tracheobronchial secretions. This form of IAD is

Veterinary Allergy, First Edition. Edited by Chiara Noli, Aiden Foster, and Wayne Rosenkrantz.

most prevalent in racehorses in their first years in training and decreases with age [10,11]and may be associated with certain transferrin alleles [12].

In general, IAD can be seen in horses of any age or use (pleasure, sporting, racing). No breed or sex predilection is seen and non-infectious causes are likely to be central to its development [2]. Both in young and in older horses, stabling in conventional management conditions and hay feeding have been identified as risk factors [13–15]. Various non-specific organic and inorganic particulate and gaseous irritants (e.g. debris from plants, micro-organisms, mites, inorganic dusts, ultrafine particles) are likely to be responsible for the predominantly neutrophilic form [2]. This form of IAD is often accompanied by coughing [16]. A large proportion of horses affected with this form of IAD are otherwise asymptomatic [13–15]. One could argue that in these asymptomatic horses, neutrophilic IAD is a 'normal' physiological response to increased inhaled dust loads.

While there are currently no clearly defined criteria to distinguish between subtypes of IAD, some authors have pointed out interesting associations based on the predominant cell type observed in BALF. The neutrophilic form of IAD, more often seen in older horses, differs in its cytokine profile from IAD with increased BALF mast cells, indicating that different and distinct pathophysiological mechanisms can cause equine IAD [17]. Some reports speculate that increased mast cell and eosinophil counts may indicate that aeroallergens and parasites, respectively, play a role in these IAD cases [8,9].

Pathogenesis of recurrent airway obstruction

Clinical signs of RAO are caused by airflow obstruction, which in turn is due to airway mucus accumulation and inflammation, bronchial hyper-reactivity, and bronchospasm [1,18–20]. Bronchospasm is the main contributor to airway obstruction during clinical exacerbation. Airway wall thickening, as well as mucus and inflammatory cell accumulation in the airway lumen, further exacerbate airflow obstruction and ventilation/perfusion mismatch [18–20].

Immunology of recurrent airway obstruction

RAO is generally believed to be due to an allergic sensitization/hypersensitivity to airborne antigens (see section 'Environmental triggers'), but it does not immunologically behave like a 'simple allergy'. It appears that T helper Th1-type andTh2-type profiles, as well as defects in innate immunity pathways, all may play a role in this disease.

Some studies have provided evidence for IgE-mediated type I hyper-reactivity [21,22](see also section 'Environmental triggers'), for a Th2-type bias with increased numbers of interleukin (IL)-4 and IL-5 positive cells [23], and for increased mRNA levels of IL-4 and IL-13 in BALF of RAO horses [24,25]. Other reports, however, did not find any evidence for a role of systemic IgE in RAO [20](see also section 'Environmental triggers'). Furthermore, Th1-type cytokines, such as interferon (IFN)-γ, can also be increased in RAO and are responsible for neutrophil recruitment (e.g. IL-8, IL-17)[26–28]. Additionally, non-specific responses to endotoxins also play a role, alone and by potentiating reactions to mould allergens [29]. Endotoxin increases Toll-like receptor (TLR)-4 and TLR2 mRNA in horse lungs [30]. Thus, the relative importance of IgE-mediated reactions, Th1-type and Th2-type profiles, innate immunity, and individual cytokines in the pathogenesis of RAO is still unclear.

To better explain the contradictory results regarding RAO immunopathology, a recent review [20] has introduced the concept of 'entopy' (a local allergic reaction limited to the airways, rather than systemic allergy) instead of 'atopy' in RAO. According to this concept, the site of sampling could strongly influence results. Furthermore, temporal differences in sampling can also have significant effects on the observed immunological profiles [25]. Finally, contradictory findings may also be due to investigations of different groups of RAO-affected horses displaying the same clinical phenotype, but with differing immunogenetic make-ups.

Recurrent airway obstruction genetics and relationship with defence against parasites and with other allergic diseases

RAO has a strong genetic basis with a complex mode of inheritance [7,31]. Segregation and genomic analyses performed on two Swiss warmblood families showed that the mode of inheritance and the main candidate chromosomal regions differ. In the first of these families, RAO was transmitted in an autosomal recessive mode and the major association was found on equine chromosome 13 (main candidate gene: IL-4 receptor [32,33]), whereas in the second, it was transmitted in an autosomal dominant mode and the major association was found to equine chromosome 15 [32–35]. Genetics also differentially influences allergen-specific IgGa and IgE levels [36]. Clinical expression of RAO did not differ between the two families [37]. These results suggest genetic heterogeneity for the clinical phenotype RAO: different genotypes converge within immunological pathways to result in a clinically indistinguishable RAO phenotype [38].

The identification of IL-4 receptor as a main candidate gene and preliminary clinical observations have led to

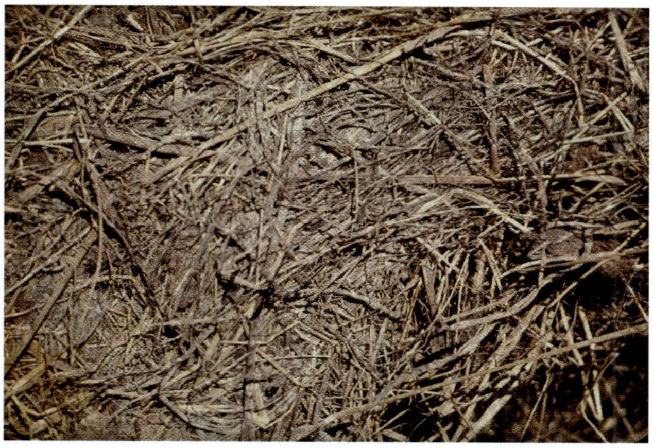

Figure 55.1 Hay of very poor quality—very dusty and mouldy. (Reprinted with permission from Swiss Institute of Equine Medicine.)

the investigation of novel aspects of RAO; affected horses show an increased risk for developing insect bite hypersensitivity and urticaria (Gerber, unpublished results), 'in exchange' they seem to be less susceptible to strongylid nematodes [39,40].

Environmental triggers

The composition of inhaled dust from hay (Figure 55.1), bedding, and other indoor sources is very heterogeneous. Even though the role of specific allergens and irritants has been studied much more intensively in RAO than in IAD, the identity of the exact inciting antigens has largely remained elusive; over 50 types of mould spores, mite particles, endotoxins, inorganic particles, and gases, all of which potentially contribute to RAO, have been identified [4,20,29].

Some of the inciting agents studied in RAO include:

- *Aspergillus fumigatus* and *Faenia rectivirgula* mould extracts can experimentally trigger signs of RAO [41].
- Histamine release by pulmonary mast cells from RAO-affected horses is increased in response to whole preparations and extracts of *A. fumigatus* and *Alternaria tenuis* moulds [42].
- Various potential mould allergens (e.g. *Micropolyspora faeni, A. fumigatus* and *Thermoactinomyces vulgaris*) have been used in intradermal testing. Dermal reactivity appears to significantly differ from pulmonary reactivity in RAO, however, greatly limiting its diagnostic value [43,44] (see also section 'Diagnostic methods').
- Endotoxin amplifies the pulmonary inflammatory and functional response to *A. fumigatus* extract inhalation [29].
- Other agents in stable dust (e.g. mite allergens such as from *Tyrophagus putrescentiae, Lepidoglyphus destructor, Acarussiro, Dermatophagoides pteronyssinus, D. farinae, Glycophagus domesticus* [43]; beta-glucans, spores, noxious gas [20,45]) and from other sources (e.g. air pollution [46]) may also play a role.
- Besides the well-established role of hay exposure, a recent epidemiological study found that RAO was associated with respiratory infection in early life [46].
- *Thermoactinomyces vulgaris* and hay pollen failed to experimentally trigger signs of RAO [18,41].

Outdoor sources of inciting agents play a role in 'summer-heaves' or 'summer pasture-associated obstructive pulmonary disease (SPAOPD)', a rarer, much less extensively studied form of RAO [47]. The seasonal pattern in affected horses in the south-east of the USA suggests that fungal spores and grass pollen grains together with hot and humid conditions are associated with SPAOPD in this region [48]. It is important to note that SPAOPD can affect horses in other regions of the world as well and that sensitization to both indoor and outdoor agents can occur together in the same affected horse [18,20].

Clinical aspects and diagnosis

Clinical signs of inflammatory airway disease

The definition of IAD currently relies on the demonstration of lower airway inflammation and/or mild lung function deficits [2](see also section 'Guidelines'). Thus, horses with IAD may also be asymptomatic, i.e. may not show any clinical signs like coughing, nasal discharge, and/or poor performance. Clinical signs may be absent and, even when present, can be difficult to interpret, since they are non-specific and do not allow a diagnosis of IAD by themselves.

Respiratory rate and expiratory effort at rest may be slightly increased and a rebreathing examination may reveal increased breathing sounds in some IAD affected horses, but a markedly elevated respiratory rate and altered breathing pattern as well as clearly abnormal sounds (in particular wheezes) at rest are all considered signs of RAO [1]. We have recently found that nasal discharge (Figure 55.2) and/or occasional coughing may indicate an increased risk that such individuals develop RAO within 2–4 years (Gerber, unpublished results). This is a first step towards answering the important, but still unresolved, question: which horses with IAD eventually will progress to the severe clinical signs of RAO?

Signs of exercise intolerance related to IAD may be relatively subtle, such as delayed recovery of respiratory rate after exercise and exaggerated respiratory effort during work. IAD is associated with decreased performance

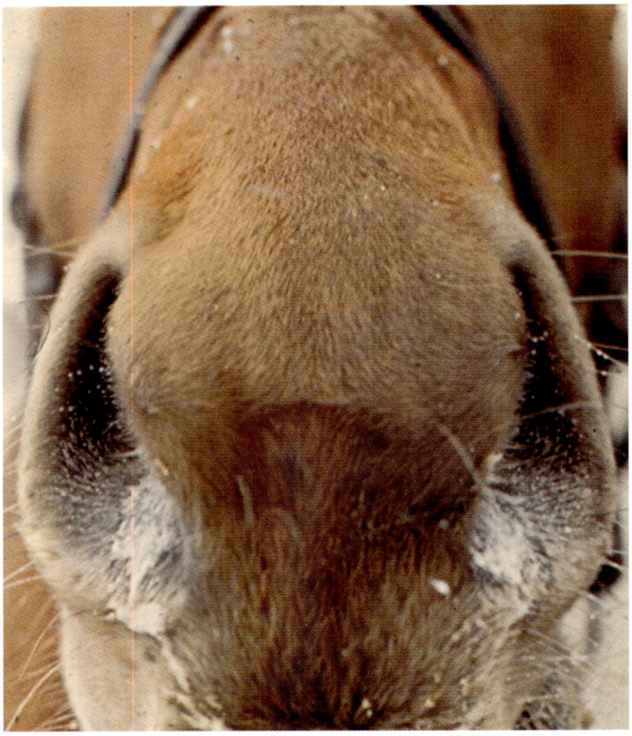

Figure 55.2 Serous to seromucous nasal discharge. (Reprinted with permission from Swiss Institute of Equine Medicine.)

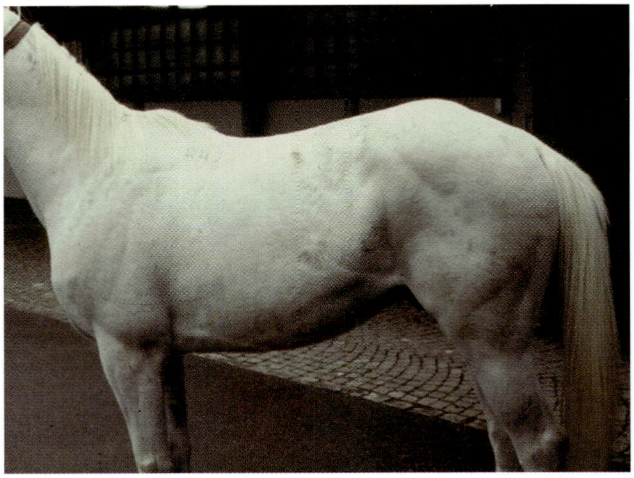

Figure 55.3 'Heave-line' typical of severe recurrent airway obstruction. (Reprinted with permission from Swiss Institute of Equine Medicine.)

particularly in racehorses [2]. In contrast, the role of IAD in 'poor performance' of sport and leisure horses is at present unclear, even though many horses with a presenting complaint of 'poor performance' are diagnosed with and treated for IAD. Increased mucus accumulation in the airways (which is not part of the ACVIM consensus definition of IAD [2]), but not increased neutrophils in tracheobronchial secretions are linked to decreased performance in show-jumpers and dressage horses [49]. It must be kept in mind, that 'poor performance' can be due to a wide variety of medical (orthopaedic, respiratory, muscular, cardiac, etc.) and management (training, feeding, etc.) factors and thus presents a particular diagnostic challenge. A thorough work-up, including all body systems and additional diagnostic tests, is often necessary to confirm a presumptive diagnosis of IAD as a cause of decreased performance.

Clinical signs of recurrent airway obstruction

RAO is characterized by intermittent to chronic cough, serous to mucopurulent bilateral nasal discharge, and, more specifically, an increased respiratory effort at rest [1,18–20]. RAO occurs in mature horses with a clinical onset rarely before 6 or 7 years of age. Both sexes are equally frequently affected and even though there is a clear genetic predisposition (see section 'Recurrent airway obstruction genetics and relationship with defence against parasites and with other allergic diseases'), there is no obvious breed predilection. Although the inciting factors differ (see section 'Environmental triggers'), RAO and SPAOPD are clinically indistinguishable [1,19,20].

In clinical exacerbation, the increased respiratory effort manifests itself with an increased respiratory rate (>18/min at rest) and in severe cases with a prolonged, exaggerated expiratory phase visible through abdominal muscles assisting with expiration ('heave-line'; Figure 55.3), flared nostrils, and a 'pumping' movement of the anus during respiration. More mildly affected horses may only show moderately increased abdominal effort at rest without an obvious nasal flare. Most RAO-affected horses cough regularly, especially during feeding and exercise. Coughing is associated with airway inflammation and mucus accumulation [50]. Chronic coughing is the clinical sign most easily recognized by owners to identify horses at risk for RAO [7]. Because of its sporadic nature, coughing cannot be assessed accurately by counting during brief periods [50]. Mucous nasal discharge and abnormal respiratory noises during auscultation (wheezes, crackles, rales, and rhonchi) are also characteristic, but less consistent clinical findings. Exercise intolerance is moderate to severe with an exaggerated respiratory effort during and after work and delayed recovery of the respiratory rate. Rarely, severely affected horses may lose weight.

Clinical signs are often best recognized by people who most consistently observe the horse. A standardized questionnaire and grading system can be helpful when collecting the history. The Horse Owner Assessed Respiratory Signs Index (HOARSI) [7], for instance, identifies RAO-affected horses with a high reliability [35], and standardized owner assessment before and after treatment (including performance, breathing effort, coughing, and nasal discharge scored using a visual analogue scale) was even superior to clinical, cytological, and endoscopic examinations made by a veterinarian [51]. These studies not only underline the importance and value of thorough history taking in RAO, they also illustrate that it is of paramount importance to inquire about changes over time in the clinical status. As a function of the exposure to the inciting environment, clinical signs during exacerbation (mostly typical and obvious) can differ greatly from those during clinical remission.

In complete remission, these clinical signs disappear within days to weeks, depending on the environment and the individual case. If clinical signs persist despite efforts to remove the inciting environmental factors, further diagnostic efforts should be taken to rule out diseases other than RAO, such as bronchiectasis, interstitial lung diseases/pulmonary fibrosis, or bronchitis of infectious origin/pneumonia.

Further diagnostic investigation

Guidelines

Numerous ancillary diagnostic methods have been described for IAD and RAO [1,2,20]. While the choice often depends on the situation (e.g. field vs. hospital setting), the availability of equipment, and the expectations of the client, some basic guidelines can be helpful:

- The definition and diagnosis of IAD is currently based on the evaluation of BALF-cytology and/or lung function testing [2].
    - This definition has been criticized because it is difficult to apply in a practical setting [52]. In the field, IAD is often diagnosed based on clinical presentation, endoscopic visualization of increased tracheal mucus, and tracheobronchial secretion (TBS) cytology.
    - This definition is also of debatable usefulness when evaluating older (asymptomatic and well-performing) horses kept in conventional stable environment: mild, subclinical increases of BALF neutrophils, eosinophils, and/or mast cells can then be very common [13] and their significance questionable.
    - When poor performance is the only presenting complaint, a systematic approach to identify differential diagnoses for decreased performance is important.
- RAO is often easier to diagnose than IAD and a working diagnosis can be reached in many cases based on the typical history and characteristic clinical signs (see section 'Diagnostic methods'). Exceptions warranting further diagnostic efforts include:
    - Cases with an unclear history that are presented with mild to moderate clinical signs and may be in (partial) remission.
    - Cases that do not respond to standard treatment (see section 'Therapy').
    - Establishment of an objective 'baseline' to evaluate the success of a planned therapy.

Diagnostic methods

In order to provide an overview, diagnostic methods are briefly discussed; for detailed descriptions of techniques and methodology the reader is referred elsewhere [1,2,20]:

- Clinical hay challenge is mostly used in research settings to differentiate IAD from RAO; in IAD clinical signs may worsen, but no obviously increased respiratory effort is observed at rest.
- Endoscopy (Figure 55.4): mucus accumulation (mucus grades 0–5 [53]) increases after work, correlates with cough, and decreased willingness to perform, and often resolves only incompletely in remission of RAO [20,35,49,51,54]. IAD-affected horses often have multiple specks to pools of mucus accumulation (grades 2–3/5), while large pools and continuous

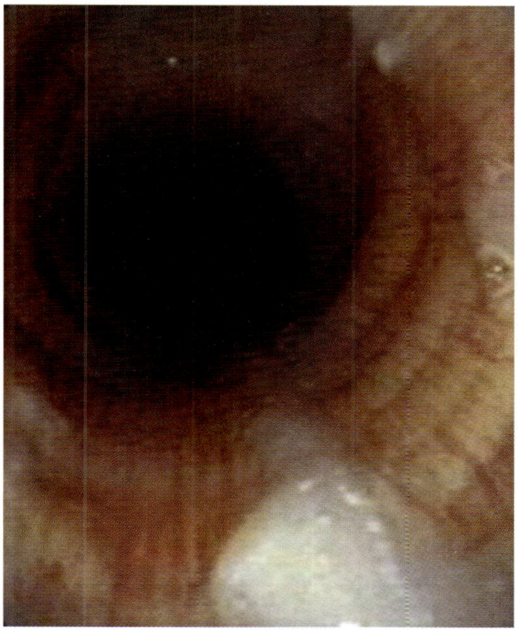

Figure 55.4 Endoscopic image of moderate to large tracheal mucus accumulation (grade 3–4/5). (Reprinted with permission from Swiss Institute of Equine Medicine.)

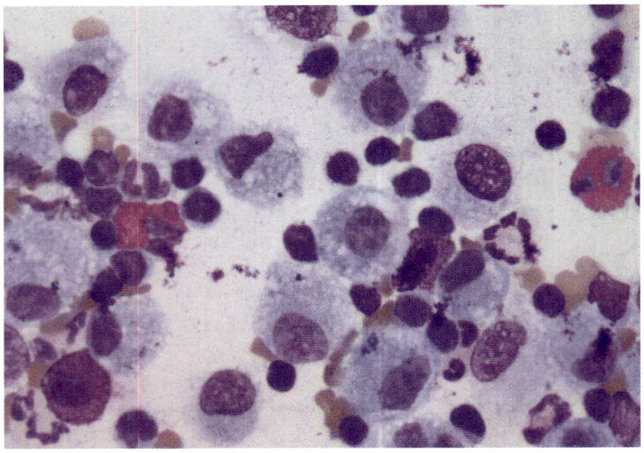

Figure 55.5 Various cell types (macrophages, lymphocytes, neutrophils, eosinophils, mast cells, and erythrocytes) in a bronchoalveolar lavage cytospin preparation (May–Grünwald–Giemsa stain; magnification 630×). (Reprinted with permission from Swiss Institute of Equine Medicine.)

streams (grades 4–5/5) are typically only seen in RAO exacerbation [13,53,54]. Endoscopy also enables evaluation for various upper airway conditions that are important as differential diagnoses for poor performance and occasional coughing. The assessment of septum thickness at the tracheal bifurcation is not helpful in the diagnosis of RAO and IAD [55].

- Cytology from tracheal wash or directly aspirated tracheobronchial secretion (TBS) is widely used because it is easy to perform in the field [51], but it has been judged insufficient for the diagnosis of IAD [2]. Instead, using BALF cytology (Figure 55.5) with cut-off values of >5% neutrophils, >2% mast cells, and/or 0.1% eosinophils was proposed to diagnose IAD. In contrast, in RAO exacerbation BALF neutrophils typically exceed 25% [1]. In clinical remission, the proportion of neutrophils decreases more completely in BALF than in TBS [37], and TBS cytology is generally less specific [1,2,20]. Airway secretion cytology can also be useful in unclear cases to identify differential diagnoses, e.g. lungworm infection (history of contact with donkeys) or eosinophilic pneumonitis.
- Lung function: standard lung mechanics are used to document changes in RAO in research settings [1,20], but are not sensitive enough to detect lung function deficits in RAO remission and in IAD. Unfortunately, more sensitive techniques, e.g. forced oscillation and forced expiration mechanics [2,20], are still mostly unavailable and are often impractical in clinical settings. As a surrogate marker, arterial oxygen tension can be readily measured in a practical setting to evaluate improvement in gas exchange in RAO before and after treatment [50]. A recently established method using flow metric plethysmography combined with histamine bronchoprovocation allows reproducible evaluation of airway hyper-responsiveness, even under field conditions [56]. In IAD, hyper-responsiveness is prominent, especially in horses with increased BALF mast cells and eosinophils. In RAO, it precedes clinical signs in exacerbation and may persist when horses are kept in low-dust environment (see section 'Environmental control of inciting agents'), but resolves at pasture [2].
- Allergen testing: the prospect of specifically avoiding and even targeting inciting agents causing exacerbation of RAO has made allergen testing the subject of numerous studies [20] (see sections 'Environmental triggers' and 'Immunotherapy'). Several factors render successful identification of causative allergens difficult, including the very heterogeneous nature of stable and hay dusts; the fact that healthy horses also frequently respond to common test antigens; and the lack of a correlation between local pulmonary allergic reactions and dermal as well as serological responses. To date, no method and protocol allows evidence-based and reliable testing of allergens in RAO or IAD [1,2,20,43]. Thus, even though 'allergen testing' is still relatively popular and wide-spread in clinical practice, controlled scientific studies demonstrating reliability and practical usefulness are lacking.
- Further diagnostic tests: thoracic radiography typically shows increased bronchointerstitial (peribronchial) patterns in IAD and more markedly in RAO [1,2]. In the latter, an overinflated lung (air trapping) with flattening of the diaphragmatic border is often also visible. These findings are of little benefit in the diagnosis of IAD and RAO. Instead, thoracic radiography (and ultrasound) can be helpful to identify or rule out differential diagnoses, such as bronchiectasis, interstitial lung diseases/pulmonary fibrosis, or bronchitis of infectious origin/pneumonia. In severe, longstanding RAO cases, cardiac function may be altered [20], which can be assessed by cardiac ultrasound. Finally, haematology and serum chemistry results, which are unremarkable in IAD and RAO, can be important to detect signs of infectious disease in unclear cases.

Therapy

To date, there are no known cures for RAO. Spontaneous desensitization appears to be very rare and affected horses recurrently develop clinical signs when exposed to the inciting environmental stimuli. Thus, environmental control is currently the fundamental therapeutic and prophylactic approach. In some horses, when environmental modification is not practically possible or when control of clinical signs is insufficient, medical therapy is necessary. In IAD, even though controlled studies are widely lacking, a combination of environmental measures and medical treatment is also often the chosen approach.

Environmental control of inciting agents

Inflammatory airway disease

Even though results from controlled clinical trials are sorely lacking, environmental control of inhaled dust loads, in particular from hay and bedding (see section 'Pathogenesis of inflammatory airway disease'), is a rational approach to IAD therapy and prevention [2,57]. Depending on the situation, practical measures may include decreasing the dust load by:

- Turning horses out to pasture without hay feeding and stabling provides the most complete dust control, but it is often not possible.
- Enhancing ventilation in the stable to reduce inhalable particles and irritant gases may improve the overall air quality in a stable, but the particle load in the breathing zone of the horses is more directly influenced by the 'dustiness' of feeds and bedding.
- Replacing hay with haylage or pelleted feed. This may in many cases be the most promising approach, but cost and availability, as well as risks of botulism (haylage) and potential gastrointestinal and behavioural problems (full pelleted feeds) must be considered.
- Replacing straw bedding with 'low-dust' alternatives such as cleaned wood shavings, cardboard, shredded paper, or peat moss. Great care should be taken to assure that these alternative bedding materials, which often cost more than straw, are indeed of good 'low-dust' quality.
- Reduce dust load by avoiding sweeping the floor and mucking-out when horses are indoors and storing hay in barn lofts above the stalls.

In our experience, clinical results after replacing hay with haylage and straw with 'low-dust' bedding vary considerably from case to case. Based on limited evidence [54,58], we can expect better short to mid-term (days to weeks) improvement regarding neutrophilic inflammation than mucus accumulation.

Long-term housing in a more dusty environment is associated with increased neutrophilic inflammation (smaller particles $\leq 2.5\,\mu m$) as well as increased tracheal mucus accumulation (larger particles 2.5–10 μm diameter) [59]. Thus, for IAD prevention, careful consideration should be given to stabling and management practices in order to reduce dust loads.

Recurrent airway obstruction

Environmental improvement is the mainstay of RAO therapy and currently the only therapeutic strategy that promises long-term relief. Basically, all the options to remove offending sources of inhalants mentioned for IAD (see section 'Inflammatory airway disease') are also valid for RAO. Specific options and protocols are chosen depending on the severity of disease, patient-specific hypersensitivities (see section 'Environmental triggers'), and management circumstances. Compared with IAD, there is considerably more evidence [1,20,57] for the efficacy of specific protocols in RAO:

- Replacing hay as the main source of inhaled allergens and irritants is central. Haylage, hay cubes, and pelleted feeds seem to be similarly effective, but each has its drawbacks (see section 'Inflammatory airway disease').
- Within days to weeks permanent turn-out at pasture (without hay feeding) is more effective in improving clinical signs, airway inflammation, and lung function measures compared to modified indoor environments.
- Housing in a 'low-dust' indoor environment (replacing hay and straw bedding, see section 'Inflammatory airway disease'), where clinical signs at rest are alleviated, but airway inflammation and hyper-reactivity persist at a lower level.

Due to budgetary and management (e.g. housing in boarding stables) constraints it is often not possible to implement permanent turn-out without hay feeding or even housing in a 'low-dust' environment. Depending on the severity and duration of disease, partial measures can in some cases provide a workable compromise:

- If hay feeding cannot be avoided, it should at least not be offered in the form of round bales. Round bale hay is associated with increased airway inflammation in horses at pasture [60].
- Replacing hay by alternative feeds in just one stall of an affected horse, while other animals in the same stable are still fed with hay, provides at least partial improvement [61], but may be insufficient in more severely affected cases.
- Similarly, the effectiveness of the relatively common practice of soaking hay prior to feeding is highly variable [62] and likely depends on both the severity of hyper-responsiveness and the feeding behaviour of the individual.
- Improve bedding, ventilation, and management practices (see section 'Inflammatory airway disease') as adjunct measures.

For SPAOPD-affected individuals, the inciting factors are found outdoors (see section 'Environmental triggers'), accordingly SPAOPD must be controlled by removing affected horses from pasture and keeping them in a clean, well-ventilated, 'low-dust' indoors environment, except for the winter months [47,48].

When control of the environment is not or only partially possible, temporary or even life-long medical treatment may be necessary.

Symptomatic therapy

Medical therapy can effectively relieve clinical signs of RAO temporarily, but once it is discontinued, housing in an unchanged environment will exacerbate the disease again, and clinical signs will promptly return. IAD in contrast, may spontaneously remiss within weeks to months, especially in younger horses, and medical therapy is also more likely to result in lasting improvement than in RAO. These statements and much of the following recommendations for IAD therapy are based on clinical experience and anecdotal evidence rather than scientific proof regarding effectiveness. There is substantially more evidence-based data on the medical therapy of RAO [1,20], and most recommendations for IAD [2] are extrapolated from proven regimens for RAO.

Anti-inflammatory medication

Of the medications that are based on a strong body of evidence for efficacy in RAO, corticosteroids are regarded as the most potent [1,20,62]. Improvements in clinical signs and lung function are apparent within hours and are maximal after 1–2 weeks of medication. Effects on airway neutrophilia and mucus accumulation are less consistent [20,50,51]. Serious adverse effects are feared (in particular laminitis), but occur very rarely. Both dexamethasone (e.g. 0.05–0.1 mg/kg once daily) and prednisolone (e.g. 1–2 mg/kg once daily or every other day) are effective when administered orally, and are well tolerated over several weeks [50,62]. Because they cause fewer side effects than systemic corticosteroids, inhaled alternatives (e.g. fluticasone and beclomethasone, both by metered-dose inhaler) are often given for long-term treatment of RAO and also IAD [2,20,62]. They are less potent than systemic dexamethasone treatment, however, and may thus be better suited for prevention of exacerbation rather than primary treatment of severely affected horses [62,63].

Mast cell stabilizers (e.g. cromolyn sodium/sodium cromoglycate or inhaled nedocromil sodium) have shown some, if variable, efficacy. They can be used to prevent clinical exacerbation in RAO and are recommended by some authors for the treatment of IAD-affected horses with elevated numbers of mast cells in BALF [2,20,62]. Other anti-inflammatory medications such as non-steroidal anti-inflammatory drugs, leukotriene-receptor antagonists, and antihistamines, are of limited or no efficacy in RAO.

Bronchodilators

β2-agonists are the most widely used bronchodilators and their effectiveness, both when given systemically (e.g. clenbuterol usually at a 'low-dose' of 0.8 μg/kg twice daily) and inhaled (both short-acting, albuterol, fenoterol, and longer-acting, salmeterol, pirbuterol) is well documented in RAO [1,20,62]. Bronchodilators are particularly helpful for short-term relief of severe clinical signs because of their rapid onset of action (e.g. albuterol: 5 minutes). Efficacy generally increases with dosage, but so do side effects. Clenbuterol also increases mucociliary clearance and has anti-inflammatory effects [20,62,64]. Because of their relatively short duration of action, β2-agonists are often combined with corticosteroids, which may prevent down-regulation of β2-adrenoceptors. Furthermore, administration of bronchodilators can improve the pulmonary distribution of inhaled corticosteroids and other aerosolized medications. Again, most recommendations and dosages for the use of β2-agonists in IAD, for which they are advocated in combination with corticosteroids and sometimes prior to strenuous work to avoid exercise-induced bronchoconstriction, are extrapolated from RAO (reviewed in [2]).

Systemic anticholinergic (parasympatholytic) drugs (e.g. atropine 0.01–0.02 mg/kg intravenously) are very effective, but their practical use is limited because of severe side effects. Inhaled anticholinergics like ipratropium bromide are better tolerated, but their duration of action is similarly limited (4–6 hours) to that of 'long-lasting' β2-agonists. Methylxanthine derivatives, non-specific phosphodiesterase (PDE) inhibitors, have bronchodilator effects, but with a relatively low therapeutic index and are sometimes used as an adjunctive therapy [20].

Other medication and symptomatic therapies

Different types of secretolytics and mucolytics are often used for horses with excessive amounts of mucus present in the airways. Unfortunately, their clinical efficacy in RAO and IAD is poorly documented [62,64].

Also wide-spread in practice is the use of complementary and alternative approaches. Unfortunately, there is very limited scientific data on their efficacy and side effects. Benefits of some herbal medicine preparations [62] as well as acupuncture treatment [65] have been investigated in RAO-affected horses, but clinical improvement could not be demonstrated.

Immunotherapy

Anecdotal reports suggests that allergen-specific immunotherapy (ASIT) is practiced relatively frequently in IAD and RAO, and some cases appear to benefit from ASIT as an adjunctive therapy (W. Rosenkrantz, personal communication). To our knowledge, no controlled studies exist on ASIT use and efficacy in IAD or RAO. The pathogenesis of IAD is very poorly understood and there is no evidence for a role of allergens; the immunological background of RAO, on the other hand, is very complex (see sections 'Pathogenesis of inflammatory airway disease' and 'Pathogenesis of recurrent airway obstruction'), and specific inciting allergens are very difficult to identify (see section 'Diagnostic methods').

Other, non-allergen-specific immunotherapeutic approaches have been documented for the treatment of IAD and RAO. In racehorses with IAD, low-dose interferon-α (oral human interferon-alpha 50–150 units once daily for 5 days; higher doses were less effective) was demonstrated to attenuate airway inflammation [66,67].

One study has reported results that show the potential of cytosine phosphate guanine oligodeoxynucleotides (CpG-ODN) in RAO. The immunostimulating agent increased IL-10 and IFN-γ and decreased IL-4 expression in cultured BALF cells [68] and aerosolized nanoparticle-bound CpG-ODN increased IL-10 expression *in vivo*. RAO-affected horses also showed clinical improvement after five consecutive inhalations [68]. Three to five consecutive nanoparticle-bound CpG-ODN inhalation treatments appeared to have a beneficial effect lasting several months in RAO-affected horses that were otherwise only in partial remission (H. Gehlen, personal communication).

Important note

Acknowledgements

The author wishes to thank Eliane Marti, University of Bern, and W. Rosenkrantz, Animal Dermatology Clinic, Tustin, California, for their valuable comments and suggestions. Much of the work reviewed in section 'Recurrent airway obstruction genetics and relationship with defence against parasites and with other allergic diseases' was supported by the Swiss Institute of Equine Medicine (ISMEquine Research) and the Swiss National Science Foundation grants No. 310000-116502 and 310030-138295.

References

1. Robinson NE. Chairperson's introduction: International Workshop on Equine Chronic Airway Disease, Michigan State University, 16–18 June 2000. *Equine Veterinary Journal* 2001; **33**: 5–19.
2. Couëtil LL, Hoffman AM, Hodgson J, *et al.* Inflammatory airway disease of horses. *Journal of Veterinary Internal Medicine* 2007; **21**: 356–361.
3. Woods P, Robinson N, Swanson M, *et al.* Airborne dust and aeroallergen concentration in a horse stable under two different management systems. *Equine Veterinary Journal* 1993; **25**: 208–213.
4. McGorum BC, Ellison J, Cullen RT. Total and respirable airborne dust endotoxin concentrations in three equine management systems. *Equine Veterinary Journal* 1998; **30**: 430–434.
5. Clarke A. A review of environmental and host factors in relation to equine respiratory disease. *Equine Veterinary Journal* 1987; **19**: 435–441.
6. Davis M, Foster W. Inhalation toxicology in the equine respiratory tract. In: Lekeux P, ed. *Equine Respiratory Diseases*. Ithaca, NY: International Veterinary Information Services (www.ivis.org, accessed July, 2013).
7. Ramseyer A, Gaillard C, Burger D, *et al.* Effects of genetic and environmental factors on chronic lower airway disease in horses. *Journal of Veterinary Internal Medicine* 2007; **21**: 149–156.
8. Hoffman AM, Mazan MR, Ellenberg S. Association between bronchoalveolar lavage cytologic features and airway reactivity in horses with a history of exercise intolerance. *American Journal of Veterinary Research* 1998; **59**: 176–181.
9. Hare JE, Viel L. Pulmonary eosinophilia associated with increased airway responsiveness in young racing horses. *Journal of Veterinary Internal Medicine* 1998; **12**: 163–170.
10. Chapman P, Green C, Main J, *et al.* Retrospective study of the relationships between age, inflammation and the isolation of bacteria from the lower respiratory tract of thoroughbred horses. *Veterinary Record* 2000; **146**: 91–95.
11. Wood JL, Newton JR, Chanter N, *et al.* Association between respiratory disease and bacterial and viral infections in British racehorses. *Journal of Clinical Microbiology* 2005; **43**: 120–126.
12. Newton JR, Woodt JL, Chanter N. Evidence for transferrin allele as a host-level risk factor in naturally occurring equine respiratory disease: a preliminary study. *Equine Veterinary Journal* 2007; **39**: 164–171.
13. Gerber V, Robinson NE, Luethi S, *et al.* Airway inflammation and mucus in two age groups of asymptomatic well-performing sport horses. *Equine Veterinary Journal* 2003; **35**: 491–495.
14. Holcombe S, Jackson C, Gerber V, *et al.* Stabling is associated with airway inflammation in young Arabian horses. *Equine Veterinary Journal* 2001; **33**: 244–249.
15. Tremblay GM, Ferland C, Lapointe JM, *et al.* Effect of stabling on bronchoalveolar cells obtained from normal and COPD horses. *Equine Veterinary Journal* 1993; **25**: 194–197.
16. Bedenice D, Mazan MR, Hoffman AM. Association between cough and cytology of bronchoalveolar lavage fluid and pulmonary function in horses diagnosed with inflammatory airway disease. *Journal of Veterinary Internal Medicine* 2008; **22**: 1022–1028.

17. Lavoie JP, Cesarini C, Lavoie-Lamoureux A, *et al.* Bronchoalveolar lavage fluid cytology and cytokine messenger ribonucleic acid expression of racehorses with exercise intolerance and lower airway inflammation. *Journal of Veterinary Internal Medicine* 2011; **25**: 322–329.
18. Lowell FC. Observations on heaves an asthma-like syndrome in the horse. *Journal of Allergy and Clinical Immunology* 1964; **35**: 322–330.
19. Robinson NE, Derksen FJ, Olszewski MA, *et al.* The pathogenesis of chronic obstructive pulmonary disease of horses. *British Veterinary Journal* 1995; **152**: 283–306.
20. Leclere M, Lavoie-Lamoureux A, Lavoie JP. Heaves, an asthma-like disease of horses. *Respirology* 2011; **16**: 1027–1046.
21. Halliwell RE, McGorum BC, Irving P, *et al.* Local and systemic antibody production in horses affected with chronic obstructive pulmonary disease. *Veterinary Immunology and Immunopathology* 1993; **38**: 201–215.
22. Hare JE, Viel L, Conlon PD, Marshall, JS. In vitro allergen-induced degranulation of pulmonary mast cells from horses with recurrent airway obstruction (heaves). *American Journal of Veterinary Research* 1999; **60**: 841–846.
23. Lavoie JP, Maghni K, Desnoyers M, *et al.* Neutrophilic airway inflammation in horses with heaves is characterized by a Th2-type cytokine profile. *American Journal of Respiratory and Critical Care Medicine* 2001; **164**: 1410–1413.
24. Cordeau ME, Joubert P, Dewachi O, *et al.* IL-4, IL-5 and IFN-gamma mRNA expression in pulmonary lymphocytes in equine heaves. *Veterinary Immunology and Immunopathology* 2003; **97**: 87–96.
25. Horohov DW, Beadle RE, Mouch S, *et al.* Temporal regulation of cytokine mRNA expression in equine recurrent airway obstruction. *Veterinary Immunology and Immunopathology* 2005; **108**: 237–245.
26. Giguere S, Viel L, Lee E, *et al.* Cytokine induction in pulmonary airways of horses with heaves and effect of therapy with inhaled fluticasone propionate. *Veterinary Immunology and Immunopathology* 2002; **85**: 147–158.
27. Ainsworth DM, Wagner B, Franchini M, *et al.* Time-dependent alterations in gene expression of interleukin-8 in the bronchial epithelium of horses with recurrent airway obstruction. *American Journal of Veterinary Research* 2006; **67**: 669–677.
28. Debrue M, Hamilton E, Joubert P, *et al.* Chronic exacerbation of equine heaves is associated with an increased expression of interleukin-17 mRNA in bronchoalveolar lavage cells. *Veterinary Immunology and Immunopathology* 2005; **105**: 25–31.
29. Pirie RS, Dixon PM, McGorum BC. Endotoxin contamination contributes to the pulmonary inflammatory and functional response to Aspergillus fumigatus extract inhalation in heaves horses. *Clinical and Experimental Allergy* 2003; **33**: 1289–1296.
30. Singh Suri S, Janardhan KS, Parbhakar O, *et al.* Expression of Toll-like receptor 4 and 2 in horse lungs. *Veterinary Research* 2006; **37**:541–551.
31. Marti E, Gerber H, Essich G, *et al.* On the genetic basis of equine allergic diseases. I. Chronic hypersensitivity bronchitis. *Equine Veterinary Journal* 1991; **23**: 457–460.
32. Jost U, Klukowska-Rötzler J, Dolf G, *et al.* A region on equine chromosome 13 is linked to recurrent airway obstruction in horses. *Equine Veterinary Journal* 2007; **39**: 236–241.
33. Klukowska-Rötzler J, Swinburne JE, Drögemüller C, *et al.* The interleukin 4 receptor gene and its role in recurrent airway obstruction in Swiss Warmblood horses. *Animal Genetics* 2012; **43**: 450–453.
34. Gerber V, Baleri D, Klukowska-Rötzler J, *et al.* Mixed inheritance of equine recurrent airway obstruction. *Journal of Veterinary Internal Medicine* 2009; **23**: 626–630.
35. Swinburne JE, Bogle H, Klukowska-Rötzler J, *et al.* A whole-genome scan for recurrent airway obstruction in Warmblood sport horses indicates two positional candidate regions. *Mammalian Genome* 2009; **20**: 504–515.
36. Scharrenberg A, Gerber V, Swinburne JE, *et al.* IgE, IgGa, IgGb and IgGT serum antibody levels in offspring of two sires affected with equine recurrent airway obstruction. *Animal Genetics* 2010; **41** (Suppl. 2): 131–137.
37. Laumen E, Doherr MG, Gerber V. Relationship of horse owner assessed respiratory signs index to characteristics of recurrent airway obstruction in two Warmblood families. *Equine Veterinary Journal* 2010; **42**: 142–148.
38. Racine J, Gerber V, MiskovicFeutz M, *et al.* Comparison of genomic and proteomic data in recurrent airway obstruction affected horses using ingenuity pathway analysis®. *BMC Veterinary Research* 2011; **7**: 48.
39. Bründler P, Frey CF, Gottstein B, *et al.* Lower shedding of strongylid eggs by Warmblood horses with recurrent airway obstruction compared to unrelated healthy horses. *Veterinary Journal* 2011; **190**: 12–15.
40. Neuhaus S, Bruendler P, Frey CF, *et al.* Increased parasite resistance and recurrent airway obstruction in horses of a high-prevalence family. *Journal of Veterinary Internal Medicine* 2011; **24**: 407–413.
41. McGorum BC, Dixon PM, Halliwell RE. Responses of horses affected with chronic obstructive pulmonary disease to inhalation challenges with mould antigens. *Equine Veterinary Journal* 1993; **25**: 261–267.
42. Hare JE, Viel L, Conlon PD, *et al.* In vitro allergen-induced degranulation of pulmonary mast cells from horses with recurrent airway obstruction (heaves). *American Journal of Veterinary Research* 1999; **60**: 841–847.
43. Tahon L, Baselgia S, Gerber V, *et al.* In vitro allergy tests compared to intradermal testing in horses with recurrent airway obstruction. *Veterinary Immunology and Immunopathology* 2009; **127**: 85–93.
44. McGorum BC, Dixon PM, Halliwell RE. Evaluation of intradermal mould antigen testing in the diagnosis of equine chronic obstructive pulmonary disease. *Equine Veterinary Journal* 1993; **25**: 273–275.
45. Pirie RS, Dixon PM, McGorum BC. Evaluation of nebulised hay dust suspensions (HDS) for the diagnosis and investigation of heaves. 3: Effect of fractionation of HDS. *Equine Veterinary Journal* 2002; **34**: 343–347.
46. Hotchkiss JW, Reid SW, Christley RM. A survey of horse owners in Great Britain regarding horses in their care. Part 2: Risk factors for recurrent airway obstruction. *Equine Veterinary Journal* 2007; **39**: 301–308.
47. Seahorn TL, Beadle RE. Summer pasture-associated obstructive pulmonary disease in horses: 21 cases (1983–1991). *Journal of the American Veterinary Medical Association* 1993; **202**: 779–782.
48. Costa LR, Johnson JR, Baur ME, *et al.* Temporal clinical exacerbation of summer pasture-associated recurrent airway obstruction and relationship with climate and aeroallergens in horses. *American Journal of Veterinary Research* 2006; **67**: 1635–1642.
49. Widmer A, Doherr MG, Tessier C, *et al.* Association of increased tracheal mucus accumulation with poor willingness to perform in show-jumpers and dressage horses. *Veterinary Journal* 2009; **182**: 430–435.

50. Robinson NE, Berney C, Eberhart S, *et al.* Coughing, mucus accumulation, airway obstruction, and airway inflammation in control horses and horses affected with recurrent airway obstruction. *American Journal of Veterinary Research* 2003; **64**: 550–557.
51. Gerber V, Schott II HC, Robinson NE. Owner assessment in judging the efficacy of airway disease treatment. *Equine Veterinary Journal* 2011; **43**: 153–158.
52. Cardwell JM, Christley RM, Gerber V, *et al.* What's in a name? Inflammatory airway disease in racehorses in training. *Equine Veterinary Journal* 2011; **43**: 756–758.
53. Gerber V, Straub R, Marti E, *et al.* Endoscopic scoring of mucus quantity and quality: observer and horse variance and relationship to inflammation, mucus viscoelasticity and volume. *Equine Veterinary Journal* 2004; **36**: 576–582.
54. Gerber V, Lindberg A, Berney C, *et al.* Airway mucus in recurrent airway obstruction—short-term response to environmental challenge. *Journal of Veterinary Internal Medicine* 2004; **18**: 92–97.
55. Koch C, Straub R, Ramseyer A, *et al.* Endoscopic scoring of the tracheal septum in horses and its clinical relevance for the evaluation of lower airway health in horses. *Equine Veterinary Journal* 2007; **39**: 107–112.
56. Nolen-Walston RD, Kuehn H, Boston RC, *et al.* Reproducibility of airway responsiveness in horses using flow metricplethysmography and histamine bronchoprovocation. *Journal of Veterinary Internal Medicine* 2009; **23**: 631–635.
57. Art T, McGorum BC, Lekeux P. Environmental control of respiratory disease. In: Lekeux P, ed. *Equine Respiratory Diseases.* Ithaca, New York: International Veterinary Information Service, 2002 (www.ivis.org, accessed October 24, 2012).
58. Boog C. Benefits of feeding haylage instead of hay for upper and lower airway health in horses affected with inflammatory airway disease Inaugural-Dissertation, Universität Bern, 2004; 31–39.
59. Millerick-May ML, Karmaus W, Derksen FJ, *et al.* Local airborne particulate concentration is associated with visible tracheal mucus in Thoroughbred racehorses. *Equine Veterinary Journal* 2013; **45**: 85–90
60. Robinson NE, Karmaus W, Holcombe SJ, *et al.* Airway inflammation in Michigan pleasure horses: prevalence and risk factors. *Equine Veterinary Journal* 2006; **38**: 293–299.
61. Jackson CA, Berney C, Jefcoat AM, *et al.* Environment and prednisone interactions in the treatment of recurrent airway obstruction (heaves). *Equine Veterinary Journal* 2000; **32**: 432–438.
62. Lavoie JP. Recurrent airway obstruction (heaves) and summer-pasture-associated obstructive pulmonary disease In: McGorum BC, Dixon PM, Robinson NE, *et al.*, eds. *Equine Respiratory Medicine and Surgery*, 1st edn. Amsterdam: Saunders Elsevier, 2007: 565–589.
63. Robinson NE, Berney C, Behan A, *et al.* Fluticasone propionate aerosol is more effective for prevention than treatment of recurrent airway obstruction. *Journal of Veterinary Internal Medicine* 2009; **23**: 1247–1253.
64. Gerber V, Robinson NE. Airway secretions and mucociliary function. In: McGorum BC, Dixon PM, Robinson NE, *et al.*, eds. *Equine Respiratory Medicine and Surgery*, 1st edn. Amsterdam: Saunders Elsevier, 2007: 55–69.
65. Wilson DV, Berney CE, Peroni DL, *et al.* The effects of a single acupuncture treatment in horses with severe recurrent airway obstruction. *Equine Veterinary Journal* 2004; **36**: 489–494.
66. Moore B, Krakowka S, Cummins J. Changes in airway inflammatory cell populations in Standard bred racehorses after interferon administration. *Veterinary Immunology and Immunopathology* 1996; **49**: 347.
67. Klier J, May A, Fuchs S, *et al.* Immunostimulation of bronchoalveolar lavage cells from recurrent airway obstruction-affected horses by different CpG-classes bound to gelatin nanoparticles. *Veterinary Immunology and Immunopathology* 2011; **144**: 79–87.
68. Klier J, Fuchs S, May A, *et al.* A nebulized gelatin nanoparticle-based CpG formulation is effective in immunotherapy of allergic horses. *Pharmaceutical Research* 2012; **29**: 1650–1657.

Section 4

Contact and Other Allergic Diseases

56

Equine allergic contact dermatitis

Chris Reeder and Joya Griffin

Animal Dermatology Clinic, Louisville, KY, USA

Conflict of interest: none declared.

Pathogenesis

While the knowledge about allergic and irritant contact dermatitis is vast in human medicine, there is a paucity of information in veterinary species, most reports are anecdotal. Firstly, there are two distinct types of contact dermatitis, 'irritant' and 'allergic'. By definition, an 'irritant' contact dermatitis is from a substance that causes direct damage to the keratinocytes. Many of these substances are acids, alkalis, solvents, enzymes, etc. The most severe irritant contact dermatitis is considered to be a 'chemical burn' [1]. Genetic influence is thought to be involved in sensitizing humans but this has not been proven in animals. The pathophysiology of irritant contact dermatitis is the result of phospholipase activation through keratinocyte damage from the offending substance. The arachidonic acid cascade is activated, resulting in numerous proinflammatory cytokines and chemokines. No sensitization phase is required to elicit an irritant contact dermatitis, which is in contrast to allergic contact dermatitis.

Allergic contact dermatitis (ACD; or contact hypersensitivity) is defined as contact dermatitis due to allergic sensitization. In this type of contact dermatitis 'contact allergens' (haptens) are low molecular weight, usually lipid-soluble, substances that are non-immunologic until coupled with epidermal proteins. German shepherd dogs have been shown to have an increased incidence of contact hypersensitivity [2]. Other breeds of dogs have also been involved in increased incidences; however, horses have not been associated with any breed predispositions to date [3]. There are three phases of ACD: (1) sensitization phase, (2) elicitation phase, and (3) resolution phase (Figure 56.1). The pathophysiology of ACD begins when a new hapten enters through the epidermis and binds to epidermal proteins, which act as carrier molecules. The hapten–carrier complex is pinocytosed by Langerhans cells, which then migrates from the epidermis to the parafollicular cortex of a regional lymph node. Naïve T cells are presented the new antigen (hapten) through accessory signals, interleukin-1(IL-1) secretion for example. The hapten is conjugated into a new antigen molecule complex and expressed on the surface of the Langerhans cell. An unprimed T cell must recognize the new complex and antigen components on the Langerhans cell to become activated. The activated T cell will produce IL-2, which will create a proliferation of a primed T-cell clone. These are known as 'memory cells' and will circulate throughout the body.

The elicitation phase of allergic contact dermatitis starts with hapten penetration into the epidermis and conjugation into cell surface–antigen complexes. Langerhans cells remain in the skin and efficiently process antigens for presentation to primed T helper cells. Stimulated memory T cells secrete cytokines like IL-2R, promoting local lymphocyte proliferation, and gamma-interferon, which induces keratinocytes to generate new cell surface molecules. Intercellular adhesion molecule 1 (ICAM-1) and other cytokines create more leukocyte interactions, along with keratinocytes, to likely directly present antigens to effector T cells. Stimulated keratinocytes secrete eicosanoids and recruit basophils, mast cells, and macrophages, adding to the inflammatory phase. The resolution phase results in the increased

Veterinary Allergy, First Edition. Edited by Chiara Noli, Aiden Foster, and Wayne Rosenkrantz.

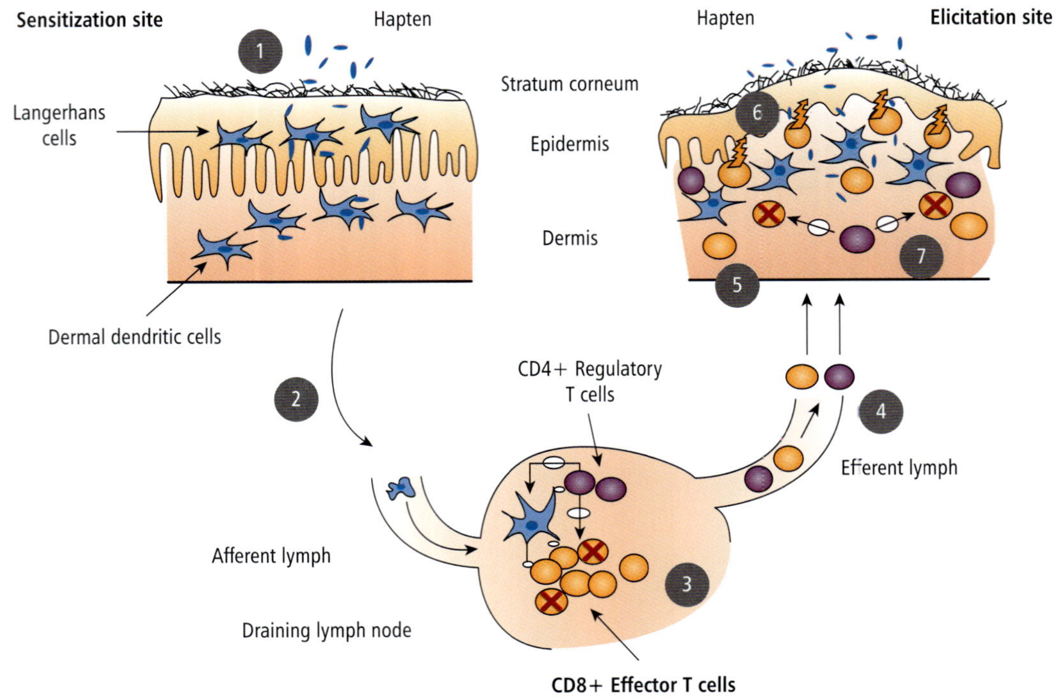

Figure 56.1 Pathophysiology of allergic contact hypersensitivity. Sensitization step: haptens penetrate the stratum corneum. Hapten loading by skin dendritic cells (step 1) parallels activation and migration of DC through the afferent lymphatic vessels to the draining lymph nodes (step 2). Migrating dendritic cells are located in the para-cortical area of the draining lymph node where they can present haptenated peptides on MHC class I and II molecules to $CD8^+$ and $CD4^+$ T cells, respectively (step 3). Specific T-cells precursors expand clonally in the draining lymph node and diffuse to the bloodstream through the efferent lymphatic vessels and the thoracic duct (step 4). During this process they acquire skin-specific homing antigens (CLA and CCR4) and become memory T cells. Primed T cells preferentially diffuse in the skin after transendothelial migration. At the end of the sensitization step everything is ready for the development of a contact sensitivity reaction upon challenge with the relevant hapten. Elicitation phase: when the hapten is painted for a second (and subsequent) time, it diffuses through the epidermis and could be loaded by Langerhans cells or other skin cells expressing MHC molecules, such as keratinocytes and dermal dendritic cells, which are then able to activate trafficking specific T cells (step 5). $CD8^+$ cytotoxic T-cell activation initiates the inflammatory process through keratinocyte apoptosis and cytokine/chemokine production (step 6). This is responsible for the recruitment of leukocytes (including regulatory T cells) from the blood to the skin leading to the development of skin lesions (step 7). Reprinted from [4] © 2004, with the permission of John Libbey Eurotext.

expression of the anti-inflammatory cytokine IL-10 being released from keratinocytes [4].

Allergic contact dermatitis

Allergic contact dermatitis has been reported in horses with exposure to various substances. Shampoos and parasiticidal sprays have been linked to possible ACD and may be an aetiology of contact urticaria, through a systemic antibody response [5,6]. There has been a report of ACD occurring in horses fed hay made from grass treated previously with an herbicide (the type of herbicide was not reported) [7]. Five horses developed swollen, cracked lips, and serous nasal discharge. Within 48 hours of removing the hay, all horses returned to normal. Weeks later the owner of the horses experimented by re-feeding the suspected causative hay and all five horses had a recurrence of the signs within 24 hours. Common tack items, blankets, and grooming supplies may also be a source of allergic contact dermatitis. The suspected agent is a preservative or dye in the tack and not a reaction to rubber, wool, or leather materials (Figure 56.2) (W. Rosenkrantz, personal communication).

Irritant contact dermatitis

Buttercups, particularly the tall buttercup (*Ranunculus acris*), and many other *Ranunculus* species, have been shown to cause contact dermatitis in horses in their fresh state [8,9]. The causative toxin, ranunculin, is a glycoside from which protoanemonin is released when the plant is crushed by virtue of enzymatic action, which is activated by crushing. Horses may develop erosions, ulcerations, and blisters on the muzzle and in the oral cavity from this toxin. The dried buttercups (within days), frozen, or in hay are safe to be consumed and are

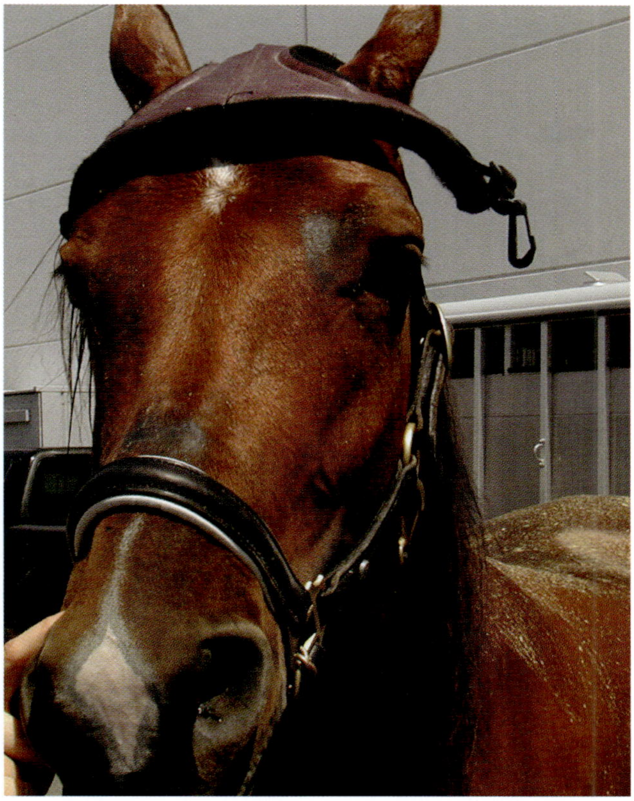

Figure 56.2 Leather racing hat and halter creating an allergic contact dermatitis on the face and supraorbital region. (Reprinted with permission from Wayne Rosenkrantz.)

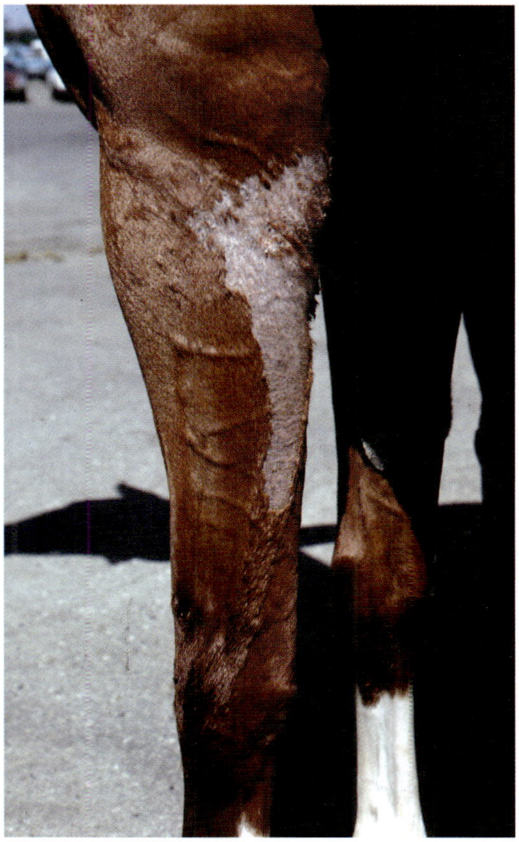

Figure 56.3 Alopecia due to contact with an unknown liquid medication; note 'drip pattern'. (Reprinted with permission from Stephen White.)

not considered toxic because the volatile chemical dissipates. Oil, pine tar, and other petroleum products have been thought to cause irritant contact dermatitis in horses [10,11]. Hoof paints and many insecticidal sprays have also been implicated as irritants [12,13]. Irritant contact allergy to tack has also been suspected from the leather itself or any products used on the leather, such as cleaners, solvents, polishing agents, or water-proofing substances (W. Rosenkrantz, personal communication).

Many practitioners and dermatologists report that some allergens or irritants may cause contact urticaria in horses. This phenomenon has been difficult to establish and has been reported as a 'rare' condition in horses [6,12].

Clinical features

Allergic contact dermatitis may take weeks to years for the sensitization period [12]. In both allergic and irritant contact dermatitis the features are similar, with varying degrees of pruritus, erythema, oedema, papules, scaling, alopecia, vesicles, and excoriations (Figure 56.3). Secondary pyoderma may be seen in some cases as well.

Because of sweating, horses may present with lesions distant from the point of contact of the substance. A seasonal pattern or a single horse affected when a group of horses are housed together would point more to allergic contact dermatitis. When the lesions are non-seasonal or multiple horses are affected with similar lesions, this would tend to support irritant contact dermatitis or a contagious disease [12].

Diagnosis

Diagnosis of either ACD or irritant contact dermatitis is difficult. The standard diagnostic test in humans is patch testing. Unfortunately, in animals patch testing does not come as a commercial kit and often the specific offending allergen or irritant substance is difficult to isolate.

The positive patch test reproduces an experimental contact dermatitis on a limited area of the skin. A positive reaction of the patch test indicates a contact sensitization is present. Finn Chambers on Scanpor adhesive strips (SmartPractice, Phoenix, AZ) and several other tape methods are currently in use for humans, as in the

T.R.U.E. Test (Thin-layer Rapid Use Epicutaneous Test; Mekos Laboratories AS, Hillerød, Denmark); however, their validity has not been established for animals. The typical patch test is performed for 48–72 hours then removed and read for signs of irritation, erythema, and secondary lesions (e.g. papules, pustules, etc.), or in some cases skin biopsies may be collected [4].

To perform patch testing one must rechallenge the animal with the suspected irritant/allergen. Upon re-exposure to the substance, a reaction at the site of application will usually develop within 48–72 hours. This type of patch testing is an accurate method of testing a suspected substance for contact dermatitis; however, it will not distinguish between irritant and allergic contact dermatitis. To perform patch testing properly the substance in question should be applied to the skin, a shaved patch is best, with an occlusive substance that is non-irritating (e.g. petroleum jelly or lubricating jelly), then bandaged and left to stand for the 48–72 hour period. In the horse, the best site is the lateral cervical area. It is advised to also perform a 'control' patch with only the occlusive substance. Examination of a skin biopsy from the site may provide further information about an irritant versus allergic contact dermatitis. Irritant contact dermatitis has been shown on histopathology to have a prominent spongiosis, neutrophilic exocytosis, epidermal necrosis, and neutrophils in the dermal infiltrate. This is in contrast to allergic contact dermatitis, in which there may be less spongiosis, more lymphocytic perivascular inflammation, and lymphocytic exocytosis. Both irritant and allergic contact dermatitis can occur with the same substance [1].

Treatments for contact dermatitis vary depending on the severity of the lesions. Many cases may be successfully managed with avoidance of the offending substance. Topical corticosteroids may be of value for cases where a small patch is affected. For larger lesions or multifocal lesions, oral corticosteroids may be necessary. Occasionally, oral antihistamines can be used to treat recurrent and non-specific contact dermatitis. (See antihistamine types and dosages in Chapter 54 'Equine atopic disease symptomatic therapy and allergen-specific immunotherapy'). Pentoxifylline 10–15 mg/kg twice daily has been used in horses with cutaneous vasculitis caused by photoaggravation and has been anecdotally used in horses with contact dermatitis and also in dogs and humans for ACD [14–16]. Topical tacrolimus 0.1% has been shown in human studies to aid in reduction or resolution of ACD lesions, when applied at twice daily dosing for 14 days [17]. Additionally, hyposensitization has been attempted in humans with good preliminary data to support a beneficial effect at repeated, increasing concentrations of the topically applied offending substances over a 9 to 11-month period [18]. This type of treatment is very new in human medicine and has not yet been explored beyond rodent models.

Photohypersensitivity

Photosensitivity

Photosensitivity is caused by photosensitizing agents, exogenous or endogenous, that absorb radiation energy in lightly haired, non-pigmented areas of skin. Normally, non-pigmented sites are at risk and darker pigmented skin is typically unaffected. The light energy must be within the appropriate wavelength and is usually within the ultraviolet A wavelengths [19,20]. It occurs when skin has increased susceptibility to the damaging effects of UV light because of a photodynamic agent. These photosensitizers can be agents administered systemically or topically or from endogenous porphyrias, which result from enzymatic defects in heme biosynthetic pathways. The elevated levels of porphyrins act as phototoxic agents. Exogenous agents may be ingested feed or pasture and several agents have been described [21,22].

Photosensitivity is most typically classified by being either primary or secondary. Primary photosensitivity is associated with photodynamic agents absorbed from the gastrointestinal tract that react in non-pigmented skin when exposed to UV light. Ingested compounds contain polyphenolic pigments and are in the highest concentration in green plants. St. John's wort (hypericin) is implicated in photosensitivity in horses after ingestion and represents a classic example of primary photosensitization [21,22] (Table 56.1). Recently, a case of suspected primary photosensitivity was reported in a chestnut pony mare with a crusted dermatitis on the non-pigmented skin of the lower lip, muzzle, and blaze. Hogweed was abundant in the horse's pasture and lesions resolved after removal [23]. Primary photosensitivity also includes horses with congenital abnormalities in pigment (porphyrin) synthesis [24]. Secondary or hepatogenous photosensitivity is more common than primary photosensitization, and occurs in animals with liver disease that prevents the removal of by-products such as phylloerythrin that can react with UV light causing photosensitization. Phylloerythrin is a bacterial breakdown product of chlorophyll and acts as the photosensitizing compound [25]. This compound can accumulate in the blood stream if the liver is sufficiently diseased to prevent its removal and excretion in the bile [25]. Pyrrolizidine alkaloids (PAs) from ingested plants often cause hepatotoxicity, leading to secondary photosensitization (Figures 56.4 and 56.5). PAs are bioactivated by the liver's mono-oxygenase system to

Table 56.1 Examples of exogenous primary photosensitizing agents

Common name	Scientific name	Agent
Buckwheat	*Polygonum fagopyrum*	Fabopyrin
St. John's wort	*Hypericum perforatum*	Hypericin
Perennial rye grass	*Lolium perenne*	Peroline
Bishop's weed	*Ammima jus*	Psoralen
Dutchman's breeches	*Thamnosma texana*	Psoralen
Spring parsley	*Cymopterus watsoni*	Psoralen

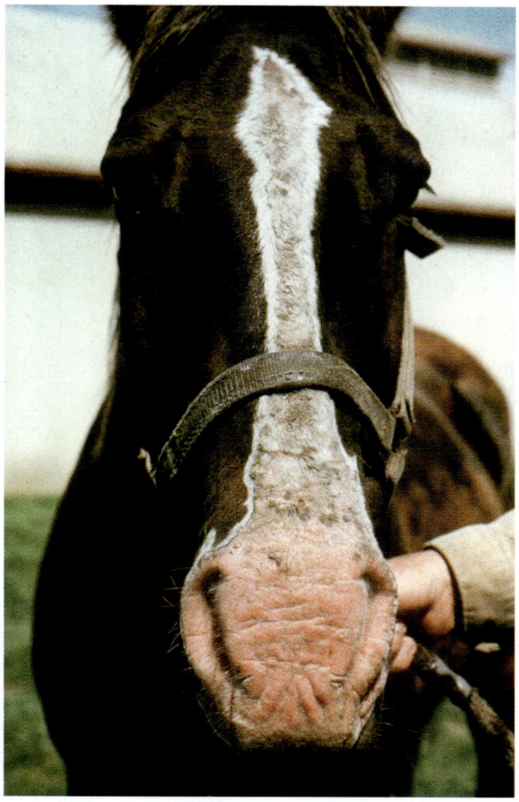

Figure 56.4 Photosensitivity due to hepatic damage from ingestion of pyrrolizidine alkaloid. (Reprinted with permission from Stephen White.)

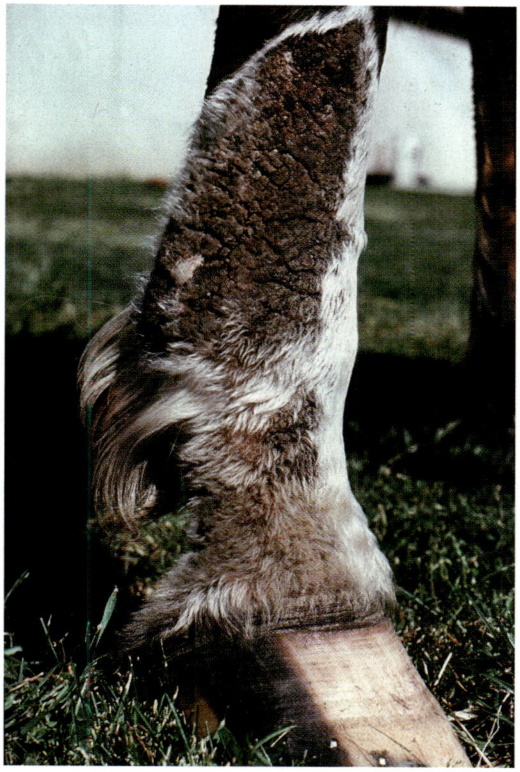

Figure 56.5 Photosensitivity due to hepatic damage from ingestion of pyrrolizidine alkaloid. (Reprinted with permission from Stephen White.)

Table 56.2 Examples of hepatogenous photosensitization agents

Common name	Scientific name	Mechanism
Common groundsel	*Senecio vulgaris*	Pyrrolizidine alkaloid
Ragwort	*Senecio jacobaea*	Pyrrolizidine alkaloid
Rattleweed	*Crotalaria* spp.	Pyrrolizidine alkaloid
Salvation Jane	*Echium lycopsis*	Pyrrolizidine alkaloid
Tarweed	*Amsinckia intermedia*	Pyrrolizidine alkaloid
Alsike clover	*Trifolium hybridum*	Unknown
Kleingrass	*Panicum coloratum*	Sapogenin

toxic pyrroles in the digestive tract. The pyrroles inhibit mitosis and replication of hepatocytes and at high doses can cause hepatocellular necrosis [26]. The effects of PAs are cumulative, with clinical signs of liver disease and photosensitization often occurring several months after the toxic agent was ingested and thus making identification of the offending toxic plant difficult [25](Table 56.2).

Exogenously induced photosensitivity can be further subdivided into two categories: phototoxicity and photoallergy. Phototoxicity is caused by direct tissue injury from the agent and radiation. This occurs in all individuals exposed to the right dose of the agent and the activating wavelengths of UVA light. It is the most common type of photosensitization in animals. Conversely, photoallergy occurs only in sensitized individuals and is a type IV delayed hypersensitivity. It only requires a small concentration of the photoallergen [19].

Phototoxicity

Phototoxicity, a non-immunological reaction, occurs through several mechanisms and is a dose-related response to light exposure. One pathway results in tissue damage after absorption of radiation energy by the photosensitizer, causing excitation of the molecule resulting, ultimately, in free radical formation. These free radicals cause cytotoxic injury through the oxidation of lipids, nucleic acids, and proteins [19,24]. Tissue injury can also result after radiation exposure generates stable photoproducts that covalently bind to pyrimidine bases of DNA. Through either mechanism, inflammatory mediators such as eicosanoids, proteases, complement, and polymorphonuclear leukocytes also participate in phototoxic tissue injury, damaging the epidermis and blood vessels [19,22].

All animals exposed to phototoxic agents under the same conditions will be affected. In humans, phototoxicity is often associated with a burning sensation. Affected horses may also experience this same sensation because they are often irritable and uncomfortable [19,21,22]. Phototoxicity in equines occurs in white, light-coloured, or damaged skin [21]. The degree and onset of the reaction is related to the duration of UV light exposure, the intensity of the sunlight and the individual animal.

Photoallergy

Photoallergy requires the presence of both the photoallergen and the activating wavelength of radiation, usually in the UVA range. The photoallergen must penetrate skin and be activated by the immune system of a previously sensitized individual [19–21]. After the UV energy is absorbed, the photoallergen is converted to an excited state molecule and may conjugate with a carrier protein to form a complete antigen [19–21]. Alternatively, the photoallergen may form a stable photoproduct that conjugates with a carrier protein to form a complete antigen. From this point, the mechanism of photoallergy is identical to that of contact allergy, a type IV delayed hypersensitivity (Figure 56.1), in which the complete antigen is taken up by Langerhans cells and presented to T lymphocytes in the regional lymph nodes. The activated T lymphocytes then circulate to the UV exposed site to initiate an inflammatory response [19]. This response can be induced by small amounts of the photoallergen [22]. Therapeutic agents, antibacterial agents, and fragrances are the most commonly documented topical products causing photoallergy in humans. This reaction is also most commonly associated with pruritus.

Pastern leukocytoclastic vasculitis

There is a specific entity in the horse termed pastern leukocytoclastic vasculitis (PLV) that in many cases appears to be a form of photoaggravated vasculitis [14,22]. Its clinical signs suggest a photoactivated aetiology because lesions are usually restricted to non-pigmented distal extremities in the majority of cases and occur most commonly in the summer months in areas with abundant sunlight. It occurs in regionally endemic areas [22]. In a few horses, direct immunofluorescence studies have shown deposition of IgG and/or C3 in the affected vessel walls. The significance of this finding is not entirely understood. The disease may have a more complicated aetiology because it may occur in only one of several non-pigmented limbs or affect only one horse in a herd while others with non-pigmented extremities are unaffected (Figures 56.6 and 56.7). PLV has also been seen in two related horses on the same farm whereas other horses with non-pigmented limbs were not affected [14]. This may suggest a genetic or familial predisposition. In addition, it has been noted that simple avoidance of sunlight is not always sufficient to control the disease [14,22–24].

Clinical lesions and diagnosis

Cutaneous lesions of photosensitivity in horses are most often restricted to the light-haired areas but can extend into darker skinned areas, especially if the lesions are severe. Erythema and oedema often progress to vesicles and bullae. These lesions can also be seen as ulceration,

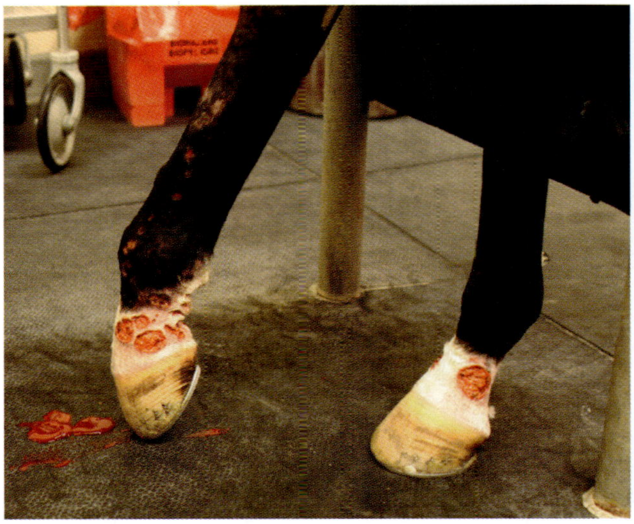

Figure 56.6 Pastern leukocytoclastic vasculitis. Erythema and punctuate ulcers in linear arrangement on light-skinned, white haired distal extremities. (Reprinted with permission from Stephen White.)

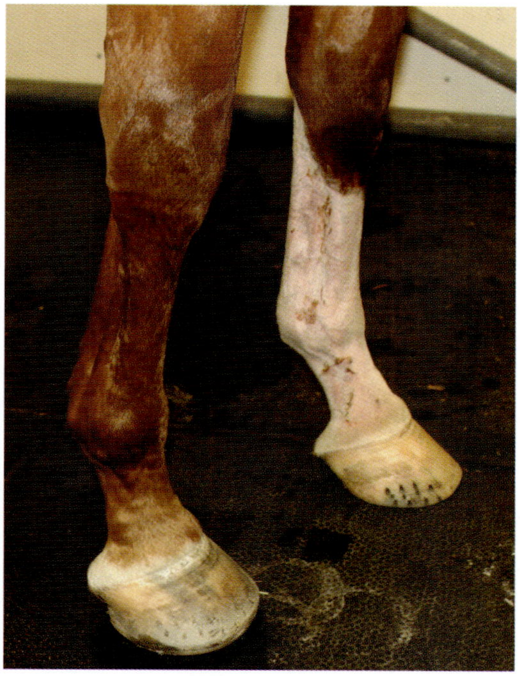

Figure 56.7 Pastern leukocytoclastic vasculitis. Erythema and erosions on light-skinned, white-haired distal extremities. (Reprinted with permission from Stephen White.)

crusting, scaling, and hairloss, with secondary infections commonly occurring [21]. The most severe and chronic lesions may result in necrosis and sloughing. Lesions affect the muzzle, face, pinnae, back, perineum, and distal limbs and can be associated with pruritus or pain. The coronets can also be affected. Some affected animals will attempt to avoid sun exposure [21].

Diagnosis of photohypersensitivity in the horse requires detailed history, thorough physical examination, and exploration of the premises. Blood work and histopathology aid in the diagnosis and confirm or exclude underlying liver disease. Lesion distribution or confinement to a specific body part that is lightly haired or non-pigmented points toward a photodynamic process. Lesions confined to the limbs or muzzle may be due to photocontact reactions or photoactivated vasculopathies. If multiple animals are affected, a photosensitizing agent may be implicated. Histopathology often reveals the chronicity of the disease and not the primary cause. Acute lesions commonly reveal epidermal or dermal oedema with intramural and perivascular amorphous eosinophilic material in the superficial dermis [21].

Treatment

Treatment relies on identifying the underlying cause and eliminating the photosensitization agent if possible. Liver disease should be treated and controlled, and direct sunlight avoided if possible. Glucocorticoids (prednisolone at 2 mg/kg once daily) and non-steroid anti-inflammatory agents such as phenylbutazone and pentoxifylline (10–15 mg/kg twice daily) are beneficial [16,21]. Topical therapies should be minimized as contact dermatitis can occur. Secondary bacterial infections should be treated systemically [22].

References

1. Walder EJ, Conroy JD. Review article: contact dermatitis in dogs and cats: pathogenesis, histopathology, experimental induction and case reports. *Veterinary Dermatology* 1994; **5**: 149–162.
2. Thomsen MK, Kristensen F. Contact dermatitis in the dog: a review and clinical study. *Nordic Veterinary Medicine* 1986; **38**: 129–147.
3. Olivry T, Prélaud P, Hériрret D, *et al.* Contact dermatitis in the dog: principles and diagnosis. *Veterinary Clinics of North America: Small Animal Practice* 1990; **20**: 1433–1456.
4. Saint-Mezard P, Rosieres A, Krasteva M, *et al.* Allergic contact dermatitis. *European Journal of Dermatology* 2004; **14**: 284–295.
5. Patterson S. Investigation of skin disease and urticaria in the horse. *In Practice* 2000; **22**: 446–455.
6. Rufenacht S, Marti E, Von Tscharner C, *et al.* Immunoglobulin E-bearing cells and mast cells in skin biopsies of horses with urticaria. *Veterinary Dermatology* 2005; **16**: 94–101.
7. Ross GD, Cranstoun KE. Herbicide-treated hay as a possible cause of dermatitis in horses. *Veterinary Record* 2009; **164**: 188.
8. University of Illinois Veterinary Medical Library. *Buttercups (Ranunculus spp.)*. Available at: http://www.library.illinois.edu/vex/toxic/butcup/butcup.htm (accessed June 2012).
9. Ministry of Agriculture, Food and Rural Affairs. *Poisoning of Horses by Plants*. Available at: http://omafra.gov.on.ca/english/livestock/horses/facts/poison.htm#Buttercups (accessed June 2012).
10. Salsbury DL. Pine tar dermatitis in a horse. *Veterinary Medicine Small Animal Clinician* 1970; **95**: 60–61.
11. Scott DW, Miller WH Jr. Skin immune system and allergic skin diseases: contact hypersensitivity. In: *Equine Dermatology*,1st edn. St. Louis: Saunders,2001: 449–452.
12. Fadok VA. Dermatology: overview of equine pruritus. *Veterinary Clinics of North America: Equine Practice* 1995; **1**: 1–10.
13. Reeves WK, Miller MM. Aqueous 2% geraniol as a mosquito repellent failed against Aedes aegyption ponies. *Journal of the American Mosquito Control Association* 2010; **26**: 340–341.
14. White SD, Affolter VK, Dewey J, *et al.* Cutaneous vasculitis in equines: a retrospective study of 72 cases. *Veterinary Dermatology* 2009; **20**: 600–606.
15. Saricaoğlu H, Tunali Ş, Bülbül E, *et al.* Prevention of nickel-induced allergic contact reactions with pentoxifylline. *Contact Dermatitis* 1998; **39**: 244–247.
16. Bruynzeel I, Stoff TJ, Willemze R. Pentoxifylline and skin inflammation. *Clinical and Experimental Dermatology* 1998; **23**: 168–172.
17. Woo DK, James WD. Topical tacrolimus: a review of its uses in dermatology. *Dermatitis* 2005; **16**: 6–21.
18. Abbas M, Hull PR. Hyposensitization and desensitization in allergic contact dermatitis. *Dermatitis* 2012; **23**: 148–152.
19. Lim HW. Abnormal responses to ultraviolet radiation: photosensitivity induced by exogenous agents. In: Wolff K, Goldsmith L, Katz S, *et al.*, eds. *Fitzpatrick's Dermatology in General Medicine*, 7th edn. New York: McGraw Hill Medical, 2003: 828–831.

20. Boord MJ. Photosensitivity. In: Robinson NE, ed. *Current Therapy in Equine Medicine*, 3rd edn. Philadelphia: WB Saunders, 2003: 174–176.
21. Scott DW, Miller WH. Environmental skin diseases. In: *Equine Dermatology*, 1st edn. St. Louis: Saunders, 2003: 619–621.
22. Stannard AA. Pastern leukocytoclastic vasculitis. *Veterinary Dermatology* 2000; **11**: 217–223.
23. Iven P. Hogweed suspected of causing primary photosensitisation in a horse. *Veterinary Record* 2011; **169**: 81–82.
24. Santoro FA, Lim HW. Update on photodermatoses. *Seminars in Cutaneous Medicine and Surgery* 2011; **30**: 229–238
25. Knight AP, Walter RG. Plants affecting the skin and liver. In: Knight AP, Walter RG, eds. *A Guide in Plant Poisoning of Animals in North America*. Ithaca, NY: International Veterinary Information Service, 2003: 1–32.
26. Swick RA. Hepatic metabolism and bioactivation of mycotoxins and plant toxins. *Journal of Animal Science* 1984; **58**: 1017–1028.

Part 4

Allergy in Other Domestic Species

(Editor: Aiden Foster)

57

Immunopathogenesis of allergic skin disease in livestock

Adri van den Broek

Royal (Dick) School of Veterinary Studies, University of Edinburgh, Easter Bush Veterinary Centre, Roslin, Midlothian, UK

Conflict of interest: none declared.

Introduction

This chapter should be read in conjunction with the Introduction: The immunological basis of allergic diseases for an overview of the immunopathogenesis of allergic diseases. In contrast to companion animal species, particularly the dog, the important allergens in livestock species are usually related to ectoparasites, consequently the following discussion focuses on ectoparasites and particularly psoroptic mange in sheep as a type example.

The outer layers of the skin provide a rich, readily accessible and continuously renewed source of nutrition—a surface lipid emulsion, tissue fluid, blood vessels, and lymphatics. Ectoparasites exploit this resource and display diverse adaptations of their mouthparts, digestive systems, and life cycles that enable them do this. As they feed, mouthparts adapted for sucking, rasping, biting, and penetrating the epidermis will traumatize cells. In addition, ectoparasites deposit secretory and excretory products on or in the epidermis or inject them intradermally. These contain a great variety of irritant, cytotoxic, and pharmacologically active substances and a diverse array of antigens and allergens and immunomodulatory compounds. It appears that it is the cytotoxic and immunopharmacological properties of these products and, to a lesser extent, the site at which they are deposited, that determines the nature of the cutaneous inflammatory response to different ectoparasites [1,2].

Histopathology at tick attachment sites has elegantly demonstrated that this diverse range of biologically active substances elicits a dynamic, multifaceted immune response, which evolves in the course of primary infestations and in successive challenge infestations [3–6]. Temporal studies have demonstrated that, with minor variations, ectoparasite-derived products provoke a stereotypic immune response. This comprises an immediate, innate inflammatory response and later, layered over this, an acquired adaptive immune response characterized by the development of isotype-specific antibody responses and, finally, a sequence of hypersensitivity responses comprising: immediate, late-phase, and delayed hypersensitivity reactions [7,8]. These acquired responses may contribute to the development of a protective immunity [8–12].

The innate response

The observation, in tick-naïve cattle, sheep, and rabbits, of significant cellular infiltration within 1 to 24 hours of infestation [3,5,6,13] and of a profound polymorphonuclear infiltrate in *Psoroptes ovis*-naïve sheep within 3 to 24 hours after infestation [14,15] is consistent with the activation of an immediate innate response. The nature

Veterinary Allergy, First Edition. Edited by Chiara Noli, Aiden Foster, and Wayne Rosenkrantz.

of the response, although non-specific, appears to be particular to the ectoparasite and its host. In cattle, neutrophils dominated the infiltrate provoked by *Ixodes holocyclus* [3] while eosinophils were the principal cells detected in infestations with *Boophilus microplus* [13]. In sheep, *P. ovis* provokes an intense eosinophil infiltrate [14], while in cattle the eosinophil response to *P. ovis* infestation is less consistent [9,16]. This preferential recruitment of cells demonstrates the plasticity of the innate response and may be attributable to a combination of differences in chemoattractants produced by ectoparasites and in the expression cytokines and chemokines induced in host epidermal and dermal cells by their products. This supposition is supported by *in vitro* studies that have demonstrated that cellular damage caused by mouthparts and the biological activity of ectoparasite-derived products will provoke immediate, antigen-independent release of cytokines from cells resident in the epidermis and dermis such as keratinocytes [17] and mast cells [18].

In vitro studies of the excretory products of *Dermatophagoides pteronyssinus* (the house dust mite (HDM) that, like *Psoroptes ovis* and *Sarcoptes scabiei*, is a member of the Order Astigmata) have shown that two products, Der p 3 and Der p 9, can stimulate the expression of eotaxin, a potent eosinophil chemoattractant, by alveolar epithelial cells [19], while HDM extract can induce the production of IL-8 and TNFα, two potent neutrophil chemoattractants, by cultured epithelial cells [20]. In addition, the eosinophil and neutrophil chemoattractant properties of another HDM product, Der p 1, have been demonstrated [21]. *Psoroptes ovis*-derived homologues of these HDM products (Pso o 1, 3, and 9) have been identified [22,23], and by analogy it is probable that they exert effects similar to those of their HDM homologues. Similarly, *in vitro* studies have demonstrated that *P. ovis* mite extract possesses eosinophil chemoattractant properties [24] and stimulates the expression of IL-8 by ovine keratinocytes [25]. It is probable that products of other ectoparasite also possess chemoattractant properties and induce cytokine and chemokine expression. This ectoparasite activity drives the release of a cascade of cytokines and chemokines [23,26], establishing the early microenvironment that regulates the preferential recruitment of effector cells through up-regulation of adhesion molecules on postcapillary venules.

In instances where surface-living and burrowing ectoparasites deposit their secretory and excretory products on or in the epidermis, the integrity of the stratum corneum is pivotal in minimizing penetration of these exogenous molecules. *In vitro* studies have demonstrated that a recombinant *Sarcoptes scabiei* serine protease, rSar s 3, a homologue of Pso o 3, cleaves recombinant human filaggrin [27]. This suggests that other proteolytic enzymes in ectoparasite products may promote transepidermal penetration of molecules through disruption of the epidermal barrier by cleavage of filaggrin and other proteins integral to the cornified envelop and by cleavage of tight junctions [28]. Studies also suggest that the inflammatory response may reduce production of proteins integral to the function of the cornified envelop [15]. These changes will facilitate the passage of bioactive ectoparasite products augmenting the innate response and will also increase the exposure of antigen-presenting cells to antigens and allergens [29,30], enhancing the development of the adaptive response.

In addition to their influence on cell recruitment, the direct activity of the diverse array of enzymes and biologically active compounds present in ectoparasite products [31] will, together with the cascade of mediators released by mast cells, basophils, neutrophils, and particularly eosinophils [32], contribute to the significant epidermal and dermal pathology observed in the early stages of ectoparasite infestation [14].

The adaptive response

Polarization of the adaptive immune response towards a Th1 or Th2 response is determined by information programmed into APCs (Langerhans and dermal dendritic cells) by antigens and allergens and the local cytokine microenvironment generated by the innate response [33,34]. In the milieu of cytokines released by keratinocytes, recruited mast cells, basophils, and eosinophils, IL-4 and IL-13 play a critical role in promoting a Th2 response in naïve antigen-specific cells in lymphoid tissue and also in Th memory and effector cells in lesional tissue [35,36]. They also promote B cell IgE isotype switching [37]. Degranulation of mast cells and basophils releases several cytokines, including IL-4 and IL-13 [35,38], while eosinophils express IL-4 [39]. *In vitro* studies have demonstrated that parasite allergens with proteolytic activity, such as Der p 1, trigger the release of IL-4 from mast cells and basophils and it is possible that the same mechanism may also trigger the release of IL-13 [18], while increased cutaneous cytokine gene expression of IL-4 and IL-13 has been documented in lambs infested with *Bovicola ovis* following intradermal challenge with crude louse antigen [40]. Analysis of ovine transcriptome (sets of RNA molecules transcribed from the genetic code) microarray data has demonstrated significant differential expression of RNA, with a bias towards a Th2 response, which included a significant increase in IL-4, in skin biopsies collected in the first 24 hours after infestation of *P. ovis*-naïve sheep [23].

Recruitment and degranulation of eosinophils, mast cells, and basophils are typically prominent in host's innate response to ectoparasites and has been well documented within hours of *P. ovis* infestation of sheep [14]. Release of IL-4 and IL-13 by these cells may contribute significantly to the polarization of the developing adaptive immune response towards an IgE-meditated Type 2 (allergic) response. Regulatory T cells are thought to play a critical role in modulating hypersensitivity responses, principally by suppressing T effector cells [41–43]. Although increased numbers of Foxp3$^+$ T cells, a subset of T regulatory cells, have been detected in the dermis of sheep following infestation with *P. ovis* [44], and possibly of humans in association with *Sarcoptes scabiei* infestation [45], their role in the development of hypersensitivity responses in ectoparasitic infestations remains to be clarified.

Acquired antigen-specific IgE antibody and hypersensitivity responses

Antigen-specific IgE antibody responses

Although antigen-specific IgE antibody responses have been reported in *P. ovis* infestations of sheep [12], they appear to have been recorded infrequently in other ectoparasite infestations. However, positive wheal reactions to intradermal tests (IDTs) and Prausnitz–Küstner (PK) tests have provided putative evidence of IgE-mediated responses to several ectoparasites [7,8,46–48]. In addition, positive passive cutaneous anaphylaxis and basophil degranulation responses have been obtained with sera from sheep infested with *Bovicola ovis* [49–51].

Hypersensitivity responses

Clinical observation of wheal responses to ectoparasite bites or intradermal injection of ectoparasite antigens has demonstrated that host responses to arthropod ectoparasites commonly include immediate and delayed hypersensitivity responses [7,8,46,47]. Late-phase and cutaneous basophil hypersensitivity responses are detected less frequently. A number of studies have revealed a distinct temporal pattern in the development of these responses in the course of exposure to ectoparasites [52–54]. Clinical responses to bites of haematophagous arthropods typically progress through five distinct phases [52,53,55,56]. These comprise: a period of induction when no response occurs; only delayed hypersensitivity responses; immediate and delayed reactions; only immediate responses; and finally a period of desensitization, when no hypersensitivity responses are elicited.

A similar sequence of hypersensitivity reactions has been demonstrated in pigs infested with the *S. scabiei* var *suis* [54,57]. In contrast to this classical pattern, the sequence in sheep infested with *P. ovis* was induction, immediate and late-phase responses, and then immediate, late-phase, and delayed responses [58]. The temporal development of responses to other ectoparasitic mites does not appear to have been reported. Lesional histopathology has provided supportive evidence of hypersensitivity reactions [46,47,59] and demonstrated that some arthropods (black flies [47], *Sarcoptes scabiei* var *suis* infestation of pigs [57], and *P. ovis* infestation of sheep [60]) provoked an eosinophil-rich delayed hypersensitivity response. These may be examples of the Th2 cytokine-mediated delayed-type hypersensitivity response [61,62], which is characterized by the preferential recruitment of eosinophils rather than mononuclear cells. Temporal studies also demonstrate that the hypersensitivity responses are layered over each other and the continuing innate response.

The innate response in many ectoparasite infestations is characterized by the preferential recruitment of eosinophils, mast cells, basophils, and neutrophils accompanied by dermal oedema. These are all features of an immediate hypersensitivity response [39,63,64] and have, for example, been reported in sheep infested with *P. ovis* [14] and pigs infested with *S. scabiei* [65]. However, temporal studies indicate that immediate hypersensitivity responses are not detected until later in the course of infestation [57,58]. Although currently available techniques may lack the sensitivity required to detect the true onset of isotype-specific IgE antibody responses, evidence suggests that the contribution of hypersensitivity reactions to lesional pathology early in primary infestations is of questionable significance.

References

1. Burns DA Diseases caused by arthropods and other noxious animals. In: Champion RH, Burton JL, Burns DA, *et al.*, eds. *Textbook of Dermatology*, Vol. 2, 6th edn. Oxford: Blackwell Science, 1998: 1423–1482.
2. Wikel SK. Immunology of the tick-host interface. In: Wikel SK, ed. *The Immunology of Host-Ectoparasite Arthropod Relationships.* Wallingford, Oxon: CAB International, 1996: 204–231.
3. Allen JR, Doube BM, Kemp DH. Histology of bovine skin reactions to *Ixodes Holocyclus* Neumann. *Canadian Journal of Comparative Medicine* 1977; **41**: 26–35.
4. Brown SJ, Barker RW, Askenase PW. Bovine resistance to *Amblyomma-Americanum* Ticks—an acquired immune-response characterized by cutaneous basophil infiltrates. *Veterinary Parasitology* 1984; **16**: 147–165.
5. Walker AR, Fletcher JD. Histological study of the attachment sites of adult *Rhipicephalus-appendiculatus* on rabbits and cattle. *International Journal for Parasitology* 1986; **16**: 399–413.
6. Abdul-Amir IM, Gray JS. Resistance of sheep to laboratory infestations of the tick, *Ixodes ricinus. Research in Veterinary Science* 1987; **43**: 266–267.
7. Wikel SK. Immune-responses to arthropods and their products. *Annual Review of Entomology* 1982; **27**: 21–48.

8. Allen JR. Host resistance to ectoparasites. *Revue Scientifique et Technique* 1994; **13**: 1287–1303.
9. Stromberg PC, Fisher WF. Dermatopathology and immunity in experimental *Psoroptes ovis* (Acari: Psoroptidae) infestation of naive and previously exposed Hereford cattle. *American Journal of Veterinary Research* 1986; **47**: 1551–1560.
10. James PJ. Do sheep regulate the size of their mallophagan louse populations? *International Journal for Parasitology* 1999; **29**: 869–875.
11. Bates P. Differences between primary and secondary infestations with the sheep scab mite, *Psoroptes ovis*. *Veterinary Record* 2000; **146**: 528–529.
12. van den Broek AH, Huntley JF, Machell J, *et al.* Cutaneous and systemic responses during primary and challenge infestations of sheep with the sheep scab mite, *Psoroptes ovis*. *Parasite Immunology* 2000; **22**: 407–414.
13. Tatchell RJ, Moorhouse DE. Feeding processes of cattle tick *Boophilus Microplus* (Canestrini). 2. Sequence of host-tissue changes. *Parasitology* 1968; **58**: 441–459.
14. van den Broek AHM, Else RW, Huntley JF, *et al.* Early innate and longer-term adaptive cutaneous immunoinflammatory responses during primary infestation with the sheep scab mite, *Psoroptes ovis*. *Journal of Comparative Pathology* 2004; **131**: 318–329.
15. Stoeckli MR, McNeilly TN, Frew D, *et al.* The effect of *Psoroptes ovis* infestation on ovine epidermal barrier function. *Veterinary Research* 2013; **44**: 11.
16. Stromberg PC, Guillot FS. Pathogenesis of psoroptic scabies in Hereford heifer calves. *American Journal of Veterinary Research* 1989; **50**: 594–601.
17. Arlian LG, The immunology of scabies. In: Wikel SK, ed. *The Immunology of Host-Ectoparasite Arthropod Relationships*. Wallingford, Oxon: CAB International, 1996: 232–258.
18. Machado DC, Horton D, Harrop R, *et al.* Potential allergens stimulate the release of mediators of the allergic response from cells of mast cell lineage in the absence of sensitization with antigen-specific IgE. *European Journal of Immunology* 1996; **26**: 2972–2980.
19. Lau LCK, Leir SH, Lackie P, *et al.* House dust mite allergen cleaves epithelial adhesion molecules and activates epithelial cells by an IgE independent pathway. *American Journal of Respiratory and Critical Care Medicine* 1999; **159**: A179.
20. Sun G, Stacey MA, Schmidt M, *et al.* Interaction of mite allergens Der P3 and Der P9 with protease-activated receptor-2 expressed by lung epithelial cells. *Journal of Immunology* 2001; **167**: 1014–1021.
21. Fahy O, Hammad H, Senechal S, *et al.* Synergistic effect of diesel organic extracts and allergen Der p 1 on the release of chemokines by peripheral blood mononuclear cells from allergic subjects: involvement of the map kinase pathway. *American Journal of Respiratory Cellular and Molecular Biology* 2000; **23**: 247–254.
22. Temeyer KB, Soileau LC, Pruett JH. Cloning and sequence analysis of a cDNA encoding Pso o II, a mite group II allergen of the sheep scab mite (Acari: Psoroptidae). *Journal of Medical Entomology* 2002; **39**: 384–391.
23. Burgess ST, Frew D, Nunn F, *et al.* Transcriptomic analysis of the temporal host response to skin infestation with the ectoparasitic mite Psoroptes ovis. *BioMed Central Genomics* 2010; **11**: 624.
24. Wildblood LA, Jones G. Stimulation of the in vitro migration of ovine eosinophils by factors derived from the sheep scab mite, *Psoroptes ovis*. *Veterinary Research Communications* 2007; **31**: 197–206.
25. Watkins CA, Mackellar A, Frew D, *et al.* Gene expression profiling of ovine keratinocytes stimulated with *Psoroptes ovis* mite antigen—a preliminary study. *Parasite Immunology* 2009; **31**: 304–11.
26. Burgess ST, McNeilly TN, Watkins CA, *et al.* Host transcription factors in the immediate pro-inflammatory response to the parasitic mite *Psoroptes ovis*. *Plos One* 2011; **6**: e24402.
27. Beckham SA, Boyd SE, Reynolds S, *et al.* Characterization of a serine protease homologous to house dust mite group 3 allergens from the scabies mite *Sarcoptes scabiei*. *Journal of Biological Chemistry* 2009; **284**: 34413–34422.
28. Wan H, Winton HL, Soeller C, *et al.* The transmembrane protein occludin of epithelial tight junctions is a functional target for serine peptidases from faecal pellets of *Dermatophagoides pteronyssinus*. *Clinical and Experimental Allergy* 2001; **31**: 279–294.
29. Wan H, Winton HL, Soeller C, *et al.* Der p 1 facilitates transepithelial allergen delivery by disruption of tight junctions. *Journal of Clinical Investigation* 1999; **104**: 123–133.
30. Strid J, Strobel S. Skin barrier dysfunction and systemic sensitization to allergens through the skin. *Current Drug Targets Inflammation and Allergy* 2005; **4**: 531–541.
31. Nisbet AJ, Billingsley PF. Hydrolytic enzymes of *Psoroptes cuniculi* (Delafond). *Insect Biochemistry and Molecular Biology* 1999; **29**: 25–32.
32. Gleich GJ, Adolphson CR. The eosinophilic leukocyte: structure and function. *Advances in Immunology* 1986; **39**: 177–253.
33. Fearon DT, Locksley RM. The instructive role of innate immunity in the acquired immune response. *Science* 1996; **272**: 50–53.
34. Medzhitov R, Janeway CA, Jr. Innate immunity: impact on the adaptive immune response. *Current Opinions in Immunology* 1997; **9**: 4–9.
35. Schwartz LB. Mast cells: function and contents. *Current Opinions in Immunology* 1994; **6**: 91–97.
36. Kapsenberg ML, Hilkens CM, Wierenga EA, *et al.* The role of antigen-presenting cells in the regulation of allergen-specific T cell responses. *Current Opinions in Immunology* 1998; **10**: 607–613.
37. Bacharier LB, Geha RS. Regulation of IgE synthesis: the molecular basis and implications for clinical modulation. *Allergy and Asthma Proceedings* 1999; **20**: 1–8.
38. Vercelli DG. Control of immunoglobulin E synthesis. In: Middleton E, Reed CE, Ellis EF, *et al.*, eds. *Allergy: Principles and Practice*, Vol. 1, 4th edn. Philadelphia: Mosby, 1993: 72–82.
39. Weller PF. Human eosinophils. *Journal of Allergy and Clinical Immunology* 1997; **100**: 283–287.
40. Shu D, Pfeffer A, Pernthaner A. Cutaneous cytokine gene expression and cellular responses in lambs infested with the louse, *Bovicola ovis*, and following intradermal injection of crude louse antigen. *Veterinary Immunology and Immunopathology* 2009; **129**: 82–92.
41. Robinson DS, Larche M, Durham SR. Tregs and allergic disease. *Journal of Clinical Investigation* 2004; **114**: 1389–1397.
42. Hawrylowicz CM, O'Garra A. Potential role of interleukin-10-secreting regulatory T cells in allergy and asthma. *Nature Reviews Immunology* 2005; **5**: 271–283.
43. Akdis M. Immune tolerance in allergy. *Current Opinions in Immunology* 2009; **21**: 700–707.
44. McNeilly TN, McIntyre J, Frew D, *et al.* Infestation of sheep with *Psoroptes ovis*, the sheep scab mite, results in recruitment of Foxp3(+) T cells into the dermis. *Parasite Immunology* 2010; **32**: 361–369.
45. Arlian LG, Morgan MS, Paul CC. Evidence that scabies mites (Acari: Sarcoptidae) influence production of interleukin-10 and the function of T-regulatory cells (Tr1) in humans. *Journal of Medical Entomology* 2006; **43**: 283–287.

46. Allen JR. Immunology, immunopathology, and immunoprophylaxis of tick and mite infestations. In: Soulsby EJL, ed. *Immune Responses in Parasite Infections: Immunology, Immunopathology, and Immunoprophylaxsis.* Florida: CRC Press, 1987: 141–174.
47. Nelson WA. Other blood-sucking and myiasis-producing arthropods. In: Soulsby EJL, ed. *Immune Responses in Parasite Infections: Immunology, Immunopathology and Immunoprophylaxis.* Florida: CRC Press, 1987: 175–209.
48. James PJ, Moon RD. Pruritis and dermal response to insect antigens in sheep infested with *Bovicola ovis. International Journal for Parasitology* 1998; **28**: 419–427.
49. Pfeffer A, Bany JS, Phegan MD, *et al.* Hypersensitivity skin testing of lambs infested with the biting louse (*Bovicola ovis*). *New Zealand Veterinary Journal* 1994; **42**: 76.
50. Pfeffer A, Phegan MD, Bany J. Detection of homocytotropic antibody in lambs infested with the louse, *Bovicola ovis*, using a basophil histamine-release assay. *Veterinary Immunology and Immunopathology* 1997; **57**: 315–325.
51. Pfeffer A, Wilson JA, Pernthaner A. Changes in morphology and key cytokine gene expression after intradermal injection of louse (*Bovicola ovis*) antigen in sheep with naturally occurring atopic dermatitis. *Journal of Comparative Pathology* 2007; **136**: 36–48.
52. Mellanby K. Man's reaction to mosquito bites. *Nature* 1946; **158**: 554.
53. Benjamini E, Feingold BF, Kartman L. Skin reactivity in guinea pigs sensitized to flea bites: the sequence of reactions. *Proceedings of the Society for Experimental Biology and Medicine* 1961; **108**: 700–702.
54. Davis DP, Moon RD. Density of itch mite, *Sarcoptes-scabiei* (Acari, Sarcoptidae) and temporal development of cutaneous hypersensitivity in swine mange. *Veterinary Parasitology* 1990; **36**: 285–293.
55. Larrivee DH, Benjamini E, Feingold BF, *et al.* Histologic studies of guinea pig skin: different stages of allergic reactivity to flea bites. *Experimental Parasitology* 1964; **15**: 491–502.
56. Feingold BF, Benjamin E, Michaeli D. Allergic responses to insect bites. *Annual Review of Entomology* 1968; **13**: 252–254.
57. Sheahan BJ. Pathology of *Sarcoptes scabiei* infection in pigs. 2. histological, histochemical and ultrastructural changes at skin-test sites. *Journal of Comparative Pathology* 1975; **85**: 97–110.
58. van den Broek AHM, Huntley JF, Halliwell REW, *et al.* Temporal development of ovine cutaneous hypersensitivity responses to *Psoroptes ovis* (sheep scab mite). In: Hillier A, Foster AP, Kwochka KW, eds. *Advances in Veterinary Dermatology*, Vol. 5. Oxford: Blackwell Science Publications, 2004: 97–103.
59. Goldman L, Rockwell E, Richfield DF. Histopathological studies on cutaneous reactions to the bites of various arthropods. 3. *American Journal of Tropical Medicine and Hygiene* 1952; **1**: 514–525.
60. van den Broek AHM, Huntley JF, Halliwell REW, *et al.* Cutaneous hypersensitivity reactions to *Psoroptes ovis* and Der p 1 in sheep previously infested with *P. ovis*—the sheep scab mite. *Veterinary Immunology and Immunopathology* 2003; **91**: 105–117.
61. Askenase PW. Effector and regulatory molecules and mechanisms in delayed-type hypersensitivity. In: Middleton E, Reed CE, Ellis EF, *et al.*, eds. *Allergy, Principles and Practice.* Vol. 1, 4th edn. Philadelphia: Mosby, 1996: 323–341.
62. Meeusen ENT. Immunology of helminth infections, with special reference to immunopathology. *Veterinary Parasitology* 1999; **84**: 259–273.
63. Barnes PJ. Pathophysiology of allergic inflammation. In: Middleton E, Reed CE, Ellis EF, *et al.*, eds. *Allergy, Principles and Practice*, 4th edn. Philadelphia: Mosby, 1996: 356–465.
64. Parrish WE, Breathnach SM. Clinical immunology and allergy. In: Champion RH, Burton JL, Burns DA, *et al.*, eds. *Textbook of Dermatology*, Vol. 1, 6th edn. Oxford: Blackwell Science, 1998: 277–336.
65. Sheahan BJ. Pathology of *Sarcoptes-scabiei* infection in pigs. 1. naturally occurring and experimentally induced lesions. *Journal of Comparative Pathology* 1975; **85**: 87–95.

58

Psoroptes ovis

Adri van den Broek[1] and Stewart T.G. Burgess[2]

[1] Royal (Dick) School of Veterinary Studies, University of Edinburgh, Easter Bush Veterinary Centre, Roslin, Midlothian, UK
[2] Moredun Research Institute, Pentlands Science Park, Edinburgh, Midlothian, UK

Conflict of interest: none declared.

Incidence and importance

Sheep scab is caused by *Psoroptes ovis*, an obligate, surface-living, astigmatid mite. Typically, it is an intensely pruritic, exudative dermatitis that can spread rapidly to affect extensive areas of the skin, resulting in severe damage to the fleece and hide, loss of condition, epileptiform seizures, and occasionally death. It is highly contagious and endemic in many flocks in the UK [1] and is prevalent in Northern Europe [2,3], Pakistan [4], and India [5], and is therefore of considerable economic and welfare importance. In the UK, it is arguably the most important ectoparasitic disease of sheep. At present, the available control measures are poor and made worse by the development of mite resistance to acaricides [6,7], the possible role of endectocides in the development of gastrointestinal/gut nematode resistance to macrocylic lactones [8,9], and concerns for human health and the environment raised by the use of organophosphates and synthetic pyrethroids [10–14].

Clinical signs

Typically, infestation is followed by a subclinical phase, which persists for a variable time, and then a rapid growth phase [15–17]. In this phase, the potentially exponential expansion of the mite population [18] and lesions [17] is determined by the interplay of host susceptibility, mite virulence, husbandry, and environmental conditions [16,19–21].

Lesions are generally first detected on the dorsum [15,22] and then may extend rapidly over the flanks to the limbs and head, while sparing areas where the hair growth is sparse. The mites provoke an intense inflammatory response characterized by papular erythema and serous exudation. Subsequently, vesicles and greenish yellow pustules develop, increase in size, and rupture, discharging their contents onto the skin surface [20,23,24]. The serocellular discharge and exudate stain the base of wool fibres yellow–orange and, as they coagulate and dry, they produce an area of yellowish scale and crust and matted fleece (Figure 58.1) [15,22]. The scab is surrounded by a moist, faintly green zone of exudation with an outer ring of inflammation that merges into normal skin. At this interface of lesional and non-lesional skin mites congregate, feed, and deposit eggs [15,17,22,25]. As mites advance centrifugally individual lesions expand, coalesce, and eventually may extend to involve most of the body. As the disease progresses the fleece overlying lesional skin becomes increasingly stained, moist, soiled with environmental debris, and matted, and secondary bacterial infection of lesions, principally with *Staphylococcus aureus*, may occur [26,27].

Initially, lesions generate a mild to moderate pruritus manifested by head tossing and scratching, rubbing, and biting at affected sites [15,22]. Tufts and clumps of fleece may be pulled out and self-trauma of exposed areas results in abrasions, ulcers, and excoriation. As lesions

Veterinary Allergy, First Edition. Edited by Chiara Noli, Aiden Foster, and Wayne Rosenkrantz.

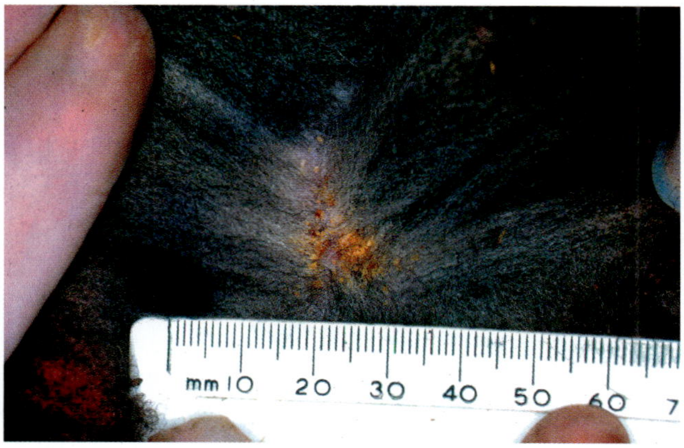

Figure 58.1 Exuberant crust and scale formation 24 hours after experimental infestation with 25 ovigerous mites.

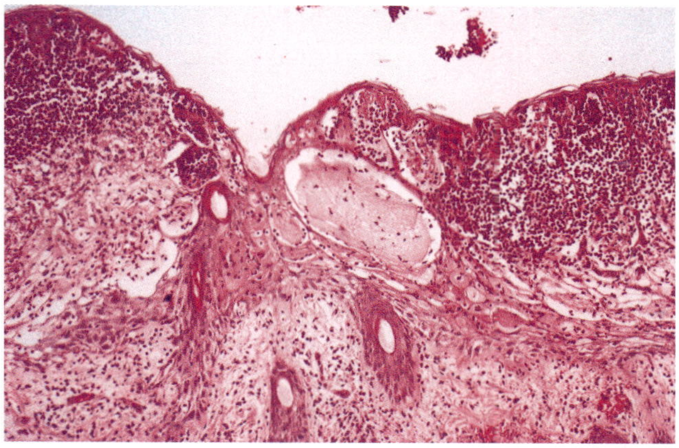

Figure 58.2 Multiple subcorneal, eosinophilic pustules and vesicles and disruption of the epidermal architecture in *Psoroptes ovis* infestation. Haematoxylin and eosin.

become more extensive the pruritus becomes more intense and affected animals may become hyperaesthetic. Consequently, when stimulated by rubbing they often exhibit a pronounced nibble reflex with protrusion of the tongue and lip smacking. Occasionally, self-trauma precipitates epileptiform convulsions and death [28].

In severe infestations productivity falls, with reduced weight gain in growing animals and weight loss in adults [29]. In pregnant ewes loss of protein causes low birth weight and high perinatal mortality, while in lactating ewes milk yield is depressed [30]. In some cases loss of condition may be extreme and result in depression, emaciation, and death.

Most animals will recover without treatment [15] and as lesions resolve new wool growth lifts the scab away from the skin, which may appear hyperkeratotic and lichenified. In some animals the mite population may die out completely, while in others mites may persist in cryptic sites such as the inguinal and infraorbital fossa and external auditory meatus [15,24,31]. Occasionally, exuberant crusts and scales persist and may be peeled back to expose an abundance of mites. These cases, described as 'flakers' [15], appear to be analogous to Norwegian scabies in man, pigs, and dogs and may be associated with immunodepression/deficiency [32].

Infestations may sometimes be limited to the external auditory meatus. These may cause head shaking and rubbing and scratching of the affected ear, which result in aural haematomata, inflammation, and excoriation of the pinna and base of the ear [33,34].

Pathology of primary infestations

Lesional histopathology indicates that mite-derived products provoke a rapid and profound cutaneous inflammatory response [35]. This occurs within 1 to 3 hours of experimental infestation and is characterized by an intense polymorphonuclear dermal infiltrate that is dominated by eosinophils [36]. By 24 hours after infestation, eosinophils in the upper dermis exhibit marked degranulation, subcorneal eosinophilic pustules are frequently detected and numerous eosinophils and smaller numbers of neutrophils and mononuclear cells are present in the overlying scab [17,35]. The dermal infiltrate of eosinophils is accompanied by variable numbers of neutrophils, macrophages, lymphocytes, and basophils (Figure 58.2) [17,35,37–40]. Marked dermal mast cell hyperplasia is observed 4 days after infestation with partial degranulation of many mast cells and basophils [17,35]. Immunohistochemical analysis has shown that the lymphocyte infiltrate comprises principally $CD4^+$ and γδ T cells and $CD45RA^+B$/naïve T cells, and smaller numbers of $CD1^+$ dendritic cells [41]. An influx of $Foxp3^+$ T regulatory cells has also been recorded [42].

In addition, within 3 hours of experimental infestation there is loss of epidermal architecture with hydropic degeneration of cells of the stratum basale and stratum spinosum [36], followed 4 days after infestation by epidermal hyperplasia with marked acanthosis, hypergranulosis, and hyperkeratosis [35]. There is also pronounced dermal oedema [35,37], disruption of collagen bundles, and occasionally arector pili muscle [35].

Haematology

Development of a circulating eosinophilia [17,43] and basophilia [17] have been recorded in the course of experimental primary infestations of sheep with *P. ovis*. Neutrophilia, lymphopenia, and a significant fall in haemoglobin concentration have also been reported in the course of experimental primary infestations of sheep with *P. ovis* but are less consistent [43].

Isotype-specific antibody responses

Psoroptes ovis antigen-specific, serum IgG [15,44] and IgM, IgE, and IgA [17,44] levels have been monitored by ELISA following experimental infestation of naïve sheep. A significant increase in IgG antibody levels was first detected 2 weeks after infestation, in IgE antibody level 6–7 weeks after infestation [17], and in IgM antibody level 7 weeks after infestation [44], but no increase in IgA antibody level was detected. In a further study, IgE antibody immunoreactivity was detected 6 weeks after infestation only in sera from *S. aureus*-positive sheep [26].

Cutaneous hypersensitivity responses

Intradermal tests (IDT), employing whole *P. ovis* mite extract, have confirmed the development of a series of hypersensitivity responses to *P. ovis* allergens [45]. An immediate IgE-mediated, type 1, hypersensitivity response (IH) was obtained after IDT in sheep that had been infested with *P. ovis* mites and after Prausnitz–Küstner (PK) tests in *P. ovis* naïve sheep [45]. This IH response was followed 6 hours after intradermal challenge by an eosinophil-rich response [45] with histopathology typical of a late-phase response (LPR)[46–48], and then, at 24 hours after challenge, by a cell-mediated eosinophil-rich delayed type hypersensitivity response (ER-DTH), which was maximal at 30 hours and sustained until 72 hours after challenge [45]. The kinetics of the delayed response was similar to that described in some cutaneous basophil hypersensitivity (CBH) reactions and the classical tuberculin-induced delayed hypersensitivity (DTH) response [49,50]. However, the eosinophil-dominated infiltrate in this delayed response was fundamentally different from the CBH and classical tuberculin-induced, mononuclear cell-dominated DTH response of sheep [51] and other animals, but has been observed in responses of sensitized ruminants to intradermal injection of helminth extracts [52,53]. The eosinophil-rich infiltrate was correlated with numbers of infiltrating $CD4^+$ T cells [54]—an observation that parallels that of ovine mammary gland responses to infused nematodes [55]. Observation of the temporal development of these hypersensitivity reactions in the course of primary infestations indicated that the IH and LPR responses first occurred at 7 weeks and the ER-DTH response at 9 weeks after infestation [54].

Although the IH, late-phase response and non-classical ER-DTH play a crucial role in selective eosinophil recruitment, it is evident from early histopathology that the innate response provoked by *P. ovis* also makes a substantial contribution to the influx of eosinophils [35].

Challenge infestations

Lesional growth after experimental challenge infestations is significantly reduced [17,56], while epidermal pathology is not as severe as in primary infestations and dermal pathology is relatively muted. However, challenge infestations provoke a rapid lesional infiltration of eosinophils and basophils, and mast cell hyperplasia [17]. They also elicit a pronounced and sustained amnestic IgE antibody response and a transient amnestic IgG antibody response, but no amnestic IgM antibody response [17,44]. Restriction of lesional growth indicates that *P. ovis* stimulates a protective response while the amnestic IgE antibody response and lesional infiltration of eosinophils and mast cell hyperplasia suggest that a hypersensitivity responses may contribute to this protective response.

Overview, including molecular aspects, of the immunopathogenesis of sheep scab

Psoroptes ovis is a surface-living mite and its mouthparts, designed to abrade and siphon surface lipid emulsion and inflammatory fluid into a preoral cavity [57–59], fail to penetrate beyond the outer layers of the stratum corneum [60]. Mite-derived products containing allergens, enzymes, chemoattractants, proinflammatory, and possibly cytotoxic substances are, therefore, deposited on the stratum corneum. The direct activity of the diverse array of enzymes and biologically active compounds present in these products [61], together with the cascade of mediators released by keratinocytes, recruited mast cells, basophils, and particularly eosinophils [62], contribute to the significant epidermal and dermal pathology observed early in ectoparasite infestations.

As these products disrupt epidermal architecture and provoke a profound innate inflammatory response within hours of infestation, it is clear that they penetrate the epidermal barrier very rapidly. The stratum corneum plays a key role in barrier function and is composed of anucleated corneocytes, embedded in an extracellular lipid matrix [63] and encased by a cornified envelope consisting of cross-linking proteins such as filaggrin, loricrin, and involucrin [64,65]. Integrity of the stratum corneum is critical in minimizing transepidermal penetration of exogenous molecules, including allergens [66] which provoke an immediate inflammatory response, and in reducing exposure of dermal antigen presenting cells (APCs) to allergens [67].

Recent studies have shown that a number of factors may contribute to compromised epidermal barrier function. Among the allergens and enzymes deposited on the stratum corneum by *P. ovis* are Pso o 1 and Pso o 3 which are, respectively, homologues of the proteolytic enzymes Der p 1 (cysteine protease) and Der p 3 (serine protease) produced by the house dust mite *Dermatophagoides pteronyssinus.* Proteolytic activity of Der p 1 and 3 disrupts the epidermal barrier by cleavage of tight junctions [68,69], and by analogy their *P. ovis* homologues may exhibit the same activity. In addition, analysis of microarray data, obtained by employing an ovine transcriptome array to evaluate the cutaneous response, demonstrated that expression of a cluster of genes located in the epidermal differentiation complex (EDC), including those for filaggrin, loricrin, and involucrin (integral components of the cornified enveloped), was significantly repressed 24 hours after infestation with *P. ovis* [70]. Recent investigations employing qPCR have confirmed these observations and also demonstrated a significant reduction in fluorescent staining of filaggrin and loricrin in the stratum corneum [36]. Earlier, microarray analyses revealed similar alterations in the expression of EDC genes in human atopic dermatitis and, notably, the repressed expression of filaggrin, loricrin, and involucrin [71,72]. The importance of these proteins in barrier function is indicated by the observation that loss-of-function mutations in filaggrin, the most intensively studied EDC gene, are associated with diseases with compromised epithelial barrier function, such as atopic dermatitis, ichthyosis, psoriasis, and asthma [73–77]. It is currently believed that loss-of-function mutations in EDC genes, such as filaggrin, affect barrier function, enabling increased allergen penetration and therefore heighten the immune response and increase the risk of allergic sensitization [78–80].

Although loss-of-function mutations have not yet been demonstrated in sheep, down-regulated expression of critical components of the epidermal barrier such as filaggrin, loricrin, and involucrin following infestation with *P. ovis* [70] may exacerbate the damage done by mite proteases, increasing mite allergen exposure and further aggravating the inflammatory response.

The mechanism for this down-regulation of EDC genes is uncertain. However, the Th2 cytokines, interleukin 4 (IL4) and IL13, are over-expressed in human atopic skin [72,81,82] and are able to trigger down-regulation of filaggrin [83], loricrin [72], and involucrin [72] in human keratinocytes. Therefore, a Th2-driven inflammatory response may contribute to decreased filaggrin production in atopic patients and consequently epidermal barrier dysfunction. A similar bias towards a Th2-dominated inflammatory response has been demonstrated by transcriptomic analysis of the ovine response to *P. ovis* infestation including up-regulation of IL4 and IL13 [70] and suggests that Th2 cytokines may also be involved in suppression of filaggrin synthesis in *P. ovis*-infested skin.

Another possible cause of reduced filaggrin and loricrin content of the stratum corneum is active cleavage of these proteins by mite proteases. *In vitro* studies have shown that a recombinant scabies mite protease, Sar s 3 (serine protease), another homologue of *Pso o 3*, is capable of cleaving recombinant human filaggrin [84]. Moreover, human filaggrin can be immunolocalized to the scabies mite digestive tract, indicating active ingestion of this protein [84]. Cleavage of tight junctions and of integral constituents of the cornified envelop, such as filaggrin, and down-regulated expression of critical EDC genes will combine to increase barrier permeability, facilitating the ingress of mite-derived products, including allergens, and establishing a vicious cycle of continued antigen exposure and inflammatory response [85].

On penetrating the epidermal barrier, in addition to any direct proinflammatory and chemoattractant influence that they exert, mite-derived products will interact initially with cells of the epidermis and then the dermis to trigger the release of a cascade of proinflammatory and immunomodulatory cytokines and chemokines. This will generate the immediate innate inflammatory response and, subsequently, layered over this, the specific adaptive immune response with isotype-specific IgM, IgG, and IgE responses [17,44], and then immediate IgE-mediated and delayed-type hypersensitivity responses [54]. Although the exact mechanisms by which the mite induces an early proinflammatory response are not fully understood, studies suggest that the initial host–parasite interactions trigger a nuclear factor kappa-B (NF-κβ) mediated proinflammatory response [86], leading to the expression of cytokines, chemokines, selectins, and adhesion molecules. The combined activity of this mite-induced proinflammatory response and mite-derived chemoattractant compounds, particularly eosinophil chemoattractants, is probably responsible for the intense, eosinophil-dominated inflammatory response observed within hours of infestation [35,36]. This rapid infiltration of polymorphonuclear cells is consistent with the presence of potent chemoattractants in *P. ovis* products.

In vitro studies have demonstrated the eosinophil and neutrophil chemoattractant properties of HDM products Der p 1, 3, and 9, and the ability of HDM extract to induce expression of two potent neutrophil chemoattractants, IL8 and tumour necrosis factor alpha (TNF), by epithelial cells [87,88]. *Psoroptes ovis* homologues of these HDM products, such as Pso o 1, 3, and 9 [70,89] and a *P. ovis*-derived eosinophil chemoattractant [90], have been identified. In addition, the ability of *P. ovis*-derived antigens to stimulate IL-8 expression by cultured ovine keratinocytes has been demonstrated [91]. Similarly, as HDM extracts induce expression of adhesion molecules and cytokines by human dermal endothelial cells [92] it is probable that homologous molecules produced by *P. ovis* will have the same effect, leading to the extravasation of leukocytes and lymphocytes at the site of infestation [41].

Although it is anticipated that the acquired immune response will involve both Th1 and Th2 $CD4^+$ T cells, the detection of an IgE antibody response and IH, LPR, and ER-DTH responses, suggests the response to *P. ovis* is dominated by the activity of $CD4^+$ lymphocytes expressing a Th2-like cytokine profile. The ability of APCs to polarize the immune response along a Th2-type pathway may also be influenced by mite-derived substances and the mite-induced release of immunomodulatory cytokines, particularly IL-4 and IL-13, histamine from mast cells, and basophils and IL-4 from eosinophils. It is also possible that, by analogy with Der p 14, some mite products act as proallergic adjuvants and promote a Th2-type response [93]. More recently, a study [94] demonstrated that the HDM allergen Der p 2 was capable of functional mimicry of MD-2, an extracellular adaptor or co-receptor of the Toll-like receptor 4 (TLR4) which is involved in the cellular response to bacterial lipopolysaccharide (LPS)[95]. *P. ovis* produces a homologue of Der p 2 (Pso o 2) which, like Der p 2, contains a conserved MD-2-related lipid-recognition (ML) domain. Previous studies in mice have shown that low levels of LPS exposure can promote the development of a Th2-type immune response [96]. It is conceivable that LPS, either from host commensal bacteria on the skin or from mite commensal/symbiotic bacteria [97], acting in conjunction with mite-derived allergens like Pso o 2, could trigger TLR4 activity, instigating an NF-κβ-mediated proinflammatory response and promoting a Th2-type response. The possible role of *S. aureus* in the pathogenesis of sheep scab lesions remains to be elucidated. Its association with the development of *P. ovis* antigen-specific IgE [26] may indicate that it enhances the IgE response to *P. ovis* and would be consistent with the observation that *S. aureus* augments allergen-specific IgE responses in atopic patients [98] and mice [99].

The acquired eosinophil-rich hypersensitivity responses are layered over the eosinophil-dominated innate response. Although the IH, late-phase response, and non-classical ER-DTH play a crucial role in selective eosinophil recruitment it is evident from early histopathology that they are layered over the eosinophil-rich innate response provoked by *P. ovis* [35]. These hypersensitivity reactions will augment the inflammatory response, exacerbate tissue damage, and increase pruritus.

It is clear that primary infestations of *P. ovis* generate a substantial protective immunity [17]. However, the mechanism for this is unclear. The temporal development of hypersensitivity responses in the course of primary infestations coincides with a plateau in lesional growth and reduction in density of the mite population. It is therefore possible that, as in *P. ovis* infestations of cattle [100], by reducing mite fecundity they make an important contribution to the significant protective response demonstrated in the challenge study. This is supported by the association of an amnestic IgE response with restricted lesional growth in challenge infestations. Ovine immunoglobulins have been detected in *P. ovis* mites harvested from infested sheep [101] and release of mast cell-mediators in IH reactions may increase epidermal permeability, facilitating transepidermal efflux of *P. ovis* antigen-specific immunoglobulins. In addition, exocytosis of basophils and of eosinophils, which have been detected in the midgut of *P. ovis* mites obtained from infested sheep [102], may also contribute to this resistance.

Diagnosis

A diagnosis of sheep scab is suggested by history and clinical signs and confirmed by identification of *P. ovis* mites in skin scrapings taken from lesional skin, particularly the periphery of the lesion where mites are concentrated. However, subclinical infestations will by their nature escape routine examination. Consequently, additional methods of detection need to be developed. A study in Switzerland has demonstrated the potential value of serodiagnostic tests to screen flocks for subclinical sheep scab and institute flock treatment on the basis of the results [103]. The sandwich ELISA test used crude *P. ovis* antigens [103]. More recently, an ELISA test employing a single recombinant *P. ovis* antigen (rPso o 2) has been developed at the Moredun Research Institute [104,105]. As it has a specificity of 0.90 and sensitivity 0.93, detects early *P. ovis* infestation before the development of obvious cutaneous lesions, and does not cross-react with antigens of the chewing louse, ticks, or gastrointestinal nematodes, it has considerable potential value for screening flocks in field conditions.

Treatment and prevention

These will be dealt with briefly.

Treatment

Plunge dipping with diazinon is an effective treatment. Mites are killed within 24 hours, residual activity persists for several weeks, and there are no adverse systemic effects. However, skilled labour is required to ensure adequate immersion, including the head, of sheep and to maintain the dip at the correct concentration with minimal contamination with soil and faeces. The use of diazinon also requires an extended withdrawal time of 70 days for slaughter (at least in the UK) and raises health and environmental concerns. An effective alternative is the use of macrocyclic lactones such as ivermectin (200 µg/kg, two subcutaneous doses 7 days apart), moxidectin (200 µg/kg, two subcutaneous doses 10 days apart), or depot moxidectin (one subcutaneous dose) and doramectin (300 µg/kg, one intramuscular dose). But it should be noted that repeated use of these will accelerate the development of resistance in the mite population and may also expose the nematode population to macrocyclic lactones, contributing to the emergence of anthelmintic resistance. Pour-on solutions, sprays, jetting races, and shower dipping are not considered to be effective. Alternative, novel control measures include the use of entomopathogenic fungi, although considerable advances need to be made before these present effective replacements for current treatments [106,107].

Prevention

Infestations can be transmitted by direct contact between susceptible sheep and animals with subclinical disease, as well as those with clinical disease. In addition, mites can be transferred by fomites and remain infective away from their host for up to 17 days [108–110]. Consequently, *P. ovis* is highly contagious and it needs the successful transfer of only one ovigerous female from an infested to susceptible sheep to establish an infestation.

The most important element in prevention is effective biosecurity. All animals introduced should be quarantined and treated to ensure any infestation is killed before mixing with the flock. Boundaries should be secure to minimize spread from potentially infested neighbouring flocks—co-operation between farmers can greatly enhance these measures. Finally, comparison of lesional growth during primary and challenge infestations has demonstrated that primary infestations of *P. ovis* generate a substantial protective immunity. This suggests that development of an effective vaccine may contribute to prevention of this disease. However, despite research over the last 10 years a commercially viable vaccine has not yet been developed. Various extracts and fractions of mite material have been employed in attempts to induce a protective immunity [111] and a soluble mite extract was identified that stimulated high titres of mite-specific serum antibodies [112]. Subsequently, by employing serum from successful vaccine trials to screen a *P. ovis* cDNA library two potential vaccine candidates have been identified [113]. These vaccine candidates have been expressed as recombinant proteins and combined with four additional recombinant allergens as components of a vaccine [113]. However, the efficacy of this vaccine has not yet been determined.

References

1. Rose H, Learmount J, Taylor M, *et al.* Mapping risk foci for endemic sheep scab. *Veterinary Parasitology* 2009; **165**: 112–118.
2. Demeler J, Schein E, von Samson-Himmelstjerna G. Advances in laboratory diagnosis of parasitic infections of sheep. *Veterinary Parasitology* 2012; **189**: 52–64.
3. Falconi F, Ochs H, Deplazes P. Serological cross-sectional survey of psoroptic sheep scab in Switzerland. *Veterinary Parasitology* 2002; **109**: 119–127.
4. Tasawar Z, Rauf B, Hayat, CS, *et al.* Prevalence of *Psoroptes ovis* in sheep around Multan, Pakistan. *Pakistan Veterinary Journal* 2007; **27**: 199–200.
5. Hagawane SD, Rajurkar, GR, Shinde SB. Ethno-veterinary drug therapy for ear mange in sheep. *Veterinary World* 2010; **3**: 295–296.
6. Synge BA, Bates PG, Clark AM, *et al.* Apparent resistance of *P-ovis* to flumethrin. *Veterinary Record* 1995; **137**: 51.
7. Clark AM, Stephen FB, Cawley GD, *et al.* Resistance of the sheep scab mite *Psoroptes ovis* to propetamphos. *Veterinary Record* 1996; **139**: 451.
8. Coles CC. Drug resistant parasites of sheep: an emerging problem in Britain? *Parasitology Today* 1998; **14**: 86–88.
9. Taylor MA. SCOPS and COWS—'Worming it out of UK farmers. *Veterinary Parasitology* 2012; **186**: 65–69.
10. Gasser B, Wuthrich A, Lis J, *et al.* Topical application of synthetic pyrethroids to cattle as a source of persistent environmental contamination. *Journal of Environmental Science and Health B* 1997; **32**: 340–343.
11. Littlejohn JW, Melvin MAL. Sheep-dips as a source of pollution of fresh-waters—a study in Grampian region. *Journal of the Institution of Water and Environmental Management* 1991; **5**: 21–27.
12. Murray VS, Wiseman HM, Dawling S, *et al.* Health effects of organophosphate sheep dips. *British Medical Journal* 1992; **305**: 1090.
13. Stephens R, Spurgeon A, Calvert IA, *et al.* Neuropsychological effects of long-term exposure to organophosphates in sheep dip. *Lancet* 1995; **345**: 1135–1139.
14. Beynon SA. Potential environmental consequences of administration of anthelmintics to sheep. *Veterinary Parasitology* 2012; **189**: 113–124.
15. Bates P. The pathogenesis and aging of sheep scab lesions—Part 1. *State Veterinary Journal* 1997; **7**: 11–15.
16. O'Brien DJ. Treatment of psoroptic mange with reference to epidemiology and history. *Veterinary Parasitology* 1999; **83**: 177–185.
17. van den Broek AH, Huntley JF, Machell J, *et al.* Cutaneous and systemic responses during primary and challenge infestations of sheep with the sheep scab mite, *Psoroptes ovis. Parasite Immunology* 2000; **22**: 407–414.
18. Wall R, Smith KE, Berriatua E, *et al.* Simulation analysis of the population dynamics of the mite, *Psoroptes ovis*, infesting sheep. *Veterinary Parasitology* 1999; **83**: 253–264.

19. Roberts IH, Meleney WP. Variations among strains of *Psoroptes-ovis* (Acarina-Psoroptidae) on sheep and cattle. *Annals of the Entomological Society of America* 1971; **64**: 105–108.
20. Bates P. The pathogenesis and aging of sheep scab lesions—Part 2. *State Veterinary Journal* 1997; **7** 13–16.
21. Fourie LJ, Kok DJ, Visagie E. Sheep scab. Effect of breed on population growth. *16th International Conference of the World Association for the Advancement of Parasitology* Sun City, Republic of South Africa, 1997: 10–15.
22. Sargison ND. Differential diagnosis and treatment of sheep scab. *In Practice* 1995; **17**: 3–9.
23. Downing W. The life history of *Psoroptes communis* var *ovis* with particular refernce to latent or suppressed scab. I Introduction and II Life history. *Journal of Comparative Pathology and Therapeutics* 1936; **49**: 162–180.
24. Spence T. The Latent phase of sheep scab—its nature and relation to the eradication of the disease. *Journal of Comparative Pathology and Therapeutics* 1949; **59**: 305–318.
25. Kirkwood AC. History, biology and control of sheep scab. *Parasitology Today* 1986; **2**: 302–307.
26. Oliveira AM, MacKellar A, Hume L, *et al.* Immune responses to *Staphylococcus aureus* and *Psoroptes ovis* in sheep infected with *P. ovis*—the sheep scab mite. *Veterinary Immunology and Immunopathology* 2006; **113**: 64–72.
27. Billingsley P. Project OD0536: Biochemical and physiological studies of *P. ovis*. In: *Sheep Scab Projects Management Meeting*. Moredun Research Institute, 2003.
28. Bygrave AC, Bates PG, Daniel NJ. Epileptiform seizure in ewes associated with sheep scab mite infestation. *Veterinary Record* 1993; **132**: 394–395.
29. Kirkwood AC. Effect of *Psoroptes ovis* on the weight of sheep. *Veterinary Record* 1980; **107**: 469–470.
30. Sargison N, Scott P, Penny C, *et al.* Effect of an outbreak of sheep scab (*Psoroptes ovis* infestation) during mid-pregnancy on ewe body condition and lamb birthweight. *Veterinary Record* 1995; **136**: 287–289.
31. Downing W. The life history of *Psoroptes communis* var *ovis* with particular reference to latent or suppressed scab. III The clinical aspect of sheep scab. *Journal of Comparative Pathology and Therapeutics* 1936; **49**: 183–209.
32. Espy PD, Jolly HW, Jr. Norwegian scabies: occurrence in a patient undergoing immunosuppression. *Archives of Dermatology* 1976; **112**: 193–196.
33. Morgan KL. Parasitic otitis in sheep associated with Psoroptes infestation—a clinical and epidemiologic-study. *Veterinary Record* 1992; **130**: 530–532.
34. Bates PG. Epidemiology of subclinical ovine psoroptic otoacariasis in Great Britain. *Veterinary Record* 1996; **138**: 388–393.
35. van den Broek AHM, Else RW, Huntley JF, *et al.* Early innate and longer-term adaptive cutaneous immunoinflammatory responses during primary infestation with the sheep scab mite, *Psoroptes ovis*. *Journal of Comparative Pathology* 2004; **131**: 318–329.
36. Stoeckli MR, McNeilly TN, Frew D, *et al.* The effect of *Psoroptes ovis* infestation on ovine epidermal barrier function. *Veterinary Research* 2013; **44**: 11.
37. Rapeanu MD. Effect of the integrity of the skin on the histolopathogical changes in psoroptic mange of sheep. *Revista de Zootehnie si Medicina Veterinara* 1972; **22**: 1002–1007.
38. Rovere RJ, Nunez, JL. Psoroptic mange in sheep. Histopathological study of the skin in acute and chronic cases. *Gaceta Veterinaria* 1977; **39**: 172–177.
39. Abu-Samra MT, Imbabi SE, Mahgoub ES. Mange in domestic animals in the Sudan. *Annals of Tropical Medicine and Parasitology* 1981; **75**: 627–637.
40. Rosa AB, Moschini G. Psoroptic mange in sheep. Histopathology of acute and chronic cases. *Veterinaria Argentina* 1988; **5**: 771–773.
41. van den Broek AHM, Huntley JF, Mackellar A, *et al.* Characterisation of lesional infiltrates of dendritic cells and T cell subtypes during primary infestation of sheep with *Psoroptes ovis*, the sheep scab mite. *Veterinary Immunology and Immunopathology* 2005; **105**: 141–150.
42. McNeilly TN, McIntyre J, Frew D, *et al.* Infestation of sheep with *Psoroptes ovis*, the sheep scab mite, results in recruitment of Foxp3(+) T cells into the dermis. *Parasite Immunology* 2010; **32**: 361–369.
43. O'Brien DJ, Robinson AB, Gray JS, *et al.* Haematology and blood biochemistry during the course of psoroptic scabies in sheep. *Veterinary Research Communications* 1995; **19**: 39–48.
44. van den Broek AHM, Huntley JF, Machell J, *et al.* Temporal pattern of isotype-specific antibody responses in primary and challenge infestations of sheep with *Psoroptes ovis*—the sheep scab mite. *Veterinary Parasitology* 2003; **111**: 217–230.
45. van den Broek AHM, Huntley JF, Halliwell REW, *et al.* Cutaneous hypersensitivity reactions to *Psoroptes ovis* and *Der p 1* in sheep previously infested with *P-ovis*—the sheep scab mite. *Veterinary Immunology and Immunopathology* 2003; **91**: 105–117.
46. Solley GO, Gleich GJ, Jordon RE, *et al.* The late phase of the immediate wheal and flare skin reaction. Its dependence upon IgE antibodies. *Journal of Clinical Investigation* 1976; **58**: 408–420.
47. Frew AJ, Kay AB. The relationship between infiltrating CD4+ lymphocytes, activated eosinophils, and the magnitude of the allergen-induced late phase cutaneous reaction in man. *Journal of Immunology* 1988; **141**: 4158–4164.
48. Tsicopoulos A, Hamid Q, Haczku A, *et al.* Kinetics of cell infiltration and cytokine messenger RNA expression after intradermal challenge with allergen and tuberculin in the same atopic individuals. *Journal of Allergy and Clinical Immunology* 1994; **94**: 764–772.
49. Dvorak HF. Cutaneous basophil hypersensitivity. *Journal of Allergy and Clinical Immunology* 1976; **58**: 229–240.
50. Parrish WEB, Breathnach SM. Clinical immunology and allergy. In: Champion RH, Burton JL, Burns DA, *et al.*, eds. *Textbook of Dermatology*, 6th edn, Vol. 1. Oxford: Blackwell Science, 1996: 277–336.
51. Pyrah IT, Watt NJ. Immunohistological study of the cutaneous delayed type hypersensitivity reaction in sheep. *Veterinary Immunology and Immunopathology* 1995; **48**: 299–312.
52. Meeusen E, Barcham GJ, Gorrell MD, *et al.* Cysticercosis: cellular immune responses during primary and secondary infection. *Parasite Immunology* 1990; **12**: 403–418.
53. Starke WA, Machado RZ, Bechara GH, *et al.* Skin hypersensitivity tests in buffaloes parasitized with *Toxocara vitulorum*. *Veterinary Parasitology* 1996; **63**: 283–290.
54. van den Broek AHM, Huntley JF, Halliwell REW, *et al.* Temporal development of ovine cutaneous hypersensitivity responses to *Psoroptes ovis* (sheep scab mite). In: Hillier A, Foster AP, Kwochka KW., eds. *Advances in Veterinary Dermatology*, Vol. 5. Oxford: Blackwell Science, 2004: 97–103.
55. Meeusen ENT. Immunology of helminth infections, with special reference to immunopathology. *Veterinary Parasitology* 1999; **84**: 259–273.

56. Bates P. Differences between primary and secondary infestations with the sheep scab mite, *Psoroptes ovis*. *Veterinary Record* 2000; **146**: 528–529.
57. Blake BH, Bay DE, Meola SM, *et al.* Morphology of mouthparts of sheep scab mite, *Psoroptes-ovis*. *Annals of the Entomological Society of America* 1978; **71**: 289–294.
58. Sinclair AN, Kirkwood AC. Feeding-behaviour of *Psoroptes-Ovis*. *Veterinary Record* 1983; **112**: 65.
59. Rafferty DE, Gray JS. The feeding-behavior of Psoroptes spp mites on rabbits and sheep. *Journal of Parasitology* 1987; **73**: 901–906.
60. Sinclair AN, Filan SJ. Lipid ingestion from sheep epidermis by *Psoroptes-ovis* (Acari, Psoroptidae). *Veterinary Parasitology* 1989; **31**: 149–164.
61. Nisbet AJ, Billingsley PF. Hydrolytic enzymes of *Psoroptes cuniculi* (Delafond). *Insect Biochemistry and Molecular Biology* 1999; **29**: 25–32.
62. Gleich GJ, Adolphson CR. The eosinophilic leukocyte: structure and function. *Advances in Immunology* 1986; **39**: 177–253.
63. Feingold KR. Thematic review series: skin lipids. The role of epidermal lipids in cutaneous permeability barrier homeostasis. *Journal of Lipid Research* 2007; **48**: 2531–2546.
64. Candi E, Schmidt R, Melino G. The cornified envelope: a model of cell death in the skin. *Nature Reviews Molecular Cell Biology* 2005; **6**: 328–340.
65. Suter MM, Schulze K, Bergman W, *et al.* The keratinocyte in epidermal renewal and defence. *Veterinary Dermatology* 2009; **20**: 515–532.
66. Elias P, Schmuth M. Abnormal skin barrier in the etiopathogenesis of atopic dermatitis. *Current Allergy and Asthma Reports* 2009; **9**: 265–272.
67. Nakamura T, Hirasawa Y, Takai T, *et al.* Reduction of skin barrier function by proteolytic activity of a recombinant house dust mite major allergen *Der f 1*. *Journal of Investigative Dermatology* 2006; **126**: 2719–2723.
68. Wan H, Winton HL, Soeller C, *et al. Der p 1* facilitates transepithelial allergen delivery by disruption of tight junctions. *Journal of Clinical Investigation* 1999; **104**: 123–133.
69. Wan H, Winton HL, Soeller C, *et al.* The transmembrane protein occludin of epithelial tight junctions is a functional target for serine peptidases from faecal pellets of *Dermatophagoides pteronyssinus*. *Clinical and Experimental Allergy* 2001; **31**: 279–294.
70. Burgess ST, Frew D, Nunn F, *et al.* Transcriptomic analysis of the temporal host response to skin infestation with the ectoparasitic mite *Psoroptes ovis*. *BMC Genomics* 2010; **11**: 624.
71. Sugiura H, Ebise H, Tazawa T, *et al.* Large-scale DNA microarray analysis of atopic skin lesions shows overexpression of an epidermal differentiation gene cluster in the alternative pathway and lack of protective gene expression in the cornified envelope. *British Journal of Dermatology* 2005; **152**: 146–149.
72. Kim BE, Leung DY, Boguniewicz M, *et al.* Loricrin and involucrin expression is down-regulated by Th2 cytokines through STAT-6. *Clinical Immunology* 2008; **126**: 332–327.
73. Irvine AD, McLean WH. Breaking the (un)sound barrier: filaggrin is a major gene for atopic dermatitis. *Journal of Investigative Dermatology* 2006; **126**: 1200–1202.
74. Segre JA. Epidermal differentiation complex yields a secret: mutations in the cornification protein filaggrin underlie ichthyosis vulgaris. *Journal of Investigative Dermatology* 2006; **126**: 1202–1204.
75. Weidinger S, Rodriguez E, Stahl C, *et al.* Filaggrin mutations strongly predispose to early-onset and extrinsic atopic dermatitis. *Journal of Investigative Dermatology* 2007; **127**: 724–726.
76. Hoffjan S, Stemmler S. On the role of the epidermal differentiation complex in ichthyosis vulgaris, atopic dermatitis and psoriasis. *British Journal of Dermatology* 2007; **157**: 441–449.
77. McGrath JA, Uitto J. The filaggrin story: novel insights into skin-barrier function and disease. *Trends in Molecular Medicine* 2008; **14**: 20–27.
78. Elias PM, Steinhoff M. 'Outside-to-inside' (and now back to 'outside') pathogenic mechanisms in atopic dermatitis. *Journal of Investigative Dermatology* 2008; **128**: 1067–1070.
79. Marsella R, Samuelson D. Unravelling the skin barrier: a new paradigm for atopic dermatitis and house dust mites. *Veterinary Dermatology* 2009; **20**: 533–540.
80. Hudson TJ. Skin barrier function and allergic risk. *Nature Genetics* 2006; **38**: 399–400.
81. Hamid Q, Boguniewicz M, Leung DY. Differential *in situ* cytokine gene expression in acute versus chronic atopic dermatitis. *Journal of Clinical Investigation* 1994; **94**: 870–876.
82. Homey B, Steinhoff M, Ruzicka T, *et al.* Cytokines and chemokines orchestrate atopic skin inflammation. *Journal of Allergy and Clinical Immunology* 2006; **118**: 178–189.
83. Howell MD, Kim BE, Gao P, *et al.* Cytokine modulation of atopic dermatitis filaggrin skin expression. *Journal of Allergy and Clinical Immunology* 2009; **124**: R7–R12.
84. Beckham SA, Boyd SE, Reynolds S, *et al.* Characterization of a serine protease homologous to house dust mite group 3 allergens from the scabies mite *Sarcoptes scabiei*. *Journal of Biological Chemistry* 2009; **284**: 34413–34422.
85. Rawlings AV, Harding CR. Moisturization and skin barrier function. *Dermatologic Therapy* 2004; **17** (Suppl. 1): 43–48.
86. Burgess ST, McNeilly TN, Watkins CA, *et al.* Host transcription factors in the immediate pro-inflammatory response to the parasitic mite *Psoroptes ovis*. *Plos One* 2011; **6**: e24402.
87. Lau LCK, Leir SH, Lackie P, *et al.* House dust mite allergen cleaves epithelial adhesion molecules and activates epithelial cells by an IgE independent pathway. *American Journal of Respiratory and Critical Care Medicine* 1999; **159**: A179.
88. Fahy O, Hammad H, Senechal S, *et al.* Synergistic effect of diesel organic extracts and allergen Der p 1 on the release of chemokines by peripheral blood mononuclear cells from allergic subjects: involvement of the map kinase pathway. *American Journal of Respiratory Cellular and Molecular Biology* 2000; **23**: 247–254.
89. Temeyer KB, Soileau LC, Pruett JH. Cloning and sequence analysis of a cDNA encoding Pso o II, a mite group II allergen of the sheep scab mite (Acari : Psoroptidae). *Journal of Medical Entomology* 2002; **39**: 384–391.
90. Wildblood LA, Jones G. Stimulation of the in vitro migration of ovine eosinophils by factors derived from the sheep scab mite, *Psoroptes ovis*. *Veterinary Research Communications* 2007; **31**: 197–206.
91. Watkins CA, Mackellar A, Frew D, *et al.* Gene expression profiling of ovine keratinocytes stimulated with *Psoroptes ovis* mite antigen—a preliminary study. *Parasite Immunology* 2009; **31**: 304–311.
92. Arlian LG, Elder BL, Morgan MS. House dust mite extracts activate cultured human dermal endothelial cells to express adhesion molecules and secrete cytokines. *Journal of Medical Entomology* 2009; **46**: 595–604.
93. Epton MJ, Dilworth RJ, Smith W, *et al.* Sensitisation to the lipid-binding apolipophorin allergen Der p 14 and the peptide Mag-1. *International Archives of Allergy and Immunology* 2001; **124**: 57–60.
94. Trompette A, Divanovic S, Visintin A, *et al.* Allergenicity resulting from functional mimicry of a Toll-like receptor complex protein. *Nature* 2009; **457**: 585–588.

95. Visintin A, Iliev DB, Monks BG, *et al.* Md-2. *Immunobiology* 2006; **211**: 437–447.
96. Eisenbarth SC, Piggott DA, Huleatt JW, *et al.* Lipopolysaccharide-enhanced, toll-like receptor 4-dependent T helper cell type 2 responses to inhaled antigen. *Journal of Experimental Medicine* 2002; **196**: 1645–1651.
97. Hogg JC, Lehane MJ. Microfloral diversity of cultured and wild strains of *Psoroptes ovis* infesting sheep. *Parasitology* 2001; **123**: 441–446.
98. Hofer MF, Harbeck RJ, Schlievert PM, *et al.* Staphylococcal toxins augment specific IgE responses by atopic patients exposed to allergen. *Journal of Investigative Dermatology* 1999; **112**: 171–176.
99. Matsui K, Nishikawa A. Lipoteichoic acid from Staphylococcus aureus enhances allergen-specific immunoglobulin E production in mice. *Clinical and Experimental Allergy* 2003; **33**: 842–848.
100. Guillot FS, Stromberg PC. Reproductive success of *Psoroptes Ovis* (Acari, Psoroptidae) on Hereford calves with a previous infestation of psoroptic mites. *Journal of Medical Entomology* 1987; **24**: 416–419.
101. Pettit D, Smith WD, Richardson J, *et al.* Localisation and characterisation of ovine immunglobulin within the sheep scab mite, *Psoroptes ovis*. *Veterinary Parasitology* 2000; **89**: 231–239.
102. Mathieson BR, Lehane MJ. Ultrastructure of the alimentary canal of the sheep scab mite, *Psoroptes ovis* (Acari: Psoroptidae). *Veterinary Parasitology* 2002; **104**: 151–166.
103. Jacober P, Ochs H, Torgerson PR, *et al.* A method for sheep scab control by applying selective treatment based on flock serology. *Veterinary Parasitology* 2006; **136**: 373–378.
104. Nunn FG, Burgess STG, Innocent G, *et al.* Development of a serodiagnostic test for sheep scab using recombinant protein Pso o 2. *Molecular and Cellular Probes* 2011; **25**: 212–218.
105. Burgess STG, Innocent G, Nunn F, *et al.* The use of a *Psoroptes ovis* serodiagnostic test for the analysis of a natural outbreak of sheep scab. *Parasites and Vectors* 2012; **5**: 7.
106. Rose H, Wall R. Pathogenicity of biological control agents for livestock ectoparasites: a simulation analysis. *Medical and Veterinary Entomology* 2009; **23**: 379–386.
107. Losson BJ. Sheep psoroptic mange: an update. *Veterinary Parasitology* 2012; **189**: 39–43.
108. Babcock OG, Black WL. The common sheep scab mite and its control. *Texas Agricultural Experiment Station Bulletin* 1933; **479**: 1–34.
109. Wilson GI, Blachut K, Roberts IH. The infectivitiy of scabies (mange) mites, *Psoroptes ovis* (Acrina: Psoroptidae) to sheep in naturally contaminated enclosures. *Research in Veterinary Science* 1977; **22**: 292–297.
110. O'Brien DJ, Gray JS, O'Reilly PF. Survival and retention of infectivity of the mite *Psoroptes ovis* off the host. *Veterinary Research Communications* 1994; **18**: 27–36.
111. Smith WD, Van den Broek A, Huntley J, *et al.* Approaches to vaccines for *Psoroptes ovis* (sheep scab). *Research in Veterinary Science* 2001; **70**: 87–91.
112. Smith WD, Pettit DM. Immunization against sheep scab: preliminary identification of fractions of *Psoroptes ovis* which confer protective effects. *Parasite Immunology* 2004; **26**: 307–314.
113. Nisbet AJ, Halliday AM, Parker L, *et al.* *Psoroptes ovis*: identification of vaccine candidates by immunoscreening. *Experimental Parasitology* 2008; **120**: 194–199.

59

Allergic diseases of livestock species

Aiden P. Foster

Animal Health and Veterinary Laboratories Agency, Shrewsbury, Shropshire, UK

Conflict of interest: Aiden Foster is editor in chief of the journal *Veterinary Dermatology* published by Wiley.

Introduction

This chapter is primarily devoted to cutaneous manifestations of allergic disease and will provide some comments on respiratory and gastrointestinal diseases in several livestock species.

The investigation of suspected allergic skin diseases in livestock is similar to that in companion animals in so far as the history and observations about the clinical signs, especially details about the nature, distribution, and pattern of pruritus, are important. Given the manner in which the skin can react to a variety of agents, the differential diagnoses may include microbial infections, including dermatophilosus, bacterial infections especially staphylococcal spp. and, given that the haired skin is often affected, dermatophytosis. Ectoparasites are the main cause of pruritus in livestock and where several animals are affected one should consider lice and mites as possible factors. The number of animals in a group with allergic disease will usually be much lower than the number with signs of ectoparasite infestation.

Camelids

South American camelids (SACs), notably alpacas and llamas, have been exported from their native countries to be farmed in various western countries since the early 1990s [1]. They are susceptible to a variety of ectoparasites [2–5]; the immunopathogenesis of ectoparasitic conditions has not been studied in detail.

Sarcoptic mange

The clinical signs associated with sarcoptic mange in camelids may include alopecia, crusting, skin thickening (Figure 59.1), and severe pruritus; infestation may lead to death/euthanasia, with severely affected individuals also showing severe weight loss. It is unclear if there are any predisposing factors for severely affected animals, such as poor nutrition, gastrointestinal diseases, or intercurrent infection, for example pestivirus or mycobacterial infection.

Sarcoptic mange is usually, in other species, difficult to diagnose because mites are present in small numbers; in some camelids there may be large numbers of mites that are easy to detect with superficial skin scrapes. The potential for zoonotic spread to people handling affected camelids should always be considered. It is important to establish an accurate diagnosis before embarking on treatment because this can be arduous, involving repeated and protracted treatment of all of the animals in a group using a combination of topical and systemic therapies. The response to treatment protocols used in other livestock species with sarcoptic mange may be variable and disappointing. The limitations on treatment options include the lack of lanolin in camelid fibre, which may reduce the efficacy of topical products, the reported reduced absorption of both subcutaneous and oral ivermectin compared to ruminants [6], and the lack of licensed products. Success has been reported using repeated subcutaneous injections of ivermectin at 200 μg/kg [7] and at 400 μg/kg [8]. Topical treatment with amitraz [9] may be beneficial.

Veterinary Allergy, First Edition. Edited by Chiara Noli, Aiden Foster, and Wayne Rosenkrantz.

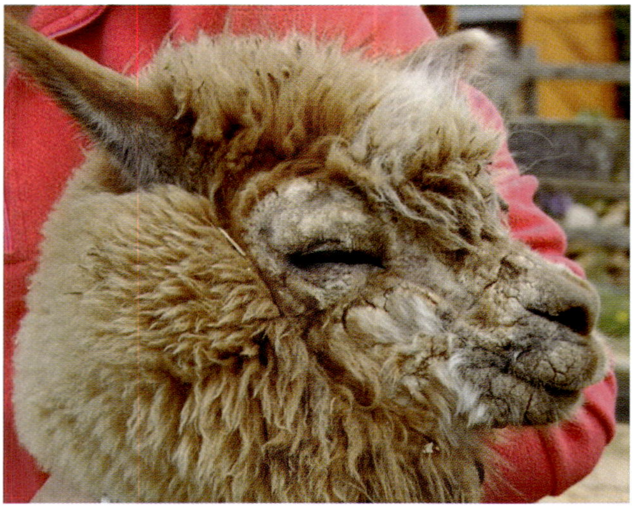

Figure 59.1 Young alpaca with chronic severe sarcoptic mange with periocular and perinasal alopecia and crusting and thickening of the skin. (Reprinted with permission from Natalie Jewell.)

Cases that relapse with skin disease due to scabies may be hypersensitive to the activity of the mites or perhaps to mite antigen/allergens but this is speculative given the lack of studies. Cutaneous changes observed in skin biopsies are similar to those seen in other livestock species with ectoparasite infestations [10].

Chorioptic mange

Chorioptic mange in SACs is usually assumed to involve *Chorioptes bovis*. Clinical signs may include mild pruritus, alopecia, and scaling of the feet and tail base with extension to the ventral abdomen, medial limbs, and the ears. The alpaca may be more susceptible than the llama. *Chorioptes* mites may be found by collecting superficial skin scrapings from SACs with or without skin disease. While the distribution of clinical signs may be similar to sarcoptic mange, some authors propose that one difference is that the skin can be very thickened in sarcoptic mange. However, like many chronic skin problems, thickening may also be a feature of idiopathic hyperkeratosis syndromes and chronic chorioptic mange. Ideally, all animals in the group should be sampled because, like horses with chorioptic mange, there may be mild or absent clinical signs but mites could still be present—consistent with asymptomatic or subclinical carriage. This may reflect that some animals, like horses, may harbour low level infestations with no ill effect, while some other animals with severe skin problems may be suffering from a hypersensitivity response.

Treatment of chorioptic mange in camelids can be a challenge and in many cases control rather than eradication may be a pragmatic aim. A variety of topical and systemic therapies have been reported, which may variably reduce numbers of mites but relapses are common. While many camelids seem to cope with mild infestation, some develop severe skin problems and underlying predisposing disease may need to be considered—as for sarcoptic mange. Macrocyclic lactones (MLs) have been shown to have some affect although they may need to be combined with topical therapies, including fipronil spray once monthly or selenium sulphide-based shampoos applied every other week; treatment courses can last months rather than weeks; all animals in a group should be considered as infested; particular attention should be paid to the distal limbs where the mites tend to reside [2,3,11].

Danny Scott in New York State, USA, described five cases of presumptive **insect-bite hypersensitivity** in alpacas [10] where *Culicoides* spp. may have been involved. Affected animals were the only ones from the herd to show signs on a recurrent seasonal basis that improved in the winter or with housing and insect control measures. Lesions included crusts, alopecia, and lichenification with some papules on the pinnae, periocular area, bridge of the nose, axillae, groin, and ventral trunk, extending to the distal legs; pruritus was a major feature. Some of these findings are consistent with mange but there was no response to treatment for mites and none found from diagnostic samples. Histopathological findings were consistent with an allergic aetiology with eosinophilic interstitial dermatitis, there was also eosinophilic epidermal microabscesses and eosinophilic infiltrative mural and luminal folliculitis. There are anecdotal reports, from clinicians in other parts of North America, of alpacas and llamas with similar suspected allergic skin disease (W. Rosenkrantz, personal communication).

Further investigations are required to characterize alpacas with suspected allergic skin disease.

Cattle

Allergic diseases of cattle have been studied in terms of the IgE response to a variety of antigens, including aerosolized antigens, bacteria, parasites, protozoa, and viruses; reviewed by Gershwin [12]. The prevalence of many of these diseases is unknown and the documentation of naturally occurring allergic diseases is generally limited; there are detailed reviews of the literature by Halliwell and Gorman [13] and Scott [14]. Although photosensitization is mentioned for other species in this book, it will not be covered here and the reader is directed to other sources of information such as Ginn *et al.* [15].

Enzootic nasal granuloma (allergic rhinitis)

Early reports of this condition initially came from Australia and it has since been reported widely; the clinical signs consist of a serous nasal discharge, which may become mucopurulent, nasal pruritus, and lacrimation associated with conjunctivitis; facial swelling, sneezing, and snuffling with increased respiratory effort. Large numbers of small (1–2 mm) white nodules may be observed within the nasal vestibules; histopathological findings include squamous metaplasia and goblet cell hyperplasia of the nasal gland duct and surface epithelium, with a dense infiltrate of eosinophils and lymphocytes. Signs may be observed from 6 months of age and usually improve or disappear when cattle are housed; however, they may recur in the spring and summer months year on year [16,17]. A type 1 hypersensitivity response is presumed to exist although the allergens involved have not been identified [16–18].

Hypersensitivity pneumonitis (extrinsic allergic alveolitis)

In cattle, anaphylactoid reactions usually involve the respiratory tract with signs of apnoea associated with bronchoconstriction and pulmonary oedema, which may lead to blood-stained froth and emphysema. Cattle that are housed may develop an allergic reaction to the spores of actinomycetes, especially *Saccharopolyspora rectivirgula* (formerly known as *Micropolyspora faeni*), which is the cause of farmer's lung in humans. Several hypersensitivity mechanisms may be involved in the bovine form of this disease, including immune-complex formation and delayed reactions. Histopathological findings may include granulomatous lesions, comprising a mixed cell infiltrate within the alveoli and associated with oedema. Experimental reproduction of the disease with parenteral immunization and aerosol exposure has shown clinical signs of apnoea as well as IgE responses and immediate cutaneous reactions after injection of *M. faeni* allergens [12,19,20].

Urticaria

This condition has also been called hives, blaine, heat bumps, and angioedema; it is poorly understood and the allergens are usually unknown [21]. The history may suggest that infections, injectable medications, and agents such as antibacterial agents, vaccines (Figure 59.2), and blood transfusions may be implicated; insects and arthropods through feeding (biting) and stinging may be involved; feed components have also been suggested as possible allergens [22]. As such, urticaria is one of the cutaneous manifestations of a drug reaction that may concurrently present with pruriginous urticaria and necrotic dermatitis [23]; urticaria in general can be regarded as a cutaneous reaction pattern that is triggered or exacerbated by a variety of immunological and non-immunological factors, making the determination of a definitive cause potentially very difficult.

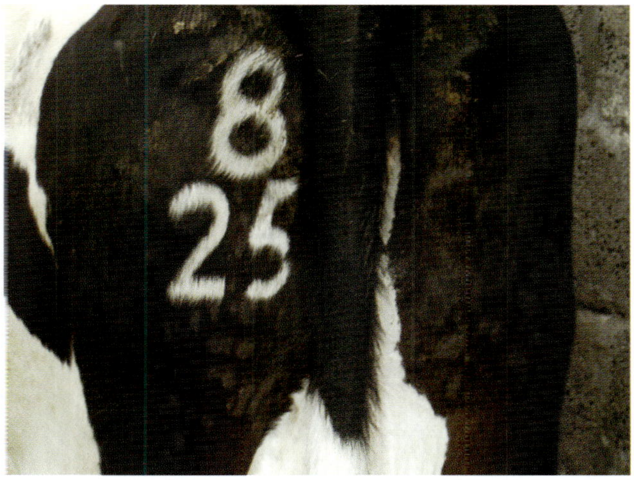

Figure 59.2 Multifocal, firm, flat, variably sized plaque-like skin lesions in a dairy cow suggestive of urticaria. Histopathological findings from a skin biopsy from another cow with similar lesions in the herd were consistent with an allergic type 1 hypersensitivity reaction, with a diffuse subacute eosinophilic dermatitis and limited oedema, as may be seen in early urticaria. Five out of 120 dairy cows were affected; a form of drug reaction was suspected to vaccines administered two weeks prior to lesion development, although there had also been a change in diet and a new milking parlour introduced at the same time. This demonstrates the difficulties of investigating this sort of skin disease where a detailed history and histopathological findings may support but not necessarily definitively diagnosis a presumed allergic skin disease, which may include urticarial changes. (Reprinted with permission from Mick Millar and Mark Hinds.)

Clinical signs may include multiple wheals of variable size, almost anywhere on the body. Some cattle make a rapid, uneventful recovery, while others may develop systemic signs with pyrexia, pain, and erythema, followed by localized sloughing of skin. Lesions may be present around the anus, eyes, lips, muzzle, and vulva.

A distinct form of urticaria was reported by Campbell in the 1970s and has not been substantially reported since. This was seen mainly in Channel Isles breeds and was associated with drying off adult cattle that appeared to develop an urticarial reaction to their own milk. Intradermal and passive cutaneous anaphylaxis tests with autologous milk extracts were indicative of a type 1 hypersensitivity response [24].

Contact dermatitis

This skin disease is uncommonly reported in cattle and it is difficult to distinguish allergic from irritant forms. The history may suggest an irritant reaction when there are large numbers of animals affected, while allergic animals are likely to be small in number [22]. In two reports patch testing was utilized to define the allergens.

In one study, four cows were patch tested with calcium cyanamide, which had been added to the bedding material to reduce bacteria in the environment. Up to 9/250 cows in the herd had shown signs of skin disease, initially involving the ventral body surfaces including the mammary gland, teats, lower abdomen, and brisket; skin lesions consisted of alopecia, erythema, and crusts with pruritus (marked licking); lesions spread to the head and neck. Three of the four cows had variably positive patch tests to calcium cyanamide and cyanamide and not to urea or bicarbonate, presented in Finn chambers applied to the rump (gluteal region) for a 72-hour period. Histopathological findings were consistent with an allergic response for an affected cow that was provocatively challenged with calcium cyanamide [25].

In the second case report, a single cow with chronic skin lesions mainly involving the teats was shown to have immediate and delayed patch test reactions to *N*-isopropyl-*N*-phenyl diamine, which was a constituent of the rubber cluster used to milk the cow. The signs improved when milking was stopped or when a silicon cluster was employed. The histopathological findings were suggestive of an immediate type hypersensitivity reaction [26].

Goats

Chorioptes

This form of mange is due to the surface-dwelling mite *Chorioptes* spp., which resemble morphologically those seen on cattle; *C. bovis* and *C. texanus* have been reported in goats. It has been stated that chorioptic mange is a form of allergic skin disease due to the mites or mite by-products [27]. There appears to be no definitive evidence that goats are allergic to mites and the diagnosis of an allergic response is made on the basis of the cases that present with severe pruritus and lesions, together with histopathological findings consistent with a hypersensitivity reaction [14].

Evidence of infestation is usually apparent on the caudal aspect of the distal limbs with alopecia, erythema, and crusting (Figure 59.3); lesions may also be seen on the udder and hind limbs. The diagnosis can sometimes be difficult in severely affected cases and it can be helpful to clip away hair from the margin of the affected areas

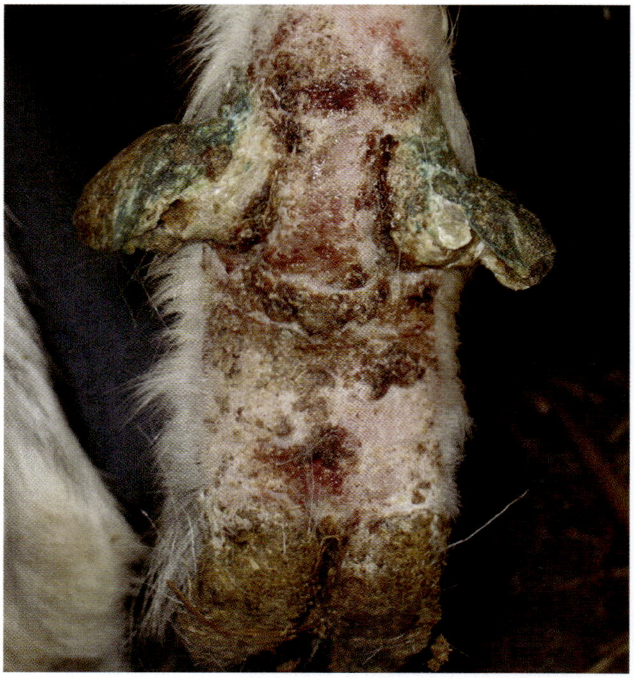

Figure 59.3 The caudal aspect of the distal limb of an adult dairy goat with chronic chorioptic mange with alopecia, erythema, and crusting.

in order to collect superficial skin scrapings for microscopic examination from the leading edge of the affected skin and find the characteristic mites with their short, sucker-like (some times called wine glass shaped) pulvillus with a short, unsegmented stalk.

While the diagnosis can be established relatively quickly the management of the condition can be challenging because these mites can survive off the host for many weeks in the environment, and many infested animals are not severely affected and so act as a major reservoir. It may be the case that some goats are particularly susceptible to infestation and develop a severe hypersensitivity response, leading to significant self-trauma and clinical signs; the same has been postulated for camelids (see section 'Camelids'). Consideration should be given to the management of the environment in housed goats and this may include attention to disposal of bedding, although most of the mites will be on the goats and a whole group should be treated, with accurate knowledge of the body weight if systemic treatments are being given.

Topical therapies are important for these surface-dwelling mites and may include fipronil-based sprays (once a month) and selenium sulphide shampoos (applied every other week). In some countries, products based on lime sulphur are used for ectoparasite control in a variety of species and although they may smell and stain surfaces, they are safe and can be used weekly. Other topical agents used elsewhere include amitraz, which is available as a dip for small and, in some countries, large animal, use and may cause changes in blood glucose and blood pressure; it is potentially valuable for surface treatment on a monthly basis for goats. The main drawback in dairy goats is the need for a minimum statutory with-holding period for milk, which in the UK is 7 days; for some products there is no safety data and so they can not be administered to milking goats. Readers are reminded of their obligation to adhere to the national regulations pertaining to the use of veterinary drugs. Treatment should be pursued for up to two mite life cycles, i.e. up to 6 weeks. Systemic treatments based on macrocyclic lactones have been the mainstay of treatment for large numbers of goats but consideration must always be given to the drawback in milking goats with long milk with-holding periods and on some farms the impact on enteric parasites, notably nematodes [4].

It has been suggested that goats require higher (double) dosages of MLs because they metabolize the drugs in a different manner from other ruminants [28]. This may be partially true but with *Chorioptes* in other host species there may be very limited exposure of the mite to such drugs when administered systemically, which may partially explain why trials have shown limited efficacy. Even topical application of MLs can be problematic with suggestions that drug absorption may be influenced by degradation on the surface of the skin or that it is trapped within skin surface layers. Generally, all MLs have shown limited efficacy for the control of *Chorioptes* mites in goats. One should consider combinations of therapies where practical—although large dairy goat groupings may prohibit this approach, in practical terms, with respect to regular topical applications. In severely affected animals some owners will consider culling because some cases become intractable and there is a poor response to various treatments.

Other causes of allergic skin disease, where parasites have been ruled out, are rarely described in goats and include a case report of a 5-year-old castrate with generalized skin lesions and pruritus, where skin testing was performed but significant allergens were not identified even with changes of housing and feed [29].

Pigs

Experimental studies in pigs have shown that they are capable of showing allergic responses, including anaphylaxis, with signs that may involve the skin, gut, and respiratory tract. Antigens used to explore allergic responses have included *Escherichia coli* and parasites including *Metastrongylus apri* (lungworm), *Trichinella spiralis*, and *Ascaris suum*. In-depth studies have been carried out using peanut, hen egg ovalbumin, and ovomucoid allergens to sensitize pigs. Interestingly, the indices used to define sensitization, such as direct skin test reactivity to allergens, heat-labile serum-induced passive cutaneous anaphylaxis, and reverse cutaneous anaphylaxis, serum IgG, and IgE antibodies, are not always consistently correlated with clinical signs on allergen challenge [30]. Such signs may include generalized erythema (Figure 59.4a,b), pruritus manifest as scratching, vomiting, diarrhoea, and breathing difficulty (reviewed by Rupa *et al.* [31]). There is no doubt that pigs have the mechanisms for allergic disease including, notably, IgE production, which may be detected by skin and serology testing. The clinical manifestations of an allergic response, given the presence

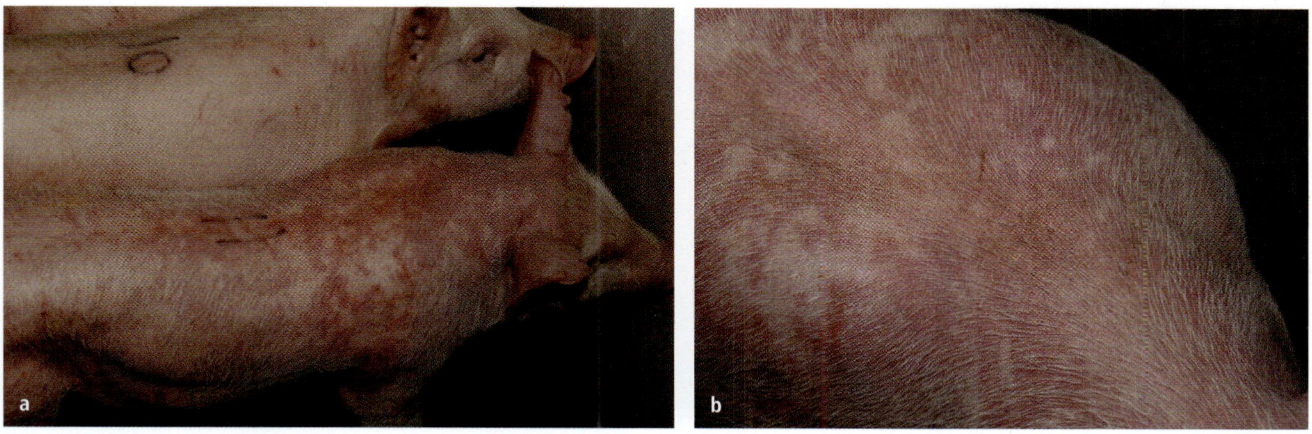

Figure 59.4 (a,b) Pigs receiving egg white orally, after experimental sensitization with ovomucoid, develop erythema within 2 hours of challenge, with small foci coalescing into lesions that sometimes covered all of the surface and regressing within 2 hours. Lesions begin on the snout, ears, perineum, and dorsal mid-line before progressing to the lateral and ventral aspects of the trunk. (Reprinted with permission from Bruce N. Wilkie.)

of IgE, may be controlled by environmental factors which may influence T reg cell activity and facilitate clinical tolerance [30].

Experimental studies have also been performed using pig skin as a model for induced allergic contact dermatitis in humans given the similarities of their skin to human skin and the knowledge of their immune system [32,33].

Food allergy has been reported as a generalized erythematous reaction in response to exposure to plant allergens [14]; it is assumed that this is a very rare dermatosis in pigs.

In the past pigs, have rarely been reported to show signs of urticaria, particularly involving the trunk and proximal limbs, associated with feedstuffs, infection (erysipelas), insect and arthropod bites and stings, plants, and systemic and topical medications and biological agents [14].

There are four types of hypersensitivity reaction described by Day (see the Introduction), including immune complex formation (type III). Porcine dermatopathy and nephropathy syndrome (PDNS) has been associated, not exclusively, with porcine circovirus type 2 (PCV-2) infection; this can be a fatal disease. Skin lesions in PDNS include raised purpuric lesions progressing to multifocal erythematous crusts with a black centre (Figure 59.5); pigs may also show signs of lethargy and pyrexia. The skin lesions are due to necrotizing and neutrophilic leukocytoclastic vasculitis involving the dermal and hypodermal capillaries and the arterioles with immune complex formation [34]; this leads to thrombosis and infarction of the skin. Greasy pig disease has been associated with PCV-2 infection; another differential diagnoses for the cutaneous lesions associated with PCV-2 is infection with *Erysipelas rhusiopathiae*, which can also cause thrombosis and vasculitis. Thus PDNS is a form of porcine allergic skin disease; it has been reducing as a problem in recent years following the introduction of vaccines for PCV-2.

A herd with signs of intense cutaneous and systemic hypereosinophilia was reported by Ted Clark (personal communication), where multiple animals were affected with cutaneous signs (Figure 59.6). It was presumed that the signs were a form of type 1 hypersensitivity reaction, although the trigger was not identified. The herd was diagnosed with PCV-2 and porcine parvovirus around the time the skin lesions were observed but these viruses were not implicated as the likely cause of the cutaneous eosinophilia.

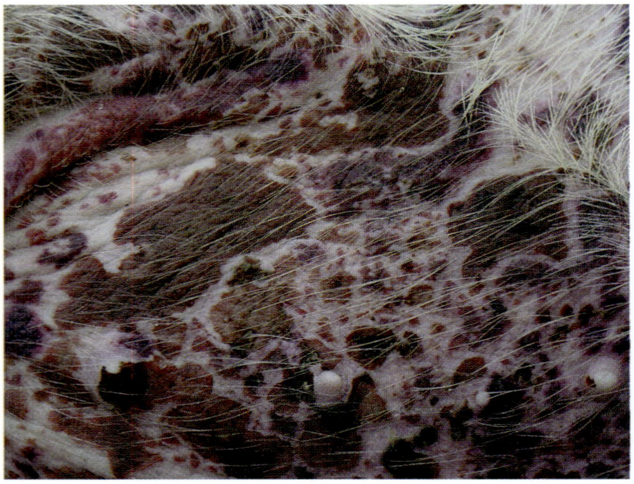

Figure 59.5 Skin lesions in porcine dermatopathy and nephropathy syndrome (PDNS) include raised purpuric lesions progressing to multifocal erythematous crusts with a black centre. (Reprinted with permission from Ted Clark.)

Scabies

The most significant skin disease of pigs is sarcoptic mange and there is only limited evidence that this involves an allergic reaction. This disease is considered to be common, widely spread, and well recognized; it causes significant disease and requires control measures to reduce the impact on production. There have been numerous reviews of this condition and the aim here is to review the evidence that infestation may lead to an allergic response [14,35,36].

The clinical signs of sarcoptic mange are primarily related to pruritus, with excessive rubbing and scratching. Mites are particularly likely to be found in the ear canals and with progression of the infestation secondary lesions of crusting and excoriation on the pinnae may be observed. This is followed by a generalized erythematous macular–papular eruption over the whole of the trunk, particularly on the rump, flank, and abdomen

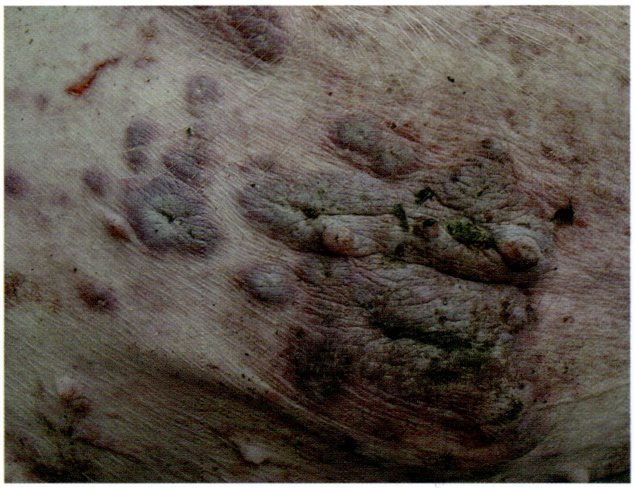

Figure 59.6 Intense cutaneous and systemic hypereosinophilia. (Reprinted with permission from Ted Clark.)

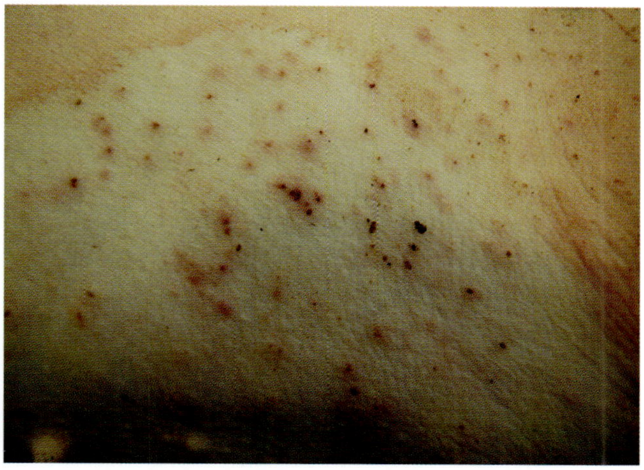

Figure 59.7 Erythematous macular-papular eruption on the trunk of a fattening pig with chronic sarcoptic mange.

(Figure 59.7). Histopathological findings include variable numbers of eosinophilic pustules within the epidermis associated with focal areas of erosion and ulceration, accompanied by mixed inflammatory cell infiltrates at the viable interface. In some pigs, especially when untreated and pigs debilitated with other diseases, lesions may progress to severe crusting of the ears, neck, and head, with large to enormous numbers of mites. In general terms, the younger growing pigs are likely to present with the pruritic hypersensitive form of scabies, with small numbers of mites, while older pigs such as sows may present with the chronic hyperkeratotic form with many mites. There is a third group of pigs that seem to harbour small numbers of mites in their ear canals. They show limited clinical signs of infestation and may act as an important reservoir of infection in chronically infected herds; this is a chronic-subclinical form.

The presence of scabies has been assessed at the farm level from the visual inspection of fattened pigs at the abattoir using a sarcoptic mange severity score based on the number and distribution of erythematous papules. The scoring system is correlated with clinical signs, particularly pruritus and the burden of mite infestation, although mites are mainly found in the ears and not on the trunk [37]. Similar lesions may, on some farms, be associated with biting flies, lice infestation, and even fleas; so it is important to assess the potential importance of other agents that can cause skin lesions. Other differential diagnoses that may be considered include environmental factors such as sunburn or photosensitization; dietary factors such as niacin or biotin deficiency, infectious agents such as dermatophytosis, swine pox, and exudative dermatitis (greasy pig disease); also some forms of parakeratosis [14,34,35].

Early experimental studies reported histopathological findings that were consistent with immediate and delayed hypersensitivity responses when mites were injected into the skin of infested pigs [38]. These studies were extended and led to the presumption that pigs with scabies responded in a similar manner to guinea pigs with fleas. Intradermal test reactions to scabies mite extracts were observed at 15 minutes and 24 hours in piglets at 3, 7, 17, and 20 weeks after infection. This suggested that there was an initial induction phase, followed by a stage of delayed reactions only, then later by immediate and delayed reactions [39]. These findings were extended by Davis and Moon [40] who infested piglets with two doses of scabies mites and then injected intradermally a scabies mite extract. Immediate skin test reactions were observed after 15 minutes as erythematous lesions; after 24 hours delayed hypersensitivity reactions were presumed when oedematous indurated lesions were observed. Over a 9-week study period there appeared to be four phases to the skin test reactions: phase one was one of induction; followed by delayed hypersensitivity reactions only; phase three saw immediate and delayed reactions; and phase four was associated with immediate reactions only. This latter phase was not associated with the dose of scabies mite exposure.

In recent years, pigs have been used as a model to explore the pathogenesis and immune responses in scabies infestations; this has included repeated passage of mites through several litters using oral dexamethasone to suppress the immune system. Interestingly, as in dogs infested with scabies when receiving steroids, mite numbers can increase substantially with such therapy, albeit in some but not other pigs, enabling collection of sufficient material to carry out detailed molecular and genetic studies [41]. *Sarcoptes scabiei* antigens have been studied in order to find candidate genes to provide better diagnostic tools and even candidate antigens for vaccines. Some of these antigens, as in psoroptic mange in sheep, are homologous to house dust mite allergens and may have a role in immune evasion by the parasite [42–45].

Control of porcine scabies can be established by taking into account three key factors: piglets become infested after birth from their dam or contact with other infested pigs; mites have a limited lifespan off the host; and acaricides are highly effective [36]. Careful attention to biosecurity, hygiene, treatment of all animals in a management group, and an all-in then all-out system of management can prove effective and economic for the eradication of scabies in pig herds.

Sheep

There are various experimental studies that report on allergic responses of sheep involving the gastrointestinal and respiratory tracts and skin. Reagents have been developed to detect serum IgE [46]. Studies of the immunopathogenesis of skin diseases have focused on psoroptic mange (covered by van den Broek and Burgess in Chapter 58) and pediculosis. There have been suggestions that sheep may be afflicted with atopic dermatitis although in other species this is assumed to have a genetic basis, which has never been clearly documented in sheep. The term atopic dermatitis has been used in association with skin disease involving *Culicoides* midges and *Bovicola* chewing lice.

*Insect bite (*Culicoides*) hypersensitivity in sheep*

Hypersensitivity reactions to the allergens presented to sheep and possibly goats through the biting activity of *Culicoides* spp. are well recognized wherever there are such midges. Cases are usually sporadic and in some flocks up to 40% of ewes may be affected [47,48]; seasonal recurrence may be seen year after year in some individuals. Skin lesions are associated with pruritus, which is typically apparent from spring to the summer months and particularly September to October [49]. The non-wool areas of the body are usually affected, including especially the ventral trunk, also the head, including the periocular, peribuccal, and nasal regions, pinnae including the inner and outer aspects of the tips, medial aspect of the legs, udder, and teats (Figure 59.8). Lesions can vary from small crusts to marked thickening of the skin with ulceration and crust formation. Pruritus may be manifest as foot stamping and dropping to the ground and sternal recumbency. Studies have found that exposure to *Culicoides* spp. can be documented and help to explain the prevalence of disease in certain geographical areas.

Histopathological findings may include acanthosis, spongiosis, orthokeratotic hyperkeratosis, perivascular dermatitis with eosinophils, mast cells, and mononuclear cells. There can be oedema, eosinophilic pustules, and changes due to secondary microbial infection [50]; all of

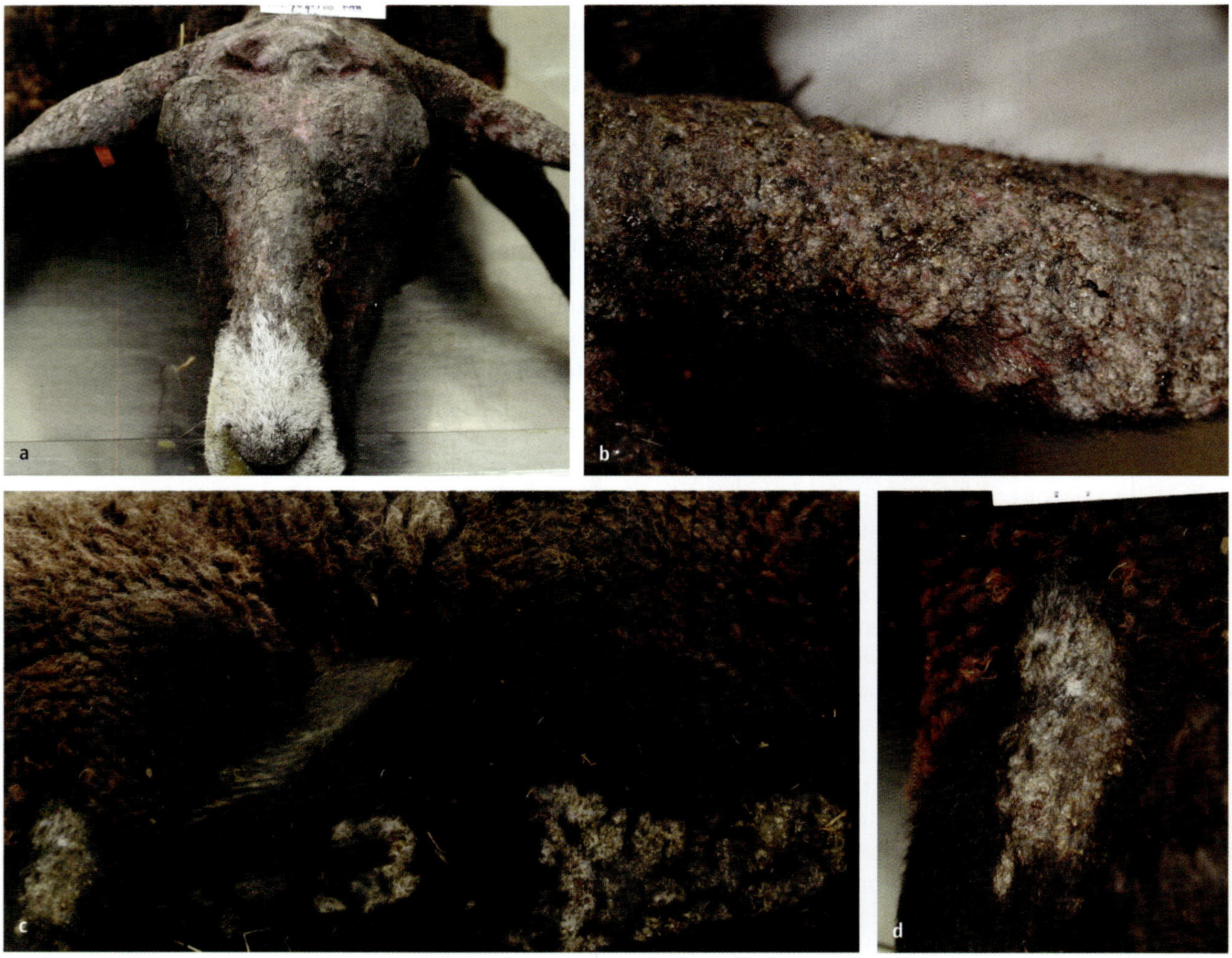

Figure 59.8 Views of (a) the face, (b) the pinna, (c) the ventral trunk, and (d) the mid foreleg of a Zwarbles ewe with severe chronic seasonal pruritic dermatosis presumed to be insect bite hypersensitivity. (Reprinted with permission from Kate Whitaker.)

these changes are consistent with an allergic response to ectoparasite activity although in themselves they do not establish hard evidence for an allergic disease process. An early description of this condition was given by Scott and Campbell [51] which included intradermal testing of an affected and several unaffected sheep using allergens employed for testing dogs, with positive reactions to pollen and mould allergens observed only in the affected ewe. One can also see a peripheral eosinophilia with routine haematology [49]. In a study carried out in 1978 and reported in 1987, Rambouillet and Columbia ewes and lambs were naturally and experimentally exposed to mosquitoes and shown to have positive skin test reactions to mosquito extracts from *Aedes dorsalis* and *A. aegypti*; passive cutaneous anaphylaxis tests were negative. It was concluded that the sheep had immediate type hypersensitivity reactions [52].

Treatment may rely on topical and systemic glucocorticoids, with antimicrobial agents as required. Housing affected sheep to reduce exposure and fly avoidance measures are important for both prevention and treatment. Regular application of topical insecticides and repellents may be useful adjunct measures.

Lice

The chewing louse *Bovicola ovis* has been associated with allergic skin disease in sheep [53]. Louse infestation has been referred to as scatter cockle and the papular lesions are a result of the feeding activity of the lice. Histopathological findings may include superficial perivascular dermatitis, particularly with an infiltrate of eosinophils. Histological analysis of intradermal injections of louse antigens and analysis of cytokine expression point to an immediate and late-phase hypersensitivity response in lambs that are infested with lice. The concentrations of IgE antibodies, both total and antigen-specific for *B. ovis*, are greater in infected compared with naïve lambs. Infected lambs also have more IgE^{+} cells and IgE staining in the dermis. The cutaneous findings suggest that IgE may play a significant role in the skin compared with circulating IgE. The specific and total IgE concentrations are not correlated with louse infestation scores and there is no clear evidence that immune responses are protective [46,54].

Chorioptes

A well recognized clinical presentation for chorioptes mite infestation is scrotal mange, which is assumed to be a form of hypersensitivity reaction. Typically, the lower part of the scrotum will have weeping shallow sores, alopecia, crusting, and there will be signs of pruritus; lesions can extend to the distal limbs (which is the usual presentation for chorioptic mange in most species of livestock) and the poll. Small numbers of mites may be found with multiple superficial skin scrapings. Histopathological findings are typical of those associated with ectoparasite infestation and may be construed to reflect an allergic reaction. Treatment usually relies on topical agents such as diazinon-based dips (see also Chorioptes in camelids and goats). If the condition is left untreated then the chronically affected skin will lead to a rise in scrotal temperature and potentially this may have an impact on fertility [55]. Macrocyclic lactones such as ivermectin and doramectin may have some impact on mite numbers.

The prevalence of chorioptes mite infestation in sheep (ewes and rams) may be influenced by measures used to control psoroptic mange. In general, disease is considered to be uncommon and mites may be carried with no clinical signs. Mites feed on epidermal debris and can cause exudative dermatitis of the wool-less areas especially on the lower limbs including the pasterns and poll [56].

Scabies

Although sarcoptic mange is uncommon in sheep it is possible that an allergic response develops when sheep are infested and there is some experimental evidence that an IgE response has a role to play in resistance to reinfection. It has been suggested that further studies are indicated to determine the value of allergens that incite IgE and IgG responses for the diagnosis of scabies and possibly for vaccination [57].

Flea bite hypersensitivity in livestock species

Fleas have been reported to infest a wide variety of livestock species [14,58]. Allergic responses to such infestation has been inferred from the severe clinical signs, which may include pruritus (which may be manifest as restlessness, rubbing, and chewing), excoriations, alopecia, and scaling, particularly of the lower limbs, also the neck and shoulder regions, in lambs, kids, and calves [59,60]. In a Libyan study, companion animals were shown to harbour *Ctenocephalides felis felis* while livestock had *Ct. felis stongylus*, thus suggesting some host adaptation of the *Ct. felis* spp., although other studies have reported *Ct. felis felis* and *Pulex irritans* on calves, kids, and lambs [61–63].

The histopathological findings are consistent with an allergic response and may include acanthosis, orthokeratotic hyperkeratosis, oedema, and a marked dermal infiltrate of eosinophils and lymphocytes [59,61]. Reports from Libya and Israel may reflect that disease is particularly seen in Mediterranean countries and this may be due to livestock living in close proximity with farm cats and dogs [64]. Heavy infestations may be associated with anaemia. There are no definitive studies of the allergic response of livestock to flea bites in terms of the investigation of the immunopathogenesis including serological or intradermal testing.

In the future, studies of ectoparasites in livestock species (particularly cattle and sheep) will focus on developing better diagnostic tests that can quickly and with high specificity screen a flock or herd for ectoparasites exposure, particularly for psoroptes and scabies [65,66], and they may be based on recombinant allergens. Such studies may also lead to candidate genes for vaccines given that alternative approaches to the control of ectoparasites are required beyond the reliance on products, particularly MLs, which are also used to control endoparasites. With growing resistance of nematodes to anthelmintics and concerns about environmental impact there will be pressure to reduce reliance on such products for the control of ectoparasites [67,68]. For the individual allergic livestock case, the study of significant allergens may facilitate not only improved diagnosis but maybe a route to immunotherapy and better control of the skin disease process. This approach may be more likely to be adopted for those animals where the resources are available to treat it in a similar fashion to a companion animal such as an atopic dog.

Acknowledgements

The author wishes to thank:

- Bruce Wilkie and colleagues (University of Guelph, Canada) for permission to reproduce their figures of allergic skin reactions in pigs.
- Kate Whitaker (formerly of AHVLA, Preston, UK) for the images of the sheep with *Culicoides* hypersensitivity.
- Natalie Jewell (AHVLA, Carmarthen, UK) for the figure of the young alpaca with scabies.
- The pig with scabies and the goat with chorioptic mange were case material from AHVLA, Shrewsbury.
- Ted Clark (University of Saskatoon, Canada) for the figures of porcine hypereosinophilia and PDNS.
- Mick Millar and Mark Hinds, AHVLA, Langford, UK and the local private vet, respectively, for the figure of a cow with suspected allergic skin lesions and to Jan Bradshaw for the histopathology report.

References

1. Bonacic C. South American Camelids. In: Webster J, ed. *Management and Welfare of Farm Animals: The UFAW Farm Handbook*, 5th edn. Oxford: Wiley Blackwell, 2011: 477–499.
2. Bornstein S. Important ectoparasites of alpaca (*Vicugna pacos*) *Acta Veterinaria Scandinavica* 2010; **52** (Suppl. 1): S17.
3. Foster A, Jackson A, D'Alterio GL. Skin diseases of South American camelids. *In Practice* 2007; **29**: 216–223.
4. Lusat J, Morgan ER, Wall R. Mange in alpacas, llamas and goats in the UK: incidence and risk. *Veterinary Parasitology* 2012; **163**: 179–184.
5. Schlögl C, Bork-Mimm S, Pfister K. Investigation on the infestation of South American camelids with external parasites. *Tierarztliche Praxis. Ausgabe G, Grosstiere/Nutztiere* 2010; **38**: 293–296.
6. Jarvinen JA, Miller JA, Oehler DD. Pharmacokinetics of ivermectin in llamas (*Lama glama*). *Veterinary Record* 2002; **150**: 344–346.
7. Twomey DF, Birch ES, Schock A. Outbreak of sarcoptic mange in alpacas (*Vicugna pacos*) and control with repeated subcutaneous ivermectin injections. *Veterinary Parasitology* 2009; **159**: 186–191
8. Vine NJ, Keevill G, Foster AP. Sarcoptic mange in alpacas. *Veterinary Record* 2010; **167**: 946–947.
9. Lau P, Hill PB, Rybníček J, *et al.* Sarcoptic mange in three alpacas treated successfully with amitraz. *Veterinary Dermatology* 2007; **18**: 272–277.
10. Scott DW, Vogel JW, Fleis RI, *et al.* Skin diseases in the alpaca (*Vicugna pacos*): a literature review and retrospective analysis of 68 cases (Cornell University 1997–2006). *Veterinary Dermatology* 2011; **22**: 2–16.
11. D'Alterio GL, Jackson AP, Knowles TG, *et al.* Comparative study of the efficacy of eprinomectin versus ivermectin, and field efficacy of eprinomectin only, for the treatment of Chorioptes mange in alpacas. *Veterinary Parasitology* 2005; **130**: 267–275.
12. Gershwin LJ. Bovine immunoglobulin E. *Veterinary Immunology and Immunopathology* 2009; **132**: 2–6.
13. Halliwell REW, Gorman NT. Hypersensitivity lung disease. In: Halliwell REW, Gorman NT, eds. *Veterinary Clinical Immunology*. Philadelphia, PA: WB Saunders, 1989: 359–377.
14. Scott DW. *Large Animal Dermatology*. Philadelphia: WB Saunders Company, 1988: 207–283 (parasites); 288–333 (allergy).
15. Ginn PE, Mansell JL, Rakich PM. Skin and appendages. In: Maxie MG, ed. *Jubb, Kennedy and Palmer's Pathology of Domestic Animals*, 5th edn. Philadelphia, PA: Elsevier Saunders, 2007; 623–626.
16. Wiseman A, Gibbs HA, McGregor AB. Bovine nasal granuloma (atopic rhinitis) in Britain. *Veterinary Record* 1982; **110**: 420–421.
17. Radostits OM, Gay CC, Hincliff KW, *et al. Veterinary Medicine: a Textbook of the Diseases of Cattle, Horses, Sheep, Pigs and Goats*, 10th edn. Edinburgh: Saunders Elsevier, 2007: 1935–1936.
18. Pemberton DH, White WE, Hore DE. Bovine nasal granuloma (atopic rhinitis) in Victoria. Experimental reproduction by the production of immediate type hypersensitivity in the nasal mucosa. *Australian Veterinary Journal* 1977; **53**: 201–207.
19. Caswell JL, Williams KJ. Respiratory system. In: Maxie MG, ed. *Jubb, Kennedy and Palmer's Pathology of Domestic Animals*, Vol. 2, 5th edn. Philadelphia, PA: Elsevier Saunders, 2007: 568–569.
20. Wilkie BN. Hypersensitivity pneumonitis: experimental production in calves with antigens of *Micropolyspora faeni*. *Canadian Journal of Comparative Medicine* 1976; **40**: 221–227.
21. Blowey RW, Weaver AD. *Color Atlas of Diseases and Disorders of Cattle*, 3rd edn. Edinburgh: Mosby Elsevier, 2011: 29–51.
22. Scott DW. Skin diseases. In: Divers TJ, Peel SF, eds. *Rebhun's Diseases of Dairy Cattle*, 2nd edn. St Louis, MO: Saunders Elsevier, 2008: 295–326.
23. Yeruham I, Yadin H, Haymovich M, *et al.* Adverse reactions to FMD vaccine. *Veterinary Dermatology* 2001; **12**: 197–201.
24. Campbell SG. Milk allergy, an autoallergic disease of cattle. *Cornell Veterinarian* 1970; **60**: 684–721.
25. Onda K, Yagisawa T, Matsui T, *et al.* Contact dermatitis in dairy cattle caused by calcium cyanamide. *Veterinary Record* 2008; **163**: 418–422.
26. Holzhauer M, Sampimon OC, Sol J, *et al.* Allergic contact dermatitis of bovine teat skin caused by milking machine cluster rubber. *Veterinary Record* 2004; **154**: 208–209.

27. Bates P. *External Parasites of Small Ruminants: a Practical Guide to their Prevention and Control*. Wallingford, Oxford, UK: CAB International, 2012: 15–48.
28. Lespine A, Chartier C, Hoste H, *et al*. Endectocides in goats: pharmacology, efficacy and use conditions in the context of anthelmintics resistance. *Small Ruminant Research* 2012; **103**: 10–17.
29. Humann-Ziehank E, Ganter M, Egen S, *et al*. Differential diagnostic, treatment trial and course of an allergic dermatitis in a goat. *Tierarztliche Praxis Ausgabe Grosstiere Nutztiere* 2001; **29**: 356–360.
30. Wilkie BN, Rupa P, Schmied J. Practical immunoregulation: neonatal immune response variation and prophylaxis of experimental food allergy in pigs. *Veterinary Immunology and Immunopathology* 2012; **148**: 110–115.
31. Rupa P, Schmied J, Wilkie BN. Porcine allergy and IgE. *Veterinary Immunology and Immunopathology* 2009; **132**: 41–45.
32. Bode G, Clausing P, Gervais F, *et al*. (Steering Group of the RETHINK Project). The utility of the minipig as an animal model in regulatory toxicology. *Journal of Pharmacological and Toxicological Methods* 2010; **62**: 196–220.
33. Vana G, Meingassner JG. Morphologic and immunohistochemical features of experimentally induced allergic contact dermatitis in Göttingen Minipigs. *Veterinary Pathology* 2000; **37**: 565–580.
34. Opriessnig T, Langohr I. Current state of knowledge on porcine circovirus type 2-associated lesions. *Veterinary Pathology* 2013; **50**: 23–38.
35. Bornstein S. Sarcoptic mange in pigs. *Pig News and Information* 2004; **25**: 11N–24N.
36. Greve JH, Davies P. External parasites. In: Zimmerman JJ, Karriker LA, Ramirez A, *et al*., eds. *Diseases of Swine*, 10th edn. Ames, IA: John Wiley, 2012: 885–894.
37. Pointon AM, Mercy AR, Backstrom L, *et al*. Disease surveillance at slaughter. In: Leman AD, Straw BE, Mengeling WL, *et al*., eds. *Diseases of Swine*, 7th edn. Ames, IA: Iowa State University Press, 1992: 968–981.
38. Sheahan BJ. Pathology of *Sarcoptes scabiei* infection in pigs: I. Naturally occurring and experimentally induced lesions. *Journal of Comparative Pathology* 1975; **85**: 87–95.
39. Sheahan BJ. Pathology of *Sarcoptes scabiei* infection in pigs: II. histological, histochemical and ultrastructural changes at skin test sites. *Journal of Comparative Pathology* 1975; **85**: 97–100.
40. Davis DP, Moon RD. Density of itch mite, *Sarcoptes scabiei* (Acari: Sarcoptidae) and temporal development of cutaneous hypersensitivity in swine mange. *Veterinary Parasitology* 1990; **36**: 285–293.
41. Mounsey KM, Ho MF, Kelly A, *et al*. A tractable experimental model for study of human and animal scabies. *PLoS Neglected Tropical Diseases* 2010; **4**: e756.
42. Hejduk G, Hofstätter K, Löwenstein M, *et al*. Characterisation of Sarcoptes scabiei antigens. *Parasitology Research* 2011; **108**: 309–315.
43. Kuhn C, Lucius R, Matthes HF, *et al*. Characterisation of recombinant immunoreactive antigens of the scab mite Sarcoptes scabiei. *Veterinary Parasitology* 2008; **153**: 329–337.
44. Mika A, Goh P, Holt DC, *et al*. Scabies mite peritrophins are potential targets of human host innate immunity. *PLoS Neglected Tropical Diseases* 2011; **5**: e1331.
45. Zhang R, Jise Q, Zheng W, *et al*. Characterization and evaluation of a *Sarcoptes scabiei* allergen as a candidate vaccine. *Parasites and Vectors* 2012; **5**: 176.
46. Shaw R, Pfeffer A, Bischof R. Ovine IgE and its role in immunological protection and disease. *Veterinary Immunology and Immunopathology* 2009; **132**: 31–40.
47. Connan RM, Lloyd S. Seasonal allergic dermatitis in sheep. *Veterinary Record* 1988; **123**: 335–337.
48. Winter A, Dawson S. Apparent hypersensitivity to *Culicoides* species in sheep. *Veterinary Record* 2000; **147**: 427–428.
49. Yeruham I, Perl S, Braverman Y. Seasonal allergic dermatitis in sheep associated with *Ctenocephalides* and *Culicoides* bites. *Veterinary Dermatology* 2004; **15**: 377–380.
50. Corrêa TG, Ferreira JM, Riet-Correa G, *et al*. Seasonal allergic dermatitis in sheep in southern Brazil caused by *Culicoides insignis* (Diptera: Ceratopogonidae). *Veterinary Parasitology* 2007; **145**: 181–185.
51. Scott DW. Campbell SG. A seasonal pruritic dermatitis resembling atopy in sheep. *Agri-Practice* 1987; **8**: 46–49.
52. Jones CJ, Lloyd JE. Hypersensitivity reactions and hematoloic changes in sheep exposed to mosquito (Diptera; Culicoidae) feeding. *Journal of Medical Entomology* 1987; **24**: 71–76.
53. James PJ. Do sheep regulate the size of their mallophagan louse populations? *International Journal of Parasitology* 1999; **29**: 869–875.
54. Shu D, Pfeffer A, Pernthaner A. Cutaneous cytokine gene expression and cellular responses in lambs infested with the louse, *Bovicola ovis*, and following intradermal injection of crude louse antigen. *Veterinary Immunology and Immunopathology* 2009; **129**: 82–92.
55. Heath ACG. The scrotal mange mite, *Chorioptes bovis* (Hering, 1845) on sheep: seasonality, pathogenicity and intra-flock transfer. *New Zealand Veterinary Journal* 1978; **26**: 299–310.
56. Sargison ND, Scott PR, Wilson DJ, *et al*. Chorioptic mange in British Suffolk rams. *Veterinary Record* 2000; **147**: 135–136.
57. Rodríguez-Cadenas F, Carbajal-González MT, Fregeneda-Grandes JM, *et al*. Clinical evaluation and antibody responses in sheep after primary and secondary experimental challenges with the mange mite Sarcoptes scabiei var. ovis. *Veterinary Immunology Immunopathology* 2010; **133**: 109–116.
58. Scott DW. *Color Atlas of Farm Animal Dermatology*. Oxford: Blackwell Publishing; 2007: 29, 123, 133, 165, 175, 212.
59. Kaal JF, Baker K, Torgerson PR. Epidemiology of flea infestation of ruminants in Libya. *Veterinary Parasitology* 2006; **141**: 313–318.
60. Christodoulopoulos G. Skin lesions in sheep infested with fleas. *Veterinary Parasitology* 2011; **181**: 397–398.
61. Yeruham I, Rosen S, Perl S. An apparent flea-allergy dermatitis in kids and lambs. *Journal of Veterinary Medicine. Series A* 1997; **44**: 391–397.
62. Christodoulopoulos G, Theodoropoulos G, Kominakis A, *et al*. Biological, seasonal and environmental factors associated with *Pulex irritans* infestation of dairy goats in Greece. *Veterinary Parasitology* 2006; **137**: 137–143.
63. Araújo FR, Silva MP, Lopes AA, *et al*. Severe cat flea infestation of dairy calves in Brazil. *Veterinary Parasitology* 1998; **80**: 83–86.
64. Colebrook E, Wall R. Ectoparasites of livestock in Europe and the Mediterranean region. *Veterinary Parasitology* 2004; **120**: 251–274.
65. Wells B, Burgess STG, McNeilly TN, *et al*. Recent developments in the diagnosis of ectoparasite infections and disease through a better understanding of parasite biology and host responses. *Molecular and Cellular Probes* 2012; **26**: 47–53.
66. Demeler J, Schein E, von Samson-Himmelstjerna G. Advances in laboratory diagnosis of parasitic infections of sheep. *Veterinary Parasitology* 2012; **189**: 52–64.
67. Burgess CGS, Bartley Y, Redman E, *et al*. A survey of the trichostrongylid nematode species on UK sheep farms and associated anthelmintic control practices. *Veterinary Parasitology* 2012; **189**: 299–307.
68. Beynon SA. Potential environmental consequences of administration of ectoparasiticides to sheep. *Veterinary Parasitology* 2012; **189**: 125–135.

60

Allergies in birds

Claudia S. Nett-Mettler

Vetderm.ch-Dermatologie und Allergologie fuer Tiere, c/o Ennetsee Klinik für Kleintiere AG, CH-Huenenberg, Switzerland

Conflict of interest: none declared.

Feather-picking

Feather-picking or feather-plucking is a frequently observed dermatological syndrome in birds and especially in psittaciformes [1–4]. The condition is characterized by an obsessive destructive behaviour pattern, resulting in amputated and damaged feathers or skin. Feather-picking prevents normal feather growth.

Feather-picking, feather-plucking, and automutilation are common problems of birds in captivity and in particular of caged psittacines (Figure 60.1). Complaints involving feather loss or damage are the most common reason for seeking veterinary attention [1,2,5]. Feather-picking is a result of various underlying aetiologies and thus a challenging and often frustrating problem for bird owners and veterinarians alike. Disorders of the gastrointestinal, hepatic, renal, pancreatic, and haematopoietic system have been identified in some cases. Nutritional deficiencies caused by a poor diet or chronic diseases are often underlying factors in skin and feather disorders in avian patients. A variety of infectious agents, including parasites, bacteria, fungi, and viruses, have also been associated with feather-picking [1,3–6]. Many cases are considered to be poorly defined psychological disorders or idiopathic [5,7]. Other feather-pickers are believed to be pruritic with allergies being proposed as an underlying aetiologic condition. Defining pruritus in a feather-picking bird is challenging; birds that focus on one part of the body or birds with aggressive picking behaviour are more likely to be pruritic [2]. The best results are obtained by identifying and removing the underlying cause, improving the environment, using appropriate drugs if indicated, and utilizing counter-conditioning techniques [1].

The change in the appearance of the bird can lead to a marked reduction in the aesthetic appeal of the bird; furthermore, feather-picking can result in serious health problems including feather follicle and skin infections, excoriations, and ulcerations (Figure 60.2) [2]. As in dogs and cats with pruritic behaviour, the reasons for feather-plucking can be manifold. To identify the underlying cause often involves multiple diagnostic steps and treatment trials and many cases remain undiagnosed [1,6,7].

The diagnostic evaluation of birds with skin and feather diseases corresponds to the approach used in mammalian dermatology. Taking an in-depth history is the first step in diagnosing dermatologic disorders in birds and can help to define a possible underlying cause. Specific information regarding the dietary history (types of food, amount eaten, frequency of feeding), the housing, the social environment, as well as the bird's origin, should be obtained in order to better understand the possible underlying cause. Malnutrition caused by a poor diet, changes in hormone levels (e.g. sex hormones), parasites, and chronic diseases are common underlying factors in skin diseases of pet birds. Non-medical causes are psychological and/or stress related. The dermatological expression of hypersensitivity/allergy is still poorly understood in pet birds. It is, therefore, important to

Veterinary Allergy, First Edition. Edited by Chiara Noli, Aiden Foster, and Wayne Rosenkrantz.

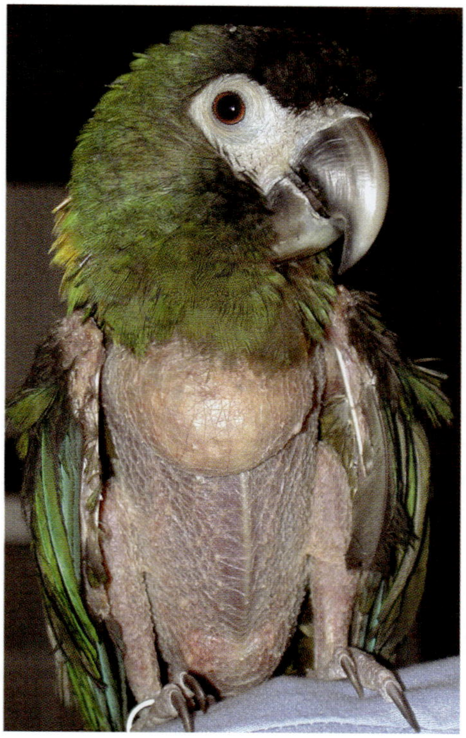

Figure 60.1 Feather-picking bird.

take a general approach and to attempt to reach a specific diagnosis.

Although feather-picking is not synonymous with pruritus, it is important for the clinician to determine whether feather and skin lesions are self-induced. The distribution of the feather lesions is a useful sign in birds with feather-picking. Typically, affected body sites are the chest, the axillary region and the rump (Figure 60.1). Picked or chewed feathers usually exhibit some damage from the beak such as a ragged, irregular appearance. Such mutilated feathers are confined to body areas where the bird can chew itself. Most commonly, flight and tail feathers are affected, while the top of the head and back of the neck are areas that are spared in birds presenting with advanced alopecia or evidence of self-mutilation [2]. In chronic cases, feather-picking results in skin excoriations and ulcerations, leading to a lack of normal insulation (Figure 60.2). Chronic feather-pickers are thus more prone to develop stress-induced disease [2].

Hypersensitivity and allergic reactions in avian species

Evidence for allergic skin conditions in birds has only been reported in recent years. Notably, some psittacines can manifest signs of pruritus and are considered to be

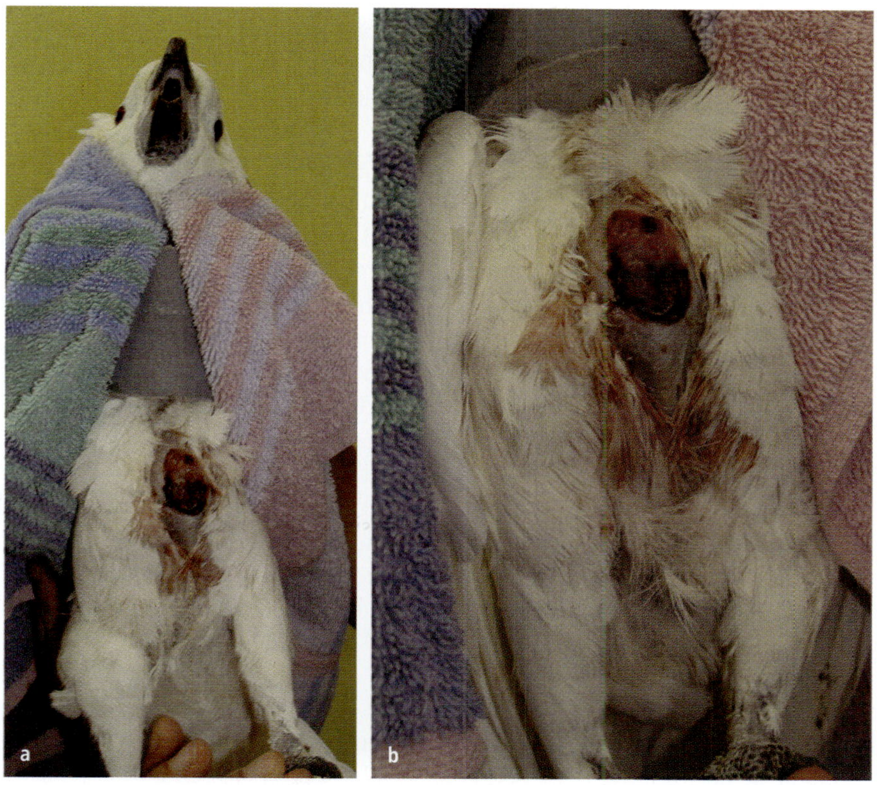

Figure 60.2 Feather-picking bird (a) with secondary deep ulceration on the proventer area (b).

susceptible to allergic skin diseases [2,7–9]. Furthermore, multiple anecdotal reports have provided evidence that antihistamines, essential fatty acids, glucocorticoids, and dietary and environmental changes might be helpful in addressing feather-picking in birds [7,8,10], just as the same treatments are used in canine allergic dermatitis [11].

Mast cells have been identified in birds and inflammatory mediators, such as histamine and serotonin, are released upon degranulation [8]. In pigeons receiving a paramyxovirus 1 vaccine, anaphylactic reactions have been documented [12]. Thus it is likely that cutaneous allergies might be an underlying cause for some feather-picking psittacines [7,8].

Several histopathological patterns of inflammation described in avian skin specimens further support the concept that allergic dermatitis could cause feather-picking [13,14]. Histological patterns described include angiocentric accumulation of mainly lymphoplasmacytic cells, a pattern similar to that seen in hypersensitivity dermatitis in mammals [13]. A recent study investigated the histologic findings in a large number of feather-picking psittacines comparing picked with normal skin [14]. The number of birds with inflammatory skin disease in the sampled population was 51%, with macaws, lorikeets, and Amazons being over represented. The diagnosis of inflammatory skin disease was based on the presence of perivascular inflammation of clinically affected and unaffected biopsy sites. The inflammatory infiltrate mainly consisted of lymphocytes, fewer plasma cells, histiocytes, and eosinophilic granulocytes. A varying degree of oedema, epidermal and follicular hyperkeratosis, and perivascular pulpitis were present in some cases [14]. The pattern and the cellular constituents of the inflammation were considered to be suggestive of a cutaneous hypersensitivity disorder.

In chickens sensitized to *Mycobacterium tuberculosis*, repeated exposure resulted in oedema at the injection site and subsequent infiltration of heterophils and mononuclear cells, indicating acute inflammation compatible with hypersensitivity [15]. Another study in chickens reported an early up-regulation of cytokine genes (interleukin (IL)-4, IL-6, IL-10 and interferon-gamma) and infiltration of eosinophils along with macrophages, $CD8^+$, and $CD4^+$ T cells at the site of induction of skin contact hypersensitivity with dinitrofluorobenzene [16].

Intradermal testing in normal and feather-picking psittacines was investigated and allergies were considered as a possible underlying cause in feather-picking [7].

All of these observations have led to the commonly accepted view that cutaneous allergies exist in avian species and that they might be an underlying cause for feather-picking.

Allergen testing in avian species

Allergen testing is the mainstay of detecting potentially significant allergens in mammalian species, including dogs, cats, horses, sheep, and humans. The results may be used to prescribe immunotherapy, which is an important treatment for atopic dermatitis [11,17,18].

Serology testing

In dogs, cats, and horses, serum allergen-specific IgE tests are widely used to identify clinically relevant allergens in atopic animals and to select allergens for allergen-specific immunotherapy. Immunotherapy is the only therapy for which there is evidence of efficacy in canine atopic dermatitis resulting in modulation of the immunological response [19].

In contrast to mammals, birds possess an immunoglobulin isotype called IgY which is functionally analogous to IgG of mammals; both isotypes are present in the serum at high concentrations and provide defence against microbial infection. During the evolution of mammals, IgY evolved into both IgG and IgE; the latter is involved in antiparasitic responses and hypersensitivity. This divergence did not occur in avians and the ancestral isotype has been conserved. Although IgY is functionally similar to IgG, its structure appears to have conserved features of both IgG and IgE [20]. In birds, serum allergen testing is currently not available. If such a serum test were to be developed it would need to detect allergen-specific IgY. The role of allergen-specific IgY antibodies in allergic diseases remains to be established in birds.

Intradermal testing

In dogs, cats, horses, and sheep intradermal testing has been commonly used to identify potentially significant allergens, particularly for atopic dermatitis [21,22]; furthermore, it has been used to select allergens for immunotherapy.

Intradermal testing is increasingly used by avian practitioners to aid in the diagnosis of allergic conditions in feather-picking birds. However, some studies reported difficulties in providing convincing evidence of positive reactions to injected allergens [7,9]. Furthermore, there are no defined protocols for intradermal testing. To the author's knowledge, only three studies have been reported evaluating intradermal testing in avian species [7,9,23].

Macwhirter *et al.* attempted to establish an intradermal test in normal and feather-picking psittacines [7]. Due to the variable response to empirical therapies in presumed allergic psittaciformes, the author attempted to elucidate if specific allergens were associated with self-mutilation. The study investigated immediate intradermal test reactivity to a limited number of environmental allergens in normal birds and self-mutilating psittaciformes. Forty-one birds without any evidence of self-mutilation, were used for the study. The skin test was performed on each bird's chest on each side along the keel with a 26-gauge needle injecting 0.02 mL of fluid. Control solutions and allergens included saline, histamine, canary, rye, oat, wheat, maize, grain mill dust, *Dermatophagoides pteronyssinus*, *D. farinae*, and sunflower. The allergen concentration was 4000 protein nitrogen units (PNU)/mL, except for dust mites, which were tested at 120 PNU/mL. Fifteen feather-picking psittaciformes, which were negative for ectoparasites, internal disease, and did not show any signs of sexual or psychological conditions, underwent the same procedure.

The results indicated that the response to histamine was inconsistent, both in normal and clinically affected birds. Only 32% of the normal and 67% of feather-picking birds showed wheal formation at the histamine site. Further, only 1/41 (2%) of the normal birds showed a response to any of the allergens tested whereas 14/15 (93%) of the self-mutilating birds showed a reaction to one or more of the allergens tested. Overall reactions were subtle and short lived. The results of this study suggested that allergens might play a role as causative agents in feather-picking birds, that histamine might not be the ideal positive control for intradermal testing, and that the wheal and flare reaction in birds is faint and inconsistent. These findings resulted in Colombini's attempt to develop and standardize a protocol for skin testing in birds [9].

Colombini *et al.* examined six potential positive control agents in 40 clinically healthy Amazon parrots [9]. The optimal site for intradermal testing was found to be the proventer region adjacent to the keel because this region has no feather follicles allowing for enough space and there is no need to pluck feathers, thus avoiding trauma to the skin. The optimal volume for injections was found to be 0.02 mL. As positive control agents histamine phosphate (1 : 100 000) and compound 48/80 at two different concentrations, codeine phosphate at two different concentrations, deionized water, and antiavian IgG were investigated. Phosphate-buffered saline served as negative control. The injection sites were measured with digital callipers at 5, 10, and 15 minutes for immediate reactions and at 4–6, 24, and 48 hours for late-phase reactions [9]. As in the previous study similar findings were observed [7]. Positive skin test sites lacked erythema and induration, and the proventer region was the best suited area for intradermal testing using 0.02 mL volume per injection. The best reading time was defined at 5 minutes after injecting the control agents. Compared to saline the reaction sites for codeine phosphate 1 : 100 000 w/v were significantly and consistently greater and did not change over time.

The protocol used by Colombini [9] failed to allow subjective grading based on wheal and flare reactions. The difference in wheal diameter—even though statistically significant—was too small to be reliable for clinical use. Consequently, the aim of the third and most recent study was to develop an intradermal testing protocol that could be used for clinical studies [23]. The study investigated the use of intravenous fluorescein as a contrast medium to enhance intradermal test reactions in a practical setting. In cats, which also have faint reactions to intradermal allergen injections, intravenous fluorescein has been used [24,25]. Positive reactions sites could easily be distinguished by the accumulation of fluorescein, which were readily visible with the aid of an ultraviolet light such as a Wood's lamp. This lamp produces light at the appropriate wavelength to excite fluorescein, resulting in green-bluish fluorescence.

Twenty-five Hispaniolan Amazon parrots were anaesthetized and the skin on each side of the keel was chosen as the test site [7,9]. Tested compounds included codeine and histamine phosphate, both at 1 : 100 000 w/v as potential positive controls, with phosphate-buffered saline as the negative control. For each compound 0.02 mL was intradermally injected in duplicate in each bird (Figure 60.3). Fluorescein-sodium 1% was injected into the superficial ulnar vein immediately prior to intradermal testing at a dose of 10 mg/kg. No side effects were recorded. Test sites were read at 5 and 10 minutes using digital callipers under daylight conditions and with a Wood's lamp. Subjective reading under ultraviolet light was based on a scoring system with fluorescence at an untouched skin site serving as a negative control (graded '0'), and fluorescence at a plucked feather follicle

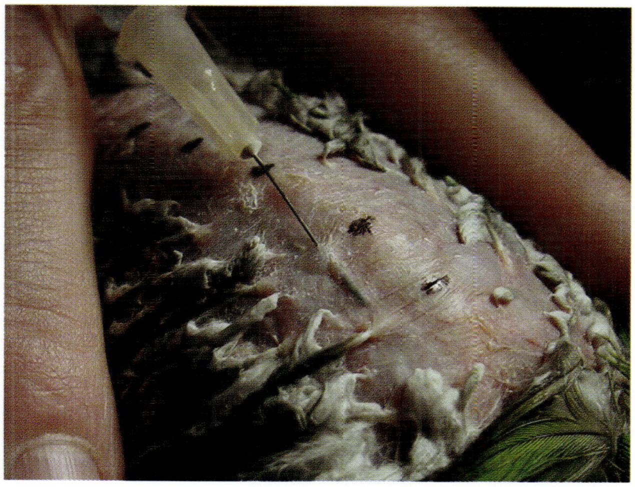

Figure 60.3 Intradermal injection into avian skin.

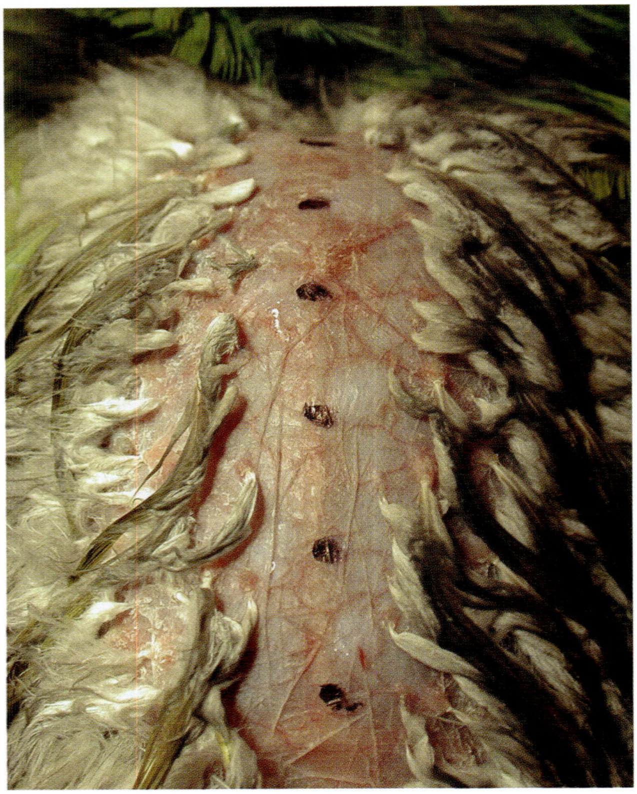

Figure 60.4 Skin test reactions with normal daylight.

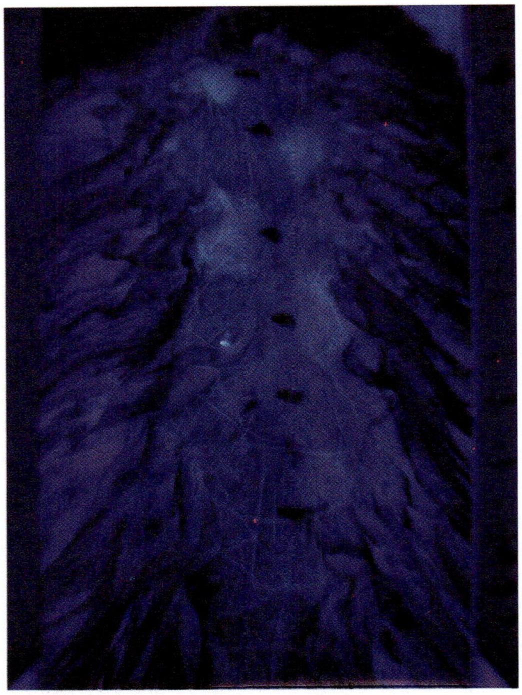

Figure 60.5 Fluorescence of skin test sites observed under a Wood's lamp.

served as a positive control (graded '2'). Under daylight, test sites lacked erythema or induration, two parameters commonly used to subjectively grade positive reactions in mammalian intradermal testing (Figure 60.4) [26,27]. Most reactions were easily detectable under ultraviolet light (Figure 60.5). However, when skin test evaluation was based on subjective reading only, the sensitivity was 84% and specificity was 42% (if saline was accounted as a negative and histamine as a positive control), which are unacceptable for a positive and negative control [23]. Even though codeine phosphate and histamine sites were significantly larger than saline sites at 5 and 10 minutes, in individual birds, saline was often larger than histamine and codeine phosphate independent of light condition or time. These findings lessen the usefulness of the employed compounds as valid positive and negative controls in intradermal testing in psittacines. Subjective reading alone under both light conditions can therefore not be recommended for the grading of intradermal tests in psittacines.

Intravenous fluorescein prior to skin testing in psittacines facilitated the reading of the test; however, subjective assessment produced poor sensitivity and specificity and none of the injected compounds raised consistent reactions neither in size, erythema, induration, or fluorescence [23]. Therefore intradermal testing with or without previous intravenous fluorescein cannot be recommended for practical clinical use.

To date none of the described protocols are sensitive or specific enough to recommend intradermal testing in birds. Future studies should possibly aim at injecting the compounds into or around feather follicles or patch testing at feather follicles sites because these are not only the main target of feather-picking birds but also possess a higher vascular and nerve fibre density than non-feathered areas. Alternatively, *in vitro* serology testing may be investigated based on IgY as the major circulating antibody in avian species.

Treatment options

Because in many feather-picking birds a definitive underlying cause cannot be established and most cases are considered to be idiopathic or poorly defined psychological disorders, there is no easy or single solution to prevent or treat this condition.

Collars can be applied to prevent the bird from further picking but they do not eliminate the cause. Secondary infections should be treated with appropriate antibacterial therapy.

Birds experiencing stress or boredom may benefit from an increased environmental enrichment (e.g.

various foods and toys offered, social contact with the bird keeper, acoustic stimulation) [3].

In many cases behavioural modification is required, including pharmacological interventions such as hormones, antidepressants, tranquilizers, and antihistamines. However, there is scant evidence for drug therapies working for what is speculatively called allergic disease in birds.

In summary, there is limited evidence that hypersensitivity reactions occur in birds and that allergic processes are the cause of feather-picking in psittacines.

References

1. Jenkins JR. Feather picking and self-mutilation in psittacine birds. *Veterinary Clinics of North America: Exotic Animal Practice* 2001; **4**: 651–667.
2. Nett C, Tully T. Anatomy, clinical presentation, and diagnostic approach to feather-picking pet birds. *Compendium for Continuing Education for the Practising Veterinarian* 2003; **25**: 1–11.
3. Rosskopf WJ, Woerpel R. Feather-picking and therapy of skin and feather disorders. In: Rosskopf W, Woerpel R, eds. *Diseases of Cage and Aviary Birds*, 3rd edn. Baltimore: Williams and Wilkins, 1996: 397–405.
4. Rosenthal K. Differential diagnosis of feather-picking in pet birds. *Proceedings of the Association of Avian Veterinarians*, 1993: 108–112.
5. Gill JH. Avian skin diseases. *Veterinary Clinics of North America: Exotic Animal Practice* 2001; **4**: 463–492.
6. Perry RA, Gill J, Cross GM. Disorders of the avian integument. *Veterinary Clinics of North America: Small Animal Practice* 1991; **6**: 1307–1327.
7. Macwhirter PJ, Mueller R. Comparison of immediate skin test reactions in clinically normal and self-mutilating psittaciformes. In: Latimer KS, Steffens WL, eds. *Proceedings of International Virtual Conferences in Veterinary Medicine: Diseases of Psittacine Birds*, May 15–June 30, 1998. University of Georgia, College of Veterinary Medicine.
8. Johnson-Delaney C, Nye RR. Allergies in pet birds. In: Rosskopf W, Woerpel R, eds. *Diseases of Cage and Aviary Birds*, 3rd edn. Baltimore: Williams and Wilkins, 1996: 507–510.
9. Colombini S, Foil CS, Hosgood G, *et al.* Intradermal skin testing in Hispaniolan parrots (*Amazona ventralis*). *Veterinary Dermatology* 2000; **11**: 271–276.
10. Cooper J, Harrison G. Dermatology. In: Ritchie B, Harrison G, Harrison I, eds. *Avian Medicine: Principles and Application*. Lake Worth, FL, USA: Wingers, 1994: 607–639.
11. Olivry T, DeBoer DJ, Favrot C, *et al.* Treatment of canine atopic dermatitis: 2010 clinical practice guidelines from the International Task Force on Canine Atopic Dermatitis. *Veterinary Dermatology* 2010; **21**: 233–248.
12. Wallis AS. Mortality associated with vaccination of pigeons against paramyxovirus type 1. *Veterinary Record* 1984; **114**: 51–52.
13. Schmidt R. Avian skin diseases: a pathologist's perspective. In: Proceedings of the 1st International Conference on Zoological and Avian Medicine, American Association of Zoo Veterinarians, 1987: 117–123. Available at: http://www.aazv.org/?page=318&hhSearchTerms=proceeding
14. Garner MM, Clubb SL, Mitchell MA, *et al.* Feather-picking psittacines: histopathology and species trends. *Veterinary Pathology* 2008; **45**: 401–408.
15. Corrier DE, DeLoach JR. Interdigital skin test for evaluation of delayed hypersensitivity and cutaneous basophil hypersensitivity in young chickens. *American Journal of Veterinary Research* 1990; **51**: 950–954.
16. Abdul-Careem MF, Hunter DB, Thanthrigen-Don N, *et al.* Cellular and cytokine responses associated with dinitrofluorobenzene-induced contact hypersensitivity in the chicken. *Veterinary Immunology Immunopathology* 2008; **122**: 275–284.
17. Olivry T, Mueller RS, International Task Force on Canine Atopic Dermatitis. Evidence-based veterinary dermatology: a systematic review of the pharmacotherapy of canine atopic dermatitis *Veterinary Dermatology* 2003; **14**: 121–146.
18. Loewenstein C, Mueller RS. A review of allergen-specific immunotherapy in human and veterinary medicine. *Veterinary Dermatology* 2009; **20**: 84–98.
19. Olivry T, for the International Task Force of Canine Atopic Dermatitis. New diagnostic criteria for canine atopic dermatitis. *Veterinary Dermatology* 2010; **21**: 124–127.
20. Taylor AI, Sutton BJ, Calvert RA. Mutations in an avian IgY-Fc fragment reveal the locations of monocyte Fc receptor binding sites. *Developmental and Comparative Immunology* 2010; **34**: 97–101.
21. Hillier A, DeBoer DJ. The ACVD task force on canine atopic dermatitis (XVII): intradermal testing. *Veterinary Immunology Immunopathology* 2001; **81**: 289–304.
22. Hillier A. Allergy testing and treatment for canine atopic dermatitis. *Veterinary Medicine* 2002; **97**: 210–224.
23. Nett CS, Hosgood G, Heatley JJ, *et al.* Evaluation of intravenous fluorescein in intradermal allergy testing in psittacines. *Veterinary Dermatology* 2003; **14**: 323–332.
24. Schleifer SG, Willemse T. Evaluation of skin test reactivity to environmental allergens in healthy cats and cats with atopic dermatitis. *American Journal of Veterinary Research* 2003; **64**: 773–778.
25. Kadoya-Minegishi M, Park SJ, Sekiguchi M, *et al.* The use of fluorescein as a contrast medium to enhance intradermal skin tests in cats. *Australian Veterinary Journal* 2002; **80**: 702–703.
26. Hubbard TL, White PD. Comparison of subjective and objective intradermal allergy test scoring methods in dogs with atopic dermatitis. *Journal of the American Animal Hospital Association* 2011; **47**: 399–405.
27. Koebrich S, Nett-Mettler C, Wilhelm S, *et al.* Intradermal and serological testing for mites in healthy beagle dogs. *Veterinary Dermatology* 2012; **23**: 192–e39.

61

Allergic diseases in other pets (rodents, rabbits, and ferrets)

Ian Sayers

South Devon Exotics, ℅ Silverton Veterinary Practice, Paignton, Devon, UK

Conflict of interest: none declared.

Small mammals are used extensively in the laboratory setting and are becoming increasingly popular as pets; indeed rabbits are the third most popular mammalian pet in the UK [1], with estimated numbers between 1 and 1.7 million. As such, it is important that the possibility of allergic disease be considered when presented with appropriate clinical signs. Unfortunately, there are few published data relating to allergic disease in these species or its incidence in clinical practice.

A number of factors may contribute to this lack of data. The low level of presentation of these species to veterinary practices (it is thought that at least 45% of pet rabbits are never registered with a veterinary surgeon in the UK) results in a lack of familiarity with the species. Financial pressures, either absolute or relating to an animal's 'value', can be another significant factor preventing thorough investigation. A pets 'value' is hard to determine, but an animal's presumed/perceived 'value' should not influence what level of service is offered. The range of diagnostic and treatment options available should be discussed with an owner and then a suitable plan elected—the whole time considering animal welfare as paramount. It is the author's experience that the majority of owners tend to 'value' an animal in relation to the lifespan and interactive nature of the owner/pet relationship; thus they are often least inclined to fund diagnostic investigation and treatment for smaller rodents (rats, mice, hamster, and gerbil), but more so for larger rodents (guinea pigs and chinchilla) or lagomorphs. The scenario is a little harder to quantify when considering mustelids, as there is marked variation depending upon whether the ferret is considered as a family pet or more of a working animal.

It is beyond doubt that these species have the mechanisms to demonstrate allergic reactions because they are frequently used as models for human disease responses. No single species can reproduce all features of human asthma [2], thus rabbits [2], guinea pigs [3], mice [4], and ferrets [5] are all used in the studies of human allergic disease and are considered vital, even though the findings of studies can be of questionable relevance [6]. How these allergic responses are induced may have a significant bearing on the type of disease seen, or rather not seen, in clinical practice. Frequently, studies use particular phenotypes of animal and the methodology of sensitization is unlikely to occur in a clinical setting, indeed the use of adjuvants are required in most models [6], even for studies involving allergens that are likely to be met naturally, e.g. pollens [7].

There are a number of texts that refer to allergic respiratory problems in small mammals, but are not substantiated by literature references. Without published data it is important to maintain a critical view so that mere repetition, particularly in non-peer-reviewed texts, does not circumvent scientific stringency and become perceived as fact. However, this does not mean that such disease does not occur.

Veterinary Allergy, First Edition. Edited by Chiara Noli, Aiden Foster, and Wayne Rosenkrantz.

Respiratory disease

The high incidence of respiratory disease in small mammals may be another factor that prevents the true incidence of respiratory allergies being recognized. Aetiological agents are numerous and, whilst a great deal of disease remains subclinical, a clinical picture of chronic recurrent disease is recognized. Frequently dispensed therapeutics are aimed at 'secondary invaders', e.g. *Pasteurella* spp., even where the primary pathogen is viral. The clinical response may improve signs sufficiently such that possible underlying allergic disease, that may be a 'trigger' factor for recrudescence, does not get investigated. Clinically it is important to differentiate causes to enable appropriate therapeutics to avoid worsening a problem, or indeed result in iatrogenic disease, e.g. inappropriate use of corticosteroids for presumed allergic disease in rabbits [8] causing immunosuppression and resultant clinical/exacerbation of subclinical respiratory disease.

Evidence for allergic responses to various substrates remains anecdotal. Respiratory and skin effects have been reported in small mammals. It has been shown that cedar shavings can affect microsomal oxidative liver enzymes in rats and mice; however, no clinical signs associated with these changes have been documented [9,10]. Anecdotally reported allergy to pine-scented sawdust or shavings may be an irritant response to the aromatic oils rather than an allergic response, particularly when proximity of the respiratory tract of small mammals to the substrate and ventilation factors are considered. Alleviation of clinical signs in response to substrate change does not confirm or exclude an allergic reaction.

Investigation of allergic respiratory disease can be difficult due to a number of factors, of which size is possibly the most limiting. Radiography is one of the diagnostic procedures used in the investigation of allergic respiratory disease in other species such as cats and it is possibly one of the easiest to apply to small mammals. The diagnostic value of such a procedure, however, has not been studied in these species and the interpretation of the images is more complex. For small rodents, rapid respiratory rates make it difficult to ensure that exposure occurs at peak inspiration. The difficulty of intubation of small rodents because of a lack of commonly available equipment and frequent use of gaseous anaesthesia means 'inflated' views are not practicable. This can be similarly difficult when the larger rodents (guinea pig and chinchilla) are considered as they posses a palatal ostium, thus rigid endoscopy is often required to enable intubation. Rabbits and ferrets are much more easily intubated but interpretation of the image can still be difficult. Rabbits have a relatively small lung volume (4–6 mL/kg in comparison to 10–15 mL/kg for cats and dogs) thus the area of interest is smaller. For rodents the area of interest is smaller in absolute terms. The increasing use of high-quality digital radiography means that enlarging/'zooming' into the lungs is more easily performed and more detail is evident, but this still relies on good radiographic technique and appropriate exposure in the first instance. The small size of rats and mice mean that it may be more appropriate to use equipment primarily intended for dental use. A further complicating factor is that subclinical (infectious) respiratory disease is common in a number of these species, thus the radiographic changes themselves, e.g. a bronchial pattern (as expected with feline asthma), may not be typically seen, or masked by other changes, e.g. interstitial pattern or areas of consolidation due to concurrent chronic disease.

Bronchoscopy may also be limited by size factors and is only really an option for the larger rabbit breeds, i.e. similar in size or larger than a cat. Ferrets and rabbits that are below this size may still have tracheoscopy performed, via rigid endoscopes, but changes may not be as overt. Certainly, bronchoalveolar lavage (BAL) is preferred to tracheal washes in cats. Again, due to a lack of data, interpretation of findings will be difficult initially, in much the same way that it was for cats (the mere presence of eosinophils in BAL samples does not necessarily indicate asthma).

Gastrointestinal disease

Similar to respiratory disease, allergic gastrointestinal disease is not common or the true incidence is unknown. However, potential food allergies appear to be frequently 'referred' to in relation to ferrets, particularly via internet sites or discussion groups. Invariably there has been little or no investigation of cases, or no evidence to suggest this, but various foodstuffs get 'labelled' as causing 'food allergies'. It is important that the clinician be aware of this potential when dealing with unfamiliar species, particularly when faced with a confident 'discussion-group-educated' client. There are diseases in ferrets where an underlying food allergy may be attributable to the cause, but this in itself does not constitute a diagnosis.

Inflammatory bowel disease (IBD) is a common cause of gastroenteritis in ferrets [11]. Eosinophilic granulomatous disease ('eosinophilic gastroenteritis') is an uncommon disease [12–14]. Both diseases may present with typical signs of gastroenteritis (diarrhoea, weight loss, vomiting, and lethargy) and whilst the cause of both conditions is unknown, dietary intolerance/hypersensitivity is a potential underlying aetiology, as it is in humans and some dogs [15]. Diagnosis can be difficult for both diseases. IBD cases may be subclinical (up to 50% of cases at one US clinic) and initial suspicion may be based on findings of blood biochemistry results (elevated liver enzymes and serum globulins). The inflammatory process in eosinophilic granulomatous disease does not appear to originate in the gut mucosa. Abdominal lymphatics and other organs are involved; the gut is usually involved by the time cases are recognized. Definitive diagnosis of both diseases requires histological examination of full thickness gastric and intestinal biopsies as well as any visibly enlarged mesenteric lymph nodes. Treatment is aimed at suppressing the immune response and dietary management. Good responses to novel protein source or hypoallergenic/hydrolysed diets may be seen.

Dermatological disease

There are no published scientific studies of proven allergic skin diseases implicating environmental or dietary allergens, with dermatological signs, in pet ferrets or other small mammal species. Ferrets with hair loss are reported as having food allergies, rather than the more commonly expected adrenal disease, but these remain anecdotal reports.

Bedding changes may be considered and, anecdotally at least, have been reported to be clinically important in some cases, but in itself this does not prove an allergic condition. For smaller rodents it is relatively easy to alter bedding to shredded paper rather than more typically used substrates, but it is a rather different situation for 'fibrevores'. Eliminating exposure to potential trophoallergens, e.g. grasses, in some fibrevore rodents, is not a possibility as inadequate dietary fibre provision is likely to result in life-threatening ileus.

It is far more likely that small mammal species are infested with an ectoparasite and that skin lesions and signs of pruritus are due to such parasites rather than an allergic response to diet or environmental allergens. It is important to investigate pruritus in small mammals with ectoparasites, including fleas, lice, and mites, as the most likely diagnosis.

In multi-pet households, rabbits and ferrets may be exposed to fleas particularly when sharing a home with cats and/or dogs. While severe pruritus may be associated with flea infestation, there are no substantive studies to definitively demonstrate that ferrets or rabbits are allergic to fleas although this is often inferred. Some flea control products licensed for cats and dogs are also licensed for use in ferrets and rabbits. Ectoparasites of rodents can cause marked pruritus and they frequently present with areas of self trauma that may also have secondary microbial infection. Diagnostic samples for a number of ectoparasites can be easily obtained via tape strips or coat brushings, or via otoscopy. These are easy and quick to perform in the consulting room with little extra discomfort for the patient, other than the pre-existing pruritus. Parasite eggs or adults are easily seen on low to medium power (×40 to ×100) microscopy (Figures 61.1, 61.2, and 61.3). A degree of caution may be necessary when sampling guinea pigs. The most significant ectoparasite of this species is the sarcoptic mite *Trixacarus caviae*, a potential zoonosis. It is a burrowing mite that can cause such extreme pruritus that seizures may occur, thus anaesthesia may be indicated to allow appropriate skin scrapes to be obtained without stressing the patient further.

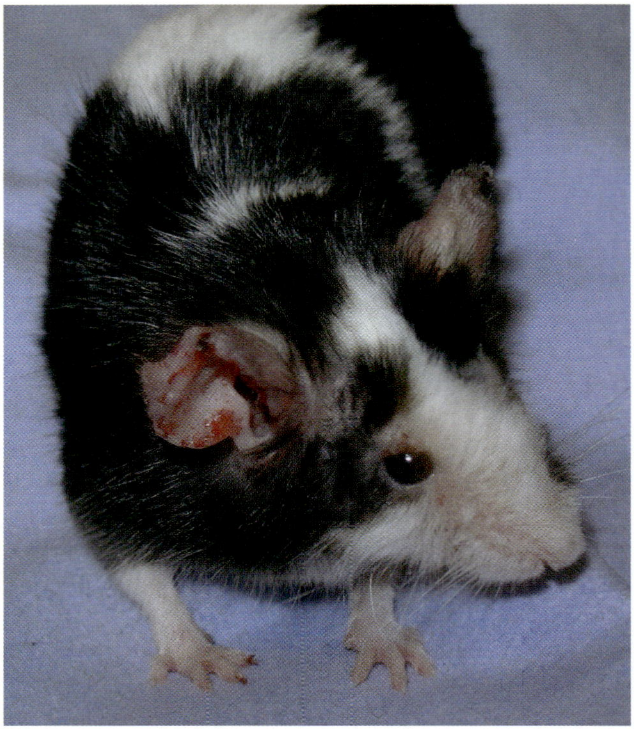

Figure 61.1 Mouse that was demonstrating marked pruritus with lesions on the pinnae.

Identifying the presence of an ectoparasite may only be part of the problem. In rabbits, cheyletiellosis, another potential zoonosis, is frequently a sign of disease rather than a diagnosis, and results from an inability to groom properly caused by numerous conditions, e.g. dental disease, obesity, spondylosis, or due to immunosuppression [16]. A survey of laboratory rabbits found that 43.2% had inapparent *Cheyletiella* infestations [17], a more recent survey of pet rabbits [18] had similar findings (57.1%). As such, appropriate investigation is indicated, not just ectoparasite therapy.

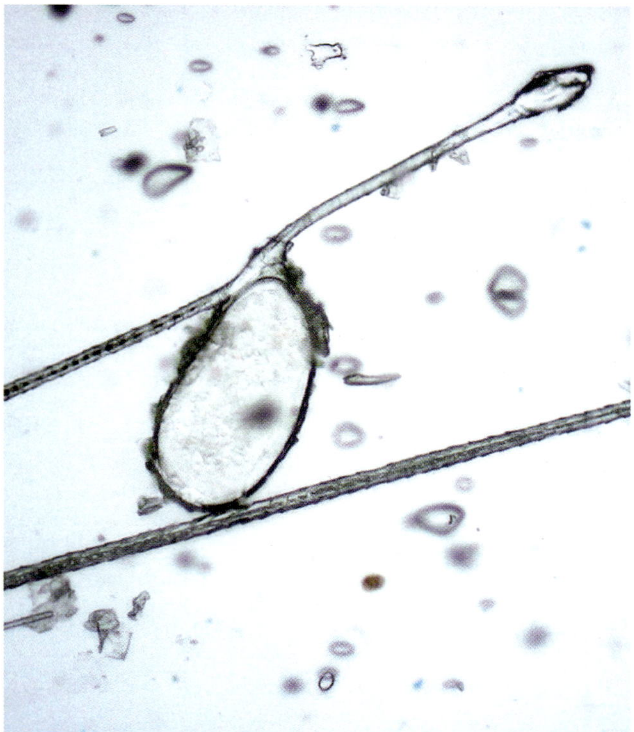

Figure 61.2 Fur mite eggs, taken from the mouse in Figure 61.1, demonstrated via tape strips and ×10 microscopy.

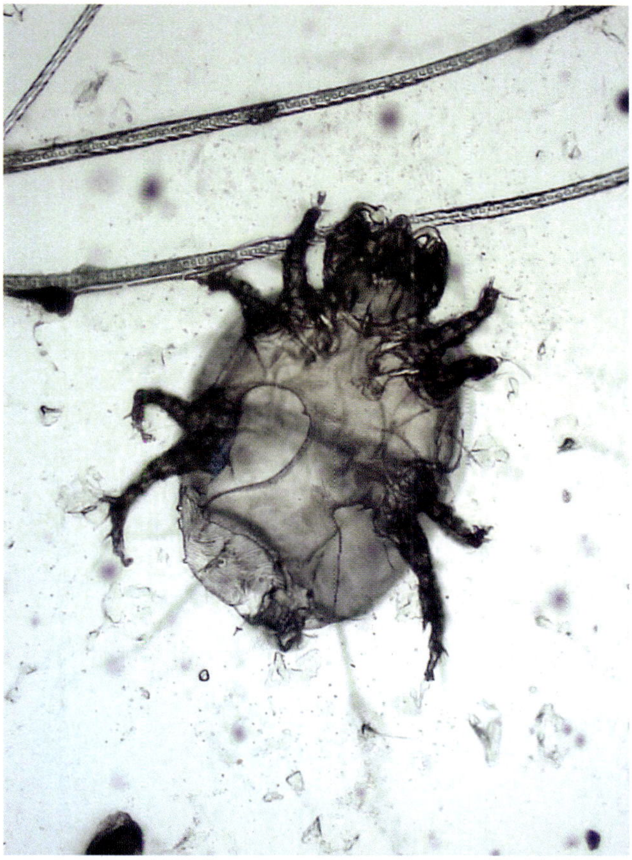

Figure 61.3 *Cheyletiella parasitivorax* demonstrated via tape strip and ×10 microscopy.

The author believes in the importance of identifying the presence of ectoparasites and monitoring the patient for response to treatments. Whilst this may not be necessary in all situations, e.g. *Cheyletiella parasitivorax* in rabbits, due to potential inapparent infestation rates, it is extremely important in those cases where pruritus is marked, e.g. where self-trauma occurs or the potential for seizures. Typically, the use of macrocylic lactones are indicated, but the author prefers to administer treatments orally (generally more readily accepted than injections) rather than use topical preparations. Repeat visits for oral administration enables close monitoring of clinical improvement, generally does not appear to be particularly stressful for the animals, and allows decision making as to the length of treatment required.

The majority of cases resolve with a course of three treatments (at an appropriate dose), given at intervals of 8–10 days; however, there are a number of cases that require longer courses. In the author's experience, these protracted cases usually relate to guinea pigs where up to six or seven treatments have been required before full resolution. The author prefers to use 'high-end' doses (i.e. 400 μg/kg) for these species. Without direct veterinary assessment, use of 'over the counter' preparations may not result in full resolution, thus extending the period of pruritus and adversely affecting patient welfare.

The author has seen several cases where the condition is ongoing despite use of, aforementioned, topical preparations and is aware of similar experiences from other colleagues. Frequently, in-contact animals will have clinically silent infestations, thus group investigation/treatment is to be recommended.

Once ectoparasites have been ruled out and when an allergic reaction to environmental allergens is suspected, the investigation and identification of clinically significant allergens is much more complex than for dogs and cats. Serological testing for IgE, whilst potentially attractive for rabbits or ferrets related to relative ease of blood sampling, is not currently available because tests rely on species-specific reagents and/or have not been validated in these species. The use of intradermal allergens may be more of a possibility because allergens are not species-specific. Positive test reactions to allergens are likely to be similar to those seen in other species and thus immunotherapy may be a possibility, but what induction and maintenance protocols are required, or success rate, is unknown. Certainly, if this route was to be considered, it would be important that a clinician familiar with intradermal testing was responsible for performing the tests. At present, it is not known what concentrations of allergens would be required to avoid confusion with possible irritant rather than allergic reactions. Choosing which allergens to test, in the first instance, may also be a challenge. Subsequent immunotherapy protocols would have to be extrapolated from other species. For most clinicians the identification of significant allergens may only be inferred from clinical improvement when bedding, housing/accommodation, or food items are changed and an improvement is observed.

It is recognized that rabbits benefit from same-species companions [19] but there are no reports, anecdotal or otherwise, of behavioural issues as a cause of alopecia in lone individuals, that may be mistaken for pruritus, as it can be in other species, e.g. feather-plucking in birds. Indeed, in small mammals, it is far more likely that alopecia as a result of behaviour occurs when animals are kept in groups, i.e. 'barbering'.

As small mammals become more popular as pets, the need for owners to have 'something different' is ever present. As such, clinicians are likely to be presented with potentially increasingly unfamiliar species. Each of these is just as likely, as far as we know, to suffer from allergic disease, which seems to be poorly reported and recognized. There have been texts available for some time which 'reference' anecdotal reports of allergic gastrointestinal and skin diseases, with histological evidence suggestive of allergy, for example of unknown source in African pygmy hedgehogs [20]. It is important that clinicians offer the same level of service to all these species as they do to more commonly presented dogs and cats. Decision making, for all cases, should be evidence based. Undoubtedly, there will be constraints/difficulties in investigation relating to animal size or availability of tests and these should be discussed with the owner. Where the constraints are purely financial, appropriate case management should be decided upon, in conjunction with the owners. Animal welfare is of paramount importance in decision making and no different to other species.

References

1. Campbell-Ward M, Meredith A. Rabbits. In: Meredith A, Johnson-Delaney C, eds. *BSAVA Manual of Exotic Pets*, 5th edn. Gloucester: BSAVA Publications, 2010: 76–102.
2. Keir S, Page C. The rabbit as a model to study asthma and other lung diseases. *Pulmonary Pharmacology and Therapeutics* 2008; **21**: 721–730.
3. Ricciardo FL, Nijkamp F, De Rose V, *et al.* The guinea pig as an animal model for asthma. *Current Drug Targets* 2008; **9**: 452–465.
4. Wang S, Xiang YY, Ellis R, *et al.* Effects of furosemide on allergic asthmatic responses in mice. *Clinical and Experimental Allergy* 2011; **41**: 1456–1467.
5. Wilson CG, Akhter S, Mayer CA, *et al.* Allergic lung inflammation affects central noradrenergic control of cholinergic outflow to the airways in ferrets. *Journal of Applied Physiology* 2007; **103**: 2095–2104.
6. Zosky GR, Sly PD. Animal models of asthma. *Clinical and Experimental Allergy* 2007; **37**: 973–988.
7. Nabe T, Mizutani N, Shimizu K, *et al.* Development of pollen-induced allergic rhinitis with early and late phase nasal blockage in guinea pigs. *Inflammation Research* 1998; **47**: 369–374.
8. Deeb BJ. Respiratory disease and pasteurellosis. In: Quesenberry KE, Carpenter JW, eds. *Ferrets, Rabbits and Rodents Clinical Medicine and Surgery*, 2nd edn. Philadelphia: Saunders, 2004: 172–182.
9. Bihum C, Bauck L. Basic anatomy, physiology, husbandry, and clinical techniques. In: Quesenberry KE, Carpenter JW, eds. *Ferrets, Rabbits and Rodents Clinical Medicine and Surgery*, 2nd edn. Philadelphia: Saunders, 2004: 286–298.
10. Weichbrod RH, Cisar CF, Miller JG, *et al.* Effects of cage beddings on microsomal oxidative enzymes in rat liver. *Laboratory Animal Science* 1988; **38**: 296–298.
11. Burgess M, Garner M. Clinical aspects of inflammatory bowel disease in ferrets. *Exotic DVM* 2002; **4**.2: 29–34.
12. Fazakas S. Eosinophilic gastroenteritis in a domestic ferret. *Canadian Veterinary Journal* 2000: **41**: 707–709.
13. Palley LS, Fox JG. Eosinophilic gastroenteritis in the ferret. In: Kirk RW, Bonagura JD, eds. *Kirk's Current Veterinary Therapy XI: Small Animal Practice*. Philadelphia: Saunders, 1992: 1182–1184.
14. Fox JG, Palley LS, Rose R. Eosinophilic gastroenteritis with Splendore-Hoeppli material in the ferret (*Mustela putoriusfuro*). *Veterinary Pathology* 1992; **29**: 21–26.
15. Hoefer HL, Bell JA. Gastrointestinal diseases. In: Quesenberry KE, Carpenter JW, eds. *Ferrets, Rabbits and Rodents Clinical Medicine and Surgery*, 2nd edn. Philadelphia: Saunders, 2004: 25–40.
16. Scarff DH. Skin disorders of small mammals. *Journal of Small Animal Practice* 1991; **32**: 408–412.
17. Flatt RE, Wiemers J. A survey of fur mites in domestic rabbits. *Laboratory Animal Science* 1976; **26**: 343–347.
18. Kim SH, Jun HK, Song KH, *et al.* Prevalence of fur mites in pet rabbits in South Korea. *Veterinary Dermatology* 2008; **19**: 189–190.
19. Mullen SM, Main DCJ. Behaviour and personality of pet rabbits and their interactions with their owners. *Veterinary Record* 2007; **160**: 516–520.
20. Ivey E, Carpenter JW. African hedgehogs. In: Quesenberry KE, Carpenter JW, eds. *Ferrets, Rabbits and Rodents Clinical Medicine and Surgery*, 2nd edn. Philadelphia: Saunders, 2004: 339–353.

Index

Veterinary Allergy, First Edition. Edited by Chiara Noli, Aiden Foster, and Wayne Rosenkrantz.